NASM
National Academy of Sports Medicine

Optimum Performance Training for the Health and Fitness Professional

COURSE MANUAL

Second Edition
Copyright ©2004 National Academy of Sports Medicine
Printed in the United States of America

ISBN 0-9710286-2-1

Distributed by:

National Academy of Sports Medicine

26632 Agoura Road

Calabasas, CA 91302

800.460.NASM

Facsimile: 818.878.9511

http: www.nasm.org

Writers

Micheal A. Clark,
MS, PT, NASM-PES

Scott Lucett,
BS, NASM-CPT, NASM-PES

Rodney Corn,
MS, NASM-CPT, NASM-PES

Robert Cappuccio,
NASM-CPT

Reed Humphrey,
PhD, PT, FACSM

Stephen J. Kraus, PhD

Alan Titchenal, PhD

Paul Robbins, BS

Editor

Sarah Daniels

Proofreaders

Jamie Pagett, Caroline Rath

Production

Rosanne T. Wittkop

Photographer

Robert Rettmann

Chapter Models

Christy Hicks, Steven Jordan,
Susan Martens

Package Design

Persechini and Company

Page Design/Production

Angela Schill/Schill Design

Anatomical Illustrations

Primal Pictures Ltd.
www.primalpictures.com
A.D.A.M. Software, Inc.

The **NASM** Mission

The National Academy of Sports Medicine is dedicated to transforming lives and revolutionizing the health and fitness industry through its unwavering commitment to deliver innovative education, solutions and tools that produce remarkable results!

Education ■ *Application* ■ *Integrity*

Table of Contents

Table of Contents

Table of Contents

Table of Contents

Table of Contents

Table of Contents

Table of Contents

Table of Contents

Table of Contents

Table of Contents

Table of Contents

Table of Contents

Table of Contents

Table of Contents

Table of Contents

Table of Contents

Table of Contents

Table of Contents

Table of Contents

Table of Contents

Table of Contents

Table of Contents

Table of Contents

Table of Contents

Letter from the President

Congratulations and thank you for entrusting the National Academy of Sports Medicine (NASM) with your education. As the global authority in health and fitness, we are also the industry's premier provider of education and certification for fitness, performance and sports-medicine professionals. Since 1987, NASM has enjoyed international acclaim for its cutting-edge concepts and state of the art programs and products. Today, NASM is proud to serve more than 100,000 members and partners in more than 80 countries.

Our industry is on the verge of exciting changes, which will provide unlimited opportunities for qualified health and fitness professionals. Today's health club members have an increasingly high level of expectations: they want the best and the brightest, whom can provide unparalleled results. As consumers demand more, technology is rising to meet these demands. Scientific research and techniques continue to advance and, as a result, health and fitness professionals must remain on the cutting edge to remain competitive. NASM prides itself on establishing scientifically validated education, evidence-based solutions and user-friendly tools that can be put to immediate use and will keep you at the forefront of the industry.

The tools and solutions in the Optimum Performance Training (OPT™) model help put science into practice to create remarkable results for clients. OPT™ is a revolutionary program design method, used by hundreds of thousands of health and fitness professionals and athletes worldwide. NASM's techniques work, creating a dramatic difference in training programs and their results.

Welcome to NASM. We look forward to working with you to transform the health and fitness industry together.

Yours in good health,
Micheal A. Clark, MS, PT, NASM-PES
President and CEO

Code of Ethics

The following code of ethics is designed to assist certified and non-certified members of the National Academy of Sports Medicine (NASM) to uphold (both as individuals and as an industry) the highest levels of professional and ethical conduct. This Code of Ethics reflects the level of commitment and integrity necessary to ensure that all NASM members provide the uncompromised level of service and respect for all colleagues, allied professionals and the general public.

Professionalism

Each certified or non-certified member must provide optimal professional service and demonstrate excellent client care in his/her practice. Each member shall:

- Abide fully by the NASM Code of Ethics.
- Conduct him/herself in a manner that merits the respect of the public, other colleagues and NASM.
- Treat each colleague and/or client with the utmost respect and dignity.
- Not make false or derogatory assumptions concerning the practices of colleagues and/or clients.
- Use appropriate professional communication in all verbal, non-verbal and written transactions.
- Maintain a level of personal hygiene appropriate for a health and fitness setting.
- Wear clothing that is clean, modest and professional.
- Remain in good standing and maintain current certification status by acquiring all necessary continuing-education requirements (see NASM recertification information).

Safety

In addition, the certified or non-certified member is entrusted with providing and maintaining an environment that ensures client safety. At minimum, this requires that the certified or non-certified member shall:

- Not diagnose or treat illness or injury (except for basic first aid), unless the certified or non-certified member is legally licensed to do so and is working in that capacity, at that time.

- Not train clients with a diagnosed health condition, unless the certified or non-certified member has been specifically trained to do so, is following procedures prescribed and supervised by a valid licensed medical professional, or is legally licensed to do so and is working in that capacity, at that time.

- Not begin to train a client prior to receiving and reviewing a current health-history questionnaire signed by the client.

- Hold a CPR certification at all times.

- Refer the client to the appropriate medical practitioner when, at minimum, the certified or non-certified member:

  — Becomes aware of any change in the client's health status or medication.

  — Becomes aware of an undiagnosed illness, injury or risk factor.

  — Becomes aware of any unusual client pain and/or discomfort during the course the training session that warrants professional care, after the session has been discontinued and assessed.

- Refer the client to other healthcare professionals when nutritional and supplemental advice is requested, unless the certified or non-certified member has been specifically trained to do so or, holds a credential to do so and is acting in that capacity, at that time.

Confidentiality

Each certified and non-certified member shall respect the confidentiality of all client information. In his/her professional role, the certified or non-certified member must:

- Protect the client's confidentiality in conversations, advertisements and any other arena, unless otherwise agreed upon by the client in writing, or due to medical and/or legal necessity.

- Protect the interest of clients who are minors by law, or who are unable to give voluntary consent by securing the legal permission of the appropriate third party or guardian.

- Store and dispose of client records in secure manner.

Legal and Ethical

Each certified or non-certified member must comply with all legal requirements within the applicable jurisdiction. In his/her professional role, the certified or non-certified member must:

- Obey all local, state, providence and/or federal laws.

- Accept complete responsibility for his/her actions.

- Maintain accurate and truthful records.

- Respect and uphold all existing publishing and copyright laws.

Business Practice

Each certified or non-certified member must practice with honesty, integrity and lawfulness. In his/her professional role, the certified or non-certified member shall:

- Maintain adequate liability insurance.

- Maintain adequate and truthful progress notes for each client.

- Accurately and truthfully inform the public of services offered.

- Honestly and truthfully represent all professional qualifications and affiliations.

- Advertise in a manner that is honest, dignified and representative of services that can be delivered without the use of provocative and/or sexual language and/or pictures.

- Maintain accurate financial, contract, appointment and tax records, including original receipts for a minimum of four years.

- Comply with all local, state, federal or providence laws regarding sexual harassment.

NASM expects each member to uphold the Code of Ethics in its entirety. Failure to comply with the NASM Code of Ethics may result in disciplinary actions, including (but not limited to) suspension or termination of membership and/or certification. All members are obligated to report to NASM any unethical behavior or violation of the Code of Ethics by other members.

CHAPTER ONE

The Scientific Rationale for Integrated Training

Objectives

After studying this chapter, you will be able to:

- Explain the history of personal training.
- Understand today's typical client.
- Rationalize the need for integrated program design.
- Describe the Optimum Performance Training (OPT™) model.

Key Terms

- Deconditioned
- Proprioception
- Proprioceptively enriched environment
- Phase of training
- Stabilization strength
- Neuromuscular efficiency
- Prime mover
- Rate of force production
- Superset
- Plyometric

MODULE 1-1:
The Personal Training Industry

Overview of the Personal Training Industry

Personal training is one of the fastest growing occupations in the United States. A recent news release from IDEA Health and Fitness Association has noted a significant growth rate in the industry.[1] However, the origin of personal training is undocumented and anecdotal, at best. It is necessary to investigate the known beginnings of this occupation to better understand the rationale for current training concepts and their effect on clientele.

The Past

During the 1950s and 1960s, gym members were predominantly men who were training for specific goals, such as increased size (bodybuilders), strength (power lifters), explosive strength (Olympic lifters) or a combination of all of these goals (athletes). However, by the end of the 1960s, society's view of exercise began to change.

By the 1970s, going to the gym (and training to become fit) had become much more socially acceptable. It provided a structured way to achieve social interaction and health simultaneously. Fitness training did not require high levels of skill (as did sport forms of exercise) and was used to augment existing activity levels. Simply, it was an active outlet for anyone, regardless of physical ability, that could be utilized year-round, day or night and without concern for weather conditions. It was also perceived as a way to directly alter physical characteristics, in a society that had become very appearance-conscious.

Thus, the number of new gym members increased to include a large number of people who were uneducated about training and the gym environment. This brought about the desire to seek out the help and guidance from an "expert."

Essentially, the "expert" of the 1970s was the person in the gym who had been training the longest, looked the most fit or who was strongest. However, these qualities are primarily genetic in nature and are not necessarily based on training knowledge. Often, a new member would approach one of the perceived "experts" and offer that person money, in exchange for his/her training knowledge and guidance. Hence, the fitness professional was born.

While, for the most part, these individuals were probably able to provide good information on the acute variables of training such as loads, sets, reps, etc., the understanding and application of human movement science (functional anatomy, functional biomechanics and motor behavior) is something very different. It was not usual practice to assess a new client for past medical conditions, training risk factors, muscle imbalances, goals, etc. This resulted in training programs that simply mimicked those of the current fitness professional or instructor. Programs were rarely designed to meet an individual client's goals, needs and abilities.

At the time, the typical health-club member was probably better prepared for activity. The work and home environments were not as inundated with automation, personal computers, cell phones and other technology that are more prevalent today. Housekeepers, gardeners, remote controls and video games did not run a household. Furthermore, mandated activity, such as physical education in school, was not yet compromised. The activity level of daily live was still somewhat brisk.

The Present

According to the Bureau of Labor Statistics (1983 vs. 1998), more people today are spending time in office-related jobs and more hours at work.[2] This lends itself to more daily sitting, less work-related activity and less daily activity in general, which all lead to muscular dysfunction and increased incidents of injury.

From the mid-1980s to the present, the wealth of technology and automation in the United States has begun to take a toll on public health. In 1985, the International Obesity Task Force deemed the prevalence of obesity an epidemic.[3] Today, approximately two thirds of adults are considered overweight and one third (33 percent) of adults are estimated to be obese. This carries over to the adolescent population, with 15 percent of teenagers considered obese.[3]

The American population is also living longer. The U.S. Census Bureau reported that the proportion of the population over 65 is projected to increase from 12.4 percent in 2000 to 19.6 percent in 2030. The number of individuals over 80 is expected to increase from 9.3 million in 2000 to 19.5 million in 2030. This lends to the number of individuals developing chronic diseases and disability. In the United States, approximately 80 percent of all persons aged over 65 have at least one chronic condition, and 50 percent have at least two. Arthritis affects approximately 59 percent of persons over 65 and is the leading cause of disability.

Meanwhile, daily activity levels continue to decline.[2] People are less active and are no longer spending as much of their free time engaged in physical activity.[2,4] Physical education and after-school sport programs are being cut from school budgets, further decreasing the amount of physical activity in children's lives. This new environment is producing more inactive and non-functional people.

Evidence of Muscular Dysfunction and Increased Injury

Research supports the concept that decreased activity may lead to muscular dysfunction and, ultimately, injury. Some of the major topics studied include low back pain, knee injuries, chronic diseases in the adult population and musculoskeletal injuries.

LOW BACK PAIN

In 1997, a study was conducted that looked at low back pain occurrence in lower- and middle-income countries around the world.[5] It was hypothesized that the populated lower-income rural countries would exhibit higher rates of low back pain (due to harder physical labor), versus higher-income populations (where urbanized office work predominated). Quite unexpectedly, it was found that the opposite was true. Further, it was demonstrated that low back pain was significantly more predominant among workers in enclosed workspaces (such as offices). The conclusion was that low back pain may not be a result of hard physical labor. Consequently, incidents of low back pain will likely continue to rise with the progression of urbanization and industrialization.[5]

Low back pain is one the major forms of musculoskeletal degeneration seen in the adult population, affecting nearly 80 percent of all adults.[6,7] Researchers have shown that men who spend over half their workday sitting in a car have a 300-percent increased chance of disc herniation.[8-10] Other forms of degeneration, including arthritis and osteoporosis, can be seen in the elderly. It has been suggested that these degenerative conditions may result from a loss in muscle mass due to lack of use and are not necessarily the result of advanced age.[11-13]

KNEE INJURIES

The incidence of knee injuries is also a concern. An estimated 80,000 to 100,000 anterior cruciate ligament (ACL) injuries occur annually in the general U.S. population. Approximately 70 percent of these are non-contact injuries.[14,15] In addition, ACL injuries have a strong correlation to acquiring arthritis in the affected knee.[14]

Most ACL injuries between 15 and 25 years of age. This comes as no surprise when considering the lack of activity and increased obesity occurring in this age group. U.S. teenagers have an abundance of automation and technology, combined with a lack of mandatory physical education in schools.[3,4,16]

Fortunately, research suggests that enhancing neuromuscular stabilization (or body control) may alleviate the high incidence of non-contact injuries.[17]

CHRONIC DISEASES IN THE ADULT POPULATION

Physical activity has been proven to reduce the risk of chronic diseases and disorders that are related to lifestyle, such as increased triglycerides and cholesterol levels, obesity, glucose tolerance, high blood pressure, coronary heart disease and strokes.[15,17-21] More importantly, some research indicates that discontinuing (or significantly decreasing) physical activity can actually lead to a higher risk of chronic diseases that are related to lifestyle.[22,23]

MUSCULOSKELETAL INJURIES

In 1988, more than 12 percent of the American population suffered a musculoskeletal impairment.[24] More than half of these (51.7 percent) were spinal or back-related. (Shoulder and lower extremity injuries comprised 11 percent). These injuries resulted in excess of a combined 60 million days spent in bed.

Unnatural posture, due to improper sitting, results in increased neck, mid- and lower back, shoulder and leg pain.[16] Of work-related injuries, 43 percent are sprains and strains and more than 60 percent involve the trunk.[16] These work-related injuries cost workers approximately nine days per back episode or, combined, more than 39 million days of restricted activity. The monetary value of lost work time due to these musculoskeletal injuries was estimated to be approximately $120 billion dollars.[16]

It has become much more important in today's society to focus on health and well being.[16] Many individuals realize that they need to exercise. In fact, the number of people becoming involved in recreation and leisure activities has increased over the last two decades.[25] Moreover, Americans over the age of 55 are the fastest-growing age group among health-club members.

Unfortunately, however, these numbers parallel an increase in injuries to the musculoskeletal system.[26,27] It has been suggested that factors such as over- training, skeletal abnormalities, poor exercise technique and lack of warm-up can all lead to dysfunctions and injuries.[28] It is important to ensure that all components of the body are properly prepared for the stress placed on them, regardless of their perceived contribution.[29] Unfortunately, training programs and apparatus used to condition the musculoskeletal system often neglect essential parts of the body, such as the core (hips, upper and lower back and neck).[30] This results in a weakened structure.[14,29,31]

Simply put, the extent to which we condition our musculoskeletal system directly influences our risk of injury. The less conditioned our musculoskeletal systems are, the higher the risk of injury.[28] Therefore, as our daily lives include less physical activity, the less prepared we are to partake in recreational and leisure activities such as resistance training, weekend sports or simply playing on the playground.

Current Training Programs

Research has been conducted on the effectiveness of training programs on sedentary adults. It has been shown that the intensity of activity required by a sedentary person trying to improve cardiorespiratory fitness might put that person into a state of excessive overload.[28] In the initial six weeks of a study that physically trained sedentary adults, there was a 50- to 90-percent injury rate.[32] This occurred even though programs were specifically designed to minimize risk of injury. Researchers concluded that the musculoskeletal system

DECONDITIONED:
A state of lost physical fitness, which may include muscle imbalances, decreased flexibility and/or a lack of core and joint stability.

PROPRIOCEPTION:
The cumulative neural input to the central nervous system, from all mechanoreceptors that sense body position and limb movement.

PROPRIOCEPTIVELY ENRICHED ENVIRONMENT:
An unstable (but controlled) physical situation in which exercises are performed in, which causes the body to use its internal balance and stabilization mechanisms.

is very easily over-trained when it is **deconditioned**.

It is important to note that deconditioned does not simply mean a person is out of breath upon climbing a flight of stairs or that they are overweight. It is a state in which a person may have muscle imbalances, decreased flexibility and/or a lack of core and joint stability. All of these conditions can greatly affect the ability of the human body to produce proper movement and can eventually lead to injury.[33]

Most training programs do not emphasize multiplanar movements (or movement in different degrees of the various planes of the body) through the full muscle action spectrum (concentric, eccentric and isometric muscle contractions) in an environment that enriches **proprioception**.[33] A **proprioceptively enriched** environment is one that challenges the internal balance and stabilization mechanisms of the body. (Examples of this include performing a dumbbell chest press while on a stability ball or performing a single-leg squat.)

The Future

There is a general inability to meet the needs of today's client. The fitness industry has only recently recognized the trend toward non-functional living. Fitness professionals are now noticing a decrease in the physical functionality of their clients and are beginning to address it.

This is a new state of training, where the client has been physically molded by furniture, gravity and inactivity.[34] The continual decrease in everyday activity has created the postural deficiencies seen in people.[2] Today's client is not ready to begin physical activity at the same level that a typical client could 20 years ago. Therefore, today's training programs cannot stay the same as programs of the past.

The new mind-set in fitness should cater to creating programs that address functional capacity, as part of a safe program designed especially for each individual person. In other words, training programs must consider each person, their environment and the tasks that will be performed. This is best achieved by introducing an integrated approach to program design. It is upon this premise that the National Academy of Sports Medicine (NASM) presents the rationale for integrated training and the Optimum Performance Training (OPT™) model.

MODULE 1-1 Summary

The typical gym members of the 1950s were mainly athletes, and, in the 1970s, those involved in recreational sports. The first fitness professionals were physically fit individuals who did not necessarily have education in human movement science. They did not design programs to meet the specific goals, needs and abilities of their clients.

Today, more people work in offices, have longer work hours, use better technology and automation and are required to move less on a daily basis. This new environment produces more inactive and non-functional people and leads to dysfunction and increased incidents of injury including: low back pain, knee injuries, chronic diseases in the adult population and musculoskeletal injuries.

In working with today's typical client, who is likely to be deconditioned, fitness professional must take special consideration when designing programs. An integrated approach should be used to create safe programs that consider functional capacity for each individual person. They must address factors such as appropriate forms of flexibility, increasing strength and endurance and training in different types of environments. These are the basis for NASM's OPT™ model.

MODULE 1-1 Quiz

1. What problem was created in the 1970s when the number of gym members increased?

   _____

2. Today, approximately what percentage of adults is estimated to be obese?

   ☐ 15

   ☐ 22

   ☐ 33

3. Low back pain is a result of hard physical labor.

   ☐ True   ☐ False

4. A proprioceptively enriched environment is one that challenges the internal balance and stabilization mechanisms of the body.

   ☐ True   ☐ False

5. The more conditioned our musculoskeletal system is, the higher the risk of injury.

   ☐ True   ☐ False

6. What is the term for a person who has muscle imbalances, decreased flexibility and/or a lack of core and joint stability?

   _____

MODULE 1-2:
Integrated Training and the OPT™ Model

Integrated training is a concept that incorporates all forms of training in an integrated fashion as part of a progressive system. These forms of training include flexibility training, cardiorespiratory training, core training, balance training, reactive training and resistance training. This system was developed by NASM and is termed Optimum Performance Training (OPT™).[33]

What is the OPT™ Model?

The OPT™ model was conceptualized as a training program for a society that has more structural imbalances and susceptibility to injury than ever before.[17,26-30,33] It is a process of programming that systematically progresses any client to any goal.[33] The OPT™ model (Figure 1-1) is built upon a foundation of principles that progressively and systematically allow any client to achieve optimum levels of physiological, physical and performance adaptations including:

Physiological Benefits
- Improves cardiorespiratory efficiency
- Enhances beneficial endocrine and serum lipid adaptations
- Increases metabolic efficiency
- Increases tissue tensile strength
- Increases bone density

Physical Benefits
- Decreases body fat
- Increases lean body mass (muscle)

Performance Benefits
- Strength
- Power
- Endurance
- Flexibility
- Speed
- Agility
- Balance

The OPT™ model is based on the scientific rationale of human movement science.[33] Each stage has a designated purpose that provides the client with a systematic approach for progressing toward his/her individual goals, as well as addressing his/her specific needs. Now, more than ever, it is imperative that fitness professionals fully understand all components of programming as well as the right order in which those components must be addressed to help their clients achieve success.

The OPT™ Model

The OPT™ model is divided into three different building blocks — stabilization, strength and power (Figure 1-1). Each building block contains specific **phases** of training. It is imperative that the fitness professional understands the scientific rationale behind each building block in order to properly utilize the OPT™ model.

> **PHASES OF TRAINING:** Smaller divisions of training progressions that fall within the three building blocks of training.

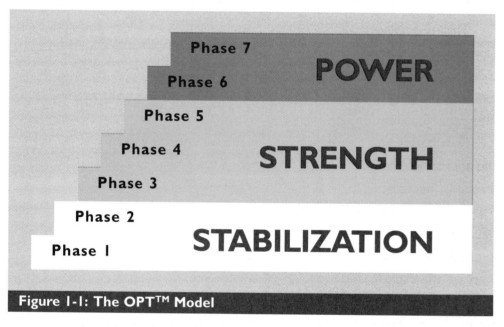

Figure 1-1: The OPT™ Model

Stabilization Training

Stabilization training consists of two phases of training — Phase 1: Corrective Exercise Training and Phase 2: Integrated Stabilization Training. The major components that make up these phases are corrective flexibility, core stabilization training, balance training, reactive training, resistance training and cardiorespiratory training.

The progression for this block of training is proprioceptively based. This means that difficulty is increased by introducing more challenge to the balance and stabilization systems of the body (versus simply increasing the load).

The main focus of stabilization training is to increase **stabilization strength** and develop optimal communication between one's nervous system and muscular system (or **neuromuscular efficiency**).[33]

If a client enters the fitness environment with active pain, has recently undergone surgery or is under the care of a medical practitioner, he/she will probably need to start in Phase 1: Corrective Exercise Training. First and foremost, the fitness professional should refer the client to a medical practitioner and consult with the current practitioner prior to initiating any workout program for that client. Following proper advice from the consulting medical practitioner, the fitness professional will initially focus on corrective exercise strategies aimed at improving:

- Muscular balance
- Increasing flexibility and extensibility
- Creating joint and postural stabilization

This is achieved by utilizing a proprioceptively enriched environment (controlled, unstable), proper flexibility techniques, followed by core and balance exercises to re-educate the neuromuscular system. Proper Corrective Exercise Training prepares and educates the kinetic chain for Phase 2: Integrated Stabilization Training.

Stabilization and neuromuscular efficiency can only be obtained by having the appropriate combination of alignment of the kinetic chain and the stability strength necessary to maintain that alignment.[35,36] Phase 2: Integrated Stabilization Training provides the needed stimuli to acquire stabilization and neuromuscular efficiency, through the use of proprioceptively enriched exercises and progressions. This is where most clients begin. The goal is to increase the client's ability to stabilize their joints and posture.

Stabilization training must be done prior to strength and power training. Research has shown that inefficient stabilization can negatively affect the way force is produced by the muscles, increase stress at the joints, overload the soft tissues and, eventually, cause injury.[37-39,41-49]

Stabilization training not only addresses the existing structural deficiencies, it also provides a superior way to alter body composition. By performing exercises in a proprioceptively enriched environment (controlled, unstable), the body is forced to recruit more muscles to stabilize itself. In doing so, more calories are expended.[50-51]

STABILIZATION STRENGTH: Ability of the body's stabilizing muscles to provide support for joints as well as maintain posture and balance, during movement.

NEUROMUSCULAR EFFICIENCY: The ability of the body's nerves to effectively send messages to the body's muscles.

Goals and Strategies of Stabilization Training

Phase 1: Corrective Exercise Training

GOALS

- Improve muscle balance
- Increase flexibility
- Enhance control of posture
- Increase neuromuscular efficiency

TRAINING STRATEGIES

- Corrective flexibility
- Core-stabilization training
- Balance-stabilization training
- Corrective resistance training in a controlled, but unstable environment
- Cardiorespiratory training

Phase 2: Integrated Stabilization Training

GOALS

- Enhance joint stability
- Increase flexibility
- Enhance control of posture
- Improve neuromuscular efficiency

TRAINING STRATEGIES

- Corrective flexibility
- Core-stabilization training
- Balance-stabilization training
- Reactive-stabilization training
- Proprioceptive resistance training
- Cardiorespiratory training

Strength Training

The strength-training phase follows the successful completion of stabilization training. The emphasis is to maintain stabilization strength while increasing **prime mover** strength. This is also the block of training an individual will progress to if his/her goals are *hypertrophy* (or muscle growth) or maximal strength (or lifting heavy loads). Strength training in the OPT™ model consists of three phases.

In Phase 3: Stabilization Equivalent Training, the goal is to enhance stabilization strength and endurance, while increasing prime mover strength.

PRIME MOVER:
The muscle that acts as the main source of motive movement.

These two adaptations are accomplished by performing two exercises per body part in a **superset** sequence (or back-to-back without rest) with similar joint dynamics (Table 1-1). One exercise is more traditional and performed in a more stable environment, while the other is an integrated exercise performed in a less stable environment. The principle behind this method is to work the prime movers predominantly in the first exercise in order to elicit prime mover strength. Then, immediately follow with an exercise that challenges the stabilization muscles. This produces an increased ability to maintain postural stabilization and dynamic joint stabilization.

> **SUPERSET:**
> Set of two exercises that are performed back-to-back, without any rest time between them.

Table 1-1: Phase 3: Stabilization Equivalent Training Exercises			
Body Part	**Strength Exercise**		**Stabilization Exercise**
Chest	Barbell Bench Press	→	Stability Ball Push-up
Back	Seated Cable Row	→	Stability Ball Dumbbell Row
Shoulders	Shoulder Press Machine	→	Single-leg Dumbbell Press
Legs	Leg Press	→	Single-leg Squat

Phase 4: Muscular Development Training is designed for individuals who have the goal of maximal muscle hypertrophy. Phase 5: Maximal Strength Training works toward the goal of maximal prime mover strength. These two components of training can be utilized as more special forms of training and as progressions within.

Goals and Strategies of Strength Training
Phase 3: Stabilization Equivalent Training
GOALS
- Improve stabilization endurance and increase prime mover strength
- Improve overall work capacity
- Enhances joint stabilization
- Increase lean body mass

TRAINING STRATEGIES
- Active flexibility
- Core-strength training
- Balance-strength training
- Reactive-strength training
- Resistance training
  - Superset one traditional strength and one stabilization exercise per body part
- Cardiorespiratory training

Phase 4: Muscular Development Training
(Phase optional, depending on client goals)
GOAL

- Achieve optimum levels of muscular hypertrophy

TRAINING STRATEGIES

- Active flexibility
- Core-strength training
- Balance-strength training *(optional)*
- Reactive-strength training *(optional)*
- Resistance training
- Cardiorespiratory training *(optional)*

Phase 5: Maximal Strength Training
(Phase optional, depending on client goals)
GOALS

- Increase motor unit recruitment
- Increase frequency of motor unit recruitment
- Improve peak force

TRAINING STRATEGIES

- Active flexibility
- Core-strength training
- Balance-strength training *(optional)*
- Reactive-strength training *(optional)*
- Resistance training
- Cardiorespiratory training *(optional)*

Power Training

Power training should only be entered upon successful completion of the two previous training blocks. This block of training emphasizes the development of speed and power. This is achieved through two major phases of training — Phase 6: Elastic Equivalent Training and Phase 7: Maximal Power Training.

The premise behind Phase 6: Elastic Equivalent Training is the execution of a more traditional strength exercise superset with a power exercise of similar joint dynamics. This is to enhance prime mover strength while also improving the **rate of force production** (Table 1-2).

RATE OF FORCE PRODUCTION: How quickly a muscle can generate force.

Table 1-2: Phase 6: Elastic Equivalent Training Exercises			
Body Part	**Strength Exercise**		**Stabilization Exercise**
Chest	Incline Dumbbell Press	→	Medicine Ball Chest Pass
Back	Pull-up	→	Soccer Throw
Shoulders	Dumbbell Overhead Press	→	Medicine Ball Scoop Toss
Legs	Barbell Squat	→	Squat Jump

Utilization of Phase 7: Maximal Power Training is a progression that produces maximal acceleration and rate of force production throughout the entire range of motion.[33] This phase of training is typically reserved for high level athletes who require maximal levels of power.

Goals and Strategies of Power Training

Phase 6: Elastic Equivalent Training
GOALS
- Enhance neuromuscular efficiency
- Increase rate of force production
- Enhance speed strength

TRAINING STRATEGIES
- Dynamic flexibility
- Core-power training
- Balance-power training
- Reactive-power training *(optional)*
- Resistance training
    — Superset one strength and one power exercise per body part
- Cardiorespiratory training

Phase 7: Maximal Power Training
GOAL
- Increase maximum speed strength and create neuromuscular adaptation throughout an entire range of motion

TRAINING STRATEGIES
- Dynamic flexibility
- Core-power training *(optional)*
- Balance-power training *(optional)*
- Reactive-power training *(optional)*
- Resistance training
    — Strictly power exercises for each body part
- Cardiorespiratory training *(optional)*
    — If this training is done, perform after the workout.

The Program Template

The uniqueness of the OPT™ model is that it packages scientific principles into an applicable form of programming. This is a direct result testing within NASM's clinical setting, used on actual clients. NASM has developed a template that provides fitness professionals with specific guidelines for creating an individualized program (Figure 1-3).

NASM — Optimum Performance Training™

NATIONAL ACADEMY OF SPORTS MEDICINE

NAME: _____   DATE: _____

TRAINER: _____   PHASE: _____

DAYS/WEEK: _____   GOAL: _____

CARDIO TRAINING:	TIME:	EQUIPMENT:

WARMUP/FLEXIBILITY	Sets	Reps	Duration	Rest	Notes
1.					
2.					
3.					
4.					

CORE & BALANCE	Sets	Reps	Tempo	Rest	Notes
1.					
2.					

REACTIVE	Sets	Reps	Tempo	Rest	Notes
1.					
2.					

SPEED, AGILITY, QUICKNESS	Sets	Reps	Time	Rest	Notes
1.					
2.					

STRENGTH	Exercise	Sets	Reps	Intensity	Tempo	Rest	Notes
TOTAL BODY							
CHEST							
BACK							
SHOULDERS							
BICEPS							
TRICEPS							
LEGS							

COOL-DOWN	
POST-WORKOUT FLEXIBILITY	

How to Utilize the OPT™ Model

Chapters later in this text will be specifically dedicated to explaining how to utilize the OPT™ model in the fitness environment and detail the necessary components of an integrated training program. They include:

- Client assessments
- Flexibility training
- Cardiorespiratory training
- Core training
- Balance training
- Reactive training
- Speed, Agility & Quickness
- Resistance training
- Program design

Each of these chapters explains how each component specifically fits into the OPT™ model and how to realistically apply the information given. Other chapters in this textbook will review:

- Basic exercise science
- Nutrition
- Supplementation
- Special populations
- Behavior modification
- Professional development

All of this combined information should provide any individual with all of the tools necessary to become a skilled and well-rounded fitness professional.

MODULE 1-2 Summary

The Optimum Performance Training (OPT™) model provides a system for properly and safely progressing any client to his/her goals, by utilizing integrated training methods. It consists of three building blocks — stabilization, strength and power.

Stabilization training addresses muscular imbalances and attempts to improve the stabilization of joints and overall posture. This is a component that most training programs leave out even though it is the most important in ensuring proper neuromuscular functioning. This training block has two phases — Phase 1: Corrective Exercise Training and Phase 2: Integrated Stabilization Training.

Strength training focuses on increasing levels of muscle size and/or maximal strength. Most traditional programs begin at this point and as a result, often lead to injury. This training block has three phases — Phase 3: Stabilization Equivalent Training, Phase 4: Muscular Development Training and Phase 5: Maximal Strength Training.

Power training that is designed to target specific forms of training that are necessary for maximal force production. This stage has two phases — Phase 6: Elastic Equivalent Training and Phase 7: Maximal Power Training.

All of these phases of training have been specifically designed to follow biomechanical, physiological and functional principles of the kinetic chain. They should provide an easy-to-follow, systematic progression that minimizes injury and maximizes results. To help ensure proper organization and structure, NASM has developed a program template that guides fitness professionals through the process.

MODULE 1-2 Quiz

1. What is the term for the combination of flexibility, cardiorespiratory, core, balance, reactive and resistance training as part of a progressive system?

   _____

2. Name the three building blocks of training in the OPT™ model.

   _____

   _____

   _____

3. In which building block does the phase of Stabilization Equivalent Training belong?

   _____

4. Which phase enhances prime mover strength and improves the rate of force production concurrently?

   _____

References

1. [Anonymous]. Trends in personal training. IDEA international fitness professional Summit 1999; Mar 5-7, Baltimore, MD.

2. [Anonymous]. Bureau of Labor Statistics 1999.

3. Caspersen CJ, Pereira MA, Curran KM. Changes in physical activity patterns in the United States, by sex and cross-sectional age. *Med Sci Sports Exerc* 2000; 32(9):1601-9.

4. [Anonymous]. International Obesity Task Force 1999. http://www.iotf.org/

5. Volinn E. The epidemiology of low back pain in the rest of the world. A review of surveys in low- and middle-income countries. *Spine* 1997 Aug; 22(15): 1747-54.

6. Wescott WL, Baechle TR. *Strength training for seniors.* Champaign, IL: Human Kinetics; 1999.

7. Whiting WC, Zernicke RF. *Biomechanics of musculoskeletal injury.* Champaign, IL: Human Kinetics; 1998.

8. Kelsey JL. An epidemiological study of acute herniated lumbar discs. *Rheumatol Rehab* 1975; 14:144-5.

9. Kelsey JL. An epidemiological study of the relationship between occupations and acute herniated lumbar discs. *Int J Epidem* 1975;4:197-204.

10. Kelsey JL, Hardy RJ. Driving motor vehicles as a risk factor for acute herniated lumbar intervertebral discs. *Am J Epidem* 1975;102:63-73.

11. Evans W, Rosenberg I. *Biomarkers.* New York: Simon and Schuster; 1992.

12. Hurley BF, Hagberg JM. Optimizing health in older persons: Aerobic or strength training? In: Holsey JO, editor. *Exerc Sports Sci Rev* Volume 26. Baltimore: Williams & Wilkins; 1998. p. 61-89.

13. Larsson L, Grimby G, Karlsson J. Muscle strength and speed of movement in relation to age and muscle morphology. *J Appl Physiol* 1979;46;451-6.

14. Gillquist J, Messner K. Anterior cruciate ligament reconstruction and the long term incidence of gonarthrosis. *Sports Med* 1999; 27:143-56.

15. Prate RR, Pratt M, Blair SN, et al. Physical activity and public health. A reccomendation from the Centers of Disease Control and Prevention and the American College of Sports Medicine. *JAMA* 1995; 273(5):402-7.

16. Chaffin DB, Andersson GJ, Martin BJ. *Occupational biomechanics.* New York: Wiley-Interscience; 1999.

17. Griffin LY, Agel J, Albohm MJ et al. Noncontact anterior cruciate ligament injuries: risk factors and prevention strategies. *J Am Acad Orthop Surg* 2000; May-Jun 8(3):141-50.

18. Wannamethee SG, Sharper AG, Whincup PH, Walker M. Role of risk factors for major coronary heart disease events with increasing length of follow-up. *Heart* 1999; 81:374-9.

19. Leon AS, Connett J. Physical activity and 10.5 year mortality in the multiple risk factor intervention trial (MRFIT). *Int J Epidemiol* 1991; 20:690-7.

20. Lee IM, Hennekens CH, Berger K, Buring JE, Manson JE. Exercise and risk of stroke in male physicians. *Stroke* 1999; 30:1-6.

21. Kiely DK, Wolf PA, Cupples LA, Beiser AS, Kannel WB. Physical activity and stroke risk: the Framingham Study. *Am J Epidemiol* 1994;140:608-20.

22. Paffenbarger MD, Kampert JB, LE IM, Hyde RT, Leung RW, Wing AI. Changes in physical activity and other lifeway patterns influencing longevity. *Med Sci Sports Exerc* 1994; 26(7):857-65.

23. Sherman SE, Agostino RBD, Silbershatz H, Kannel WB. Comparison of past versus recent physical activity in the prevention of premature death and coronary artery disease. *Am Heart J* 1999;138:900-7.

24. Praemer A, Furner S, Rice DP. *Musculoskeletal conditions in the united states.* Rosemont, IL: Academy of Orthopedic Surgeons; 1992.

25. Stephens T. Secular trends in adult physical activity: Boom or bust? *Res Q Exerc Sport* 1987;58(2):94-105.

26. Guyer B, Ellers B. Childhood injuries in the United States: Mortality, morbidity, and cost. *Am J Dis Chil* 1990;144:649-52.

27. Towner EL, Jarvis SN, Walsh SM, Aynsley-Green A. Measuring exposure to injury risk in schoolchildren aged 11-14. *Br Med J* 1994;308(6926):449-52.

28. Watkins J. *Structure and function of the musculoskeletal system.* Champaign, IL: Human Kinetics; 1999.

29. Zohar J. Preventative conditioning for maximum safety and performance. *Sport Coach* 1973; 42(9):65,113-5.

30. Gambetta V. *The gambetta method.* Sarasota, FL: Gambetta Sports Training System, Inc.; 1998.

31. Steindler A. *Kinesiology of the human body.* Springfield, IL: Charles C. Thomas; 1964.

32. Jones BH, Cowan DN, Knapik J. Exercise, training, and injuries. *Sport Med* 1994; 18(3):202-14.

33. Clark M. *Integrated training for the new millennium.* Thousand Oaks, CA: National Academy of Sports Medicine; 2000.

34. Hammer WI. Chapter 12. Muscle imbalance and postfacilitation stretch. In: Hammer WI editor. 2nd edition. *Functional soft tissue examination and treatment by manual methods.* Gaithsburg, MD: Aspen Publishers, Inc.; 1999.

35. Dominiguez RH. *Total body training*. East Dundee, IL: Moving Force Systems; 1982.

36. Jesse J. *Hidden causes of injury, prevention, and correction for running athletes*. Pasadena, CA: The Athletic Press; 1977.

37. Edgerton VR, Wolf S, Roy RR. Theoretical basis for patterning EMG amplitudes to assess muscle dysfunction. *Med Sci Sports Exerc* 1996;28(6):744-51.

38. Lewit K. Muscular and articular factors in movement restriction. *Man Med* 1985;1:83-5.

39. Sahrmann S. *Diagnosis and treatment of muscle imbalances and musculoskeletal pain syndrome*. Course manual. St. Louis, MO; 1997.

40. Borsa PA, Lephart SM, Kocher MS, Lephart SP. Functional assessment and rehabilitation of shoulder proprioception for glenohumeral instability. *J Sports Rehab* 1994; 3:84-104.

41. Hodges PW, Richardson CA. *Neuromotor dysfunction of the trunk musculature in low back pain patients*. In: Proceedings of the International Congress of the World Confederation of Physical Therapists, Washington, DC, 1995.

42. Hodges PW, Richardson CA. Inefficient muscular stabilization of the lumbar spine associated with low back pain. *Spine* 1996; 21(22):2640-50.

43. Janda V. *Muscle function testing*. London: Butterworth; 1983.

44. Janda V. *Physical therapy of the cervical and thoracic spine*. In: Grant R (ed). New York: Churchill Livingstone; 1988.

45. Janda V. *Muscle weakness and inhibition in back pain syndromes*. In: Grieve GP. Modern manual therapy of the vertebral column. New York: Churchill Livingstone; 1986.

46. Janda V. *Muscles, central nervous system regulation, and back problems*. In: Korr IM (ed). Neurobiologic mechanisms in manipulative therapy. New York: Plennum Press; 1978.

47. Janda V, Vavrova M. *Sensory motor stimulation video*. Brisbane, Australia: Body Control Systems; 1990.

48. Liebenson CL. *Rehabilitation of the spine*. Baltimore: Williams and Wilkins; 1996.

49. O'Sullivan PE, Twomey L, Allison G, Sinclair J, Miller K, Knox J. Altered patterns of abdominal muscle activation in patients with chronic low back pain. *Aus J Physiother* 1997;43(2):91-8.

50. Heus R, Wertheim AH, Havenith G. Human energy expenditure when walking on a moving platform. *Eur J Appl Physiol Occup Physiol* 1998;100(2):133-48.

51. Williford HN, Olson MS, Gauger S, Duey WJ, Blessing DL. Cardiovascular and metabolic costs of forward, backward, and lateral motion. *Med Sci Sports Exerc* 1998;30(9):1419-23.

52. Ogita F, Stam RP, Tazawa HO, Toussaint HM, Hollander AP. Oxygen uptake in one-legged and two-legged exercise. *Med Sci Sports Exerc* 2000;32(10):1737-42.

CHAPTER TWO

Basic Exercise Science

Objectives

After studying this chapter, you will be able to:

- Define the components of the kinetic chain.
- Explain the structure and function of:
  — The central and peripheral nervous systems;
  — Bones;
  — Joints and
  — Muscles.
- Describe how they all relate to human movement.

Key Terms

- Kinetic chain
- Nervous system
- Sensory function
- Integrative function
- Motor function
- Neuron
- Sensory (afferent) neurons
- Interneurons
- Motor (efferent) neurons
- Central nervous system
- Peripheral nervous system
- Mechanoreceptors
- Muscle spindles
- Golgi tendon organs
- Joint receptors
- Skeletal system
- Bones

- Joints
- Axial skeleton
- Appendicular skeleton
- Depression
- Process
- Arthrokinematics
- Synovial joints
- Non-synovial joints
- Ligament
- Muscular system
- Muscle
- Tendons
- Sarcomere
- Neural activation
- Neurotransmitter
- Pennation

Introduction to Human Movement

KINETIC CHAIN:
The combination and interrelation of the nervous, muscular and skeletal systems.

Structure allows for and provides the basis of function.[1] Therefore, the components that make up a structure have a drastic influence on how that structure ultimately functions. In the human body, the components that make up the human movement system include the nervous system, the skeletal system and the muscular system. Together, these components are known as the **kinetic chain** and are responsible for human movement (Figure 2-1).[2,3]

All systems of the kinetic chain must work together to produce movement. If one system (or component) of the kinetic chain is not working properly, it will affect the other systems and ultimately affect movement.[4-10] Therefore, it is imperative that the health and fitness professional fully understand all components of the kinetic chain and how they work together to construct efficient movement. To gain a complete understanding of the kinetic chain, it is necessary to look at the structure and function of each component.

Nervous System
Skeletal System
+ Muscular System
_____
The Kinetic Chain

Figure 2-1: The Equation for Movement

MODULE 2-1: The Nervous System

Overview of the Nervous System

The **nervous system** is a conglomeration of billions of cells forming nerves that are specifically designed to provide a communication network within the human body (Figure 2-2). It is the central command center that allows us to gather information about our internal and external environments, process and interpret the information and then respond to it.[11-14]

The three primary functions of the nervous system include sensory, integrative and motor functions.[11-13] **Sensory function** is the ability of the nervous system to sense changes in either the internal or external environment, such as a stretch placed on a muscle (internal) or the change from walking on the sidewalk to walking in the sand (external). **Integrative function** is the ability of the nervous system to analyze and interpret the sensory information to allow for proper decision making, which produces the appropriate response. The **motor function** is the neuromuscular (or nervous and muscular systems') response to the sensory information, such as causing the muscle to initially contract when stretched, or changing our walking pattern when in the sand, as opposed to the sidewalk.[11-13]

The key aspect to note here is that all movement is directly dictated by the nervous system. Thus, it becomes important to train the nervous system efficiently to ensure that proper movement patterns are being developed, which enhances performance and decreases the risk of injuries.[11,13,15] This important concept will be discussed throughout the remainder of the text.

Anatomy of the Nervous System

The Neuron

The functional unit of the nervous system is known as the **neuron** (Figure 2-2).[11] Billions of neurons make up the complex structure of the nervous system and provide it with the ability to communicate internally with itself, as well as externally with the outside environment. Collectively, the merging of many neurons together forms the nerves of the body. Neurons are comprised of three main parts: cell body, axon and dendrites.[11-13,16]

The cell body (or soma) of a neuron is much like any other cell body in that it contains a nucleus and other organelles such as lysosomes, mitochondria and a Golgi complex. The axon is a cylindrical projection from the cell body that transmits nervous impulses to other neurons or effector sites (muscles, organs, other neurons, etc.). This is the part of the neuron that provides communication from the brain and/or spinal cord to other parts of the body.

NERVOUS SYSTEM: Large groups of cells that form nerves, which provide a communication network within the body.

SENSORY FUNCTION: The ability of the nervous system to sense changes in either internal or external environments.

INTEGRATIVE FUNCTION: The ability of the nervous system to analyze and interpret sensory information to allow for proper decision making, which produces the appropriate response.

MOTOR FUNCTION: The neuromuscular response to sensory information.

NEURON: The functional unit of the nervous system.

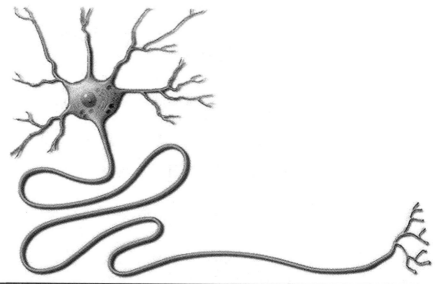

Figure 2-2: The Neuron

The dendrites are responsible for gathering information from other structures back into the neuron.[11-13,16]

Essentially, there are three main functional classifications of neurons that are determined by the direction of their nerve impulses (Table 2-1). **Sensory (afferent) neurons** transmit nerve impulses from effector sites (such as muscles and organs) via receptors to the brain and/or spinal cord. **Interneurons** transmit nerve impulses from one neuron to another.[12,16] **Motor (efferent) neurons** transmit nerve impulses from the brain and/or spinal cord to the effector sites such as muscles or glands.

A demonstration of the way these different neurons work together to produce a given response can be explained through the example of a person touching a hot object. The sensory (afferent) neurons send a signal from the hand to the brain telling the brain that the object is hot. This signal makes its way to the brain by traveling from one neuron to another via the interneurons. Once the signal has made it to the brain, the brain then interprets the information sent from the sensory neurons (the object is hot) and sends the appropriate signals down to the muscles of the hand and arm via the motor neurons, telling the muscles to contract to pull the hand away from the hot object, protecting the hand from injury.

The Central and Peripheral Nervous Systems

The nervous system is comprised of two interdependent divisions. These include the central nervous system and the peripheral nervous system.[1,11-13,16] The **central nervous system** consists of the brain and the spinal cord (Figure 2-3).[1,11-13,16] The central nervous system serves mainly to interpret information.

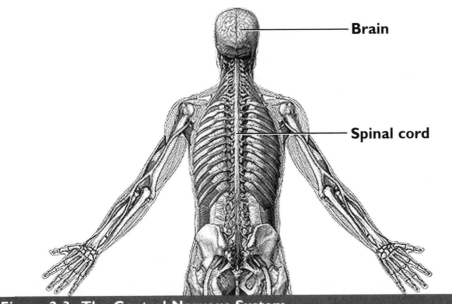

Brain

Spinal cord

Figure 2-3: The Central Nervous System

The **peripheral nervous system** consists of 12 cranial nerves, 31 pairs of spinal nerves (that branch out from the brain and spinal cord) and sensory receptors (Figure 2-4).[11-13,16]

These peripheral nerves serve two main functions. First, they provide a connection for the nervous system to activate different bodily organs, such as muscles. This is the efferent (motor) information going to an effector site (organs within the body).

Second, peripheral nerves relay information from the bodily organs back to the brain providing a constant update on the relation between the body and the environment. This is the afferent (sensory) information coming from an effector site (muscles, organs) back to the brain and/or spinal cord via sensory receptors.[11-14,16]

PERIPHERAL NERVOUS SYSTEM: Cranial and spinal nerves that spread throughout the body and serve to relay information from bodily organs to the brain and from the brain to bodily organs.

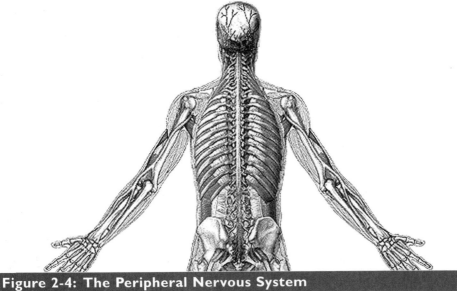

Figure 2-4: The Peripheral Nervous System

The sensory receptors are specialized structures located throughout the body that are designed to transform environmental stimuli (heat, light, sound, taste, motion, etc.) into sensory information that the brain and/or spinal cord can then interpret to produce a response. These receptors can be subdivided into four major categories. Mechanoreceptors respond to mechanical forces (touch and pressure), nociceptors respond to pain (pain receptors), chemoreceptors respond to chemical interaction (smell and taste) and photoreceptors respond to light (vision).[13,16] For relevance to this text, we will focus the attention on the mechanoreceptors.

With respect to the health and fitness professional and human movement, **mechanoreceptors** are specialized structures that are essentially responsible for sensing distortion in tissues.[18-21,23-25] This is brought about through stretch, compression, traction and/or tension to the tissue and then transmitted to the nervous system. Furthermore, it has been demonstrated that mechanoreceptors are located in muscles, tendons, ligaments and joint capsules.[23,24,26-30] Mechanoreceptors include muscle spindles, Golgi tendon organs and joint receptors.

Muscle spindles are the major sensory organs of the muscle and sit parallel to the muscle's fibers (Figure 2-5). Muscle spindles are sensitive to change in length and rate of length change.[1,5-7,10,11,13,16,20,24,30] When a muscle is stretched the spindles of that muscle are also stretched. This information is transmitted to the brain and spinal cord to update the nervous system on the status of the muscle length and the rate at which that muscle is lengthening. When excited, the muscle spindle will cause the muscle to contract. This is to prevent the muscle from stretching too far and/or too fast, either of which could otherwise cause injury.[1,5-7,10,11,13,16,20,24,30]

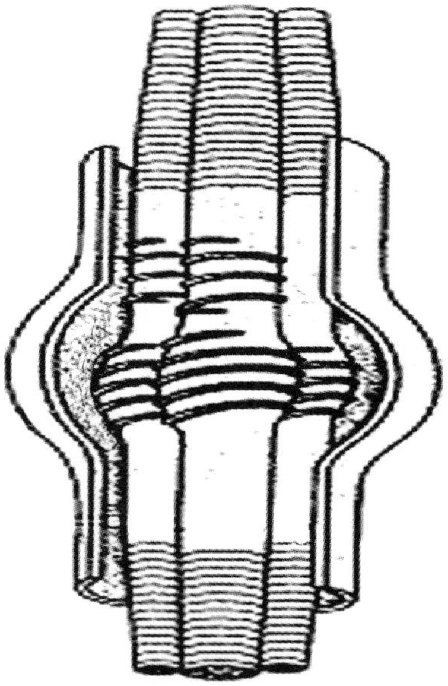

Figure 2-5: Muscle Spindles

> **MECHANO-RECEPTORS:**
> Sensory receptor responsible for sensing distortion in body tissues.

> **MUSCLE SPINDLES:**
> Fibers sensitive to change in length of the muscle and the rate of that change.

Golgi tendon organs are at the point where the muscle and tendon meet (musculotendinous junction) and are sensitive to changes in muscular tension and rate of the tension change (Figure 2-6).[1,5-7,10,11,13,16,20,24,30] When excited, the Golgi tendon organ will cause the muscle to relax. This is to prevent the muscle from being placed under excessive stress and sustaining injury.

> **GOLGI TENDON ORGANS:** Organs sensitive to change in tension of the muscle and the rate of that change.

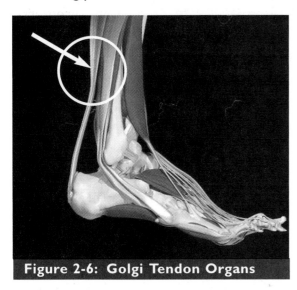

Figure 2-6: Golgi Tendon Organs

Joint receptors are located in and around the joint capsule. They respond to pressure, acceleration and deceleration of the joint (Figure 2-7). These receptors act to signal extreme joint positions and thus help to prevent injury. They can also act to initiate a reflexive inhibitory response in the surrounding muscles if there is too much stress placed on that joint.[17,23,24,32,33]

> **JOINT RECEPTORS:** Receptors sensitive to pressure, acceleration and deceleration in the joint.

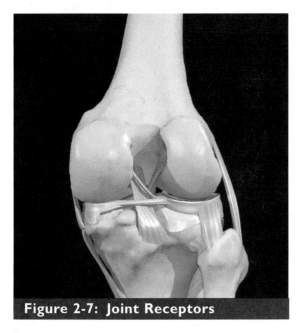

Figure 2-7: Joint Receptors

MODULE 2-1 Summary

The movement system of the human body is called the kinetic chain. The three components of the kinetic chain are the nervous system, the skeletal system and the muscular system.

The nervous system is comprised of billions of neurons that transfer information throughout the body, through two interdependent systems: the central nervous system (brain and spinal cord) and the peripheral nervous system (nerves that branch out from the brain and spinal cord). The system gathers information about our external and internal environments, processes that information and then responds to it. It has three major functions: sensory (recognizes changes), integrative (combines information and interprets it) and motor (produces a neuromuscular response).

MODULE 2-1 Quiz

1. All movement is directly dictated by the nervous system.

   ☐ True   ☐ False

2. Which part of the neuron provides communication from the brain and/or spinal cord to other parts of the body?

   ☐ Soma

   ☐ Axon

   ☐ Dendrite

3. If a woman got a splinter stuck in her finger, which neurons would transmit that pain information to her brain?

   ☐ Sensory (afferent) neuron

   ☐ Interneuron

   ☐ Motor (efferent) neuron

4. Name the two interdependent divisions of the nervous system.

   _____

5. Which kind of receptors respond to touch and pressure?

   ☐ Chemoreceptors   ☐ Mechanoreceptors

   ☐ Photoreceptors   ☐ Nociceptors

6. Match the mechanoreceptors to their functions:

   a. Muscle spindles   ____sense overtension and cause relaxation.

   b. Golgi tendon organs ____sense stress and inhibit surrounding muscles.

   c. Joint receptors   ____sense overstretching and cause contraction.

MODULE 2-2: The Skeletal System

Overview of the Skeletal System

SKELETAL SYSTEM:
The body's frame, comprised of bones and joints.

The **skeletal system** is the framework for our structure and movement (Figure 2-8). It helps to determine our stature, as the positioning of our bones will determine our size and shape.[12,34,35] Therefore, it is very important to understand that the growth, maturation and functionality of the skeletal system is greatly affected by our posture, activity (or lack thereof) and nutrition.[34]

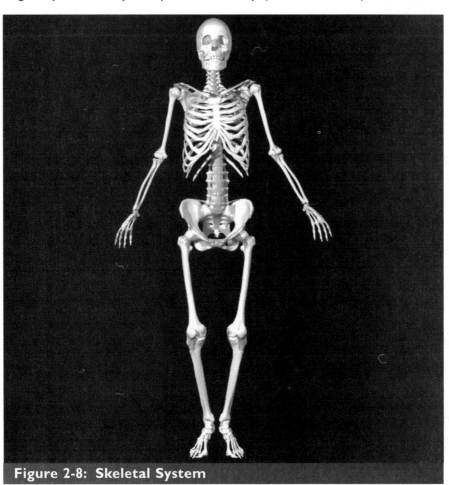

Figure 2-8: Skeletal System

BONES:
Hard connective tissues that connect to create a skeletal framework.

Further, this structure is the resting ground for the muscles of our body. **Bones** form junctions that are connected by muscles and connective tissue. These junctions are known as **joints**.[36] Joints are the sites where movement occurs as a result of muscle contraction.[36,37] Bones, joints and muscles, in conjunction with our central nervous system, make up the kinetic chain and are responsible for movement.

JOINTS:
The movable places where two or more bones meet.

Divisions of the Skeletal System

The skeletal system is divided into two divisions: the axial and appendicular skeletal systems.[12,36] The **axial skeleton** is made up of the skull, the rib cage and the vertebral column. In all, there are approximately 80 bones in the axial skeleton.[12] The **appendicular skeleton** is made up of the upper and lower extremities as well as the shoulder and pelvic girdles.[12] (Some authors, however, note that the pelvic girdle could be considered a component of either the axial or appendicular system and that it is actually a link between the two systems.)[36] The appendicular skeleton encompasses approximately 126 bones.

There are roughly 206 bones in the skeletal system with approximately 177 of these being utilized in voluntary movement. [12,35,36] In all, the bones in the body form more than 300 joints.[35]

With regard to movement, the bones (skeleton) provide two main functions. The first is leverage. The bones act and perform as levers when acted on by muscles.[34,36] The second primary function of bones (skeleton) relative to movement is to provide support.[34] This translates into posture, which is necessary for the efficient distribution of forces acting on the body.[34,37-40]

AXIAL SKELETON: Portion of the skeletal system that consists of the skull, rib cage and vertebral column.

APPENDICULAR SKELETON: Portion of the skeletal system that includes the upper and lower extremities.

Types of Bones

There are four major types of bones in the skeletal system (Table 2-1).[12] Their shape, size and proportion of bone tissue determine their classification.[34] The categories include long bones, short bones, flat bones and irregular bones.[12,34]

Table 2-1: Types of Bones		
Bone Type	**Characteristic**	**Example**
Long	Long, cylindrical shaft and irregular or widened ends	Humerus, femur
Short	Similar in length and width and appear somewhat cubical in shape	Carpals of hand, tarsals of feet
Flat	Thin, protective	Scapulae, patella
Irregular	Unique shape and function	Vertebrae

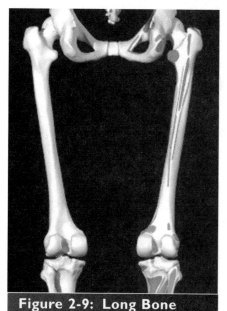

Figure 2-9: Long Bone

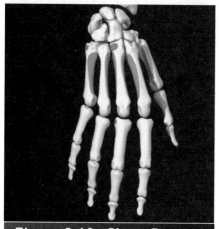

Figure 2-10: Short Bone

Long Bones

Long bones are characterized by their long cylindrical body (shaft), with irregular or widened bony ends.[12,34,36] They are shaped much like a beam and exhibit a slight curvature that is necessary for efficient force distribution (Figure 2-9).[12,34] Long bones are comprised predominantly of compact bone tissue to ensure strength and stiffness.[12,34] However, they do have considerable amounts of spongy bone tissue for shock absorption.[12,34] The long bones of the upper body include the clavicle, humerus, radius, ulna, metacarpals and phalanges, while in the lower body there are the femur, tibia, fibula, metatarsals and phalanges.

Short Bones

Short bones are similar in length and width and appear somewhat cubical in shape (Figure 2-10).[12,36] They consist predominantly of spongy bone tissue to maximize shock absorption.[12,34,36] The carpals of the hands and tarsals of the feet fit this category.[12,34,36]

Flat Bones

Flat bones are thin bones comprised of two layers of compact bone tissue surrounding a layer a spongy bone tissue (Figure 2-11).[12,34] These bones are involved in protection of internal structure and also provide broad attachment sites for muscles.[34] The flat bones include the sternum, scapulae, ribs, ilium, cranial bones and patella.[12,34,36]

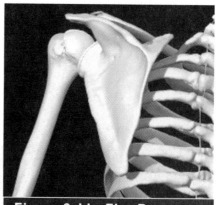

Figure 2-11: Flat Bone

Irregular Bones

Irregular bones are bones of unique shape and function that do not fit the characteristics of the other categories (Figure 2-12).[12,34,36] These include the vertebrae, pelvic bones and certain facial bones.[12,34,36]

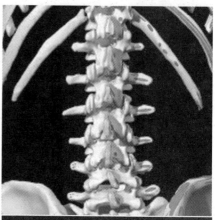

Figure 2-12: Irregular Bone

Bone Markings

The majority of all bones have specific distinguishing structures known as surface markings.[12] These structures are necessary for increasing the stability in joints as well as providing attachment sites for muscles.[12] Some of the more prominent and important ones will be discussed here. These surface markings can be divided into two simple categories: depressions and processes.[12]

Depressions

Depressions are simply flattened or indented portions of the bone.[12] One common depression is called a fossa. An example is the supraspinous or infraspinous fossa located on the scapulae (Figure 2-13). These are attachment sites for the supraspinatus and infraspinatus muscles, respectively.[12]

Another form of a depression is known as sulcus. This is simply a groove in a bone that allows a soft structure (i.e. tendon) to pass through.[12] An example of this is the intertubercular sulcus located between the greater and lesser tubercles of the humerus (Figure 2-14).[12] This is commonly known as the groove for the biceps tendon.

> **DEPRESSION:** Flattened or indented potion of bone, which can be a muscle attachment site.

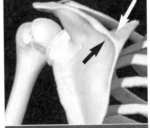

Figure 2-13: Fossa

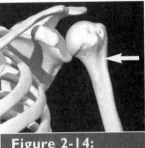

Figure 2-14: Sulcus

Processes

Processes are projections protruding from the bone to which muscles, tendons and ligaments can attach.[12] Some of the more common processes are called process, condyle, epicondyle, tubercle and trochanter.[12] Examples of a process include the spinous processes found on the vertebrae and acromion and coracoid process found on the scapula (Figure 2-15).

Condyles are located on the inner and outer portion at the bottom of the femur and top of the tibia to form the knee joint (Figure 2-16).

Epicondyles are located on the inner and outer portion of the humerus to help form the elbow joint (Figure 2-17).

> **PROCESS:** Projection protruding from the bone where muscles, tendons and ligaments can attach.

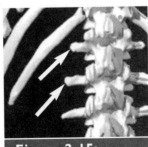

Figure 2-15: Process

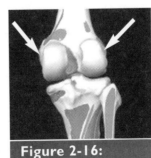

Figure 2-16: Condyle

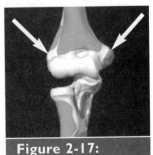

Figure 2-17: Epicondyle

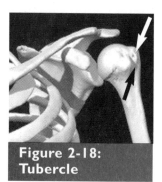

Figure 2-18: Tubercle

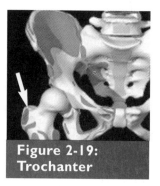

Figure 2-19: Trochanter

The tubercles are located at the top of the humerus at the glenohumeral joint (Figure 2-18). There are the greater and lesser tubercles, which are attachment sites for shoulder musculature.

Finally, the trochanters are located at the top of the femur and are attachment sites for the hip musculature (Figure 2-19).[12] The greater trochanter is commonly called the hipbone.

Joints

ARTHRO-KINEMATICS: The movements of the joints.

Joints are formed by one bone that articulates with another bone.[12] Joints can be categorized by both their structure and their function (or the way they move).[12,35,37] Joint motion is referred to as **arthrokinematics** with the three major motion types being roll, slide and spin.[7,37,41] It must be noted that these motions rarely occur, if ever, as an isolated, true motion. As is typically the case with the human body, variations and combinations of these joint motions take place during functional movement.[41]

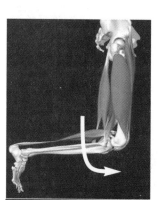

Figure 2-20: Rolling Joint

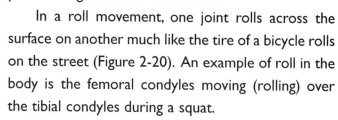

Figure 2-21: Sliding Joint

In a roll movement, one joint rolls across the surface on another much like the tire of a bicycle rolls on the street (Figure 2-20). An example of roll in the body is the femoral condyles moving (rolling) over the tibial condyles during a squat.

In a slide movement, one joint's surface slides across another much like the tire of a bicycle skidding across the street (Figure 2-21). An example of slide in the human body is the tibial condyles moving (sliding) across the femoral condyles during a knee extension.

In a spin movement, one joint surface rotates on another much like twisting the lid off of a jar (Figure 2-22). An example of spin in the human body is the head of the radius rotating on the end of the humerus during pronation and supination of the forearm.

Classification of Joints

Synovial joints are the joints most associated with movement in the body. They comprise approximately 80 percent of the joints in the body and have the greatest capacity for motion.[12,34,35,37] The synovial joint is characterized by the absence of fibrous or cartilaginous tissue directly connecting the bones (Figure 2-23). Rather, they are loosely held together by a joint capsule and ligaments.[12,34,35,37] This gives synovial joints their increased mobility.[37] Synovial

Figure 2-22: Spinning Joint

joints also have another unique quality in that they produce synovial fluid. Synovial fluid resembles egg whites and works much like engine oil. It is secreted within the joint capsule from synovial membrane.[12,35,37] Synovial fluid is essential for lubrication of the joint surfaces to reduce excessive wear and to nourish the cartilage cells that line the joint.[12,34,35,37]

There are several types of synovial joints in the body. They include gliding (plane), condyloid (condylar or ellipsoidal), hinge, saddle, pivot and ball-and-socket.[12,34,35]

A gliding (plane) joint is a non-axial joint that has the simplest movement of all joints.[12,34] It moves either back and forth or side to side. An example is the joint between the navicular bone and the second and third cuneiform bones in the foot or the carpals of the hand and in the facet joints (Figure 2-24).[12,34,35]

Condyloid (condylar or ellipsoidal) joints are termed so based upon the condyle of one bone fitting into the elliptical cavity of another bone to form the joint.[12] Movement predominantly occurs in one plane (flexion/extension in the sagittal plane) with minimal movement in the others (rotation in the transverse plane; adduction/abduction in the frontal plane). These joints are seen in the wrist between the radius and carpals and the knee joint (Figure 2-25).[34]

The hinge joint is a uniaxial joint allowing movement predominantly in only one plane of motion, the sagittal plane. Joints such as the elbow, interphalangeal and ankle are considered hinge joints (Figure 2-26).[12,34]

The saddle joint is named after its appearance. One bone looks like a saddle with the articulating bone straddling it like a rider. This joint is only found in the carpometacarpal joint in the thumb.[12,34] It allows movement predominantly in two planes of motion (flexion/extension in the sagittal plane; adduction/abduction in the frontal plane) with some rotation to produce circumduction (Figure 2-27).[12,34]

Pivot joints allow movement in predominantly one plane of motion (rotation, pronation/supination in the transverse plane). These joints are found in the alantoaxial joint at the base of the skull (top of spine) and between the radioulnar joint (Figure 2-28).[12,34]

> **SYNOVIAL JOINTS:** Joints which are held together by a joint capsule and ligaments and are most associated with movement in the body.

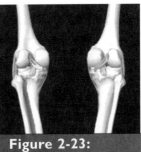
Figure 2-23: Synovial Joint

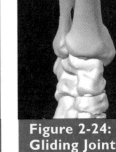
Figure 2-24: Gliding Joint

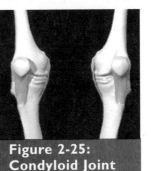
Figure 2-25: Condyloid Joint

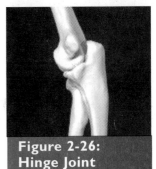
Figure 2-26: Hinge Joint

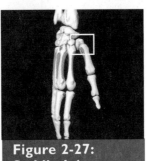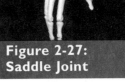
Figure 2-27: Saddle Joint

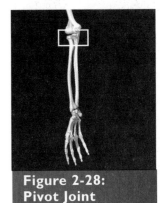
Figure 2-28: Pivot Joint

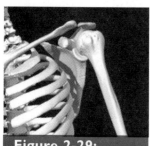

Figure 2-29: Ball-and-Socket Joint

NON-SYNOVIAL JOINTS:
Joints which do not have a joint cavity, connective tissue or cartilage.

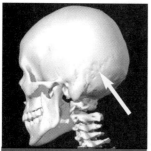

Figure 2-30: Non-Synovial Joint

Ball-and-socket joints are the most mobile of the joints. They allow movement in all three planes. Examples of these joints are the shoulder and hip (Figure 2-29).[12,34]

Non-synovial joints are named as such because they have no joint cavity, fibrous connective tissue or cartilage in the uniting structure. They can be structured in either a fibrous or cartilaginous manner. These joints exhibit little to no movement. Examples of this joint type are seen in the sutures of the skull, the distal joint of the tibia and fibula (ankle) and the symphysis pubis (Figure 2-30).[12,37]

See Table 2-2 for a full description of the characteristics of these types of joints and examples of each.

Table 2-2: Types of Joints		
Joint Type	**Characteristic**	**Example**
NON-SYNOVIAL	No joint cavity and fibrous connective tissue; little or no movement	Sutures of the skull
SYNOVIAL	Produce synovial fluid, have a joint cavity and fibrous connective tissue	Knee
Gliding	No axis of rotation; moves by sliding side-to-side and/or back and forth	Vertebrae
Condyloid	Formed by the fitting of condyles of one bone into elliptical cavities of another; moves predominantly in one plane	Knee
Hinge	Uniaxial; moves predominantly in one plane of motion (sagittal)	Elbow
Saddle	One bone fits like a saddle on another bone; moves predominantly in two planes (sagittal, frontal)	Only: Carpometacarpal joint of thumb
Pivot	Only one axis; moves predominantly in one plane of motion (transverse)	Radioulnar
Ball-and-socket	Most mobile of joints; moves in all three planes of motion	Hip

Function of Joints

First and foremost, joints provide the bones a means to be manipulated, allowing for movement throughout segments of the body.[36,37] Joints also provide stability, allowing for movement to take place without unwanted movement.

All joints in the human body are linked together. This implies that movement of one joint directly affects the motion of others.[7-9,19,37] This is an essential concept for a health and fitness professional to understand because it creates an awareness of how the body functionally operates and is the premise behind kinetic chain movement.[7-9,19,37]

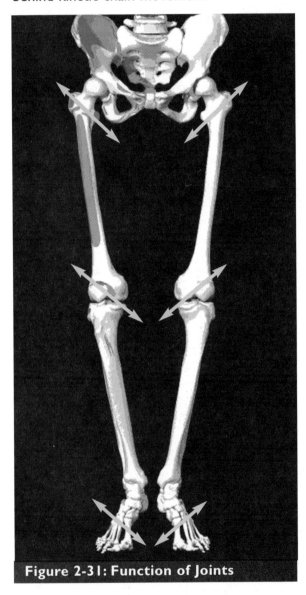

Figure 2-31: Function of Joints

This concept is very easy to demonstrate. First, start by standing with both feet firmly on the ground. Next, roll your feet inward and outward. (Figure 2-31). Notice what your knee and hips are doing. Keep your feet stationary and rotate your hips. Notice what your knees and feet are doing. Moving one of these joints will inevitably move the others. If you understand this concept, then you are well on your way to understanding true kinetic chain movement. Moreover, it should be easy to see that if one joint is not working properly, it will affect the other joints it works with. This is extremely important when looking at establishing proper client observation, flexibility, programming and exercise technique.[7-9,10,19]

LIGAMENT: Primary connective tissue that connects bones together and which provides stability, input to the nervous system, guidance and the limitation of improper joint movement.

Joint Connective Tissue

The primary connective tissue for a joint is the **ligament**. Ligaments connect bone to bone and provide static and dynamic stability as well as input to the nervous system (proprioception) (Figure 2-32).[42,43] Ligaments are primarily made up of a protein called collagen with varying amounts of another protein called elastin. Collagen fibers are situated in a more parallel fashion to the forces that are typically placed upon the ligament. Thus they provide the ligament with the ability to withstand tension (tensile strength). Elastin gives a ligament some flexibility or elastic recoil to withstand the bending and twisting it may have to endure. Not all ligaments will have the same amount of elastin.

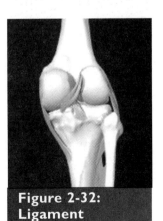

Figure 2-32: Ligament

For example, the anterior cruciate ligament of the knee contains a very low amount of elastin and is predominantly comprised of collagen. Because of this, it is much better suited for resisting strong forces and makes a good stabilizing structure of the knee.[42,43]

Each synovial joint has a joint capsule that is much like a compartment for fluid and tissues that surround the joint. Much of the tissue of the joint capsule is also ligamentous in nature.

Finally, it is important to note that ligaments are characterized by poor vascularity (or blood supply), meaning that that ligaments do not heal or repair very well and may be slower to adapt.[42,43,45,47]

MODULE 2-2 Summary

The skeletal system is the body's framework and is made up of bones and joints in two divisions: axial and appendicular. The four main types of bones are long, short, flat and irregular, which all have markings of depressions and/or processes. Bones are connected (via ligaments) by either synovial or non-synovial joints, which both provide movement as well as stability. Joints are interconnected and movement of one will affect the others.

MODULE 2-2 Quiz

1. Which portion of the skeleton includes the upper and lower extremities?

   _____

2. Match up bones with their type:
   a. Tarsals   ____ Long bone
   b. Vertebrae   ____ Short bone
   c. Femur   ____ Flat bone
   d. Patella   ____ Irregular bone

3. Which joints are most associated with movement in the body?
   ☐ Synovial
   ☐ Non-synovial

4. Match the synovial joint with an example.
   a. Gliding joint   ____ Knee
   b. Condyloid joint   ____ Radioulnar
   c. Hinge joint   ____ Vertebrae
   d. Saddle joint   ____ Elbow
   e. Pivot joint   ____ Hip
   f. Ball-and-socket joint ____ Carpometacarpal joint of thumb

5. Joints allow bone to be manipulated, which allows for movement.
   ☐ True   ☐ False

6. Joints inhibit stability.
   ☐ True   ☐ False

7. The primary connective tissue for joints is collagen.
   ☐ True   ☐ False

8. All joints in the human body are interconnected.
   ☐ True   ☐ False

MODULE 2-3: The Muscular System

Overview of the Muscular System

The nervous system is the control center for movement production and the skeletal system provides the structural framework for our bodies. However, in order to complete the cycle of movement production, the body must have a device that the nervous system can command to move the skeletal system. This is the **muscular system** (Figure 2-33). Muscles generate internal tension that, under the control of the nervous system, manipulates the bones of our body to produce movements. Muscles are the movers and stabilizers of our bodies.

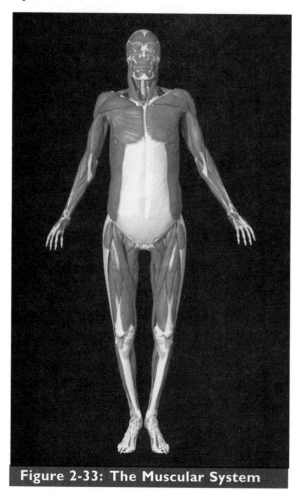

Figure 2-33: The Muscular System

> **MUSCULAR SYSTEM:**
> Series of muscles that moves the skeleton.

The Structure of Skeletal Muscle

The structure of skeletal muscle is an important piece of this complex system. It provides the health and fitness professional with a foundation of knowledge that will help to illuminate the function of the muscular system as well as the kinetic chain. The following section will discuss the structure of muscle tissue and its connective tissues as well as the microscopic view of the muscle fiber and its contractile elements.

> **MUSCLE:**
> Tissue consisting of long cells that contract when stimulated, to produce motion.

Muscle and its Connective Tissue

A **muscle** is the compilation of many individual muscle fibers that are neatly wrapped together with connective tissue that forms different bundles, much like a cable is made up of bundles of wires encased in an outer covering (Figure 2-34).[36] Breaking the bundles down into layers from outer to innermost, the first bundle is the actual muscle itself wrapped by an outer layer of connective tissue called fascia and an inner layer immediately surrounding

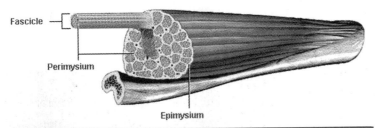

Figure 2-34: Structure of the Skeletal Muscle

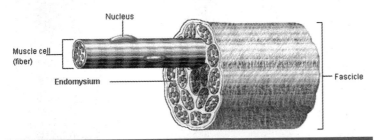

Figure 2-35: Muscle Cell

the muscle called the epimysium. The fascia and epimysium are also intimately connected with the bone and help to form the muscle's tendon.[11-13,16,20,34-37,42,48] The next bundle of muscle fiber is called a fascicle. Each fascicle is wrapped by connective tissue called perimysium. Each fascicle is in turn made up of many individual muscle fibers that are wrapped by connective tissue called endomysium (Figure 2-35).[11-13,16,20,34-37,42,48]

The connective tissues within the muscle play a vital role in movement. They allow the forces generated by the muscle to be transmitted from the contractile components of the muscle (discussed next) to the bones, creating motion. Each layer of connective tissue extends the length of the muscle helping to form the tendon.

Tendons are the structures that attach muscles to bone and provide the anchor from which the muscle can exert force and control the bone and joint.[11-13,16,20,34-37,42,48] They are very similar to ligaments in that they have poor vascularity (blood supply) which leaves them susceptible to slower repair and adaptation.[45,49]

TENDONS:
Connective tissues that attach muscle to bone and provide an anchor for muscles to produce force.

Muscle Fibers and Their Contractile Elements

Muscle fibers are encased by a plasma membrane known as the sarcolemma and contain typical cell components like cellular plasma called sarcoplasm (which contains glycogen, fats, minerals and oxygen binding myoglobin), nuclei and mitochondria (that transform energy from food into energy for the cell). However, unlike typical cells they also have structures called myofibrils. Myofibrils contain myofilaments that are the actual contractile components of muscle tissue. These myofilaments are known as actin (thin string-like filaments) and myosin (thick filaments).

The actin (thin) and myosin (thick) filaments form a number of repeating sections within a myofibril. Each one of these particular sections is known as a **sarcomere** (Figure 2-36). A sarcomere is the functional unit of the muscle much like the neuron is for the nervous system. It lies in the space between two Z lines. Each Z line denotes another sarcomere along the myofibril. [11-13,16,20,34-37,42,48]

> **SARCOMERE:**
> The functional unit of muscle that produces muscular contraction and which consists of repeating sections of actin and myosin.

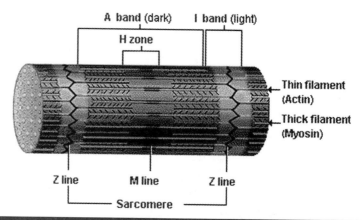

Figure 2-36: Sarcomere

Two protein structures that are also important to muscle contraction are tropomyosin and troponin. Tropomyosin is located on the actin filament and blocks myosin binding sites located on the actin filament keeping myosin from attaching to actin while the muscle is in a relaxed state. Troponin, also located on the actin filament, plays a role in muscle contraction by providing binding sites for both calcium and tropomyosin when a muscle needs to contract. (For further information, see the Excitation-contraction Coupling section of this chapter.)

Generating Force in a Muscle

Muscles generate force through a variety of methods. These methods, which include neural activation, the sliding filament theory and excitation-contraction-coupling mechanism, will be reviewed. Muscle fiber types, recruitment, firing rate and arrangement will also be discussed as they relate to force production.

Neural Activation

Neural activation is essential for a muscle to contract, for movement and/or stabilization. This activation is generated by the communication between the nervous system and the muscular system. The motor neurons of the body are connected to the muscle fibers. A motor neuron and the muscle fibers with which it connects (innervates) is known as a motor unit. The point where the neuron meets an individual muscle fiber is called the neuromuscular junction (nerve to muscle). This junction is actually a small gap between the nerve and muscle fiber often called a synapse (Figure 2-37).

NEURAL ACTIVATION: The contraction of a muscle generated by a communication between the nervous system and muscular system.

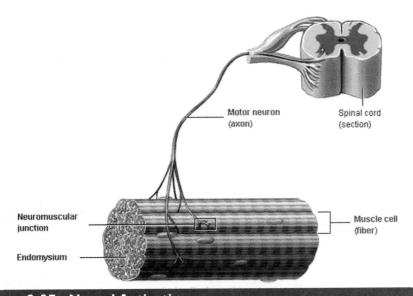

Motor neuron (axon)

Spinal cord (section)

Neuromuscular junction

Endomysium

Muscle cell (fiber)

Figure 2-37: Neural Activation

Electrical impulses (also known as action potentials) are transported from the central nervous system down the axon of the neuron. When the impulse reaches the end of the axon (axon terminal), chemicals called **neurotransmitters** are released.

Neurotransmitters are chemical messengers that cross the synapse between the neuron and muscle fiber, transporting the electrical impulse from the nerve to the muscle (much like a boat carries people from one side of a river to the other). The neurotransmitters fall into receptor sites on the muscle fiber, specifically designed for their attachment, much like a square peg fits into a square hole. The neurotransmitter used by the neuromuscular system is termed acetylcholine (ACh). Once attached, ACh stimulates the muscle fibers to go through a series of steps that produce muscle contractions.[11-13,16,20,34-37,42,48]

NEURO-TRANSMITTER: Chemical messengers that cross synapses to transmit electrical impulses from the nerve to the muscle.

Sliding Filament Theory

Sliding Filament Theory is the proposed process of how the contraction of the filaments within the sarcomere takes place, after a muscle has been given the order to contract via neural activation (Table 2-3) (Figure 2-38).

Table 2-3: Steps in the Sliding Filament Theory

Steps in the Sliding Filament Theory are summarized as follows:[11,13,16,48]

1. A sarcomere shortens as a result of the Z lines moving closer together.

2. The Z lines converge as the result of myosin heads attaching to the actin filament and asynchronously pulling (power strokes) the actin filament across the myosin, resulting in shortening of the muscle fiber.

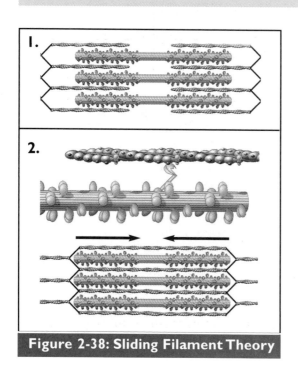

Figure 2-38: Sliding Filament Theory

Excitation-contraction Coupling: Putting It All Together

Excitation-contraction coupling is the process of neural stimulation creating a muscle contraction. It involves a series of steps that start with the initiation of a neural message (neural activation) and end up with a muscle contraction (Sliding Filament Theory) (Table 2-4) (Figure 2-39).

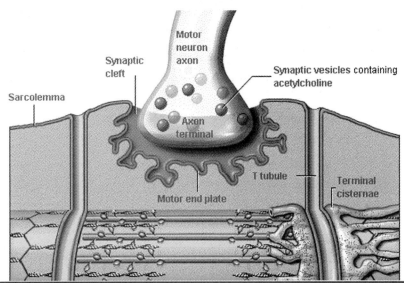

Figure 2-39: Excitation-Contraction Coupling

Table 2-4: Steps in Excitation-Contraction Coupling

Steps in excitation-contraction coupling are summarized as follows:[11,13,16,48]

1. A nerve impulse (action potential) is transmitted through the neuron and down the axon to where the axon meets the muscle fiber (neuromuscular junction) and releases ACh (acetylcholine).

2. ACh transports across the synapse and binds to its receptor on the muscle fiber.

3. This continues the neural message (action potential) to the muscle fiber that triggers the release of calcium (Ca++) into the sarcoplasm (where the actin and myosin are located).

4. Ca++ binds to the protein troponin. This forces the protein tropomyosin to move away from the myosin binding site and allowing for myosin to attach to actin.

5. Myosin attaches to actin creating a pull of the filaments across each other (Sliding Filament Theory), causing the muscle to shorten (contract).

6. Once the neural impulse for contraction subsides, calcium concentration in the sarcoplasm decreases, forcing myosin to unbind with the actin ending the muscle contraction.

Muscle Fiber Types

Muscle fiber types vary in their chemical and mechanical properties. Essentially they have been delineated into two main categories: type I and type II fibers (Table 2-5).[11-13,16,20,34-37,42,48]

Table 2-5: Muscle Fiber Types	
Type	**Characteristic**
Type I *(Slow twitch)*	■ Higher in capillaries, mitochondria and myoglobin ■ Increased oxygen delivery ■ Smaller in size ■ Produce less force ■ Slow to fatigue ■ Long-term contractions (stabilization) ■ Slow twitch
Type II *(Fast twitch)*	■ Lower in capillaries, mitochondria and myoglobin ■ Decreased oxygen delivery ■ Larger in size ■ Produce more force ■ Quick to fatigue ■ Short-term contractions (force and power) ■ Fast twitch

Type I (slow twitch) muscle fibers contain a higher number of capillaries, mitochondria (transform energy from food into ATP, or "cellular energy") and myoglobin that allows for improved delivery of oxygen. Myoglobin is similar to hemoglobin, the red pigment found in red blood cells and therefore type I muscle fibers are often referred to as red fibers.[11,13,16,48]

Type II (fast twitch) muscle fibers are sub-divided into type IIa and type IIb based again on their chemical and mechanical properties. They generally contain fewer capillaries, mitochondria and myoglobin. Type II muscle fibers are often referred to as white fibers. Type IIb muscle fibers have a low oxidative capacity (ability to use oxygen) and fatigue quickly. Type IIa muscle fibers have a higher oxidative capacity and fatigue more slowly than type IIb.[11,13,16,20,48]

Looking at the whole picture, slow twitch type I muscle fibers are smaller in size (diameter), slower to produce maximal tension and are more resistant to fatigue.[50-53] These fibers are important for muscles producing long-term contractions necessary for stabilization and postural control. An example would include sitting upright, while maintaining ideal posture against gravity, for an extended period of time.

Fast twitch type II muscle fibers are larger in size, quick to produce maximal tension and fatigue more quickly than type I fibers. These fibers are important for muscles producing movements requiring force and power such as performing a sprint.

When designing a program, it becomes very important for the health and fitness professional to incorporate specific training parameters to fulfill these muscular requirements.[7] (This is seen in the OPT™ model discussed in Chapter 13.)

It is important to note that all muscles have a combination of slow and fast twitch fiber that will vary depending on the function of the muscle.[11,13,16,20,48] For example, it has been shown that the human anterior tibialis muscle (muscle on the shin) has approximately 73 percent slow twitch type I muscle fibers while the lateral head of the gastrocnemius (superficial calf muscle) has an approximated 49 percent type I muscle fibers.[54,55]

Muscle Fiber Arrangement

Muscle fiber arrangement refers to the manner in which the fibers are situated, in relation to the tendon. Many muscles of the body have fibers that run in the same direction as the tendon they are attached to. Some examples include the rectus abdominis and the biceps brachii. However, there are many muscles in the body whose fibers run obliquely (at an angle) to the tendon. This is termed **pennation**, which comes from the Latin word penna, meaning feather.[34,37] Examples of other muscle fiber arrangement patterns include nonpennate fusiform, fan-shaped, longitudinal and quadrilateral and the pennate unipenniform, bipenniform and multipenniform (Table 2-6).

PENNATION: Muscle fibers that run at an angle to the tendon, instead of in the same direction.

Table 2-6: Muscle Types and Fiber Arrangement		
Type	**Fiber Arrangement**	**Example**
Fusiform	Parallel to direction of tendon	Biceps brachii
Fan-shaped	From broad attachment to narrow	Pectoralis major
Longitudinal	Parallel to line of pull	Sartorius
Quadrilateral	Parallel to line of pull	Rhomboid
Unipenniform	Oblique to the line of pull	Posterior tibialis
Bipenniform	Oblique to the line of pull	Rectus femoris
Multipenniform	Oblique to the line of pull	Deltoid

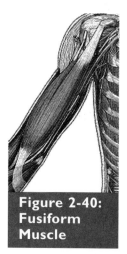

**Figure 2-40:
Fusiform
Muscle**

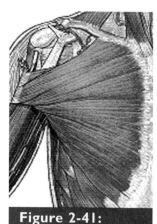

**Figure 2-41:
Fan-Shaped Muscle**

Fusiform or spindle shaped muscles have a full muscle belly (center of the muscle) and taper off at either end (Figure 2-40).[12,20,34-37] The fiber arrangement parallels the direction of the muscle and tendon (line of pull) and enables the force produced by the fibers to pull in the same direction as the line of pull.[34] An example of a fusiform muscle would be the biceps brachii.

Fan-shaped (also known as convergent or radiate) muscles have muscle fibers that span out from a narrow attachment at one end to a broad attachment at the other end (Figure 2-41).[35,36] The fiber arrangement diverges from the broad attachment to the narrow one creating various angles of pull. An example of a fan-shaped muscle is the pectoralis major.

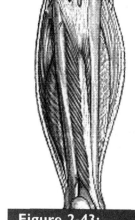

Longitudinal muscles are long strap-like muscles.[35,36] Their muscle fibers run parallel to the line of pull.[35,36] An example of a longitudinal muscle is the sartorius.

Quadrilateral muscles are four-sided and usually flat (Figure 2-42).[35,36] Their muscle fiber arrangement is parallel to the line of pull.[36] An example of a quadrilateral muscle is the rhomboid.

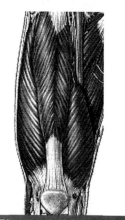

**Figure 2-42:
Quadrilateral
Muscle**

**Figure 2-43:
Unipenniform
Muscle**

Unipenniform muscles have short, oblique (diagonal) muscle fibers that extend from one side of a long tendon (Figure 2-43).[12,20,34-37] The fiber arrangement dictates that the pull of the muscle fibers runs obliquely to the line of pull of the muscle and tendon.[34] An example of a unipenniform muscle is the posterior tibialis.

Bipenniform muscles have short, oblique (diagonal) muscle fibers that extend from both sides of a long tendon (Figure 2-44).[12,20,34-37] The fiber arrangement dictates that the pull of the muscle fibers runs obliquely to the line of pull of the muscle and tendon.[34] An example of a bipenniform muscle is the rectus femoris.

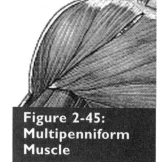

**Figure 2-44:
Bipenniform
Muscle**

**Figure 2-45:
Multipenniform
Muscle**

Multipenniform muscles have multiple tendons with obliquely running muscle fibers (Figure 2-45).[12,20,34-37] The fiber arrangement dictates that the pull of the muscle fibers runs obliquely to the line of pull of the muscle and tendon.[34] An example of a multipenniform muscle is the deltoid.

The significance of pennation lies in its ability to increase the force output of a muscle. The force that a muscle can exert is proportional to the cross-sectional area (diameter or thickness) of all of its fibers.[11,13,16,34-37] Thus a broad, thick, lengthwise muscle will produce more force than a thin one. However, in a penniform muscle, the oblique arrangement of the muscle allows a larger number of muscle fibers to be placed in a smaller space. This creates a greater cross-sectional area of a muscle that would appear to be smaller and thus, produce a greater force output.[11,13,16,34-37]

Muscles as Movers

Muscles provide the human body with a variety of functions that allow for the manipulation of forces placed on the body and to produce and slow down movement. These muscle functions categorize the muscle as an agonist, synergist, stabilizer and/or antagonist (Table 2-7).[7,10,19,34]

Agonist muscles are muscles that act as prime movers or in other words, they are the muscles most responsible for a particular movement. For example, the gluteus maximus is an agonist for hip extension.

Table 2:7: Muscle Types and Fiber Arrangement			
Muscle Type	**Muscle Function**	**Exercise**	**Muscle(s) Used**
Agonist	Prime mover	Chest press	Pectoralis major
		Overhead press	Deltoid
		Row	Latissimus dorsi
		Squat	Gluteus maximus, Quadriceps
Synergist	Assist prime mover	Chest press	Anterior deltoid, triceps
		Overhead press	Triceps
		Row	Posterior deltoid, biceps
		Squat	Hamstrings
Stabilizer	Support, while prime mover and synergist work	Chest press	Rotator cuff
		Overhead press	Rotator cuff
		Row	Rotator cuff
		Squat	Transversus abdominis
Antagonist	Oppose prime mover	Chest press	Posterior deltoid
		Overhead press	Latissimus dorsi
		Row	Pectoralis major
		Squat	Psoas

Synergist muscles assist prime movers during movement. For example, the hamstrings and the erector spinae are synergistic with the gluteus maximus during hip extension.

Stabilizer muscles support or stabilize the body while the prime movers and the synergists perform the movement patterns. For example, transversus abdominis, internal oblique and multifidus (deep muscles in the low back) stabilize the low back, pelvis and hips (lumbo-pelvic-hip complex) during hip extension.

Antagonist muscles perform the opposite action of the prime mover. For example, the psoas (a deep hip flexor) is antagonistic to the gluteus maximus during hip extension.

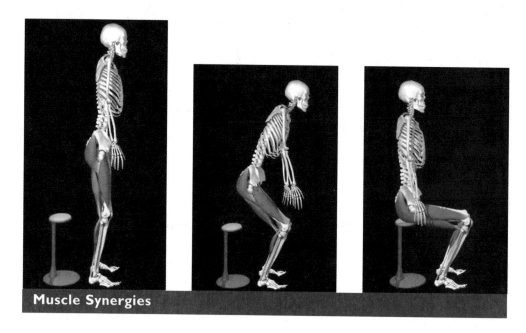

Muscle Synergies

MODULE 2-3 Summary

The muscular system is made up of many individual fibers and attaches to bones by way of tendons. There are different muscle fiber types and arrangements of them that affect how they move. Muscles generate force through neural activation, sliding filament theory and excitation-contraction coupling.

The nervous system receives and delivers information throughout the body, by way of neurons. The stimulation of the nervous system activates sarcomeres, which generates tension in the muscles. This tension is transferred through tendons to the bones and this produces motion.

MODULE 2-3 Quiz

1. What is the functional unit of the muscle that acts similarly to the neuron in the nervous system?

   _____

2. Myofibrils contain myofilaments that are the components that contract muscle tissue.

   ☐ True   ☐ False

3. What is it called when filaments within the sarcomere contract, after a muscle has been given the order to contract via neural activation?

   ☐ Sliding Filament Theory

   ☐ Excitation-contraction Coupling

4. Which kind of muscle fibers are "fast twitch"?

   ☐ Type I

   ☐ Type II

5. Which three of the following muscle fiber arrangements run parallel to the line of pull (or tendon)?

   ☐ Fusiform

   ☐ Fan-shaped

   ☐ Longitudinal

   ☐ Quadrilateral

   ☐ Unipenniform

   ☐ Bipenniform

   ☐ Multipenniform

6. Match the muscle with its appropriate action during a squat.
   a. Gluteus maximus and quadriceps   ____ Synergist
   b. Hamstrings   ____ Stabilizer
   c. Transversus abdominis   ____ Antagonist
   d. Psoas   ____ Agonist

References

1. Cohen H. *Neuroscience for rehabilitation.* 2nd edition. Philadelphia: Lippincott Williams & Wilkins; 1999.

2. Panjabi MM. The stabilizing system of the spine. Part I. Function, dysfunction, adaptation, and enhancement. *J Spin Disord* 1992;5:383-9.

3. Liebenson CL. Active muscle relaxation techniques. Part II. Clinical Application. *J Manip Physiol Ther* 1990;13(1):2-6.

4. Edgerton VR, Wolf S, Roy RR. Theoretical basis for patterning EMG amplitudes to assess muscle dysfunction. *Med Sci Sports Exerc* 1996;28(6):744-51.

5. Liebension C. Active rehabilitation protocols. Chapter 18. In: Liebension C (ed). *Rehabilitation of the spine.* Baltimore: Williams & Wilkins; 1996.

6. Chaitow L. *Muscle energy techniques.* New York: Churchill Livingstone; 1997.

7. Clark MA. *Integrated training for the new millennium.* Thousand Oaks, CA: National Academy of Sports Medicine; 2001.

8. Clark MA. *Integrated kinetic chain assessment.* Thousand Oaks, CA: National Academy of Sports Medicine; 2001.

9. Clark MA. *A scientific approach to understanding kinetic chain dysfunction.* Thousand Oaks, CA: National Academy of Sports Medicine; 2001.

10. Clark MA, Corn RJ, Parracino LA. *Integrated program design for the fitness professional.* Thousand Oaks, CA: National Academy of Sports Medicine; 2000.

11. Milner-Brown A. *Neuromuscular physiology.* Thousand Oaks, CA: National Academy of Sports Medicine; 2001.

12. Tortora GJ. *Principles of human anatomy.* 7th edition. New York: Harper Collins College Publishers; 1995.

13. Fox SI. *Human physiology.* 5th edition. Dubuque, IA: Wm. C. Brown Publishers; 1996.

14. Brooks GA, Fahey TD, White TP. *Exercise physiology: human bioenergetics and its application.* 2nd edition. Mountain View, CA: Mayfield Publishing Company; 1996.

15. Drury DG. Strength and proprioception. *Ortho Phys Ther Clin* 2000;9(4):549-61.

16. Vander A, Sherman J, Luciano D. *Human physiology: the mechanisms of body function.* 8th edition. New York: McGraw-Hill; 2001.

17. Lephart SM, Rieman BL, Fu FH. Introduction to the sensorimotor system. In: Lephart SM, Fu FH (eds). *Proprioception and neuromuscular control in joint stability.* Champaign, IL: Human Kinetics; 2000.

18. Biedert RM. Contribution of the three levels of nervous system motor control: Spinal cord, lower brain, cerebral cortex. In: Lephart SM, Fu FH (eds). *Proprioception and neuromuscular control in joint stability.* Champaign, IL: Human Kinetics; 2000.

19. Clark MA. *Human movement science.* Thousand Oaks, CA: National Academy of Sports Medicine; 2001.

20. Enoka RM. *Neuromechanical basis of kinesiology.* 2nd edition. Champaign, IL: Human Kinetics; 1994.

21. Rose DJ. *A multi level approach to the study of motor control and learning.* Needham Heights, MA: Allyn & Bacon; 1997.

22. Flowers K. Visual closed-loop and open-loop characteristics of voluntary movement in patients with parkinsonism and intention. *Brain* 1976;99:260-310.

23. Barrack RL, Lund PJ, Skinner HB. Knee proprioception revisited. *J Sport Rehab* 1994;3:18-42.

24. Grigg P. Peripheral neural mechanisms in proprioception. *J Sport Rehab* 1994;3:2-17.

25. Wilkerson GB, Nitz AJ. Dynamic ankle stability: mechanical and neuromuscular interrelationships. *J Sport Rehab* 1994;3:43-57.

26. Boyd IA. The histological structure of the receptors in the knee joint of the cat correlated with their physiological response. *J Physiol* 1954;124:476-88.

27. Edin B. Quantitative analysis of static strain sensitivity in human mechanoreceptors from hairy skin. *J Neurophysiol* 1992;67:1105-13.

28. Edin B, Abbs JH. Finger movement responses of cutaneous mechanoreceptors in the dorsal skin of the human hand. *J Neurophysol* 1991;65:657-70.

29. Gandevia SC, McClosky DI, Burke D. Kinesthetic signals and muscle contraction. *Trends Neurosci* 1992;15:62-5.

30. McClosky DJ. Kinesthetic sensibility. *Physiol Rev* 1978;58:763-820.

31. Sady SP, Wortman M, Blanke D. Flexibility training: ballistic, static, or proprioceptive neuromuscular facilitation? *Arch Phys Med Rehabil* 1982 Jun;63(6):261-3.

32. Lephart SM, Pincivero D, Giraldo J, Fu F. The role of proprioception in the management and rehabilitation of athletic injuries. *Am J Sports Med* 1997;25:130-7.

33. Proske U, Schaible HG, Schmidt RF. Joint receptors and kinaesthesia. *Exp Brain Res* 1988;72:219-24.

34. Hamill J, Knutzen JM. *Biomechanical basis of human movement.* Baltimore, MD: Williams & Wilkins; 1995.

35. Watkins J. *Structure and function of the musculoskeletal system.* Champaign, IL: Human Kinetics; 1999.

36. Luttgens K, Hamilton N. *Kinesiology: scientific basis of human motion.* 9th edition. Dubuque, IA: Brown & Benchmark Publishers; 1997.

37. Norkin CC, Levangie PK. *Joint structure and function: a comprehensive analysis.* 2nd edition. Philadelphia: FA Davis Company; 1992.

38. Chaffin DB, Andersson GJ, Martin BJ. *Occupational biomechanics.* New York: Wiley-Interscience; 1999.

39. Whiting WC, Zernicke RF. *Biomechanics of musculoskeletal injury.* Champaign, IL: Human Kinetics; 1998.

40. Bogduk N. *Clinical anatomy of the lumbar spine and sacrum.* 3rd edition. New York: Churchill Livingstone; 1997.

41. Hertling D, Kessler RM. *Management of common musculoskeletal disorders.* Philadelphia: Lippincott Williams & Wilkins; 1996.

42. Alter MJ. *Science of flexibility.* 2nd edition. Champaign, IL: Human Kinetics; 1996.

43. Gross J, Fetto J, Rosen E. *Musculoskeletal examination.* Malden, MA: Blackwell Sciences, Inc.; 1996.

44. Johns RJ, Wright V. The relative importance of various tissues in joint stiffness. *J App Physiol* 1962;17(5):824-8.

45. Nordin M, Lorenz T, Campello M. Biomechanics of tendons and ligaments. Ch 4. In: Nordin M, Franklel VH (eds). *Basic biomechanics of the musculoskeletal system.* 3rd edition. Philadelphia: Lippincott Williams & Wilkins; 2001.

46. Miyatsu M, Atsuta Y, Watakabe M. The physiology of mechanoreceptors in the anterior cruciate ligament: and experimental study in de-cerebrate-spinalized animals. *J Bone Joint Surg* 1993;75B:653-7.

47. Solomonow M, Baratta R, Zhou BH, Shoji H, Bose W, Beck C, D'Ambrosia R. The synergistic action of the anterior cruciate ligament and thigh muscles in maintaining joint stability. *Am J Sports Med* 1987;15:207-13.

48. McComas AJ. *Skeletal muscle: form and function.* Champaign, IL: Human Kinetics; 1996.

49. Kannus P. Structure of the tendon connective tissue. *Scand J Med Sci Sports* 2000; 10(6):312-20.

50. Al-Amood WS, Buller AJ, Pope R. Long-term stimulation of cat fast twitch skeletal muscle. *Natur* 1973;244:225-7.

51. Buller AJ, Eccles JC, Eccles RM. Interaction between motorneurons and muscles in respect of the characteristic speeds of their responses. *J Physiol* 1960;150:417-39.

52. Dubowitz V. Cross-innervated mammalian skeletal muscle: histochemical, phyusiological and biomechanical observations. *J Physiol* 1967;193:481-96.

53. Hennig R, Lomo T. Effects of chronic stimulation on the size and speed of long-term denervated and innervated rat fast and slow skeletal muscles. *Acta Physiologica Scand* 1987;130:115-31.

54. Johnson MA, Polgar J, Weightman D, Appleton D. Data on the distribution of fiber types in thirty-six human muscles. *J Neurological Sci* 1973;18:111-29.

55. Green HJ, Daub B, Houston ME, Thomson JA, Fraser I, Ranney D. Human vastus lateralis and gastrocnemius muscles. A comparative histochemical analysis. *J Neurological Sci* 1981;52:200-1.

CHAPTER THREE

The Cardiorespiratory System

Objectives

After studying this chapter, you will be able to:

- Describe the structure and function of:
  — The cardiorespiratory system,
  — The cardiovascular system and
  — The respiratory system.
- Explain how each of those systems relates to human movement.
- Go through oxygen testing procedures.
- Understand how oxygen is related to energy expenditure, as well as the influence that dysfunctional breathing can have on the kinetic chain.
- Outline the bioenergetic continuum.

Key Terms

- Cardiorespiratory system
- Cardiovascular system
- Heart
- Mediastinum
- Atrium
- Ventricle
- Blood
- Blood vessel
- Arteries
- Veins
- Arterioles
- Capillaries
- Venules
- Respiratory system
- Inspiration
- Expiration
- Aerobic
- Anaerobic
- Bioenergetics
- Adenosine triphosphate

Introduction to the Cardiorespiratory System

CARDIO-RESPIRATORY SYSTEM:
A system of the body comprised of the cardiovascular and respiratory systems.

t has been established that the kinetic chain is the primary system for movement production, under the direct control of the nervous system. In order to maintain a constant state of efficient operation, however, it needs to have support systems. One such support system is known as the cardiorespiratory system. The **cardiorespiratory system** is comprised of the cardiovascular and respiratory systems. Together they provide the tissues of the kinetic chain with oxygen (O^2), nutrients, protective agents and a means to remove waste by-products.[1-5] This ensures optimal cellular function within the kinetic chain. This chapter will focus on the structure and function of the cardiovascular and respiratory systems.

MODULE 3-1: The Cardiovascular System

CARDIO-VASCULAR SYSTEM:
A system of the body comprised of the heart, blood and blood vessels.

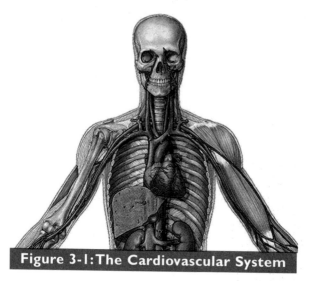

Figure 3-1: The Cardiovascular System

The cardiovascular system is comprised of the heart, the blood it pumps and the blood vessels that transport the blood from the heart to the tissues of the body (Figure 3-1). A basic understanding of the structure and function of the cardiovascular system is necessary to understand the kinetic chain.

The Heart

HEART:
A hollow muscular organ that pumps a circulation of blood through the body by means of rhythmic contraction.

The **heart** is a muscular pump that rhythmically contracts to push blood throughout the body. It is positioned obliquely in the center of the chest (or thoracic cavity) lying anteriorly to the spine and posteriorly to the sternum.[4] It is flanked laterally by the lungs.[4] This area is called the **mediastinum**.[6] The adult heart is approximately the size of a typical adult fist and weighs roughly 300 grams (approximately 10 ounces).[4,6]

Heart muscle is termed cardiac muscle and has similar characteristics to skeletal muscle. It is made up of myofibrils containing actin and myosin that crossbridge to cause contractions and is surrounded by a sarcolemma.[1-3,6] Cardiac muscle is for the most part considered an involuntary muscle, meaning that it cannot typically be consciously controlled.

Cardiac Muscle Contraction

Cardiac muscle fibers are shorter and more tightly connected than skeletal muscle, thus enabling the contraction of one fiber to stimulate the others to contract synchronously.[1-3] The conduction system (or means by which the muscle fibers are activated) is much different than in skeletal muscle. All cardiac muscle fibers have a built in contraction rhythm, and the fibers with the highest rhythm determine the heartbeat or heart rate.[1-3] The typical discharge rate and thus, heart rate, is between 70-80 beats per minute.[3,4,6,7]

The specialized conduction system of cardiac muscle that provides the rhythm for heart rate includes several items (Figure 3-2).[1-4,6,7] The sinoatrial (SA) node, which is located in the right atrium is termed the "pacemaker" for the heart, because it initiates the heartbeat. Internodal pathways transfer the impulse from the SA node to the atrioventricular (AV) node. The AV node delays the impulse before moving on to the ventricles. The atrioventricular (AV) bundle passes the impulse to the ventricles for contraction via the left and right bundle branches of the Purkinje fibers.

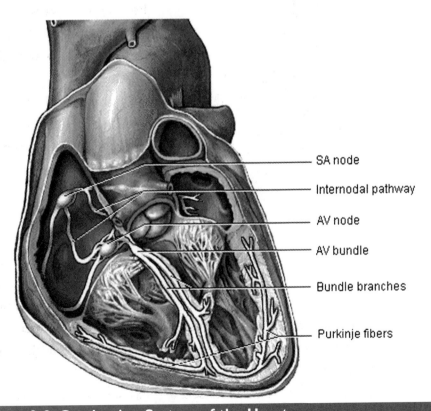

SA node
Internodal pathway
AV node
AV bundle
Bundle branches
Purkinje fibers

Figure 3-2: Conduction System of the Heart

Structure of the Heart

The heart is comprised of four hollow chambers that are delineated into two interdependent (but separate) pumps on either side. These two pumps are separated by the interatrial septum (separates the atria) and interventricular septum (separates the ventricles).[4-6] Each side of the heart has two chambers: an atrium and a ventricle (Figure 3-3).[1-4,6,7]

The **atriums** are smaller chambers, located superiorly on either side of the heart. They essentially gather blood coming to the heart, much like a reservoir. The right atrium gathers deoxygenated blood returning to the heart from the entire body, while the left atrium gathers re-oxygenated blood coming to the heart from the lungs (Figure 3-3).[1-4,6-7]

ATRIUM:
Either of the two chambers of the heart that receives blood from the veins and forces it into the ventricles.

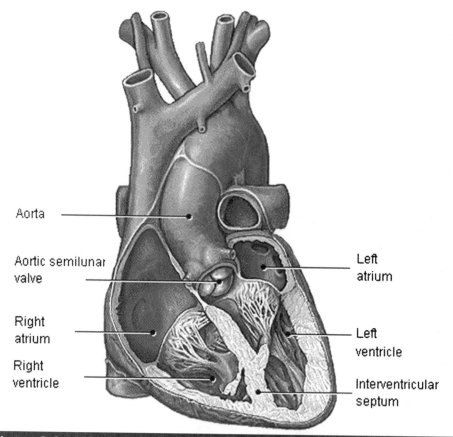

Aorta

Aortic semilunar valve

Right atrium

Right ventricle

Left atrium

Left ventricle

Interventricular septum

Figure 3-3: Atriums and Ventricles

VENTRICLE:
Either of the two chambers of the heart that receive blood from their corresponding atrium and, in turn, force blood into the arteries.

The **ventricles** are larger chambers located inferiorly on either side of the heart. They are the main pumps in the heart, as they pump blood out to the rest of the body. The right ventricle receives the deoxygenated blood from the right atrium and then pumps it to the lungs to be saturated with incoming oxygen. The left ventricle receives the re-oxygenated blood from the left atrium and proceeds to pump it to the entire body (Figure 3-3).[1-4,6,7]

Each chamber of the heart is separated from one another and major veins and arteries via valves in order to prevent a back flow or spillage of blood back into the chambers. These valves include the atrioventricular valves and the semilunar valves (Figure 3-3).[1-4,6,7]

Function of the Heart

As previously mentioned, the heart is a hollowed mass of muscle that encompasses two separate pumps (left and right ventricles), each of which distributes blood to specific parts of the body.[1-4,6,7]

Each contraction of a ventricle pushes blood from the heart into the body. The amount of blood that is pumped out with each contraction of a ventricle is the stroke volume (SV). The stroke volume of a typical adult is approximately 75-80 milliliters per beat (ml/beat).[1-3,5]

The rate with which the heart pumps, is referred to as the heart rate (HR). The heart rate of the typical person is approximately 70-80 beats per minute (bpm).[1-3,5]

Together, the heart rate and the stroke volume make up the overall performance of the heart and are collectively termed cardiac output (Q). Cardiac output is the combination of how many times the heart beats per minute and how much blood is being pumped out with each beat (Table 3-1).

Table 3-1: Functions of the Heart		
Terminology	**Action**	**Average Measurement**
Stroke Volume	The amount of blood that is pumped out with each contraction of a ventricle	For a typical adult, approximately 75-80 milliliters per beat (ml/beat)
Heart Rate	The rate with which the heart pumps	For a typical adult, approximately 70-80 beats per minute (bpm)
Cardiac Output	The combination of how many times the heart beats per minute and how much blood is being pumped out with each beat	

While it is next to impossible for a health and fitness professional to gauge the stroke volume of a client, it is relatively easy to determine the heart rate. Monitoring heart rate during exercise provides a good gauge as to the amount of work the heart is doing at any given time.[3,8] The proper procedure for manually monitoring heart rate can be seen in Figure 3-4. Another procedure commonly used is the heart rate monitor, which is worn on the body and automatically derives the beats per minute.

How To Manually Monitor Heart Rate

1. Place index and middle fingers around the palm side of the wrist (about one inch from the top of wrist, on the thumb side).
   a. The carotid artery at the neck can also be used, but with caution as it can cause dizziness and/or an inaccurate measurement if too much pressure is applied.

2. Locate the artery by feeling for a pulse with the index and middle fingers. Apply light pressure to feel the pulse. Do not apply excessive pressure as it may distort results.

3. When measuring the pulse during rest, count the number of beats in 60 seconds.
   a. There are some factors that may affect resting heart rate, including digestion, mental activity, environmental temperature, biological rhythms, body position and cardiorespiratory fitness. Because of this, resting heart rate should be measured upon waking (or, at the very least, after you have had five minutes of complete rest).

4. When measuring the pulse during exercise, count the number of beats in six seconds and add a zero to that number. Adding the zero will provide an estimate on the number of beats in 60 seconds. Or one can simply multiple the number by 10 (17 x 10 = 170) and that will provide the health and fitness professional with the same number.
   a. Example: Number of beats in six seconds = 17. Adding a zero = 170. This gives a pulse rate of 170 BPM.

Figure 3-4: How to Manually Monitor Heart Rate

BLOOD:
Fluid that circulates in the heart, arteries, capillaries and veins, which carries nutrients and oxygen to all parts of the body and also rids the body of waste products.

Blood

A properly functioning heart transports **blood** efficiently throughout the body. Blood acts as a medium to deliver and collect essential products to and from the tissues of the body.[1,2,5] Blood is thicker and heavier than water and constitutes approximately eight percent of total body weight.[1,2,5] The average person holds about five liters (roughly one and one-half gallons) of blood in his/her body at any given time.[1,2,5] Blood is a vital support mechanism, which provides an internal transportation, regulation and protection system for the kinetic chain (Table 3-1).

Transportation

Blood transports life-giving oxygen to and collects waste products from all tissues. It also transports hormones that act as chemical messengers to various organs and tissues in the body. Nutrients from the gastrointestinal tract are delivered to specific tissues by way of the bloodstream as well. Blood also conducts heat throughout the body.[1-2,5]

Regulation

Blood provides a means to regulate body temperature, due to the properties of its water content and its path of flow. As blood travels close to the skin it can give off heat or can be cooled depending on the environment.[1-3,6] Blood is essential in the regulation of the pH levels (acid balance) in the body as well as water content of bodily cells.[6]

Protection

Blood provides protection from excessive blood loss through its clotting mechanism, which seals off damaged tissue.[1,2,5] It also provides specialized immune cells to fight against foreign toxins within the body, decreasing disease and sickness.[1-3,5] Ironically, however, by this same mechanism, blood can also spread diseases and sickness.[5]

Table 3-2: Support Mechanisms of the Blood	
Mechanism	**Function**
Transportation	■ Transports oxygen and nutrients to tissues ■ Transports waste products from tissues ■ Transports hormones to organs and tissues ■ Carries heat throughout the body
Regulation	■ Regulates body temperature and acid balance in the body
Protection	■ Protects the body from excessive bleeding by clotting ■ Contains specialized immune cells to help fight disease/sickness

Blood Vessels

With each pump of each ventricle, blood is dispersed throughout the body. Concurrently, blood is also re-entering the heart. In order to circulate blood properly throughout the body and back to the heart, it must have a network through which it can travel. This network is comprised of **blood vessels**.[1,2,4-7]

Blood vessels form a closed circuit of hollow tubes that allow blood to be transported to and from the heart (Figure 3-5). Vessels that transport blood away from the heart are termed **arteries**. Vessels that transport blood back to the heart are termed **veins**.[1,2,4-7]

Arteries

Arteries leaving the heart are initially large and elastic.[4,6] These large arteries then branch out into medium-sized muscular arteries that extend to various areas throughout the body.[1,2,4-6] The medium-sized arteries further divide into smaller arteries that are called **arterioles**.[1,2,4-7] In turn, arterioles branch out into a multitude of microscopic vessels known as **capillaries**.[1,2,4-7] It is here in the capillaries that substances such as oxygen, nutrients, hormones and waste products are exchanged between tissues.[1,2,4-7]

Veins

Once substances are exchanged in the capillaries and waste products are gathered, they must then be transported to the proper area for cleaning and eventually back to the heart. The vessels that collect blood from the capillaries to perform this duty are called **venules**.[1,2,4-7] Venules progressively merge with other venules and form veins. Veins then transport all of the blood from the body back to the heart.[1,2,4-7]

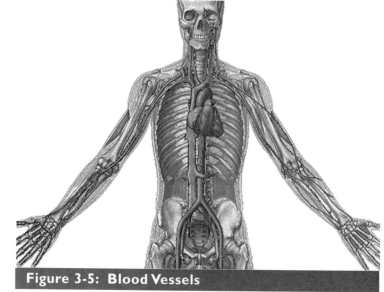

Figure 3-5: Blood Vessels

MODULE 3-1 Summary

The cardiorespiratory system is comprised of the cardiovascular system and the respiratory system. Together, they provide the body with oxygen, nutrients, protective agents and a means to remove waste products.

The cardiovascular system is comprised of the heart, blood and blood vessels. The heart is located in the mediastinum and is made up of involuntary cardiac muscle, which contracts according to a built-in rhythm in order to regularly pump blood throughout the body. It is divided into four chambers: two atriums (which gather deoxygenated blood from the body) and two ventricles (which pump blood out to the body) on each side.

The heart rate and the stroke volume make up the overall performance of the heart. Cardiac output is the combination of how many times the heart beats per minute and how much blood is being pumped out with each beat. Heart rate can be monitored manually.

Blood acts as a medium to deliver and collect essential products to and from the tissues of the body, providing an internal transportation, regulation and protection system.

The blood vessels that transport blood away from the heart are called arteries (which have smaller components called arterioles). The vessels that bring blood back to the heart are called veins (which have smaller components called venules). Capillaries are the smallest blood vessels and connect venules with arterioles.

MODULE 3-1 Quiz

1. What are the three components of the cardiovascular system?

_____

2. Which node of the cardiac system is referred to as the pacemaker?

_____

3. The ☐ **right** ☐ **left** atrium gathers deoxygenated blood returning to the heart from the entire body, while the ☐ **right** ☐ **left** atrium gathers re-oxygenated blood coming to the heart from the lungs.

4. The ☐ **right** ☐ **left** ventricle pumps blood back to the lungs.

5. Name three things that blood transports through the body.

_____

6. What is the name of the blood vessel that collects blood from the capillaries?

_____

MODULE 3-2: The Respiratory System

The second functional component of the cardiorespiratory system is the **respiratory system**, often referred to as the pulmonary system (Figure 3-6). The primary role of this system is to ensure proper cellular function.[9,10] The respiratory system works intimately with the cardiovascular system to

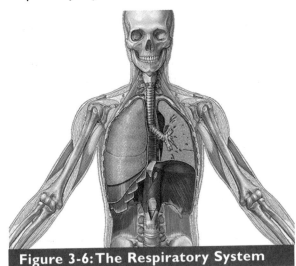

accomplish this by providing a means to collect oxygen from the environment and transport it to the bloodstream.[10] In order for this to be effectively accomplished, there must be an integrated functioning of the respiratory pump to move air in and out of the body and respiratory passageways to channel the air (Table 3-3).[10]

Figure 3-6: The Respiratory System

> **RESPIRATORY SYSTEM:**
> A system of organs (the lungs and their nervous and circulatory supply) that collects oxygen from the external environment and transports it to the bloodstream.

Respiratory Pump

The respiratory pump is located in the thorax or the thoracic (chest and abdominal) cavity. It is comprised of skeletal structures (bones) and soft tissue (muscles and pleural membranes). These systems, together with the nervous system, must work synergistically to allow for proper respiratory mechanics to occur much the same way as these systems work together to produce everyday functional movements. The skeletal structures provide the framework for the muscles to attach to as well as protection for the organs within the thorax (Table 3-3). While being strong enough to provide support, they are also flexible enough to allow for the expansion and compression needed for proper breathing.[1,2,5,6,10]

Breathing (or ventilation) is the actual process of moving air in and out of the body. It is divided into two phases: **inspiration** (or inhalation) and **expiration** (or exhalation). Inspiratory ventilation is active. This means that it requires active contraction of inspiratory muscles to increase the thoracic cavity volume, which decreases the intrapulmonary pressure (or pressure within the thoracic cavity) (Table 3-3). When the intrapulmonary pressure decreases below that of the atmospheric pressure (or the everyday pressure in the air), air is drawn into the lungs.[1-3,10,11]

> **INSPIRATION:**
> The process of actively contracting inspiratory muscles in order to move air into the body.

> **EXPIRATION:**
> The process of actively or passively relaxing inspiratory muscles in order to move air out of the body.

Table 3-3: Structures of the Respiratory Pump		
Bones	Sternum	Ribs
		Vertebrae
Muscles	Inspiration	Diaphragm
		External intercostals
		Scalenes
		Sternocleidomastoid
		Pectoralis minor
	Expiration	Internal intercostals
		Abdominals

Inspiratory ventilation occurs in two forms: normal resting state (quiet) breathing and/or heavy (deep, forced) breathing. Normal breathing requires the use of the primary respiratory muscles while heavy breathing requires the additional use of the secondary respiratory muscles.[1,2,5,6,10,12]

Expiratory ventilation can be both active and passive. During normal breathing, expiratory ventilation is passive as it results from the relaxation of the contracting inspiratory muscles. During heavy or forced breathing, the expiratory ventilation relies on the activity of expiratory muscles to compress the thoracic cavity and force air out.[1,2,5,6,10,13]

Respiratory Passageways

The purpose of ventilation is to move air in and out of the body. However, the air must have passageways to funnel it in and out of the lungs for proper utilization. These respiratory passageways are divided into two categories, the conduction passageway and the respiratory passageway.

The conduction passageway consists of all the structures that air travels through before entering the respiratory passageway (Table 3-4). The nasal and oral cavities, mouth, pharynx, larynx, trachea and bronchioles provide a gathering station for air and oxygen to be funneled into the body (Figure 3-7). These structures also allow the incoming air to be purified, humidified (or moisture added) and warmed or cooled to match body temperature.[1-3,5,7,9,10]

The respiratory passageway collects the channeled air coming from the conducting passageway (Figure 3-7).[1,2,5,6,9] At the end of the bronchioles sit the alveoli, which are made up of clusters of alveolar sacs (Table 3-4).[1,2,5,6,9] It is here, in the alveolar sacs, that gases such as oxygen and carbon dioxide (CO_2) are transported in and out of the bloodstream through a process known as diffusion.[1-3,6,9] This is how oxygen gets from the outside environment to the tissues of the body.

Table 3-4: Structures of the Respiratory Passageways	
Conduction	Nasal cavity
	Oral cavity
	Pharynx
	Larynx
	Trachea
	Right/left pulmonary bronchi
Respiratory	Alveoli
	Alveolar sacs

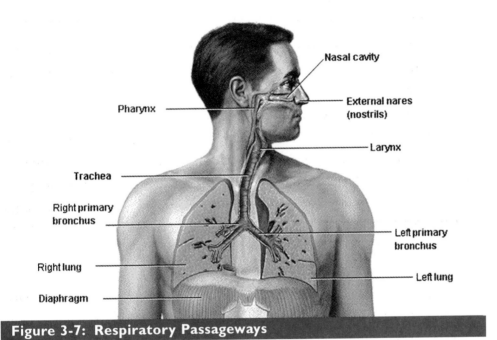

Figure 3-7: Respiratory Passageways

MODULE 3-2 Summary

The respiratory system collects oxygen from the environment and transports it to the bloodstream. The respiratory pump moves air in and out of the body and respiratory passageways to channel the air.

Breathing is divided into the inspiratory phase (or inhalation) and expiratory phase (or exhalation). Inspiratory ventilation is active, while expiratory ventilation can be both active and passive (as during normal breathing, when it results from the relaxation of the contracting inspiratory muscles).

There are two respiratory passageways. The first is the conduction passageway, which consists of all the structures that air travels through before entering the respiratory passageway. These structures purify, humidify, warm and cool air to match body temperature. The second passageway is the respiratory passageway, which collects the channeled air coming from the conduction passageway and allows gases such as oxygen and carbon dioxide to be transported in and out of the bloodstream.

MODULE 3-2 Quiz

1. The primary role of this system is to ensure proper cellular functioning.

   ☐ True   ☐ False

2. The external intercostals are muscles that act in which phase of breathing?

   ☐ Inspiration

   ☐ Expiration

3. In which structure does diffusion (oxygen and carbon dioxide being transported in and out of the bloodstream) occur?

_____

MODULE 3-3:
Cardiorespiratory Function

Together, the cardiovascular and respiratory systems make up the cardiorespiratory system. They form a vital support system to provide the kinetic chain with many essential elements (such as oxygen), while removing waste products that can cause dysfunction in the body.

The primary element for proper body function is oxygen.[3] The respiratory system provides the means to gather oxygen from the environment and transfer it into our bodies. It is inhaled through the nose and/or mouth, conducted through the trachea, down through the bronchi, where it eventually reaches the lungs and alveolar sacs.[1-3,5,6,9] Pulmonary capillaries surround the alveolar sacs and as oxygen fills the sacs it is diffused across the capillary membranes and into the alveolar sacs.[3] The oxygenated blood then returns to the left atrium through the pulmonary veins where it is pumped into the left ventricle and out to the tissues of the body (Figure 3-8).

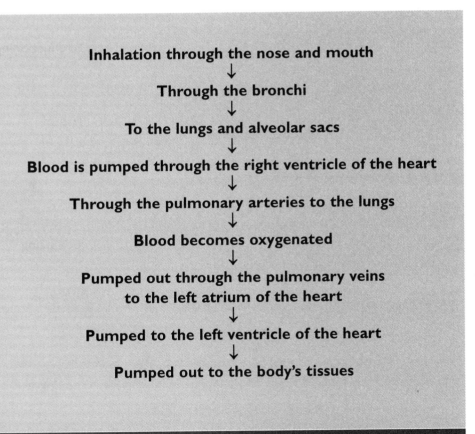

Inhalation through the nose and mouth
↓
Through the bronchi
↓
To the lungs and alveolar sacs
↓
Blood is pumped through the right ventricle of the heart
↓
Through the pulmonary arteries to the lungs
↓
Blood becomes oxygenated
↓
**Pumped out through the pulmonary veins
to the left atrium of the heart**
↓
Pumped to the left ventricle of the heart
↓
Pumped out to the body's tissues

Figure 3-8: The Cardiorespiratory Process

Concurrently, as the cells of the body are using oxygen, they produce an oxygen waste by-product known as carbon dioxide.[1-3,5,6,9] Carbon dioxide is transported from the tissues back to the heart and eventually to the lungs in the de-oxygenated blood. In the alveolar sacs, it is diffused into the pulmonary capillaries and released through exhalation.[1-3,5,6,9] In a simplistic overview, oxygen and carbon dioxide trade places in the tissues of the body, blood and lungs. As one is coming in, the other is going out.

Oxygen Consumption

The cardiovascular and respiratory systems work together to transport oxygen to the tissues of the body. Our capacity to efficiently use oxygen is dependent upon the respiratory system's ability to collect oxygen and the cardiovascular system's ability to absorb and transport it to the tissues of the body.[14] The usage of oxygen by the body is known as oxygen uptake (or oxygen consumption).[1-3,5,6,9,10]

At rest, oxygen consumption (VO_2) is estimated to be approximately 3.5 milliliters of oxygen per kilogram of body weight per minute (3.5 ml/kg-1/min-1), typically termed 1 metabolic equivalent or 1 MET.[3,5,7,10,14-16] It is calculated as:

$$VO_2 = Q \times a - VO_2 \text{ difference}$$

In the equation, VO_2 is oxygen consumption, Q is cardiac output (HR × SV) and a - VO_2 difference is the difference in the O_2 content between the blood in the arteries and the blood in the veins.

From this equation, it is very easy to see how influential the cardiovascular system is on the body's ability to consume oxygen, and that heart rate plays a major factor in VO_2.

Maximal oxygen consumption (VO_2 max) is generally accepted as the best means of gauging cardiorespiratory fitness.[3,5,7,15] Essentially, VO_2 max is the highest rate of oxygen transport and utilization achieved at maximal physical exertion.[10,14,15] VO_2 max values can range anywhere from 40-80 ml/kg-1/min-1, or approximately 11-23 METs.[7,15]

Maximal testing, however, is not very practical for most clientele and, as such, many sub-maximal testing procedures have been established to estimate VO_2 max.[14,16] These include the treadmill, cycle ergometer, stepping and field protocols.[14,16] While these protocols deliver a good generalization of a client's overall cardiorespiratory fitness level, they are based upon several assumptions that are rarely met and can contribute to estimate errors.[14,16] However, given repeatedly over a period of weeks and/or months they may show a cardiorespiratory trend.

Oxygen and Energy

Oxygen is the necessary catalyst for sustaining many bodily functions when activity is prolonged for periods of greater than 30 seconds.[3,5,16,17] In these situations, activity is said to be **aerobic**, meaning it requires oxygen.[3,17,18] Many activities, however, last for only a few seconds and are not dependent upon oxygen for proper execution. These activities are described as **anaerobic**, meaning they do not require oxygen.[3,17,18] To generate either form of activity, however, the body must still produce sufficient amounts of energy.

Energy is essentially the capacity to do work.[3,18] The study of energy in the human body, known as **bioenergetics**, looks at how chemical energy (food) is converted into mechanical energy (work).[3,18,19] During this conversion process, chemical bonds are broken, and this releases energy that is utilized to produce work (muscle contractions). This process is termed energy-yielding, as it produces energy much like a fruit tree yields fruit.[3,18,19] This energy can only be productive, however, if it can be captured and transferred to a place where it can be used. When the energy is used it is termed an energy-utilizing reaction.[3,18,19] In other words, energy is gathered from an energy-yielding source (the breakdown of food) by some storage unit and then transferred to a site that can utilize this energy (muscle contraction). Typically, the storage and transfer unit within the cells of the body is **adenosine triphosphate (ATP)**.[3,18,19]

ATP is structurally composed of a nitrogen-based compound, adenine, a five-carbon sugar called ribose, and three phosphates. ATP has the ability to store large amounts of energy in the chemical bonds of the phosphates. Essentially, this is the energy needed for muscle contraction, which performs physical activity. The supply of ATP in each cell is limited, however, and therefore cells must have a means of producing more. There are three main bioenergetic pathways that produce ATP.[3,15,18] These include the ATP-CP (Creatine Phosphate) and the Glycolysis (Lactate Acid) pathways, which are categorized as anaerobic (without oxygen) systems, and the Oxidative (Oxygen) pathway, classified as an aerobic (with oxygen) system. Collectively, these systems are known as the bioenergetic continuum (Table 3-5).[20]

AEROBIC:
An action that occurs only in the presence of oxygen.

ANAEROBIC:
An action in which the body incurs an oxygen debt.

BIOENERGETICS:
The biology of energy transformations and exchanges within the body, and between it and the environment.

ADENOSINE TRIPHOSPHATE (ATP):
A cellular structure that supplies energy for many biochemical cellular processes by undergoing enzymatic hydrolysis.

Table 3-5: The Bioenergetic Continuum

Pathway	System	Use	Time
ATP-CP (Creatine Phosphate)	Anaerobic	High-intensity, short-duration activity such as heavy weight training	Up to approximately 10 seconds of activity
Glycolysis (Lactic Acid)	Anaerobic	Moderate- to high-intensity, moderate-duration activities such as a typical set of 8-12 repetitions	30-50 seconds of activity
Oxidative (Oxygen)	Aerobic	Lower intensity, longer duration activities such as walking on the treadmill for 20-30 minutes	Activities greater than 2 minutes

ATP-CP (Creatine Phosphate)

Together, ATP and CP are called phosphagens and therefore, this system is sometimes referred to as the Phosphagen System.[18] The ATP-CP system provides energy for primarily high intensity, short duration bouts of exercise or activity. This would be seen in power and strength forms of training where heavy loads are used with only a few repetitions, or during short sprinting events. However, this system is activated at the onset of activity, regardless of intensity, due to its ability to produce energy very rapidly in comparison to the other systems.[3,18,21]

This bioenergetic system provides energy through the interactions of ATP and CP with enzymes (chemical catalysts that cause a change) such as myosin-ATPase and creatine kinsase.

The enzyme myosin ATPase causes the breaking off of one of the phosphate bonds from ATP. This results in ADP (adenosine diphosphate, meaning that there are now two phosphates instead of three). By breaking one of the high-energy phosphate bonds, energy is released.[3,18,21] This system is limited in its capacity to sustain energy production (approximately 10 seconds) because it must rely on the minimal storage of ATP and CP within the cells (Table 3-5).[3,18,21]

Glycolysis (Anaerobic/Lactic Acid)

Glycolysis (anaerobic system) utilizes the breakdown of carbohydrates (glucose) to rapidly produce ATP.[3,18,21]

Here, one glucose molecule will produce 2 ATP through anaerobic glycolysis. One of the byproducts of this process is pyruvate. If pyruvate cannot be utilized fast enough by the muscle cell, a buildup of lactic acid will occur. Excess lactic acid causes an increase in the acidity of the muscle cell and will interfere with muscle contractions.[3,18,21]

While this system can produce a significantly greater amount of energy than the ATP-CP system, it too is limited to approximately 30-50 seconds of duration.[3,18,21] Most fitness workouts will place a greater stress on this system than the other systems because a typical repetition range of eight to 12 falls within this timeframe (Table 3-5).

Oxidative (Oxygen)

The oxidative system relies primarily on carbohydrates and fats for the production of ATP. This system is the slowest producing of the three systems because it requires increased amounts of oxygen to match the muscular requirement of the exercise. Oxygen must be supplied through respiration and it takes a while to elevate the respiration rate to consume appropriate amounts of oxygen. Needless to say, this system results in a greater amount of ATP. The oxidative system uses a somewhat similar process to anaerobic glycolysis. Glucose supplied from the glycogen stores within the body is broken down in the presence of oxygen. With the presence of oxygen, pyruvate is not converted to lactic acid and becomes a usable substrate for ATP production.[3,18,21]

Here, one glucose molecule will produce 36 ATP. Depending on the specific substrates and pathways, it is possible for one glucose molecule to produce 38 ATP.[3,18,21] This system becomes more involved in activities longer than 30 seconds and is the predominant system in activities over two minutes (Table 3-5).[3]

Dysfunctional Breathing

The importance of all systems in the body working synergistically can be further demonstrated in the intimacy between the cardiorespiratory system and the kinetic chain. The cardiorespiratory system is a major support system for the kinetic chain. However, it is also the kinetic chain that provides essential support for the cardiorespiratory system. Muscles, bones and the nervous system are all essential components of the cardiorespiratory system that enable it to function optimally. Thus, if there is a dysfunction in the cardiorespiratory system, this can directly impact the components of the kinetic chain and perpetuate further dysfunction. Alterations in breathing patterns are a prime example of this relationship.

Breathing dysfunction is a very common predecessor to kinetic chain dysfunction.[22] It often results from breathing associated with high stress and/or anxiety. As a result of this altered breathing pattern, the following scenarios can occur:[23]

- The breathing pattern becomes more shallow, using the secondary respiratory muscles more predominantly than the diaphragm. This shallow, upper-chest breathing pattern becomes habitual causing overuse to the secondary respiratory muscles such as the scalenes, sternocleidomastoid, levator scapulae and upper trapezius.

- These muscles also play a major postural role in the kinetic chain, all connecting directly to the cervical and cranial portions of the body. Their increased activity and excessive tension often result in headaches, lightheadedness and dizziness.

- Excessive breathing (short shallow breaths) can lead to altered carbon dioxide/oxygen blood content that stimulates various sensors.

- This can lead to feelings of anxiety that further initiate an excessive breathing response.

- Increased nociceptor activity (pain receptors) can create increased pain.

- Inadequate oxygen and retention of metabolic waste within muscles can create fatigued stiff muscles.

- Inadequate joint motion of the spine and rib cage, due to improper breathing, causes joints to become restricted and stiff.

All of these situations can lead to a decreased functional capacity that may result in headaches, feelings of anxiety, fatigue, poor sleep patterns, as well as poor circulation. As a health and fitness professional, it is not your job to try to diagnose these problems. If a client presents any of these scenarios, refer them immediately to a medical professional for assistance.

MODULE 3-3 Summary

The respiratory system gathers oxygen from the environment, inhales it through the nose and/or mouth and processes it to be delivered to the tissues of the body. As cells use oxygen, they produce carbon dioxide, which is transported back to the heart and lungs in the de-oxygenated blood, to be released through exhalation.

The usage of oxygen by the body is known as oxygen consumption. Maximal oxygen consumption (VO_2 max) is the highest rate of oxygen transport and utilization achieved at maximal physical exertion. It is generally accepted as the best means of gauging cardiorespiratory fitness. Values can range anywhere from 11-23 METs.

Oxygen is the necessary catalyst for aerobic activity prolonged for periods of greater than 30 seconds. Anaerobic activities that last for only a few seconds are not dependent upon oxygen for proper execution. To generate either form of activity, however, the body must still produce sufficient energy.

The study of how chemical energy (food) is converted into mechanical energy (work) is known as bioenergetics. Typically, energy is gathered by adenosine triphosphate (ATP) and is transferred to a site that can utilize this energy (muscle contraction).

ATP has the ability to store large amounts of energy needed for muscle contraction in order to perform physical activity. However, the supply of ATP in each cell is limited, and cells must produce more through the bioenergetic continuum, which consists of ATP-Creatine Phosphate and the Glycolysis pathways (anaerobic systems), and the Oxidative pathway (aerobic system).

The ATP-CP system provides energy for high intensity, short bouts of activity. This system relies on the minimal storage of ATP and CP within the cells and thus is limited to energy production of approximately 10 seconds. Glycolysis uses the breakdown of carbohydrates to rapidly produce ATP. This system is limited to 30-50 seconds of duration. The oxidative system relies primarily on carbohydrates and fats and results in a higher production of ATP, allowing for activities longer than 30 seconds.

Alterations in breathing patterns can directly impact the components of the kinetic chain and lead to further dysfunction. If the breathing patterns become more shallow, the body uses secondary respiratory muscles more than the diaphragm, which can negatively impact posture. This may create excessive muscular tension, resulting in headaches, lightheadedness and dizziness. Short shallow breaths can also lead to altered carbon dioxide/oxygen blood content which causes feelings of anxiety. Inadequate oxygen and retention of metabolic waste within muscles can create stiff muscles and joints. If a client complains of headaches, feelings of anxiety, fatigue, poor sleep patterns or poor circulation, refer them immediately to a medical professional for assistance.

MODULE 3-3 Quiz

1. Number these components of the respiratory process in the correct order:

    ____ Blood becomes oxygenated

    ____ Blood is pumped through the right ventricle of the heart

    ____ Pumped out to the body's tissues

    ____ Inhalation through the nose and mouth

    ____ To the lungs and alveolar sacs

    ____ Pumped out through the pulmonary veins to the heart's left atrium

    ____ Through the pulmonary arteries to the lungs

    ____ Where blood is de-oxygenated

    ____ Through the bronchi

    ____ Pumped out to the left ventricle of the heart

2. What is the waste product of oxygen? _____

3. VO_2 max values can range anywhere from 11-23 METs.

    ☐ True   ☐ False

4. Which system(s) of the bioenergetic continuum is/are aerobic?

    ☐ ATP-CP

    ☐ Glycolysis

    ☐ Oxidative

5. Which pathway of the bioenergetic continuum would most likely be used during heavy weight training? _____

    _____

6. When a breathing pattern becomes more shallow, the body may use secondary respiratory muscles more than the _____.

References

1. Fox SI. *Human physiology*. 5th edition. Dubuque, IA: Wm. C. Brown Publishers; 1996.

2. Vander A, Sherman J, Luciano D. *Human physiology: the mechanisms of body function*. 8th edition. New York: McGraw-Hill; 2001.

3. Brooks GA, Fahey TD, White TP. *Exercise physiology: human bioenergetics and its application*. 2nd edition. Mountain View, CA: Mayfield Publishing Company; 1996.

4. Murray TD, Murray JM. Cardiovascular anatomy. Chapter 7. In: American College of Sports Medicine (ed). *ACSM's resource manual for guidelines for exercise testing and prescription*. 3rd edition. Baltimore, MD: Williams & Wilkins; 1998.

5. Hicks GH. *Cardiopulmonary anatomy and physiology*. Philadelphia: W.B. Saunders Company; 2000.

6. Tortora GJ. *Principles of human anatomy*. 7th edition. New York: Harper Collins College Publishers; 1995.

7. Williams MA. Cardiovascular and respiratory anatomy and physiology: responses to exercise. Chapter 7. In: Baechle TR (ed). *Essentials of strength training and conditioning*. Champaign, IL: Human Kinetics; 1994.

8. Holly RG, Shaffrath JD. Cardiorespiratory endurance. Chapter 52. In: American College of Sports Medicine (ed). *ACSM's resource manual for guidelines for exercise testing and prescription*. 3rd edition. Baltimore, MD: Williams & Wilkins; 1998.

9. Mahler DA. Respiratory Anatomy. Chapter 8. In: American College of Sports Medicine (ed). *ACSM's resource manual for guidelines for exercise testing and prescription*. 3rd edition. Baltimore, MD: Williams & Wilkins; 1998.

10. Brown DD. Pulmonary responses to exercise and training. Chapter 9. In: Garrett WE, Kirkendall DT (eds). *Exercise and sport science*. Philadelphia: Lippincott Williams & Wilkins; 2000.

11. Leech JA, Ghezzo H, Stevens D, Becklake MR. Respiratory pressures and function in young adults. *Am Rev Respir Dis* 1983;128:17.

12. Farkas GA, Decramer M, Rochester DF, De Troyer A. Contractile properties of intercostal muscles and their functional significance. *J Appl Physiol* 1985; 59:528-35.

13. Sharp T, Goldberg NB, Druz WF, Danon J. Relative contributions of rib cage and abdomen to breathing in normal subjects. *J Appl Physiol* 1975;39:601.

14. McConnell TR. Cardiorespiratory assessment of apparently healthy populations. Chapter 41. In: American College of Sports Medicine (ed). *ACSM's resource manual for guidelines for exercise testing and prescription*. 3rd edition. Baltimore, MD: Williams & Wilkins; 1998.

15. Franklin BA. Cardiovascular responses to exercise and training. Chapter 8. In: Garrett WE, Kirkendall DT (eds). *Exercise and sport science.* Philadelphia: Lippincott Williams & Wilkins; 2000.

16. American College of Sports Medicine. *ACSM's guidelines for exercise testing and prescription.* 5th edition. Philadelphia: Williams & Wilkins; 1995.

17. Greenhaff PL, Timmons JA. Interaction between aerobic and anaerobic metabolism during intense muscle contraction. In: Holsey JO (ed). *Exercise and sport science reviews.* Volume 26. Baltimore: Williams & Wilkins; 1998. pp 1-30.

18. Stone MH, Conley MS. Bioenergetics. Chapter 5. In: Baechle TR (ed). *Essentials of strength training and conditioning.* Champaign, IL: Human Kinetics; 1994.

19. Volek JS. Enhancing exercise performance: nutritional implications. Chapter 32. In: Garrett WE, Kirkendall DT (eds). *Exercise and sport science.* Philadelphia: Lippincott Williams & Wilkins; 2000.

20. Clark MA. *Integrated training for the new millennium.* Thousand Oaks, CA: National Academy of Sports Medicine; 2001.

21. Billeter R, Hoppeler H. Muscular basis of strength. Chapter 3. In: Komi PV (ed). *Strength and power in sport.* London: Blackwell Scientific Publications; 1992.

22. Chaitow L. *Cranial manipulation theory and practice: osseous and soft tissue approaches.* London: Churchill Livingstone; 1999.

23. Timmons B. *Behavioral and psychological approaches to breathing disorders.* New York: Plenum Press; 1994.

CHAPTER FOUR

Human Movement Science

Objectives

After studying this chapter, you will be able to:

- Understand the concepts and theories of motor behavior.
- Explain, in terms of training:
  - Why sensory information is important to human movement and
  - What internal and external feedbacks are.
- Describe how muscle actions and outside forces relate to human movement.
- Define the three stages of motor learning as well as basic biomechanical terminology.

Key Terms

- Motor behavior
- Motor control
- Synergies
- Proprioception
- Sensorimotor integration
- Motor learning
- Feedback
- Internal feedback
- External feedback
- Biomechanics
- Medial
- Lateral
- Contralateral
- Ipsilateral
- Anterior (or ventral)
- Posterior (or dorsal)
- Proximal
- Distal
- Inferior

- Superior
- Sagittal plane
- Flexion
- Extension
- Frontal plane
- Abduction
- Adduction
- Transverse plane
- Internal potation
- External potation
- Eccentric contraction
- Isometric contraction
- Concentric contraction
- Force
- Force couple
- Rotary motion
- Torque
- Momentum
- Ground reaction force

Introduction to Human Movement Science

The components and structures of the kinetic chain have now been reviewed. Although they seem separate, each system and their components must collaborate with the others to form interdependent links that create a functional chain. In turn, this entire chain must be aware of its relationship to internal and external environments, gather necessary information about them and produce the appropriate movement patterns (Figure 4-1). This process ensures optimum functioning of the kinetic chain and thus, optimum human movement (Figure 4-2).

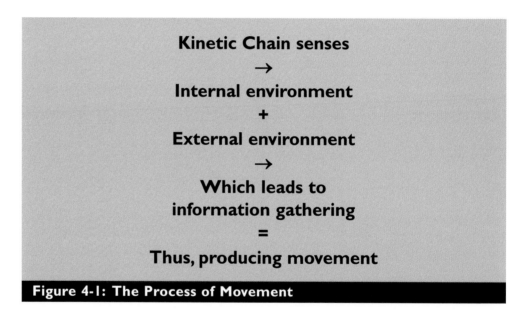

Kinetic Chain senses

→

Internal environment

+

External environment

→

**Which leads to
information gathering**

=

Thus, producing movement

Figure 4-1: The Process of Movement

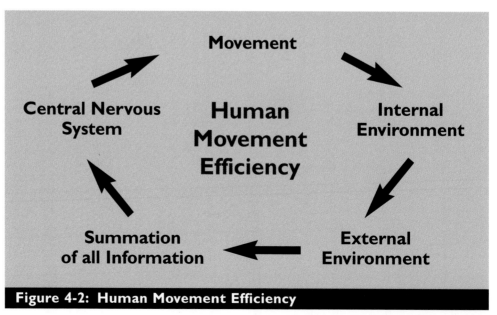

Movement

Central Nervous System

Human Movement Efficiency

Internal Environment

Summation of all Information

External Environment

Figure 4-2: Human Movement Efficiency

With this in mind, the following chapter will focus on how the kinetic chain works interdependently to learn, form and produce efficient movement. In doing so, we will discuss motor behavior and fundamental biomechanics.

MODULE 4-1: Biomechanics

Biomechanics

Biomechanics is a study that uses principles of physics to quantitatively study how forces interact within a living body. Specifically, this text focuses on the motions that the kinetic chain produces and the forces that act upon it.[1,2] This includes basic anatomical terminology, planes of motion, joint motions, muscle action, force couples, leverage, forces and the force-velocity relationship.

> **BIOMECHANICS:** A study that uses principles of physics to quantitatively study how forces interact within a living body.

Terminology

All industries have language that is specific to their needs. Because health and fitness professionals deal with human motion and the human body, it is necessary that they understand the basic anatomical terminology to allow for effective communication amongst one another. This section will include anatomical locations, planes of motion and joint motions.

Anatomical Locations

Anatomical location refers to terms that describe locations on the body (Figure 4-3). These include medial, lateral, contralateral, ipsilateral, anterior posterior proximal, distal, inferior and superior.

Superior refers to a position above a reference point. The femur is superior to the tibia. The pectoralis major is superior to the rectus abdominis.

> **SUPERIOR:** Positioned above a point of reference.

Inferior refers to a position below a reference point. The calcaneus is inferior to the talus. The gastrocnemius is inferior to the hamstrings.

> **INFERIOR:** Positioned below a point of reference.

Proximal refers to a position nearest the center of the body or point of reference. The knee is more proximal to the hip than the ankle. The lumbar spine is more proximal to the sacrum than the sternum.

> **PROXIMAL:** Positioned nearest the center of the body, or point of reference.

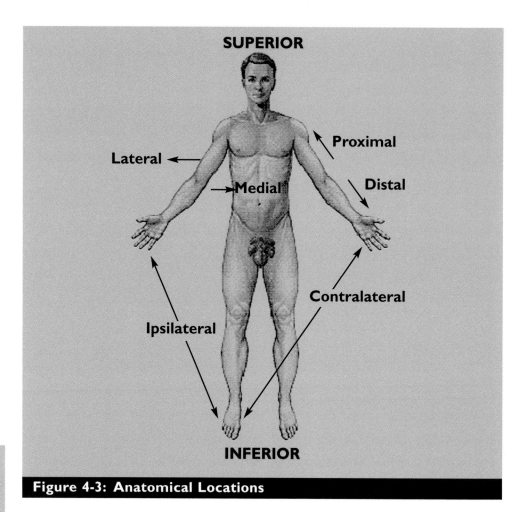

Figure 4-3: Anatomical Locations

DISTAL:
Positioned farthest from the center of the body, or point of reference.

ANTERIOR (OR VENTRAL):
On the front of the body.

POSTERIOR (OR DORSAL):
On the back of the body.

MEDIAL:
Positioned near the middle of the body.

Distal refers to a position farthest from the center of the body or point of reference. The ankle is more distal to the hip than the knee.

Anterior refers to a position on the front or toward the front of the body. The quadriceps are located on the anterior aspect of the thigh.

Posterior refers to a position on the back or toward the back of the body. The hamstrings are located on the posterior aspect of the thigh.

Medial refers to a position relatively closer to the midline of the body. The adductors are on the medial side of the thigh, since they are on the side of the limb closest to the midline of the body.

Lateral refers to a position relatively farther away from the midline of the body or toward the outside of the body. The ears are on the lateral side of the head since they are farther away from the midline of the body.

Contralateral refers to a position on the opposite side of the body. The right foot is contralateral to the left hand.

Ipsilateral refers to a position on the same side of the body. The right foot is ipsilateral to the right hand.

Planes of Motion, Axes and Joint Motions

The universally used method of describing human movements in three dimensions is based on a system of planes and axis (Figure 4-4). Three imaginary planes are positioned through the body at right angles so they intersect at the center of mass of the body. They include the sagittal, frontal and transverse planes. Movement is said to occur more predominantly in a specific plane if it is actually along the plane or parallel to it. Though

LATERAL:
Positioned farther away from the middle of the body.

CONTRALATERAL:
Positioned on the opposite side of the body.

IPSILATERAL:
Positioned on the same side of the body.

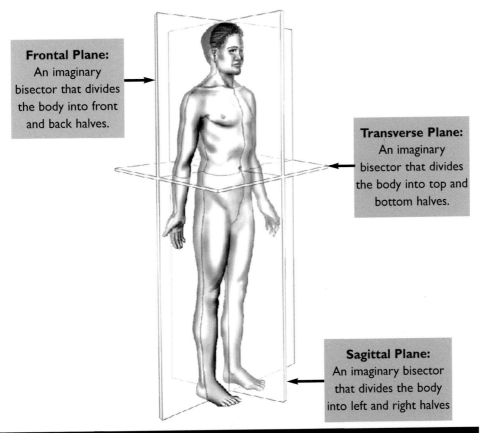

Frontal Plane:
An imaginary bisector that divides the body into front and back halves.

Transverse Plane:
An imaginary bisector that divides the body into top and bottom halves.

Sagittal Plane:
An imaginary bisector that divides the body into left and right halves

Figure 4-4: Planes of Motion

THE FRONTAL PLANE

The **frontal plane** bisects the body to create front and back halves. Frontal plane motion occurs around an anterior-posterior axis.[1,2,7] Movements in the frontal plane include abduction and adduction in the limbs (relative to the trunk), lateral flexion in the spine and eversion and inversion at the foot and ankle complex.[1,2,7,8] **Abduction** is a movement away from the midline of the body or similar to extension, it is an increase in the angle between two adjoining segments, but in the frontal plane (Figure 4-7). [1,2,7,8] **Adduction** is a movement of the segment toward the midline of the body or like flexion, it is a decrease in the angle between two adjoining segments, but in the frontal plane (Figure 4-8). [1,2,7,8] Lateral flexion is the bending of the spine (cervical, thoracic and/or lumbar) from side to side or simply side-bending. [1,2,7,8] Eversion and inversion follow the same principle, but relate more specifically to the movement of the calcaneus and tarsals in the frontal plane, during functional movements. [1,2,7,8] Examples of frontal plane movements include side lateral raises, side lunges and side shuffling (Table 4-2).

FRONTAL PLANE: An imaginary bisector that divides the body into front and back halves.

ABDUCTION: Movement of a body part away from the middle of the body.

ADDUCTION: Movement of a body part toward the middle of the body.

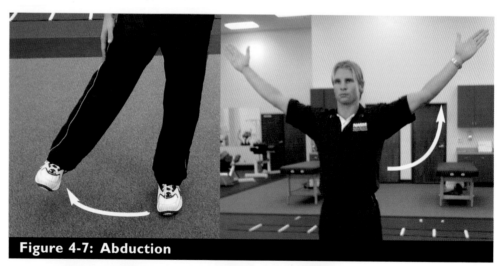

Figure 4-7: Abduction

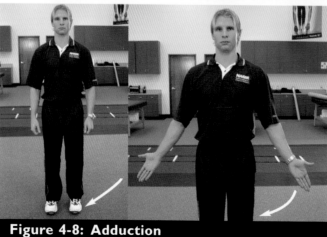

Figure 4-8: Adduction

THE TRANSVERSE PLANE

The **transverse plane** bisects the body to create upper and lower halves. Transverse plane motion occurs around a longitudinal or vertical axis.[1,2,7] Movements in the transverse plane include **internal rotation** and **external rotation** for the limbs, right and left rotation for the head and trunk and radioulnar pronation and supination (Figures 4-9 and 4-10)[1,2,7] The foot, because it is a unique entity, has transverse plane motion termed abduction (toes pointing outward, externally rotated) and adduction (toes pointing inward, internally rotated).[2-4] Examples of transverse plane movements include a single-arm cable row with rotation, alternating dumbbell shoulder press with rotation, transverse plane lunges, throwing a ball, throwing a Frisbee, golfing and swinging a bat (Table 4-2).

TRANSVERSE PLANE:
An imaginary bisector that divides the body into top and bottom halves.

INTERNAL ROTATION:
Rotation of a joint toward the middle of the body.

EXTERNAL ROTATION:
Rotation of a joint away from the middle of the body.

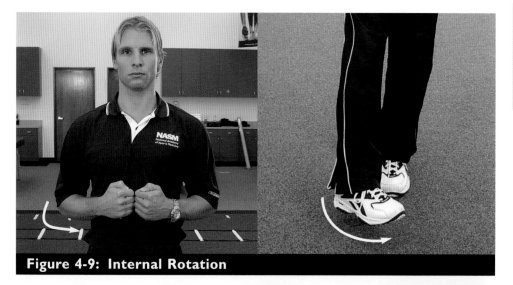

Figure 4-9: Internal Rotation

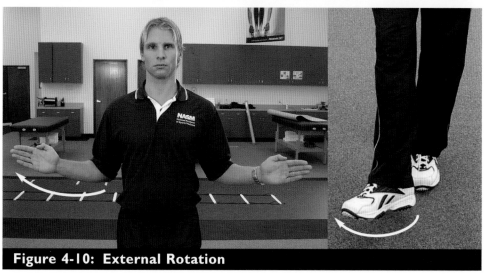

Figure 4-10: External Rotation

Muscle Actions

Muscles produce a variety of actions to effectively manipulate gravity, ground reaction forces, momentum and external resistance. There are three different actions that muscles produce:

- Eccentric
- Isometric
- Concentric

This range of muscle action is known as the muscle action spectrum and is necessary to produce efficient movement (Table 4-3).

Eccentric

When a muscle contracts **eccentrically**, it is exerting less force than is being placed upon it. This results in a lengthening of the muscle. As the muscle lengthens, the actin and myosin crossbridges are pulled apart and reattach, allowing the muscle to lengthen.[2,8] In actuality, the lengthening of the muscle usually refers to its return to a resting length and not actually increasing in its length as if it were being stretched.[8]

Eccentric muscle action is also known as "a negative" in the health and fitness industry. The term "negative" was derived from the fact that in eccentric movement, work is actually being done on the muscle (because forces move the muscle) rather than the muscle doing the work (or the muscle moving the forces).[2,8] This is due to the fact that eccentric motion moves in the same direction as the resistance is moving (known as direction of resistance).[1,2,8]

In functional activities, such as daily movements and/or sports, muscles work as much eccentrically as they do concentrically or isometrically.[3,9] Eccentrically, the muscles must decelerate or reduce the forces acting on the body (or force reduction). This is seen in all forms of resistance exercise. Whether walking on a treadmill or bench pressing, the weight of either the body or the bar must be decelerated and then stabilized in order to be properly accelerated (Table 4-3).

ECCENTRIC CONTRACTION:
The lengthening of a muscle.

Table 4-3: Muscle Action Spectrum

Action	Performance
Eccentric	Moving in the same direction as the resistance Decelerates and/or reduces force
Isometric	No visible movement with or against resistance Dynamically stabilizes force
Concentric	Moving in the opposite direction of the resistance Accelerates and/or produces force

Isometric

When a muscle contracts **isometrically**, it is exerting force equal to that placed upon it. This results in no appreciable change in the muscle length.[2,8]

In functional activities such as daily movements and/or sports, isometric actions are used to dynamically stabilize the body. This can be seen in stabilizers that are isometrically stabilizing a limb from moving in an unwanted direction. For example, the adductors and abductors of the thigh during a squat will dynamically stabilize the leg from moving too much in the frontal and transverse planes (Table 4-3).[3,8,9] During a ball crunch, the transversus abdominis and multifidus muscles stabilize the lumbar spine. During a dumbbell bench press, the rotator cuff musculature dynamically stabilizes the shoulder joint. When performing a push-up, the deep cervical flexors (longus coli, longus capitus) stabilize the cervical spine and head, keeping the head from migrating toward the ground.

> **ISOMETRIC CONTRACTION:**
> A muscle maintaining a certain length.

Concentric

When a muscle contracts **concentrically**, it is exerting more force than is being placed upon it. This results in a shortening of the muscle. As the muscle shortens, the actin and myosin crossbridges move together (known as sliding-filament theory), allowing the muscle to shorten (Table 4-3).[2,8]

> **CONCENTRIC CONTRACTION:**
> The shortening of a muscle.

Functional Anatomy

The traditional perception of muscles is that they work concentrically and predominantly in one plane of motion. However, in order to more effectively understand motion and design efficient training, reconditioning and rehabilitation programs, it is imperative to view muscles functioning in all planes of motion and through the entire muscle contraction spectrum (eccentrically, stabilization and concentrically) (Figure 4-11). The following section describes the isolated and integrated functions of the major muscles of the kinetic chain.[10-12]

Eccentric	→	Deceleration, Force Reduction
Isometric	→	Stabilization, Dynamic Support
Concentric	→	Acceleration, Force Production

Figure 4-11: Muscle Action Spectrum

Leg Musculature
Anterior Tibialis

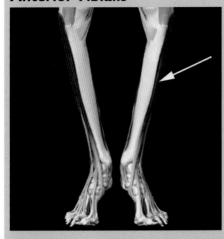

Origin
Lateral condyle and proximal two-thirds of the lateral surface of the tibia and the interosseous membrane
Insertion
Medial and plantar aspects of the medial cuneiform and the base of the first metatarsal
Isolated Function
Concentrically accelerates dorsiflexion and inversion
Integrated Function
Eccentrically decelerates plantarflexion and eversion
Isometrically stabilizes the arch of the foot
Innervation
Deep branch of peroneal nerve

Posterior Tibialis

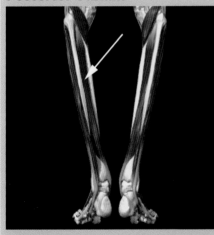

Origin
Proximal two-thirds of posterior surface of the tibia and fibula and adjacent interosseus membrane
Insertion
Every tarsal bone (navicular, cuneiform, cuboid) but the talus plus the bases of the second through the fourth metatarsal bones. The main insertion is on the navicular tuberosity and the medial cuneiform bone.
Isolated Function
Concentrically accelerates plantarflexion and inversion of the foot
Integrated Function
Eccentrically decelerates the dorsiflexion and eversion of the foot.
Isometrically stabilizes the arch of the foot.
Innervation
Tibial nerve

Leg Musculature *(Continued)*
Soleus

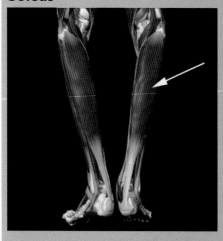

Origin
Posterior surface of the fibular head and proximal one-third of its shaft and from the posterior side of the tibia near the soleal line

Insertion
Calcaneus via the Achilles tendon

Isolated Function
Concentrically accelerates plantarflexion

Integrated Function
Decelerates ankle dorsiflexion
Isometrically stabilizes the foot and ankle complex

Innervation
Tibial nerve

Gastrocnemius

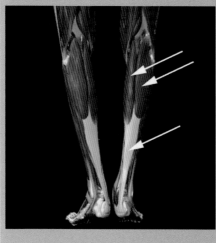

Origin
Posterior aspect of the lateral and medial femoral condyles

Insertion
Calcaneus via the Achilles tendon

Isolated Function
Concentrically accelerates plantarflexion

Integrated Function
Decelerates ankle dorsiflexion
Isometrically stabilizes the foot and ankle complex

Innervation
Tibial nerve

Peroneus Longus

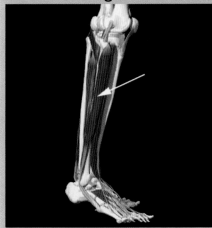

Origin
Lateral condyle of tibia, head and proximal two-thirds of the lateral surface of the fibula
Insertion
Lateral surface of the medial cuneiform and lateral side of the base of the first metatarsal
Isolated Function
Concentrically plantarflexes and everts the foot
Integrated Function
Decelerates ankle dorsiflexion
Isometrically stabilizes the foot and ankle complex
Innervation
Superficial branch of the peroneal nerve

HAMSTRING COMPLEX

Biceps Femoris — Long Head

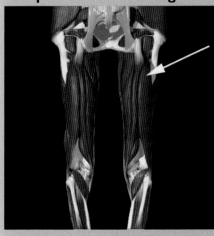

Origin
Ischial tuberosity, part of the sacrotuberous ligament
Insertion
Fibular head
Isolated Function
Concentrically accelerates knee flexion and hip extension
Tibial external rotation
Integrated Function
Eccentrically decelerates knee extension
Eccentrically decelerates hip flexion
Eccentrically decelerates tibial internal rotation at mid-stance of the gait cycle
Assists in eccentric deceleration of anterior pelvic rotation
Assists in dynamic stabilization of the lumbo-pelvic-hip complex
Innervation
Sciatic nerve

Leg Musculature (Continued)
Biceps Femoris — Short Head

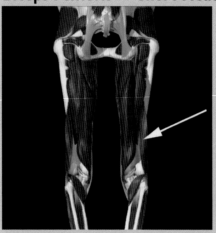

Origin
Lateral lip of the linea aspera below the gluteal tuberosity
Insertion
Fibular head
Isolated Function
Concentrically accelerates knee flexion and tibial external rotation
Integrated Function
Eccentrically decelerates knee extension
Eccentrically decelerates tibial internal rotation at mid-stance of the gait cycle
Innervation
Sciatic nerve

Semimembranosus

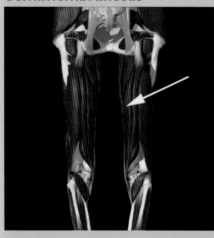

Origin
Ischial tuberosity
Insertion
Posterior aspect of the medial tibial condyle
Isolated Function
Concentrically accelerates knee flexion, hip extension and tibial internal rotation
Integrated Function
Eccentrically decelerates knee extension
Eccentrically decelerates hip flexion
Eccentrically decelerates tibial external rotation
Assists in eccentric deceleration of anterior pelvic rotation
Assists in dynamic stabilization of the lumbo-pelvic-hip complex
Innervation
Sciatic nerve

Semitendinosus

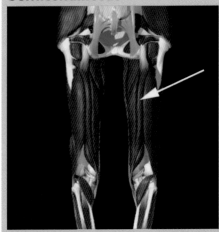

Origin
Ischial tuberosity and part of the
sacrotuberous ligament
Insertion
Proximal aspect of the medial tibial
condyle (pes anserine)
Isolated Function
Concentrically accelerates knee flexion,
hip extension and tibial internal rotation
Integrated Function
Eccentrically decelerates knee extension
Eccentrically decelerates hip flexion
Eccentrically decelerates tibial external
rotation
Assists in eccentric deceleration of
anterior pelvic rotation
Assists in dynamic stabilization of the
lumbo-pelvic-hip complex
Innervation
Sciatic nerve

QUADRICEPS COMPLEX

Vastus Lateralis

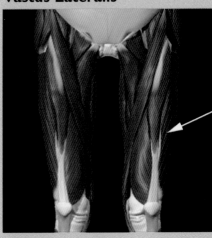

Origin
Anterior and inferior border of the
greater trochanter, lateral region of the
gluteal tuberosity, lateral lip of the linea
aspera
Insertion
Base of patella, tibial tuberosity via
ligamentum patella
Isolated Function
Concentrically accelerates knee
extension
Integrated Function
Eccentrically decelerates knee flexion,
adduction and internal rotation at heel
strike
Isometrically stabilizes the knee
Innervation
Femoral nerve

Leg Musculature *(Continued)*
Vastus Medialis

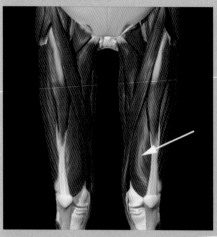

Origin
Lower region of intertrochanteric line, medial lip of linea aspera, proximal medial supracondylar line

Insertion
Base of patella, tibial tuberosity via ligamentum patella

Isolated Function
Concentrically accelerates knee extension

Integrated Function
Eccentrically decelerates knee flexion, abduction and internal rotation
Isometrically stabilizes the knee

Innervation
Femoral nerve

Vastus Intermedius

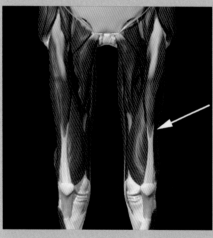

Origin
Anterior-lateral regions of the upper two thirds of the femoral shaft

Insertion
Base of patella, tibial tuberosity via ligamentum patella

Isolated Function
Concentrically accelerates knee extension

Integrated Function
Eccentrically decelerates knee flexion and internal rotation
Isometrically stabilizes the knee

Innervation
Femoral nerve

Rectus Femoris

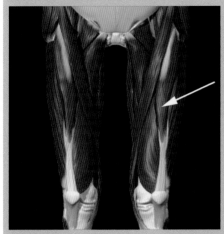

Origin
Anterior-inferior iliac spine, superior rim
of the acetabulum
Insertion
Base of patella, tibial tuberosity via
ligamentum patella
Isolated Function
Concentrically accelerates knee
extension and hip flexion
Integrated Function
Eccentrically decelerates knee flexion,
adduction and internal rotation
Isometrically stabilizes the knee
Decelerates hip extension
Innervation
Femoral nerve

Articularis Genu

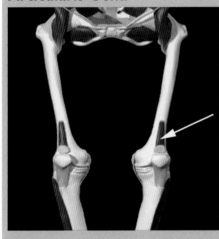

Origin
Anterior surface of the distal femoral
shaft
Insertion
Proximal synovial membrane of the knee
Isolated Function
Pulls the synovial membrane and capsule
superiorly during extension to avoid
pinching during extension
Integrated Function
Eccentrically decelerates knee flexion
and internal rotation
Isometrically stabilizes the knee
Innervation
Femoral nerve

Leg Musculature *(Continued)*
ADDUCTOR COMPLEX
Adductor Longus

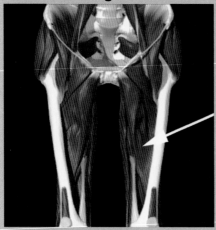

Origin
Anterior surface of the inferior pubic ramus

Insertion
Proximal one-third of the linea aspera

Isolated Function
Concentrically accelerates hip adduction, flexion and internal rotation

Integrated Function
Eccentrically decelerates hip abduction, extension and external rotation
Isometrically stabilizes the lumbo-pelvic-hip complex

Innervation
Obturator nerve

Adductor Magnus — Anterior Fibers

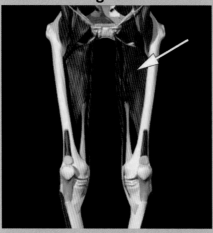

Origin
Ischial ramus

Insertion
Linea aspera of the femur

Isolated Function
Concentrically accelerates hip adduction, flexion and internal rotation

Integrated Function
Eccentrically decelerates hip abduction, extension and external rotation
Isometrically stabilizes the lumbo-pelvic-hip complex

Innervation
Obturator nerve

Adductor Magnus — Posterior Fibers

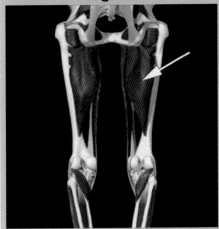

Origin
Ischial tuberosity
Insertion
Adductor tuberacle on femur
Isolated Function
Concentrically accelerates hip adduction, extension and external rotation
Integrated Function
Eccentrically decelerates hip abduction, flexion and internal rotation
Isometrically stabilizes the lumbo-pelvic-hip complex
Innervation
Sciatic nerve

Adductor Brevis

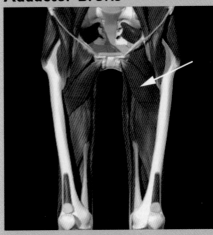

Origin
Anterior surface of the inferior pubic ramus
Insertion
Proximal one-third of the linea aspera of the femur
Isolated Function
Concentrically accelerates hip adduction, flexion and internal rotation
Integrated Function
Eccentrically decelerates hip abduction, extension and external rotation
Isometrically stabilizes the lumbo-pelvic-hip complex
Innervation
Obturator nerve

Leg Musculature *(Continued)*

Gracilis

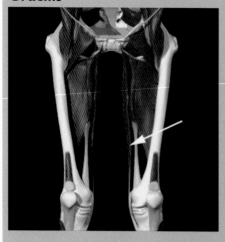

Origin
Anterior aspect of lower body of pubis and inferior ramus of pubis
Insertion
Proximal medial surface of the tibia (pes anserine)
Isolated Function
Concentrically accelerates hip adduction, flexion and internal rotation
Assists in tibial internal rotation
Integrated Function
Eccentrically decelerates hip abduction, extension and external rotation
Isometrically stabilizes the lumbo-pelvic-hip complex
Innervation
Obturator nerve

Pectineus

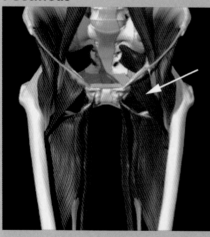

Origin
Pectineal line on the superior pubic ramus
Insertion
Pectineal line on the posterior surface of the femur
Isolated Function
Concentrically accelerates hip adduction, flexion and internal rotation
Integrated Function
Eccentrically decelerates hip abduction, extension and external rotation
Works synergistically with gluteus medius, tensor fascia latae and quadratus lumborum for frontal plane stabilization during stance phase
Innervation
Obturator nerve

HIP ABDUCTOR COMPLEX

Gluteus Medius — Anterior Fibers

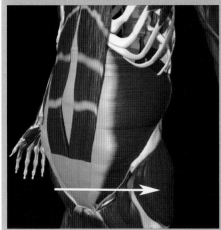

Origin
Outer surface of the ilium, above the gluteal line
Insertion
Lateral surface of the greater trochanter
Isolated Function
Concentrically accelerates hip abduction and internal rotation
Integrated Function
Eccentrically decelerates hip adduction and external rotation
Isometrically stabilizes the lumbo-pelvic-hip complex
Innervation
Superior gluteal nerve

Gluteus Medius — Posterior Fibers

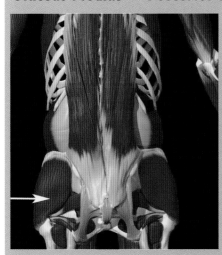

OriginOuter surface of the ilium, above the gluteal line
Insertion
Lateral surface of the greater trochanter
Isolated Function
Concentrically accelerates hip abduction and external rotation
Integrated Function
Eccentrically decelerates hip adduction and internal rotation
Isometrically stabilizes the lumbo-pelvic-hip complex
Innervation
Superior gluteal nerve

Leg Musculature *(Continued)*

Gluteus Minimus

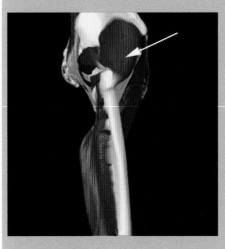

Origin
Ilium between the anterior and inferior gluteal line

Insertion
Greater trochanter

Isolated Function
Concentrically accelerates hip abduction and internal rotation

Integrated Function
Eccentrically decelerates frontal plane hip adduction and internal rotation
Isometrically stabilizes the lumbo-pelvic-hip complex

Innervation
Superior gluteal nerve

Tensor Fascia Latae

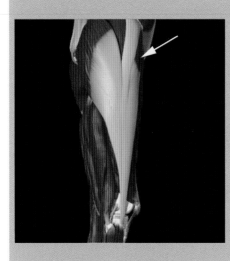

Origin
Outer surface of the iliac crest just posterior to the anterior-superior iliac spine

Insertion
Proximal one-third of the iliotibial band

Isolated Function
Concentrically accelerates hip flexion, abduction and internal rotation

Integrated Function
Eccentrically decelerates hip extension, adduction and external rotation
Isometrically stabilizes the lumbo-pelvic-hip complex

Innervation
Superior gluteal nerve

GLUTEUS MAXIMUS
Gluteus Maximus

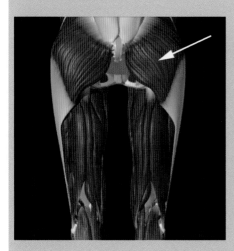

Origin
Outer ilium, posterior gluteal line, aponeurosis of the erector spinae and gluteus medius muscles, posterior side of sacrum and coccyx and part of the sacrotuberous and posterior sacro-ilac ligament

Insertion
Gluteal tuberosity and iliotibial tract

Isolated Function
Concentrically accelerates hip extension and external rotation

Integrated Function
Eccentrically decelerates hip flexion and internal rotation
Decelerates tibial internal rotation via the iliotibial band

Innervation
Inferior gluteal nerve

Psoas

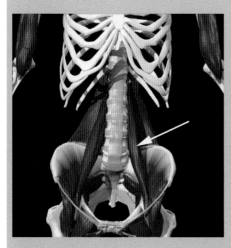

Origin
Transverse processes and lateral bodies of the last thoracic and all lumbar vertebrae including intervetebral discs

Insertion
Lesser trochanter of the femur

Isolated Function
Concentrically accelerates hip flexion and external rotation
Concentrically extends and rotates lumbar spine

Integrated Function
Eccentrically decelerates hip internal rotation
Eccentrically decelerates hip extension
Assists in stabilization of the lumbar spine during functional movements

Innervation
Spinal branches of L2-L4

Leg Musculature (Continued)

Sartorius

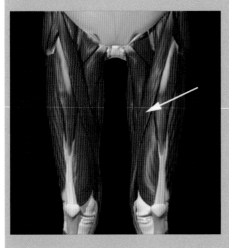

Origin
Anterior-superior iliac spine
Insertion
Proximal medial surface of the tibia
Isolated Function
Concentrically accelerates hip flexion, external rotation and abduction
Concentrically accelerates knee flexion and internal rotation
Integrated Function
Eccentrically decelerates hip extension and external rotation
Eccentrically decelerates knee extension and external rotation
Assists in stabilization of the lumbo-pelvic-hip complex and tibio-femoral joint
Innervation
Femoral nerve

HIP EXTERNAL ROTATORS

Piriformis

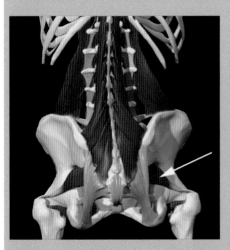

Origin
Anterior side of the sacrum between the sacral foramina; blends partially with the capsule of the sacroiliac joint
Insertion
Apex of the greater trochanter of the femur
Isolated Function
Concentrically accelerates hip external rotation, abduction and extension
Integrated Function
Eccentrically decelerates hip internal rotation, adduction and flexion
Isometrically stabilizes the hip and sacroiliac joints
Innervation
Ventral rami of S1-S2

Obturator Internus

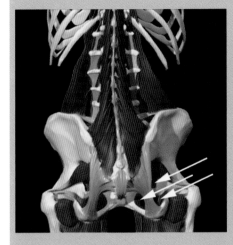

Origin
Internal side of the obturator membrane and immediate surrounding surfaces of the inferior pubic ramus and ishial ramus
Insertion
Medial surface of the greater trochanter just anterior and superior to the trochanteric fossa
Isolated Function
Concentrically accelerates hip external rotation and abduction
Integrated Function
Eccentrically decelerates hip internal rotation and adduction
Isometrically stabilizes the hip
Innervation
Nerve to obturator internus

Obturator Externus

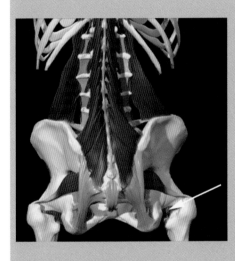

Origin
External surface of the obturator membrane and surrounding surfaces of the inferior pubic ramus and ischial ramus
Insertion
Medial surface of the greater trochanter at the trochanteric fossa
Isolated Function
Concentrically accelerates hip external rotation
Integrated Function
Eccentrically decelerates hip internal rotation
Isometrically stabilizes the hip
Innervation
Obturator nerve

Leg Musculature *(Continued)*

Gemellus Superior

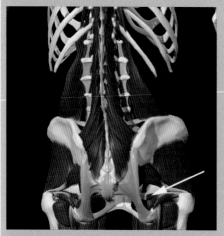

Origin
Dorsal surface of the ischial spine

Insertion
Greater trochanter via the tendon of the obturator internus

Isolated Function
Concentrically accelerates hip external rotation

Integrated Function
Eccentrically decelerates hip internal rotation
Isometrically stabilizes the hip

Innervation
Nerve to obturator internus

Gemellus Inferior

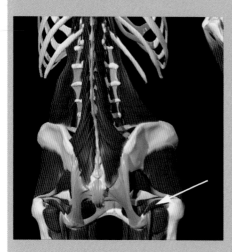

Origin
Ischial tuberosity

Insertion
Greater trochanter via the tendon of the obturator internus

Isolated Function
Concentrically accelerates hip external rotation

Integrated Function
Eccentrically decelerates hip internal rotation
Isometrically stabilizes the hip

Innervation
Nerve to quadratus femoris

Quadratus Femoris

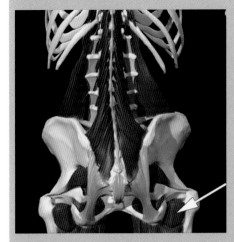

Origin
Lateral border of ischial tuberosity
Insertion
Quadrate line below intertrochanteric crest
Isolated Function
Concentrically accelerates hip external rotation
Integrated Function
Eccentrically decelerates hip internal rotation
Isometrically stabilizes the hip
Innervation
Nerve to quadratus femoris

Abdominal Musculature

Rectus Abdominis

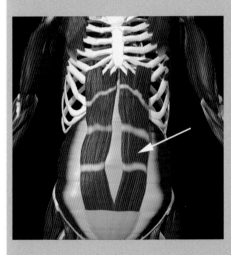

Origin
Pubic symphysis
Insertion
Ribs 5-7
Xyphoid process of the sternum
Isolated Function
Concentrically accelerates spinal flexion, lateral flexion and rotation
Integrated Function
Eccentrically decelerates spinal extension, lateral flexion and rotation
Isometrically stabilizes the lumbo-pelvic-hip complex
Innervation
Intercostal nerves (T7-T12)

Abdominal Musculature *(Continued)*
External Oblique

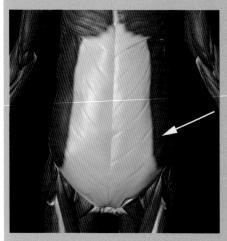

Origin
External surface of ribs 4-12
Insertion
Anterior iliac crest, linea alba and contralateral rectus sheaths
Isolated Function
Concentrically accelerates spinal flexion, lateral flexion and contralateral rotation
Integrated Function
Eccentrically decelerates spinal extension, lateral flexion and rotation
Isometrically stabilizes the lumbo-pelvic-hip complex
Innervation
Intercostal nerves (T8-T12), iliohypogastric (L1) and ilioinguinal (L1) nerves

Internal Oblique

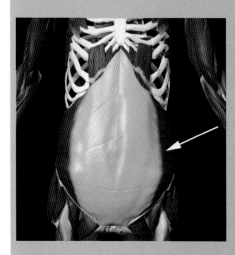

Origin
Anterior two-thirds of the iliac crest, inguinal ligament and thoracolumbar fascia
Insertion
Ribs 9-12, linea alba and contralateral rectus sheaths
Isolated Function
Concentrically accelerates spinal flexion (bilateral), lateral flexion and ipsilateral rotation
Integrated Function
Eccentrically decelerates spinal extension, rotation and lateral flexion
Works synergistically with the transversus abdominis to provide rotational and translational stability to the lumbar spine secondary to its attachment to the thoracolumbar fascia.
Innervation
Intercostal nerves (T8-T12), iliohypogastric (L1) and ilioinguinal (L1) nerves

Transversus Abdominis

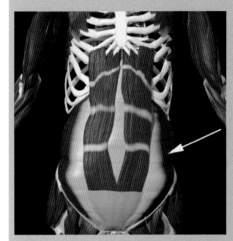

Origin
Ribs 7-12, anterior two-thirds of the iliac crest, lateral one-third of the inguinal ligament and thoraco-lumbar fascia
Insertion
Lineae alba and contralateral rectus sheaths
Isolated Function
Increases intra-abdominal pressure
Supports the abdominal viscera
Integrated Function
Works to preferentially stabilize the lumbar spine
Works synergistically with the internal oblique, multifidus and deep erector spinae to stabilize the lumbo-pelvic-hip complex
Innervation
Intercostal nerves (T7-T12), iliohypogastric (L1) and ilioinguinal (L1) nerves

Diaphragm

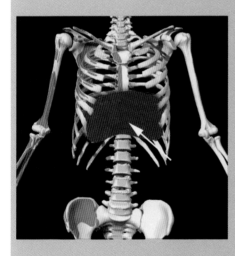

Origin
Costal part: inner surfaces of the cartilages and adjacent bony regions of ribs 6-12
Sternal part: posterior side of the xiphoid process
Crural (lumbar) part: (1) two aponeurotic arches covering the external surfaces of the quadratus lumborum and psoas major; (2) right and left crus, originating from the bodies of L1-L3 and their intervetebral discs
Insertion
Central tendon
Isolated Function
Concentrically pulls the central tendon inferiorly, increasing the volume in the thoracic cavity
Integrated Function
Isometrically stabilizes the lumbo-pelvic-hip complex
Innervation
Phrenic nerve (C3-C5)

Back Musculature

Superficial Erector Spinae: Iliocostalis, Longissimus and Spinalis

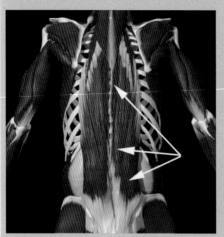

Division in the Group
Lumborum (lumbar), Thoracis (thoracic), Cervicis (cervical)

Common Origin
Iliac crest, sacrum, spinous and transverse process of T11-L5

Insertion
Iliocostalis
    Lumborum:
    Inferior border of ribs 7-12
    Thoracis:
    Superior border of ribs 1-6
    Cervicis:
    Transverse process of C4-C6
Longissimus
    Thoracis:
    Transverse process T1-T12; Ribs 2-12
    Cervicis:
    Transverse process of C6-C2
    Capitis:
    Mastoid process
Spinalis
    Thoracis:
    Spinous process of T7-T4
    Cervicis:
    Spinous process of C3-C2
    Capitis:
    Between the superior and inferior nuchal lines on occipital bone

Isolated Function
Concentrically accelerates spinal extension, rotation and lateral flexion

Integrated Function
Eccentrically decelerates spinal flexion, rotation and lateral flexion
Isometrically stabilizes the spine during functional movements

Innervation
Lumbar, thoracic and cervical spinal nerves

Quadratus Lumborum

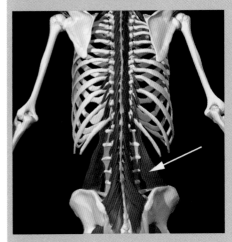

Origin
Iliolumbar ligament
Iliac crest
Insertion
12th rib
Transverse process L2-L5
Isolated Function
Spinal lateral flexion
Integrated Function
Works synergistically with the gluteus medius, tensor fascia and adductor complex as the primary frontal plane stabilization mechanism
Innervation
Spinal nerves T12-L3

TRANSVERSOSPINALIS COMPLEX

Semispinalis: Thoracis, Cervicis, Capitis

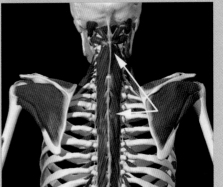

Origin
Thoracis Transverse process T12-T7
Cervicis Transverse process T6-C4
Capitis Transverse process T6-C7
      Articular process C6-C4
Insertion
Thoracis Spinous process T4-C6
Cervicis Spinous process C5-C2
Capitis Nuchal line of occipital bone
Isolated Function
Concentrically produces spinal extension and lateral flexion
Concentrically produces extension and contralateral rotation of the head
Primarily proprioception and stabilization
Integrated Function
Eccentrically decelerates and lateral flexion of the spine
Eccentrically decelerates flexion and contralateral rotation of the head
Innervation
Dorsal rami of T6-C1

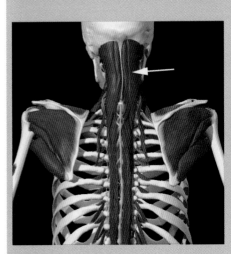

Back Musculature (Continued)
Rotatores

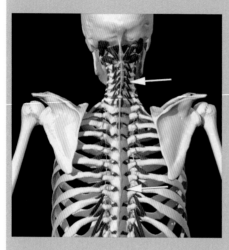

Origin
Transverse process of one thoracic vertebra below where it inserts

Insertion
Spinous process of the vertebra above

Isolated Function
Spinal extension and contralateral rotation

Integrated Function
Eccentrically decelerates spinal flexion and rotation
Provides transverse plane intersegmental stability
Provides proprioception which enhances neuromuscular efficiency

Innervation
Corresponding spinal nerves

Multifidus

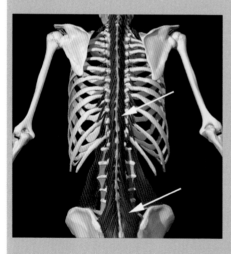

Origin
Posterior aspect of the sacrum
Mamillary processes of the lumbar spine
Transverse processes of the thoracic spine
Articular processes of the cervical spine

Insertion
Spinous processes 1-4 segments above origin

Isolated Function
Concentrically accelerates spinal extension and contralateral rotation

Integrated Function
Eccentrically decelerates spinal flexion and rotation
Works synergistically with the transversus abdominis, internal oblique, and deep erector spinae to stabilize the lumbo-sacral junction
Major stabilizer of the sacroiliac joint

Innervation
Corresponding spinal nerves

Intertransversarii

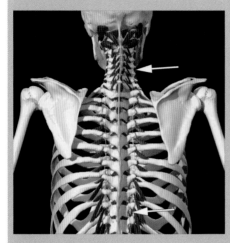

Origin
Between the transverse processes of cervical, thoracic, lumbar vertebrae

Insertion
Between the transverse processes of cervical, thoracic, lumbar vertebrae

Isolated Function
Concentrically accelerate spinal lateral flexion

Integrated Function
Eccentrically decelerates contralateral segmental spinal lateral flexion
Provides inter-segmental stability in the frontal plane
Provides proprioception during functional movements

Innervation
Spinal nerves

Interspinalis

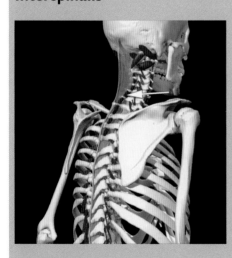

Origin
Inferior spinous process

Insertion
Superior spinous process

Isolated Function
Concentrically accelerates intersegmental spinal extension

Integrated Function
Eccentrically decelerates spinal flexion
Provides sagittal plane inter-segmental stability
Provides proprioception, which enhances spinal stabilization and neuromuscular control

Innervation
Spinal nerves

Shoulder Musculature
Latissimus Dorsi

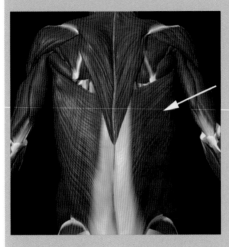

Origin
Spinous processes of T7-T12
Iliac crest
Thoracolumbar fascia
Ribs 9-12
Insertion
Inferior angle of the scapula
Intertubecular groove of the humerus
Isolated Function
Concentrically accelerates shoulder
extension, adduction and internal rotation
Bilaterally creates spinal extension
Integrated Function
Eccentrically decelerates shoulder
flexion, abduction and external rotation
Eccentrically decelerates spinal flexion
Isometrically stabilizes the
lumbo-pelvic-hip complex
Innervation
Thoracodorsal nerve (C6-C8)

Serratus Anterior

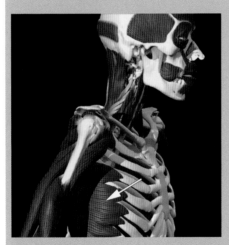

Origin
Ribs 4-12
Insertion
Medial border of the scapula
Isolated Function
Concentrically accelerates scapular
protraction
Integrated Function
Eccentrically decelerates dynamic
scapular retraction
Works synergistically with the upper and
lower trapezius to provide optimal
scapular mobility and stability during
shoulder elevation
Isometrically stabilizes to the
scapulo-thoracic joint
Innervation
Long thoracic nerve (C5-C7)

Rhomboids

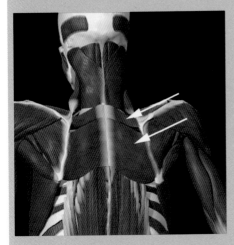

Origin
Spinous processes C7-T5
Insertion
Medial border of the scapula
Isolated Function
Concentrically produces scapular retraction and downward rotation
Integrated Function
Eccentrically decelerates scapular protraction and upward rotation
Provides stability for the rotator cuff to work efficiently
Innervation
Dorsal scapular nerve C4-C5

Lower Trapezius

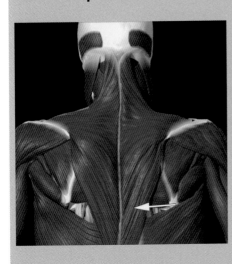

Origin
Spinous processes of T6-T12
Insertion
Spine of the scapula
Isolated Function
Concentrically accelerates scapular depression
Integrated Function
Eccentrically decelerates scapular elevation
Works synergistically with the upper trapezius and the serratus anterior to abduct the scapula during elevation
Isometrically stabilizes the scapula
Innervation
Cranial nerve XI
Ventral ramus of C2-3-4

Shoulder Musculature (Continued)

Pectoralis Minor

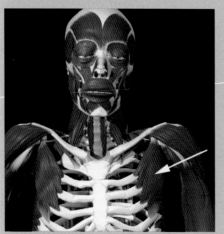

Origin
Ribs 3-5
Insertion
Coracoid process of the scapula
Isolated Function
Concentrically protracts the scapula
Integrated Function
Eccentrically decelerates scapular retraction
Dynamically stabilizes the shoulder girdle
Innervation
Medial pectoral nerve C6-T1

Deltoid — Anterior Middle and Posterior

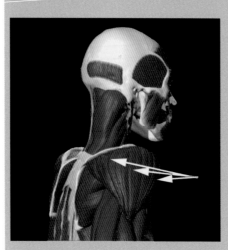

Origin
Anterior Lateral third of the clavicle
Middle Lateral and superior acromion
Posterior Spine of the scapula
Insertion
Deltoid tuberosity
Isolated Function
Anterior Concentrically accelerates shoulder flexion and internal rotation
Middle Concentrically accelerates shoulder abduction
Posterior Concentrically accelerates shoulder extension and external rotation
Integrated Function
Anterior Eccentrically decelerates shoulder extension and external rotation, works synergistically with the pectorals during functional activities
Middle Eccentrically decelerates shoulder adduction, works as a force-couple with the supraspinatus during abduction
Posterior Eccentrically decelerates shoulder flexion and internal rotation
Innervation
Axillary nerve C5-6

ROTATOR CUFF

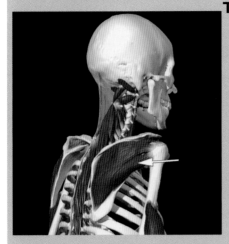

Teres Minor
Origin
Lateral border of the scapula
Insertion
Greater tubercle of the humerus
Isolated Function
Concentrically accelerates shoulder
external rotation
Integrated Function
Eccentrically decelerates shoulder
internal rotation

Works synergistically with the other
rotator cuff musculature to dynamically
stabilize the humeral head in the glenoid
fossa during dynamic activity

Works synergistically to produce a
dynamic caudal glide of the humeral head
in the glenoid fossa during elevation to
prevent impingement

Works as a ligamentous-muscular
protective reflex which enhances
proprioception during dynamic
functional activities
Innervation

Axillary nerve C5-6

Shoulder Musculature *(Continued)*

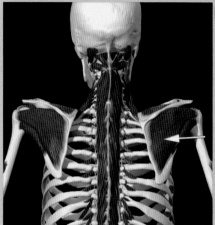

Infraspinatus

Origin

Infraspinous fossa

Insertion

Middle facet of the greater tubercle of the humerus

Isolated Function

Concentrically accelerates shoulder external rotation

Integrated Function

Eccentrically decelerates shoulder internal rotation

Works synergistically with the other rotator cuff musculature to dynamically stabilize the humeral head in the glenoid fossa during dynamic activity

Works synergistically to produce a dynamic caudal glide of the humeral head in the glenoid fossa during elevation to prevent impingement

Works as a ligamentous-muscular protective reflex which enhances proprioception during dynamic functional activities

Innervation

Suprascapular nerve C5-6

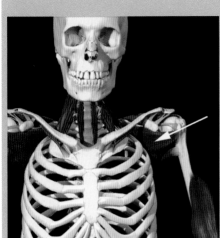

Subscapularis
 Origin
 Subscapular fossa
 Insertion
 Lesser tubercle of the humerus
 Glenohumeral shoulder capsule
 Isolated Function
 Concentrically accelerates shoulder
 internal rotation
 Integrated Function
 Eccentrically decelerates shoulder
 external rotation
 Works synergistically with the other
 rotator cuff musculature to stabilize the
 humeral head in the glenoid fossa during
 functional activities
 Innervation
 Upper and lower subscapular nerve C5-7

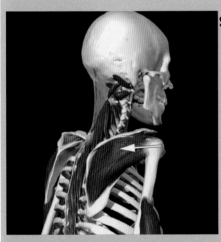

Supraspinatus
 Origin
 Supraspinous fossa
 Insertion
 Superior facet of the greater tubercle of
 the humerus
 Isolated Function
 Concentrically accelerates abduction of
 the arm
 Integrated Function
 Eccentrically decelerates adduction of
 the arm

 Works synergistically with the other
 rotator cuff musculature to dynamically
 stabilize the humeral head in the glenoid
 fossa

 Initiates abduction and dynamic caudal
 glide while the deltoid acts as the prime
 mover during shoulder abduction
 Innervation

Suprascapular nerve C5-6

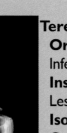

Teres Major

Origin

Inferior angle of the scapula

Insertion

Lesser tubercle of the humerus

Isolated Function

Concentrically accelerates shoulder internal rotation, adduction and extension

Integrated Function

Eccentrically decelerates shoulder external rotation, abduction and flexion

Innervation

Lower subscapular nerve C6-7

Neck Musculature

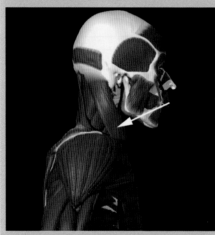

Sternocleidomastoid

Origin

Sternal head   Top of Maubrium

Clavicular head Medial one-third of the
                  clavicle

Insertion

Mastoid process, lateral superior nuchal line of the occiput

Isolated Function

Concentrically accelerates cervical flexion, rotation and lateral flexion

Integrated Function

Eccentrically decelerates cervical extension, rotation and lateral flexion Dynamically stabilizes the cervical spine and acromioclavicular joint

Innervation

Lower subscapular nerve C6-7

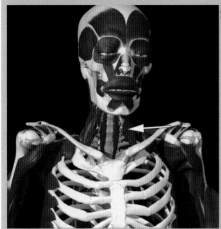

Scalenes — Anterior Fibers
Origin
Transverse processes of C3-C6
Insertion
First rib
Isolated Function
Concentrically accelerates cervical flexion, rotation and lateral flexion
Assists rib elevation during inhalation
Integrated Function
Eccentrically decelerates cervical extension, rotation and lateral flexion
Dynamically stabilizes the cervical spine
Innervation
Lower subscapular nerve C6-7

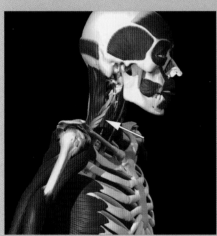

Scalenes — Middle Fibers
Origin
Transverse processes of C2-C7
Insertion
First rib
Isolated Function
Concentrically accelerates cervical flexion, rotation and lateral flexion
Integrated Function
Eccentrically decelerates cervical extension, rotation and lateral flexion
Dynamically stabilizes the cervical spine
Innervation

Lower subscapular nerve C6-7

Neck Musculature *(Continued)*

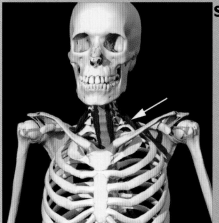

Scalenes — Posterior Fibers
Origin
Transverse processes of C5-C6
Insertion
Second rib
Isolated Function
Concentrically accelerates cervical flexion, rotation and lateral flexion
Assists rib elevation during inhalation
Integrated Function
Eccentrically decelerates cervical extension, rotation and lateral flexion
Dynamically stabilizes the cervical spine
Innervation
Lower subscapular nerve C6-7

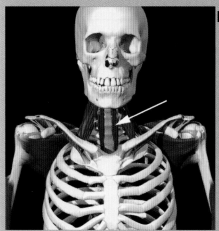

Longus Colli
Origin
Anterior portion of T1-T3
Insertion
Anterior and lateral C1
Isolated Function
Concentrically accelerates cervical flexion, lateral flexion and ipsilateral rotation
Integrated Function
Eccentrically decelerates cervical extension, lateral flexion and contralateral rotation
Dynamically stabilizes the cervical spine
Innervation

Lower subscapular nerve C6-7

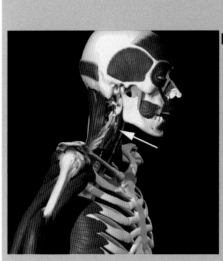

Longus Capitus
Origin
Transverse processes of C3-C6
Insertion
Inferior occipital bone
Isolated Function
Concentrically accelerates cervical
flexion and lateral flexion
Integrated Function
Eccentrically decelerates cervical
extension
Dynamically stabilizes the cervical spine
Innervation

Lower subscapular nerve C6-7

Summary of the Function Anatomy of Muscles

This review should make it clear that all muscles function in all three planes of motion (sagittal, frontal and transverse) and through the entire muscle action spectrum (eccentric, isometric and concentric). In addition, it is evident that several muscles work synergistically to produce force, stabilize the body and/or reduce force.

The more functional anatomy is understood, the more specific exercise prescription can become. A lack of understanding of the synergistic function of the kinetic chain muscles in all three planes of motion commonly leads to a lack of optimum performance and the potential of developing muscle imbalances.

Muscular Force

FORCE:
An influence applied by one object to another, which results in an acceleration or deceleration of the second object.

A **force** is defined as the interaction between two entities or bodies that result in either the acceleration or deceleration of an object.[1,2,13] Forces are characterized by magnitude (how much) and direction (which way they are moving).[1,2,13] The kinetic chain is designed to manipulate variable forces from a multitude of directions to effectively produce movement. As such, the health and fitness professional must gain an understanding of some of the concepts relating to a muscle's ability to generate force.

Length-tension Relationships

LENGTH-TENSION RELATIONSHIP:
The length at which a muscle can produce the greatest force.

Length-tension relationship refers to the length at which a muscle can produce the greatest force.[14-20] There is an optimal muscle length at which the actin and myosin filaments in the sarcomere have the greatest degree of overlap (Figure 4-12). This results in the ability of myosin to make a maximal amount of connections with actin and thus results in the potential for maximal force production of that muscle. Lengthening a muscle beyond this optimal length and then stimulating it reduces the amount of actin and myosin overlap, reducing force production (Figure 4-13). Similarly, shortening a muscle too much and then stimulating it places the actin and myosin in a state of maximal overlap and allows for no further movement to occur between the filaments, reducing its force output (Figure 4-14).[14-20]

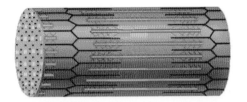

**Figure 4-12:
Optimal Length Muscle**

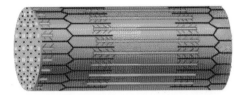

**Figure 4-13:
Lengthened Muscle**

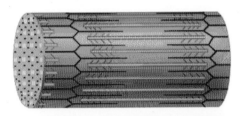

**Figure 4-14:
Shortened Muscle**

This concept is vitally important to the health and fitness professional and coincides with the previously discussed concept of joint alignment. Just as the position of one joint can drastically affect other joints, it can also affect the muscles that surround the joint. If muscle lengths are altered as a result of misaligned joints (i.e. poor posture), then they will not be able to generate proper force to allow for efficient movement. This is the beginning of understanding the kinetic chain and how it works. If one component of the kinetic chain (nervous, skeletal or muscular) is dysfunctional, it will have a direct effect on the others.[3-6,21]

Force-velocity Curve

The force-velocity curve refers to the ability of muscles to produce force with increasing velocity (Figure 4-15). As the velocity of a concentric muscle contraction increases, its ability to produce force decreases. This is thought to be the result of overlapping the actin filament that may interfere with their ability to crossbridge with myosin. Conversely, with eccentric muscle action, as the velocity of muscle action increases the ability to develop force increases. This is believed to be the result of the use of the elastic component of the connective tissue surrounding and within the muscle.[1,8,13,22]

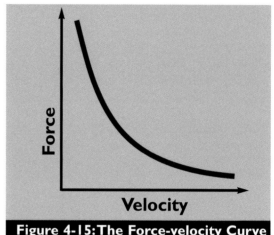

Figure 4-15: The Force-velocity Curve

Force-couple Relationships

Muscles produce a force that is transmitted to bones through their connective tissues (tendons). Because muscles are recruited as groups, many muscles will transmit force onto their respective bones, creating movement at the joints.[10,23-25] This synergistic action of muscles to produce movement around a joint is also known as a **force-couple**.[3,4,5,6,8,21] Muscles in a force-couple provide divergent pulls on the bone or bones they connect with. This is due to the fact that each muscle has different attachment sites, pull at a different angle and create a different force on that joint. The motion that results from these forces is dependent upon the structure of the joint and the collective pull of each muscle involved (Table 4-4).[2,3,8]

> **FORCE-COUPLE:**
> Muscle groups moving together to produce movement around a joint.

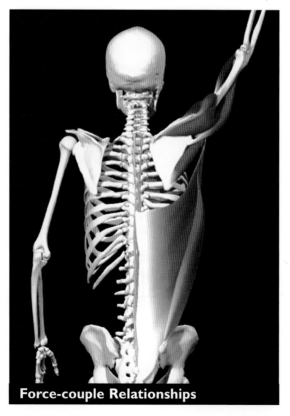

Force-couple Relationships

Table 4-4: Common Force-Couples	
Muslces	**Movement Created**
Internal and external obliques	Trunk rotation
Upper trapezius and the lower portion of the serratus anterior	Upward rotation of the scapula
Gluteus maximus, quadriceps and calf muscles	Produce hip and knee extension during walking, running, stair climbing, etc.
Gastrocnemius, peroneus longus and posterior tibialis	Performing plantarflexion at the foot and ankle complex
Deltoid and rotator cuff	Performing shoulder abduction

In reality, however, every movement we produce must involve all muscle actions (eccentric, isometric, concentric) and all functions (agonists, synergists, stabilizers and antagonists) to ensure proper joint motion as well as eliminate unwanted motion. Therefore, all muscles working together for the production of proper movement are said to be working in a force-couple.[2,3] In order to ensure that the kinetic chain moves in the right manner, it must exhibit proper force-couple relationships. This can only happen if the muscles are at the right length-tension relationships and the joints have proper arthrokinematics (or joint motion). Collectively, proper length-tension relationships, force-couple relationships and arthrokinematics allow for proper sensorimotor integration and ultimately proper and efficient movement.[2,3]

Muscular Leverage and Arthrokinematics

The amount of force that the kinetic chain can produce is not only dependent upon motor unit recruitment and muscle size, but also on the leverage of the muscles and bones.[1,2,8] In the kinetic chain, the bones act as levers that are moved by the force of the muscles. These levers are moved around different axes, which are our joints. This movement around an axis can be termed **rotary motion** and implies that the levers (bones) rotate around the axis (joints).[1,2,8] This "turning" effect of the joint is often referred to as **torque**.[1,2,8]

In resistance training, bones provide the means by which we can attach forces (or torque) to our joints. These joints must be reduced eccentrically, stabilized (or held) isometrically and/or overcome concentrically by the muscles. Since the neuromuscular system is ultimately responsible for manipulating force, the amount of leverage the kinetic chain will have (for any given movement) depends on the leverage of the muscles, in relation to the resistance. The difference between the distance that the weight is from the center of the joint and the muscle's attachment and line of pull (direction that

ROTARY MOTION:
**Movement of
the bones around
the joints.**

TORQUE:
**A force that
produces rotation.**

131

the tendon pulls) is from the joint, will determine the efficiency that the muscles will be able to manipulate the movement.[1,2,8] Since we cannot alter the attachment sites or the line of pull of our muscles, the easiest way to alter the amount of torque generated at a joint is to move the resistance. In other words, the closer the weight is to the joint, the less torque it creates. The farther away the weight is from the joint, the more torque it creates.

For example, to hold a dumbbell straight out to the side at arms length (shoulder abduction), the weight may be approximately 24 inches from the center of the shoulder joint. The prime mover for shoulder abduction is the deltoid muscle. If its attachment is approximately two inches from the joint center. That is a disparity of 22 inches (or roughly 12 times the difference). However, if the weight is moved closer to the joint center (the elbow), the resistance is only approximately 12 inches from the joint center. Now the difference is only 10 inches or five times greater. Essentially, the weight was reduced by half. Many people performing side lateral raises with dumbbells (raising dumbbells out to the side) do this inadvertently by bending their elbow and bringing the weight closer to the shoulder joint.

Health and fitness professionals can use this principle as a regression to exercises that are too demanding by reducing the torque placed on the kinetic chain, or as a progression to increase the torque and place a greater demand on the kinetic chain.

MODULE 4-1 Summary

The study of biomechanics looks at how internal and external forces affect the way the body moves. In order to understand the body and communicate about it effectively, a health and fitness professional must know the terminology for the various anatomical locations. It is also important to know how the body moves in the sagittal, frontal and transverse planes as well as the joint motions in each of these planes.

Muscles move in one of three ways: eccentrically (to decelerate force), isometrically (to stabilize), or concentrically (to accelerate force). All muscles have isolated and integrated functions to create these various actions. Each muscle should be studied at length to examine its functions as well as how it moves synergistically with others.

Muscles are influenced by outside forces from a multitude of directions. To compensate they produce corresponding forces in groups to move bones and joints, in force-couple actions. However, the amount of force that can be produced is dependent on leverage (or how far a weight being moved is from the joint). This leverage directly affects rotary motion and torque.

MODULE 4-1 Quiz

1. Match the anatomical locations to their definitions:

   a. Medial   ____ On the same side of the body

   b. Lateral   ____ Below a point of reference

   c. Contralateral ____ Farther away from the middle of the body

   d. Ipsilateral ____ Farthest from the center of the body

   e. Anterior   ____ On the back of the body

   f. Posterior   ____ On the opposite side of the body

   g. Proximal   ____ Near the middle of the body

   h. Distal   ____ Above a point of reference

   i. Inferior   ____ Nearest the center of the body

   j. Superior   ____ On the front of the body

2. Abduction and adduction occurs in which plane of motion?

   _____

3. Lowering a barbell is an example of which kind of muscle contraction?

   ☐ Eccentric   ☐ Concentric   ☐ Isometric

4. Isometric muscle contraction performs which action?

   ☐ Acceleration   ☐ Deceleration   ☐ Stabilization

5. What kind of movement is created by the force-couple of the upper trapezius and the lower portion of the serratus anterior?

   _____

6. The movement of joints and bones around an axis is_____.
   The "turning" effect of the joint is often referred to as_____.

7. As the velocity of a concentric muscle contraction ☐ **increases** ☐ **decreases**, its ability to produce force ☐ **increases** ☐ **decreases**.

MODULE 4-2: Motor Behavior

Motor behavior is the kinetic chain's response to environmental stimuli (internal and external). To study it, we must examine the manner with which the nervous, skeletal and muscular systems interact to produce movement via sensory information from internal and external environments. In this text, the study of motor behavior consists of the studies of motor control (or how the kinetic chain creates movement) and motor learning (or how the kinetic chain learns those movements).[2,3]

Internal Environment	**External Environment**
■ Length-tension Relationships	■ Stability
■ Force-couple Relationships	■ Speed
■ Arthrokinematics	■ Intensity
	■ Amplitude
	■ Frequency

Motor Control

For the kinetic chain to move in an organized and efficient manner, it must exhibit precise control over its segments. This segmental control is an integrated process involving all components of the kinetic chain (neural, skeletal and muscular) to produce appropriate motor responses. This process (and the study of these movements) is known as **motor control**. More specifically, it looks at the involved structures and mechanisms that the nervous system uses to gather all sensory information (internal and external) and integrates it all with previous experiences to produce a motor response.[2,3,10,23-26] Essentially, motor control is concerned with those neural structures that are involved with motor behavior and how they produce movement.[24]

Muscles Synergies

One of the most important concepts in motor control is that muscles are recruited by the central nervous system as groups (or **synergies**).[10,23-25] This simplifies movement by allowing muscles and joints to operate as a functional unit.[11] Through practice of proper movement patterns (proper exercise technique), these synergies become more fluent and automated (Table 4-5).

MOTOR BEHAVIOR: The process of the body responding to internal and external stimuli.

MOTOR CONTROL: The study of posture and movements and the involved structures and mechanisms that the central nervous system uses to assimilate and integrate sensory information with previous experiences.

SYNERGIES: Groups of muscles that are recruited by the central nervous system to provide movement.

Table 4-5: Common Muscle Synergies	
Exercise	**Muscle Synergies**
Lat Pulldown	Latissimus dorsi, rotator cuff, bicep brachii
Squat	Quadriceps, hamstrings, gluteus maximus
Shoulder Press	Deltoid, rotator cuff, trapezius

Proprioception

PROPRIOCEPTION:
The cumulative neural input to the central nervous system from all mechanoreceptors that sense position and limb movements.

The mechanoreceptors, discussed in the previous chapter, collectively feed the nervous system with a form of sensory information known as **proprioception**. Proprioception utilizes information from the mechano-receptors (muscle spindle, Golgi tendon organ and joint receptors) to provide information about body position, movement and sensation, as it pertains to muscle and joint force.[24] Proprioception is a vital source of information that the nervous system utilizes to gather information about the environment to produce the most efficient movement.[27] Research has demonstrated that propriocpetion is altered following injury. This becomes relevant to the health fitness professional as 85 percent of the adult population experiences low back pain, an estimated 80,000-100,000 anterior cruciate ligament (ACL) injuries occur annually as well as more than two million ankle sprains. This means that many of today's health club members many have altered proprioception due to past injuries. This provides a rationale for core and balance training to enhance one's proprioceptive capabilities, increasing postural control and decreasing tissue overload.

Sensorimotor Integration

SENSORIMOTOR INTEGRATION:
The cooperation of the nervous and muscular system in gathering information, interpreting and executing movement.

Sensorimotor integration is the ability of the nervous system to gather and interpret sensory information and to select and execute the proper motor response.[2,3,21,23,27,28-33] The definition tells us that the nervous system ultimately dictates movement. Sensorimotor integration is only as effective as the quality of incoming sensory information.[2,21,30-32] If individuals train with improper form, improper sensory information will be delivered to the central nervous system, leading to movement compensations and potential injury. Thus, it is important to design proper programs and train with correct technique. For example, if an individual consistently performs a chest press while rounding and elevating their shoulders, this can lead to altered length-tension relationships of muscles (decreased force production), altered force-couple relationships (improper recruitment pattern of muscles) and altered arthrokinematics (improper joint motion). This can ultimately lead to shoulder impingement.

Motor Learning

Motor learning is the integration of these motor control processes, with practice and experience, leading to a relatively permanent change in the capacity to produce skilled movements.[2,3,23,34] Essentially, the study of motor learning looks at how movements are learned and retained for future use. Examples would include riding a bike, throwing a baseball, playing the piano or even performing a squat. In each of these instances, proper practice and experience will lead to a permanent change in one's ability to perform the movement efficiently. For this to occur, the utilization of feedback will be necessary to ensure optimal development of these skilled movements.

Feedback

Feedback is the utilization of sensory information and sensorimotor integration to aid the kinetic chain in the development of permanent neural representations of motor patterns. This allows for efficient movement. This is achieved through two different forms of feedback. These are internal (or sensory) feedback and external (or augmented) feedback.

Internal Feedback

Internal feedback (or sensory feedback) is the process whereby sensory information is utilized by the body via length-tension relationships (posture), force-couple relationships and arthrokinematics to reactively monitor movement and the environment. Essentially, internal (sensory) feedback acts as a guide, steering the kinetic chain to the proper force, speed and amplitude of movement patterns. Thus, it is important to having proper form when exercising to ensure that the incoming sensory feedback is correct information, allowing for optimal sensorimotor integration and ideal structural and functional efficiency.

External Feedback

External feedback is simply information provided by some external source, such as a health and fitness professional, videotape, mirror or heart rate monitor. It is used to supplement internal feedback.[23,35] External feedback provides the client with another source of information that allows him/her to associate whether the achieved movement pattern was ("good" or "bad") with what he/she is feeling internally.

MOTOR LEARNING: Repeated practice of motor control processes, which lead to a change in the ability to produce complex movements.

FEEDBACK: The use of sensory information and sensorimotor integration to help the kinetic chain in motor learning.

INTERNAL FEEDBACK: The process whereby sensory information is utilized by the body to reactively monitor movement and the environment.

EXTERNAL FEEDBACK: Information provided by some external source, such as a health and fitness professional, videotape, mirror or heart rate monitor to supplement internal environment.

Two major forms of external feedback are Knowledge of Results and Knowledge of Performance (Table 4-17).[23,34-36] *Knowledge of Results* is used after the completion of a movement to help inform the client about the outcome of their performance. This should come from the health and fitness professional as well as from the client. An example of this is the fitness professional telling a client that their squats were "good" and asking the client if they could "feel" or "see" their form. By getting the client to become involved with the knowledge of results, they increase their awareness and augment the other forms of sensory feedback. This can be done after each repetition, after a few repetitions or after the set is completed. As the client becomes more familiar with the desired technique of a movement (exercise), knowledge of results from the health and fitness professional should be given less frequently. This improves neuromuscular efficiency.[35]

Knowledge of Performance provides information about the quality of the movement during an exercise. An example of this would be noticing that during a squat, the client's feet were externally rotated and the knees were excessively adducting and then, asking the client if her/she felt or saw anything different about those reps. Again, this gets the client involved in his/her own sensory process. It should be given less frequently as the client becomes more proficient.[35]

Knowledge of Results

Feedback used after the completion of a movement, to help inform the client about the outcome of his performance.

Example: Telling a client that his squats were "good" and asking the client if he could "feel" or "see" his form.

Knowledge of Performance

Feedback that provides information about the quality of the movement during exercise.

Example: Noticing that during a squat, the client's feet were externally rotated and her knees were excessively adducting. Then, asking the client if she felt or saw anything different about those reps.

Figure 4-17: Forms of External Feedback

These forms of external feedback allow for the identification of performance errors. They are also an important component in motivation. Furthermore, they give the client supplemental sensory input to help create an awareness of the desired action.[23,34,35,36] However, it is important to state that a client must not become dependent on external feedback, especially from the health and fitness professional, as this may detract from his/her responsiveness to internal sensory input.[23,34,35,36] This could alter sensorimotor integration and affect the client's motor learning and, ultimately, movement patterns (especially in the absence of a health and fitness professional).

MODULE 4-2 Summary

Each system of the kinetic chain is interdependent. The entire chain must work together to gather information from internal and external environments to create and learn movements (or motor behavior). The body uses proprioception, sensorimotor integration and muscle synergies to create efficient movement (motor control). Then, repeated practice, as well as internal and external feedback allows this efficient movement to be reproduced (motor learning).

MODULE 4-2 Quiz

1. Which is considered internal feedback utilized by the body to monitor movement?

   ☐ Length-tension Relationships

   ☐ Force-couple Relationships

   ☐ Arthrokinematics

   ☐ All of the above

2. Sensorimotor integration requires proprioception.

   ☐ True   ☐ False

3. A heart rate monitor is an example of which type of feedback?

   ☐ Internal

   ☐ External

4. Correcting a client's posture during an exercise provides:

   ☐ Knowledge of Performance

   ☐ Knowledge of Results

References

1. Hamill J, Knutzen JM. *Biomechanical basis of human movement.* Baltimore, MD: Williams & Wilkins; 1995.

2. Norkin CC, Levangie PK. *Joint structure and function: a comprehensive analysis.* 2nd edition. Philadelphia: FA Davis Company; 1992.

3. Clark MA. *Integrated training for the new millennium.* Thousand Oaks, CA: National Academy of Sports Medicine; 2001.

4. Clark MA. *An integrated approach to human movement science.* Thousand Oaks, CA. National Academy of Sports Medicine; 2001.

5. Clark MA, Corn RJ, Parracino LA. *Integrated program design for the fitness professional.* Thousand Oaks, CA: National Academy of Sports Medicine; 2000.

6. Clark MA. *A scientific approach to understanding kinetic chain dysfunction.* Thousand Oaks, CA: National Academy of Sports Medicine; 2001.

7. Kendall FP, McCreary EK, Provance PG. *Muscles testing and function.* 4th edition. Baltimore, MA: Lippincott Williams & Wilkins; 1993.

8. Luttgens K, Hamilton N. *Kinesiology: scientific basis of human motion.* 9th edition. Dubuque, IA: Brown & Benchmark Publishers; 1997.

9. Gray GW. *Chain reaction festival.* Adrian, MI: Wynn Marketing; 1996.

10. Brooks VB. *The neural basis of motor control.* New York: Oxford University Press; 1986.

11. Gel'fand IM, Gurfinkel VS, Tsetlin ML, Shik ML. Some problems in the analysis of movements. In: Gel'fand IM, Gurfinkel VS, Formin SV, Tsetlin ML (eds). *Models of the structural-functional organization of certain biological systems.* Cambridge, MA: MIT Press; 1971.

12. Gambetta V. Everything in balance. *Train Condit* 1996;1(2)15-21.

13. Enoka RM. *Neuromechanical basis of kinesiology.* 2nd edition. Champaign, IL: Human Kinetics; 1994.

14. Milner-Brown A. *Neuromuscular physiology.* Thousand Oaks, CA: National Academy of Sports Medicine; 2001.

15. Fox SI. *Human physiology.* 5th edition. Dubuque, IA: Wm. C. Brown Publishers; 1996.

16. Vander A, Sherman J, Luciano D. *Human physiology: the mechanisms of body function.* 8th edition. New York: McGraw-Hill; 2001.

17. Hamill J, Knutzen JM. *Biomechanical basis of human movement.* Baltimore, MD: Williams & Wilkins; 1995.

18. Watkins J. *Structure and function of the musculoskeletal system.* Champaign, IL: Human Kinetics; 1999.

19. Luttgens K, Hamilton N. *Kinesiology: scientific basis of human motion.* 9th edition. Dubuque, IA: Brown & Benchmark Publishers; 1997.

20. Norkin CC, Levangie PK. *Joint structure and function: a comprehensive analysis.* 2nd edition. Philadelphia: FA Davis Company; 1992.

21. Clark MA. *Integrated kinetic chain assessment.* Thousand Oaks, CA: National Academy of Sports Medicine; 2001.

22. Fleck SJ, Kraemer WJ. *Designing resistance training programs.* 2nd edition. Champaign, IL: Human Kinetics; 1997.

23. Rose DJ. *A multilevel approach to the study of motor control and learning.* Needham Heights, MA: Allyn & Bacon; 1997.

24. Newton RA. Neural systems underlying motor control. In: Montgomery PC, Connoly BH editors. *Motor control and physical therapy: theoretical framework and practical applications.* Hixson, TN: Chatanooga Group, Inc; 1991.

25. Kelso JAS. *Dynamic patterns: the self-organization of brain and behavior.* Cambridge, MA: The MIT Press; 1995.

26. Gurfinkel VS, Cordo PJ. The scientific legacy of nikolai berstein. In: Latash ML (ed). Progress in motor control. Vol 1. *Berstein's traditions in movement studies.* Champaign, IL: Human Kinetics; 1998.

27. Ghez C. The control of movement. In: Kandel E, Schwartz J, Jessel T (eds). *Principles of neuroscience.* New York: Elsevier Science; 1991.

28. Biedert RM. Contribution of the three levels of nervous system motor control: Spinal cord, lower brain, cerebral cortex. In: Lephart SM, Fu FH (eds). *Proprioception and neuromuscular control in joint stability.* Champaign, IL: Human Kinetics; 2000.

29. Boucher JP. Training and exercise science. Ch 3. In: Liebension C (ed). *Rehabilitation of the spine.* Baltimore: Williams & Wilkins; 1996.

30. Janda V, Va Vrova M. Sensory motor stimulation. Ch 15. In: Liebension C (ed). Rehabilitation of the spine. Baltimore: Williams & Wilkins; 1996.

31. Gagey PM, Gentez R. Postural disorders of the body axis. Ch 16. In: Liebension C (ed). *Rehabilitation of the spine.* Baltimore: Williams & Wilkins; 1996.

32. Drury DG. Strength and proprioception. *Ortho Phys Ther Clin* 2000;9(4):549-61.

33. Grigg P. Peripheral neural mechanisms in proprioception. *J Sport Rehab* 1994;3:2-17.

34. Schmidt RA, Lee TD. *Motor control and learning: a behavioral emphasis.* 3rd edition. Champaign, IL: Human Kinetics; 1999.

35. Swinnen SP. Information feedback for motor skill learning: a review. Chapter 3. In: Zelaznik HN (ed). *Advances in motor learning and control.* Champaign, IL: Human Kinetics; 1996.

36. Schmidt RA, Wrisberg CA. *Motor learning and performance.* 2nd edition. Champaign, IL: Human Kinetics; 2000.

CHAPTER FIVE

Fitness Assessment

Objectives

After studying this chapter, you will be able to:

- Explain the components and function of an integrated fitness assessment.
- Ask appropriate general and medical questions to gather subjective information from clients.
- Understand the importance of posture and how it relates to movement observation.
- Perform a systematic assessment to obtain objective information about clients.

Key Terms

- Fitness assessment
- Subjective information
- Objective information
- Skin fold calipers
- Posture

- Postural equilibrium
- Neuromuscular efficiency
- Functional strength
- Postural distortion patterns

MODULE 5-1:
Introduction to Fitness Assessments

Overview of Fitness Assessments

Designing an individualized, systematic fitness assessment can only be properly accomplished by having an understanding of a client's goals, needs and abilities. This entails knowing what a client wants to gain from a training program, what a client needs from their program to successfully accomplish their goal(s) and how capable they are (structurally and functionally) of performing the required tasks, within an integrated program. The information necessary to create the right program for a specific individual (or group of individuals) comes through a proper fitness assessment. The remainder of this chapter will focus on the fitness assessment for the health and fitness professional.

Definition

A fitness assessment is a systematic problem-solving method that provides the health and fitness professional with a basis for making educated decisions about exercise and acute variable selection. Assessments provide an ongoing gathering of information, allowing the health and fitness professional to modify and progress a client through an integrated training program. Fitness assessments allow the health and fitness professional to continually monitor a client's needs, functional capabilities and physiological effects of exercise, enabling the client to realize the full benefit of an individualized training program.

It is important that the health and fitness professional understand that a fitness assessment is not designed to diagnose any condition, but rather, to observe each client's individual structural and functional status. Furthermore, the fitness assessment presented by NASM is not intended to replace a medical examination. If a client exhibits extreme difficulty or pain with any observation or exercise, the health and fitness professional should refer the client to his/her physician or qualified health-care provider to identify any underlying cause.

What Information Does a Fitness Assessment Provide?

A fitness assessment provides the health and fitness professional with a three-dimensional representation of the client. It gives insight into the client's past, present and perhaps their future. The assessment covers information regarding habits, hobbies, movement abilities and past and present medical history. Essentially, a fitness assessment allows the health and fitness professional to see the current structure and function of a client.

By gathering information through the fitness assessment, a fundamental representation of a client's goals, needs and status can be created. This enables proper construction of an integrated training program that is individualized specifically for each client. When conducting a fitness assessment, it is essential to utilize a variety of observation methods in order to obtain a balanced overview of a client (Figure 5-1).

Table 5-1: Guidelines for Health Professionals

DO NOT	DO
Diagnose medical conditions.	■ Obtain exercise or health guidelines from a physician, physical therapist, registered dietitian, etc. ■ Follow national consensus guidelines of exercise prescription for medical disorders. ■ Screen clients for exercise limitations. ■ Identify potential risk factors for clients, through screening procedures. ■ Refer clients who experience pain or exhibit other symptoms to a qualified medical practitioner.
Prescribe treatment.	■ Design individualized, systematic progressive exercise programs. ■ Refer clients to a qualified medical practitioner for medical exercise prescription.
Prescribe diets or recommend specific supplements.	■ Provide clients with general information on healthy eating, according to the Food Pyramid. ■ Refer clients to a qualified dietitian or nutritionist for specific diet plans.
Provide treatment of any kind for injury or disease.	■ Refer clients to a qualified medical practitioner for treatment of injury or disease. Use exercise to help clients improve overall health. Assist clients in following the medical advice of a physician and/or therapist.
Provide rehabilitation services for clients.	■ Design exercise programs for clients after they are released from rehabilitation. ■ Provide post-rehabilitation services.
Provide counseling services for clients.	■ Act as a coach for clients. ■ Provide general information. ■ Refer clients to a qualified counselor or therapist.

Subjective Information
General and Medical History:
Occupation, Lifestyle, Medical and Personal information

Objective Information
Physiological Assessments
Body Composition Testing
Cardiorespiratory Assessments
Static and Dynamic Postural Assessments
Performance Assessments

Figure 5-1: Components of a Fitness Assessment

MODULE 5-1 Summary

A health and fitness professional's primary responsibility is to safely and effectively guide clients to successful attainment of their goals. To do so, requires a comprehensive understanding of clients' personal and professional backgrounds as well as their physical capabilities and desires. The fitness assessment is a comprehensive tool to systematically gather subjective and objective information about clients and utilize the information appropriately. It is not designed to diagnose any condition nor replace a medical examination. Health and fitness professionals should refer clients to qualified health-care providers whenever necessary.

MODULE 5-1 Quiz

1. A fitness assessment is a systematic problem-solving method that provides health and fitness professionals with a basis for making educated decisions about exercise and _____ selection.

2. A fitness assessment is designed to observe each client's individual structural and functional status and diagnose conditions.

    ☐ True   ☐ False

3. Health and fitness professionals should give clients diet plans and recommend specific supplements.

    ☐ True   ☐ False

4. The fitness assessment includes objective and _____ information such as habits, hobbies, movement abilities and medical history.

MODULE 5-2: Subjective Information Provided in the Fitness Assessment

Types of Subjective Information

Subjective information is gathered from a prospective client to give the health and fitness professional feedback regarding personal history such as occupation, lifestyle and medical background.

General and Medical History

Gathering personal background information about a client can be very valuable. It can help a health and fitness professional to understand a client's physical condition and can also provide insight to what types of imbalances they may exhibit. One of the easiest forms of gathering this information is through a questionnaire.[1] The Physical Activity Readiness Questionnaire (PAR-Q) is a questionnaire that has been designed to help qualify a person for low-to-moderate-to-high activity levels.[1,2] Furthermore, it aids in identifying people for whom certain activities may not be appropriate or who may need further medical attention.

Questions	Yes	No
1 Has your doctor ever said that you have a heart condition and that you should only perform physical activity recommended by a doctor?	☐	☐
2 Do you feel pain in your chest when you perform physical activity?	☐	☐
3 In the past month, have you had chest pain when you were not performing any physical activity?	☐	☐
4 Do you lose your balance because of dizziness or do you ever lose consciousness?	☐	☐
5 Do you have a bone or joint problem that could be made worse by a change in your physical activity?	☐	☐
6 Is your doctor currently prescribing any medication for your blood pressure or for a heart condition?	☐	☐
7 Do you know of any other reason why you should not engage in physical activity?		

If you have answered "Yes" to one or more of the above questions, consult your physician before engaging in physical activity. Tell your physician which questions you answered "Yes" to. After a medical evaluation, seek advice from your physician on what type of activity is suitable for your current condition.

Figure 5-2: Sample Physical Activity Readiness Questionnaire (PAR-Q)

The PAR-Q is directed toward detecting any possible cardiorespiratory dysfunction, such as coronary heart disease. It is a good beginning point for gathering personal background information concerning a prospective client's cardiorespiratory function. However, it is only one component of a thorough fitness assessment. While this information is extremely important for a health and fitness professional, asking other questions can provide additional information about a client. This includes questions about a client's general and medical history.

General History

Asking some very basic questions concerning a client's history and/or personal background can provide a wealth of information. Two important areas to start with are occupation and lifestyle.

Occupation

Knowing a client's occupation can provide the health and fitness professional with insight into what his/her movement capacity is and what kinds of movement patterns are performed throughout the day. Examples of typical questions are shown in Figure 5-3.

Questions	Yes	No
1 What is your current occupation?_____		
2 Does your occupation require extended periods of sitting?	☐	☐
3 Does your occupation require extended periods of repetitive movements? (If yes, please explain.) _____		
4 Does your occupation require you to wear shoes with a heel (dress shoes)?	☐	☐
5 Does your occupation cause you anxiety (mental stress)?	☐	☐

Figure 5-3: Sample Questions: Client Occupation

By obtaining this information, a health and fitness professional can begin to recognize important clues about the structure and, ultimately, the function of a client. Each question provides relevant information.

Extended Periods of Sitting

This is a very important question that provides a lot of information. First, if a client is sitting a large portion of the day, the client's hips are flexed for prolonged periods of time. This, in turn, can lead to tight hip flexors that can cause postural imbalances within the kinetic chain.[3-6] Second, if a client is sitting for prolonged periods of time, especially at a computer, there is a tendency for the shoulders and head to fatigue under the constant influence of gravity. This often leads to a postural imbalance of rounding of the shoulders and head.[3-5]

Repetitive Movements

Repetitive movements can create a pattern overload to muscles and joints and may lead to tissue trauma and eventually, kinetic chain dysfunction.[3-5,7-9] This can be seen in jobs that require a lot of overhead work such as construction, painting, etc. Working with the arms overhead for long periods of time may lead to shoulder soreness that could be the result of tightness in the latissimus dorsi and weakness in the rotator cuff. This imbalance does not allow for proper shoulder motion and/or stabilization during activity.

Dress Shoes

Wearing shoes with a heel puts the ankle complex in a plantarflexion position for extended periods of time. This can lead to tightness in the gastrocnemius and soleus causing postural imbalance, such as over-pronation at the foot and ankle complex (flattening of the foot).[3-5]

Mental Stress

Mental stress or anxiety can lead to a dysfunctional breathing pattern that can further lead to postural distortion and kinetic chain dysfunction.[10,11] Please refer to Chapter 3 (Dysfunctional Breathing) for details.

Lifestyle

Questions pertaining to a client's lifestyle will reflect what a client does in his/her free time. This is generally known as their recreation and/or hobbies. Examples of typical questions are shown in Figure 5-4.

As discussed earlier, each of the questions above provides relevant information.

Recreation

Recreation, in the context of the assessment, refers to a client's physical activities outside of the work environment. By finding out what recreational activities a client performs, a health and fitness professional can better design a program to fit these needs.

For example, many clients like to golf, ski, play tennis or a variety of other

Questions	Yes	No
1 Do you partake in any recreational activities (golf, tennis, skiing, etc.)? (If yes, please explain.) _____ _____	☐	☐
2 Do you have any hobbies (reading, gardening, working on cars, exploring the Internet, etc.)? (If yes, please explain.) _____ _____	☐	☐

Figure 5-4: Sample Questions: Client Lifestyle

sporting activities in their spare time. Proper forms of training must be incorporated to ensure that clients are trained in a manner that optimizes the efficiency of the kinetic chain, without predisposing it to injury.[3]

Hobbies

Hobbies, in the context of the assessment, refer to activities that a client may partake in regularly, but are not necessarily athletic in nature. Examples include gardening, working on cars, playing cards, reading, watching television, spending time on the Internet, etc. In many of these cases, the client does not receive a lot of physical stimulation.

In instances where clients have hobbies that require little physical activity, it is still necessary to take lifestyle choices into account in order to create a properly planned integrated training program. It should be noted, however, that these clients probably will not be at the same level of training as someone who plays a lot of tennis.

Medical History

Finding out a client's medical history is absolutely crucial. Most importantly, it provides the health and fitness professional with information about any life-threatening chronic diseases (such as coronary heart disease, high blood pressure, diabetes, etc.).[1] Furthermore, it provides information about the structure and function of the client. Some important areas to cover include past injuries, surgeries and chronic conditions.

Questions	Yes	No
1 Have you ever had any pain or injuries (ankle, knee, hip, back, shoulder, etc.)? (If yes, please explain.) _____ _____	☐	☐
2 Have you ever had any surgeries? (If yes, please explain.) _____ _____	☐	☐
3 Has a medical doctor ever diagnosed you with a chronic disease, such as coronary heart disease, coronary artery disease, hypertension (high blood pressure), high cholesterol or diabetes? (If yes, please explain.) _____ _____	☐	☐
4 Are you currently taking any medication? (If yes, please list.) _____ _____	☐	☐

Figure 5-5: Sample Questions: Client Medical History

Past Injuries

Inquiring about a client's past injuries can illuminate possible dysfunctions. There is a vast array of research that has demonstrated that past injuries affect the functioning of the kinetic chain. This is especially true of the following injuries:

1. Ankle Sprains

Ankle sprains have been shown to decrease the neural control to the gluteus medius and gluteus maximus muscles. This, in turn, can lead to poor control of the lower extremities during many functional activities, which can eventually lead to injury.[3,4,12-21]

2. Knee Injuries Involving Ligaments

Knee injuries can cause a decrease in the neural control to muscles that stabilize the patella (kneecap) and lead to further injury. Knee injuries that are not the result of contact (such as non-contact injuries), are often the result of ankle and/or hip dysfunctions, like the result of an ankle sprain.[3,4] The knee is caught between the ankle and the hip. If the ankle or hip joint begins to function improperly this results in altered movement and force distribution of the knee. Over time, this can lead to further injury.[22-37]

3. Low Back Injuries

Low back injuries can cause decreased neural control to stabilizing muscles of the core, resulting in poor stabilization of the spine. This can further lead to dysfunction in upper and lower extremities.[3,4,7,38-48]

4. Shoulder Injuries

Shoulder injuries cause altered neural control of the rotator cuff muscles, which can lead to instability of the shoulder joint during functional activities.[3,4,49-53]

5. Other Injuries

Injuries that result from kinetic chain imbalances include repetitive hamstring strains, groin strains, patellar tendonitis (jumper's knee), plantar fasciitis (pain in the arch of the foot), posterior tibialis tendonitis (shin splints), biceps tendonitis (shoulder pain) and headaches.[3,4]

All of the aforementioned past injuries should be taken into consideration while assessing clients, as the mentioned imbalances will manifest over time, unless proper care has been given.

Past Surgeries

Surgical procedures create trauma for the body and may have similar effects to those of an injury. They can create dysfunction, unless properly rehabilitated. Some common surgical procedures include:

- Foot and ankle surgery
- Knee surgery
- Back surgery
- Shoulder surgery
- Cesarean section for birth (cutting through the abdominal wall to deliver a baby)
- Appendectomy (cutting through the abdominal wall to remove the appendix)

In each case, surgery will cause pain and inflammation that can alter neural control to the affected muscles and joints if not rehabilitated properly.[54,55]

Chronic Conditions

It is estimated that more than 75 percent of the American adult population does not partake, on a daily basis, in 30 minutes of low-to-moderate physical activity.[56] The risk of chronic disease goes up significantly in individuals who are not as physically active as this minimal standard.[57,58] Some chronic diseases include:[56,59]

- Cardiovascular disease, coronary heart disease, coronary artery disease or congestive heart failure
- Hypertension (high blood pressure)
- High cholesterol
- Stroke
- Lung or breathing problems
- Obesity
- Diabetes mellitus

Table 5-2: Common Medications by Classification	
Medication	**Basic Function**
Beta-Blockers (ß-Blockers)	Generally used as anti-hypertensive (high blood pressure), may also be prescribed for arrythmias (irregular heart rate)
Calcium Channel Blockers	Generally prescribed for hypertension and angina (chest pain)
Nitrates	Generally prescribed for hypertension, congestive heart failure
Diuretics	Generally prescribed for hypertension, congestive heart failure and peripheral edema
Bronchodilators	Generally prescribed to correct or prevent bronchial smooth muscle constrictor in individuals with asthma and other pulmonary diseases
Vasodilators	Used in the treatment of hypertension and congestive heart failure
Antidepressants	Used in the treatment of various psychiatric and emotional disorders

Medications

Many clients coming into the fitness industry will be under the care of a medical professional and may be required to use any one of a variety of medications. It is not the role of any health and fitness professional to administer, prescribe or educate on the usage and effects of any of these medications.

Always consult with clients' medical professionals for their health information and any medication they may be using.

The purpose of this section is to briefly outline some of the primary classes of drugs and their proposed physiological effects (Table 5-2). The table is merely intended to present a simplistic overview of medications. It is *not* intended to serve as conclusive evidence regarding the medications and/or their effects. For more complete information regarding medications, contact a medical professional and/or refer to the *Physician's Desk Reference* (PDR).

Table 5-3: Effects of Medication on Heart Rate, Blood Pressure and Exercise Capacity		
Medication	**Heart Rate**	**Blood Pressure**
Beta-Blockers (ß-Blockers)	↓	↓
Calcium Channel	↑	↓
Blockers	↔ or ↓	
Nitrates	↑	↔
	↔	↓
Diuretics	↔ ↓	↔
Bronchodilators	↔	↔
Vasodilators	↑	↓
Antidepressants	↑ or ↔	↔ or ↓

Key: ↑ = Increase   ↔ = No Effect   ↓ = Decrease

MODULE 5-2 Summary

A health and fitness professional can gather essential information that provides insight to a client's daily physical activity by gathering subjective information about a client's personal history, including occupation, lifestyle and medical background. Asking questions can provide important clues about the structure and function of a client. It provides information about movement capacity and what kinds of movement patterns are performed throughout the day. The Physical Activity Readiness Questionnaire (PAR-Q) qualifies clients for low-to-moderate-to-high activity levels and aids in identifying people who may need medical attention.

Questions about recreation and/or hobbies will reflect what a client does in his/her free time. Proper forms of training for specific activities must be incorporated to increase the efficiency of the kinetic chain, while avoiding injury. Clients with sedentary hobbies will probably not be at the same level of training as those who participate in recreational sports.

Finding out a client's medical history is crucial. Past injuries affect the functioning of the kinetic chain and are important to ask about in order to discover possible dysfunctions. Surgical procedures have similar effects as injuries since they cause pain and inflammation that can alter neural control to the affected muscles and joints, if not rehabilitated properly. It is also important to ask about chronic conditions, which are likely to occur in individuals who are not physically active. Finally, many clients use medications. It is important to know some of their basic effects, however, health and fitness professionals should not administer, prescribe or educate on the usage and effects of any of these medications. Be sure to consult with clients' medical professionals if they use medication.

MODULE 5-2 Quiz

1. If a client spends a lot of time sitting at his/her job, it can lead to tightness in the:

   ☐ Gluteus maximus

   ☐ Rhomboids

   ☐ Hip flexors

2. Which of the following are considered recreational activities (as opposed to hobbies)?

   ☐ Golfing

   ☐ Skiing

   ☐ Gardening

   ☐ Working on cars

   ☐ Playing tennis

3. A PAR-Q is a good way to gather personal background information concerning a prospective client.

   ☐ True　　☐ False

4. It is estimated that more than _____ percent of the American adult population does not partake, on a daily basis, in 30 minutes of low-to-moderate physical activity.

MODULE 5-3: Objective Information Provided in the Fitness Assessment

Types of Objective Information

Objective information is gathered to provide the health and fitness professional with forms of measurable data. This information can be used to compare beginning numbers to those measured weeks, months or years later, denoting improvements in the client, as well as the effectiveness of the training program. Categories of objective information include:

- Physiological assessments
- Body-composition assessments
- Cardiorespiratory assessments
- Posture and movement assessments
- Performance assessments

Physiological Assessments

Physiological assessments provide the health and fitness professional with valuable information regarding the status of the client's health. By assessing and reassessing a client's *resting heart rate and blood pressure*, health and fitness professionals gather valuable information in designing a client's conditioning program. In addition, the following tests can be used as motivational tools assisting in client retention.

Heart Rate

The resting heart rate can be taken on the inside of the wrist (radial pulse) (preferred) or on the neck to the side of the windpipe (carotid pulse) (use with caution). To gather an accurate recording, it is best to teach clients how to test their resting heart rate upon rising in the morning. Instruct them to test their RHR three mornings in a row and average the three readings.

Radial Pulse

To find the radial pulse, lightly place two fingers along the arm in line and just above the thumb (Figure 5-6). Once the pulse is identified, count the pulses for 30 seconds and multiply by two. Record the 60-second pulse rate and average over three days. Points to consider:

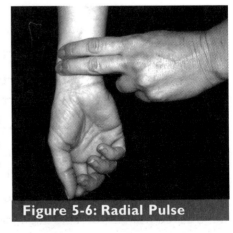
Figure 5-6: Radial Pulse

> **OBJECTIVE INFORMATION:** Measurable data about a client's physical state such as body composition, movement and cardiovascular ability.

- The touch should be gentle.

- The test must be taken when the client is calm.

- Tests must be taken the same time of the morning, to ensure accuracy.

Carotid Pulse

To find the carotid pulse, lightly place two fingers on the neck, just to the side of the larynx. Once the pulse is identified, count the pulses for 30 seconds and multiply by two. Record the 60-second pulse rate and average over three days. Points to consider:

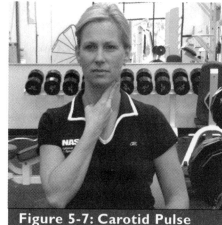

Figure 5-7: Carotid Pulse

- The touch should be gentle. Excessive pressure can decrease heart rate and blood pressure leading to possible dizziness and fainting.[1]

- The test must be taken when the client is calm.

- All three tests must be taken at the same time of the morning, to ensure accuracy.

Resting heart rates can vary. On average, the resting heart rate for a male is 70 beats per minute and 75 beats per minute for a female.[1]

The health and fitness professional can also calculate the training heart rate zone in which a client should perform cardiorespiratory exercise. There are many ways to determine heart rate zones. Create heart rate zones by first determining the client's maximum heart rate by subtracting the client's age from the number 220 (220 - age). Second, multiply the estimated maximum heart rate by the appropriate intensity (65-90 percent) in which the client should work in while performing cardiorespiratory exercise.[1]

Zone One   Maximum Heart Rate x 0.65
                    Maximum Heart Rate x 0.75

Zone Two   Maximum Heart Rate x 0.80
                    Maximum Heart Rate x 0.85

Zone Three Maximum Heart Rate x 0.86
                    Maximum Heart Rate x 0.90

The heart rate zone numbers should be combined with the various cardiorespiratory assessments (discussed later in this chapter) in order to establish which heart rate zone a client will start in. This calculation is a crude average that will most likely have to be modified. Intensity levels may need to be lowered (40-55 percent) depending on the client's physical condition.

Table 5-4: Heart Rate Training Zones	
Training Zone	**Purpose**
One	Builds aerobic base and aids in recovery
Two	Increases endurance and trains the anaerobic threshold
Three	Builds high-end work capacity

Blood Pressure

Blood pressure measurements consist of systolic and diastolic readings. The systolic reading (top number) reflects the pressure produced by the heart as it pumps blood to the body. Normal systolic pressure ranges from 120 millimeters of mercury (mmHg) to 130mmHg. The diastolic blood pressure (lower number) signifies the minimum pressure within the arteries through a full cardiac cycle. Normal diastolic pressure ranges from 80 millimeters of mercury (mmHg) to 85mmHg.[1]

Blood Pressure Testing

Blood pressure is measured using a sphygmomanometer, which consists of an inflatable cuff, a pressure meter and a bulb with a valve and a stethoscope. To record blood pressure, instruct the client to assume a comfortable seated position and place the appropriate size cuff on the client, just above the elbow (Figure 5-8). Next, rest the arm on a supported chair (or support the arm using your own arm) and place the stethoscope over the brachial artery, using a minimal amount of pressure. Continue by rapidly inflating the cuff to 20 to 30mmHg above the point when the pulse can no longer be felt at the wrist. Next, release the pressure at a rate of about 2mmHg per second, listening for the pulse. To determine the systolic pressure, listen for the first observation of the pulse. Diastolic pressure is determined when the pulse fades away. For greater reliability, repeat procedure on opposite arm.[1]

It is important for the health and fitness professional to go through formal training in taking blood pressure prior to assessing blood pressure on health club members.

Figure 5-8: Proper Sphygmomanometer Placement

Body Composition

Gathering body-composition statistics about a client provides the health and fitness professional with a measure of a client's starting point. Using body fat, circumference measurements, hip-to-waist ratio and/or body mass index to assess and then reassess can be motivating for a client. In addition, it is a good indication of how well the training program has been designed.

Body Fat Measurements

One of the most important pieces of information that can be obtained by a health and fitness professional is the client's starting body fat percentage. Body fat reduction is often the primary goal of many clients. As such, its analysis can be a powerful tool to use when discussing progress. Other methods would include asking a client how his clothes are fitting, utilizing before and after pictures and getting comments from friends.

Body fat can be measured in a variety of ways. Depending on the tools available, the most common methods are discussed below.

1. **Skin fold calipers** measure a client's amount of subcutaneous fat (or fat beneath the skin) by calculating the size of skin folds.

2. **Bioelectrical impedance** uses a portable instrument to conduct an electrical current through the body in order to measure fat. This form of assessment is based on the hypothesis that tissues high in water content conduct electrical currents with less resistance than those with little water (such as adipose tissue).

3. **Underwater weighing** is a method of determining the proportion of fat to lean tissue. This difference is determined by weighing a person through normal methods and then, weighing the person under water. Because lean tissue is denser than fat, the more lean a person is, the more he/she will weigh underwater. The results of underwater weighing indicate a person's overall density (compared to the water) and as such, are a composite of body weight to body volume.

> **SKIN FOLD CALIPER:**
> An instrument with two adjustable legs to measure thickness of a skin fold.

Skin Fold Caliper Measurements

Most health and fitness professionals do not have an exercise physiology laboratory at their disposal, so the skin fold caliper method will be the method emphasized in this text. When using caliper measurements, health and fitness professionals must be consistent with the exact areas of skin folds measured, as well as the conditions of administering the assessment. For example, if a skin fold measurement is taken before a client's workout, this agenda should remain consistent in future re-assessments.

Calculating Body Fat Percentages

NASM utilizes the Durnin formula (sometimes known as the Durnin/Womersley formula) to calculate a client's percentage of body fat.[60] This formula was chosen for its simple four-site upper body measurement process. The Durnin formula's four sites of skin fold measurement are as follows:

1. **Biceps:** A vertical fold on the front of the arm over the biceps muscle, halfway between the shoulder and the elbow (Figure 5-9).

2. **Triceps:** A vertical fold on the back of the upper arm, with the arm relaxed and held freely at the side. This skin fold should also be taken halfway between the shoulder and the elbow (Figure 5-10).

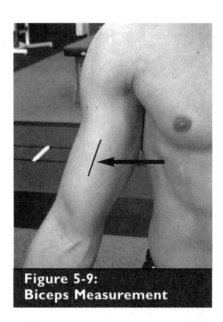

Figure 5-9:
Biceps Measurement

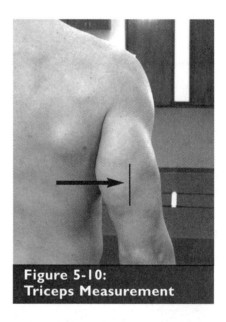

Figure 5-10:
Triceps Measurement

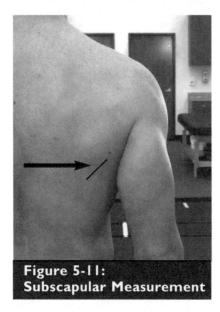

Figure 5-11:
Subscapular Measurement

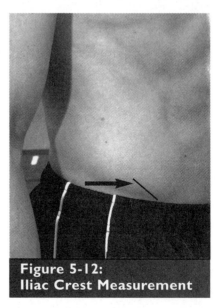

Figure 5-12:
Iliac Crest Measurement

3. **Subscapular:** A 45-degree angle fold of one to two centimeters, below the inferior angle of the scapula (Figure 5-11).

4. **Iliac Crest:** A 45-degree angle fold, taken just above the iliac crest and medial to the axillary line (Figure 5-12).

When taking these measurements, all should be taken on the right side of the body (unless otherwise noted on the assessment form).

After the four sites have been measured, add the totals of the four sites (this should be done in millimeters). Then, find the appropriate gender and age categories for the body composition on the Durnin/Wormersley Body Fat Percentage Calculation table (Table 5-5, page 164).

For example, a 40-year-old female client with the sum of the skin folds being 40, has a body fat percentage of 28.14 (or round down to 28 percent).

Circumference Measurements

Circumference measurements can also be another source of feedback used with clients who have the goal of altering body composition. They are designed to assess girth changes in the body. The most important factor to consider when taking circumference measurements is consistency. Remember when taking measurements to make sure the tape measure is taut and level around the area that is being measured.

1. **Neck:** Across the Adam's apple (Figure 5-13)
2. **Chest:** Across the nipple line (Figure 5-14)

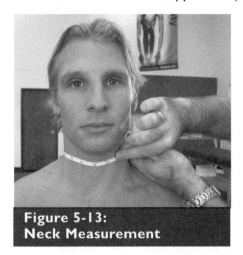

Figure 5-13:
Neck Measurement

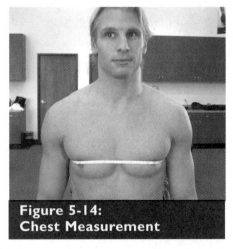

Figure 5-14:
Chest Measurement

3. **Waist:** At the narrowest point of the waist, below the rib cage and just above the top of the hipbones. If there is no apparent narrowing of the waist, measure at the naval (Figure 5-15).

4. **Hips:** With feet together, at the widest portion of the buttocks (Figure 5-16).

Table 5-5: Durnin/Wormersley Body Fat Percentage Calculation

Sum of Folds	Males <19	Males 20-29	Males 30-39	Males 40-49	Males >50	Females <19	Females 20-29	Females 30-39	Females 40-49	Females >50
5	-7.23	-7.61	-1.70	-5.28	-6.87	-2.69	-3.97	0.77	3.91	4.84
10	0.41	0.04	5.05	3.30	2.63	5.72	4.88	8.72	11.71	13.10
15	5.00	4.64	9.09	8.47	8.38	10.78	10.22	13.50	16.40	18.07
20	8.32	7.96	12.00	12.22	12.55	14.44	14.08	16.95	19.78	21.67
25	10.92	10.57	14.29	15.16	15.84	17.33	17.13	19.66	22.44	24.49
30	13.07	12.73	16.17	17.60	18.56	19.71	19.64	21.90	24.64	26.83
35	14.91	14.56	17.77	19.68	20.88	21.74	21.79	23.81	26.51	28.82
40	16.51	16.17	19.17	21.49	22.92	23.51	23.67	25.48	28.14	30.56
45	17.93	17.59	20.41	23.11	24.72	25.09	25.34	26.96	29.59	32.10
50	19.21	18.87	21.53	24.56	26.35	26.51	26.84	28.30	30.90	33.49
55	20.37	20.04	22.54	25.88	27.83	27.80	28.21	29.51	32.09	34.75
60	21.44	21.11	23.47	27.09	29.20	28.98	29.46	30.62	33.17	35.91
65	22.42	22.09	24.33	28.22	30.45	30.08	30.62	31.65	34.18	36.99
70	23.34	23.01	25.13	29.26	31.63	31.10	31.70	32.60	35.11	37.98
75	24.20	23.87	25.87	30.23	32.72	32.05	32.71	33.49	35.99	38.91
80	25.00	24.67	26.57	31.15	33.75	32.94	33.66	34.33	36.81	39.79
85	25.76	25.43	27.23	32.01	34.72	33.78	34.55	35.12	37.58	40.61
90	26.47	26.15	27.85	32.83	35.64	34.58	35.40	35.87	38.31	41.39
95	27.15	26.83	28.44	33.61	36.52	35.34	36.20	36.58	39.00	42.13
100	27.80	27.48	29.00	34.34	37.35	36.06	36.97	37.25	39.66	42.84
105	28.42	28.09	29.54	35.05	38.14	36.74	37.69	37.90	40.29	43.51
110	29.00	28.68	30.05	35.72	38.90	37.40	38.39	38.51	40.89	44.15
115	29.57	29.25	30.54	36.37	39.63	38.03	39.06	39.10	41.47	44.76
120	30.11	29.79	31.01	36.99	40.33	38.63	39.70	39.66	42.02	45.36
125	30.63	30.31	31.46	37.58	41.00	39.21	40.32	40.21	42.55	45.92
130	31.13	30.82	31.89	38.15	41.65	39.77	40.91	40.73	43.06	46.47
135	31.62	31.30	32.31	38.71	42.27	40.31	41.48	41.24	43.56	47.00
140	32.08	31.77	32.71	39.24	42.87	40.83	42.04	41.72	44.03	47.51
145	32.53	32.22	33.11	39.76	43.46	41.34	42.57	42.19	44.49	48.00
150	32.97	32.66	33.48	40.26	44.02	41.82	43.09	42.65	44.94	48.47
155	33.39	33.08	33.85	40.74	44.57	42.29	43.59	43.09	45.37	48.93
160	33.80	33.49	34.20	41.21	45.10	42.75	44.08	43.52	45.79	49.38
165	34.20	33.89	34.55	41.67	45.62	43.20	44.55	43.94	46.20	49.82
170	34.59	34.28	34.88	42.11	46.12	43.63	45.01	44.34	46.59	50.24
175	34.97	34.66	35.21	42.54	46.61	44.05	45.46	44.73	46.97	50.65
180	35.33	35.02	35.53	42.96	47.08	44.46	45.89	45.12	47.35	51.05
185	35.69	35.38	35.83	43.37	47.54	44.86	46.32	45.49	47.71	51.44
190	36.04	35.73	36.13	43.77	48.00	45.25	46.73	45.85	48.07	51.82
195	36.38	36.07	36.43	44.16	48.44	45.63	47.14	46.21	48.41	52.19
200	36.71	36.40	36.71	44.54	48.87	46.00	47.53	46.55	48.75	52.55

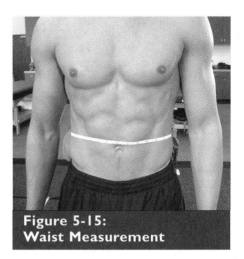
Figure 5-15:
Waist Measurement

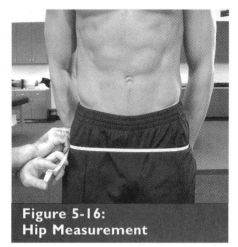
Figure 5-16:
Hip Measurement

5. **Thigh:** Just below the buttocks or 10 inches above the top of the patella (Figure 5-17).

6. **Calf:** At the maximal circumference between the ankle and the knee (Figure 5-18).

7. **Upper arm:** At the maximal circumference of the upper arm, with arm extended, palm facing forward (Figure 5-19).

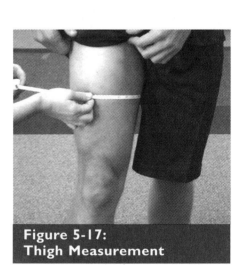
Figure 5-17:
Thigh Measurement

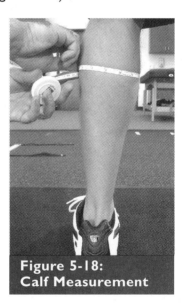
Figure 5-18:
Calf Measurement

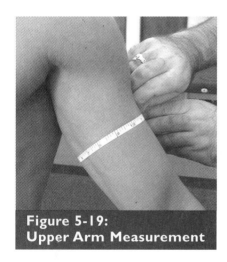
Figure 5-19:
Upper Arm Measurement

Circumference measurements can also be utilized to calculate body fat percentage. This is an important method to have available particularly when skin fold measurements are not an option. (Refer to the conversion tables in the Appendix for proper calculations.)

Waist-to-hip Ratio

The waist-to-hip ratio is one of the most used clinical applications of girth measurements. This assessment is important because there is a correlation between chronic diseases and fat stored in the midsection.[1]

The waist-to-hip ratio can be computed by dividing the waist measurement by the hip measurement by doing the following:[1]

1. Measure the smallest part of the client's waist, without instructing the client to draw in the stomach.

2. Measure the largest part of the client's hips.

3. Compute the waist-to-hip ratio by dividing the waist measurement by the hip measurement.
   a. For example, if a client's waist measures 30 inches and his hips measure 40 inches, divide 30 by 40 for a waist-to-hip ratio of 0.75.

A ratio above 0.80 for females and above 0.95 for males may put people at risk for a number of diseases.

Body Mass Index (BMI)

Although this assessment is not designed to assess body fat, the Body Mass Index (BMI) is a quick and easy method for determining if your client's weight is appropriate for his/her height. To assess weight relative to height, divide body weight (in kilograms) by height (in meters squared) or kg/m^2.[59]

It has been shown that obesity-related health problems increase when a person's BMI exceeds 25. The obesity classifications using BMI are the following:[1]

- Mild = 25-30
- Moderate = 30-35
- Severe > 35

MODULE 5-3 Summary

Objective information (such as body composition, movement observation and cardiovascular assessment) provides measurable data that tracks changes in a client. It can be motivating for a client to assess and reassess body fat, circumference measurements, hip-to-waist ratio and/or body mass index.

Many clients want to lose body fat and, as such, it is important to be able to determine starting body fat percentage. Calipers are the easiest way to do this in a gym setting. Consistency (in location and administration) is vital when measuring skin folds. Calculate a client's percentage of body fat by measuring four sites with calipers, adding the totals of all four sites and then finding the appropriate gender/age categories on the Durnin/Wormersley Body Fat Percentage Calculation table.

Circumference measurements and waist-to-hip ratio are other sources of feedback that assess girth changes in the body. Again, consistency in measurements is key. A waist-to-hip ratio above 0.80 for females and above 0.95 for males may put people at risk for a number of diseases.

Finally, the Body Mass Index (BMI) is a good way to determine if a client's weight is appropriate for his/her height. The chances of having obesity-related health problems increase when a person's BMI exceeds 25.

MODULE 5-3 Quiz

1. Name three ways to measure body fat.

_____

2. On which side of the body should measurements be taken for the Durnin/Womersley formula?

   ☐ Right

   ☐ Left

   ☐ Center

3. Which four sites of the body are used to determine a sum for the Durnin/Womersley formula?

   ☐ Thigh   ☐ Calf

   ☐ Bicep   ☐ Tricep

   ☐ Iliac crest ☐ Hips

   ☐ Subscapular ☐ Waist

4. According to obesity calculations using BMI, at what level of obesity is a person who has a BMI of 31?

   ☐ Mild

   ☐ Moderate

   ☐ Severe

MODULE 5-4:
Cardiorespiratory Assessments

Cardiorespiratory assessments provide the health and fitness professional with valuable information regarding cardiorespiratory efficiency and overall condition. They can also provide health and fitness professionals with a starting point for which zone their client should begin cardiorespiratory exercise (specific to that person's physical condition and goals). Two common forms of assessing cardiorespiratory efficiency are the Step Test and the Rockport Walk Test.

Step Test

This test is designed to estimate a cardiovascular starting point.[61] The starting point is then modified, based on ability level. Once determined, refer to the cardiorespiratory programming section of the text for specific programs.

Step One: Determine the client's maximum heart rate by subtracting the client's age from the number 220 (220 - age). Then, take the maximum heart rate and multiply it by the following figures to determine the heart rate ranges for each zone.

Zone One	Maximum Heart Rate x 0.65
	Maximum Heart Rate x 0.75
Zone Two	Maximum Heart Rate x 0.80
	Maximum Heart Rate x 0.85
Zone Three	Maximum Heart Rate x 0.86
	Maximum Heart Rate x 0.90

Step Two: Perform a three-minute step test by having a client do 24 steps per minute on an 18-inch step (may need to be lowered depending on client's physical capabilities), for a total of three minutes (72 steps total). Have the client rest for one minute. Then, measure client's pulse for 30 seconds and record the number as the recovery pulse. Determine fitness level by:

$$\frac{\text{Duration of exercise (sec) x 100}}{\text{Recovery pulse x 5.6}} = \text{CV efficiency}$$

Step Three: Locate the final number in one of the following categories:

28-38	Poor
39-48	Fair
49-59	Average
60-70	Good
71-100	Very Good

Step Four: Determine the appropriate starting program using the appropriate category:

Poor	Zone One
Fair	Zone One
Average	Zone Two
Good	Zone Two
Very Good	Zone Three

Please refer to Chapter 7 (Cardiorespiratory Training) for proper utilization of these zones through specific stage training programs.

Rockport Walk Test

This test is designed to estimate a cardiovascular starting point. The starting point is then modified, based on ability level. Once determined, refer to the cardiovascular programming section of the text for specific programs.

Step One: Determine the client's maximum heart rate by subtracting the client's age from the number 220 (220 - age). Then, take the maximum heart rate and multiply it by the following figures to determine the heart rate ranges for each zone.

Zone One	Maximum Heart Rate x 0.65
	Maximum Heart Rate x 0.75
Zone Two	Maximum Heart Rate x 0.80
	Maximum Heart Rate x 0.85
Zone Three	Maximum Heart Rate x 0.86
	Maximum Heart Rate x 0.90

Step Two: First, record the client's weight. Have the client walk one mile, as fast as he/she can control on a treadmill. Record the time it takes the client to complete the walk. Immediately record the client's heart rate (beats per minute) at the one mile mark. Use the following formula to determine the VO_2 score:[62]

$$132.853$$
$$- (0.0769 \times weight)$$
$$- (0.3877 \times age)$$
$$+ (6.315 \times 1) \text{ for men or } + (6.315 \times 0) \text{ for women}$$
$$- (3.2649 \times time)$$
$$- (.1565 \times heart\ rate)$$
$$= VO_2\ score$$

Step Three: Locate the VO_2 score in one of the following categories:

Males					
Age	Poor	Fair	Average	Good	Very Good
20-24	32-37	38-43	44-50	51-56	57-62
25-29	31-35	36-32	43-48	49-53	54-59
30-34	29-34	35-40	41-45	46-51	52-56
35-39	28-32	33-38	39-43	44-48	49-54
40-44	26-31	32-35	36-41	42-46	47-51
45-49	25-29	30-34	35-39	40-43	44-48
50-54	24-27	28-32	33-36	37-41	42-46
55-59	22-26	27-30	31-34	35-39	40-43
60-65	21-24	25-28	29-32	33-36	37-40

Females					
Age	Poor	Fair	Average	Good	Very Good
20-24	27-31	32-36	37-41	42-46	47-51
25-29	26-30	31-35	36-40	41-44	45-49
30-34	25-29	30-33	34-37	38-42	43-46
35-39	24-27	28-31	32-35	36-40	41-44
40-44	22-25	26-29	30-33	34-37	38-41
45-49	21-23	24-27	28-31	32-35	36-38
50-54	19-22	23-25	26-29	30-32	33-36
55-59	18-20	21-23	24-27	28-30	31-33
60-65	16-18	19-21	22-24	25-27	28-30

Step Four: Determine the appropriate starting program using the appropriate category:

Poor	Zone One
Fair	Zone One
Average	Zone Two
Good	Zone Two
Very Good	Zone Three

Please refer to Chapter 7 (Cardiorespiratory Training) for proper utilization of these Zones through specific stage training programs.

MODULE 5-4 Summary

There are many ways to determine heart rate zones, based on cardiovascular assessments. Once the ability level is determined, special programs can be chosen. Short descriptions of the purpose of each test follows:

- **Step Test:** Estimates a cardiovascular starting point, modified by ability level.
- **Rockport Walk Test:** Also estimates a cardiovascular starting point.

MODULE 5-4 Quiz

1. How do you calculate the heart rate for Zone Two?

_____

2. A client has completed the three-minute step test and their 30-second heart rate measures 70 bpm. In what stage of cardiorespiratory training should they begin? (Use the Step Test formula provided in the course manual.)

_____

MODULE 5-5:
Posture and Movement Assessments

General Static and Movement Observation

Every movement needs a base from which to generate (and accept) force. This is better known as posture. **Posture** is the alignment and function of all components of the kinetic chain at any given moment. It is under the control of the central nervous system (Figure 5-20). [3,4,63-65]

Posture

Posture is often viewed as being static (or without movement). However, everyday posture is constantly changing to meet the demands placed upon the kinetic chain. The main purpose of proper posture is to maintain enough **structural efficiency** to overcome constant forces placed upon the body (i.e. gravity). [3,4,64,66] Structural efficiency is defined as the alignment of the musculoskeletal system, which allows our center of gravity to be maintained over a base of support.

Any deviation from proper postural alignment can cause a change in the body's center of gravity, which affects the **functional efficiency** of the kinetic chain. [3,4,63,67] Functional efficiency is defined as the ability of the neuromuscular system to monitor and manipulate movement during functional tasks using the least amount of energy, creating the least amount of stress of the kinetic chain.

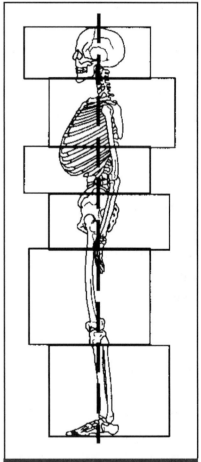

Figure 5-20: Posture

The ability to efficiently maintain balance is termed **postural equilibrium**. [3,4,68] The kinetic chain exhibits some type of posture and requires maintenance of that posture at all times. Therefore, it can be said that posture is the position from which all movement begins and ends. [69]

POSTURE:
Position and bearing of the body for alignment and function of the kinetic chain.

STRUCTURAL EFFICIENCY:
The alignment of the musculoskeletal system that allows our center of gravity to be maintained over our base of support.

FUNCTIONAL EFFICIENCY:
The ability of the neuromuscular system to monitor and manipulate movement during functional tasks using the least amount of energy, creating the least amount of stress of the kinetic chain.

POSTURAL EQUILIBRIUM:
Maintaining a state of balance in the alignment of the kinetic chain.

Importance of Posture

Proper postural alignment allows optimum **neuromuscular efficiency** (Figure 5-21).[3,4,7,9,38,63,70-73] This is particularly true with respect to the neuromuscular system. Proper posture ensures that the muscles of the body are optimally aligned at the proper length-tension relationships necessary for efficient functioning of force-couples.[3,4,9,38,63,70-72] This allows for proper joint mechanics (or arthrokinematics) and effective absorption and distribution of forces throughout the kinetic chain, alleviating excess stress on joints.[3,4,7,9,63,70-73]

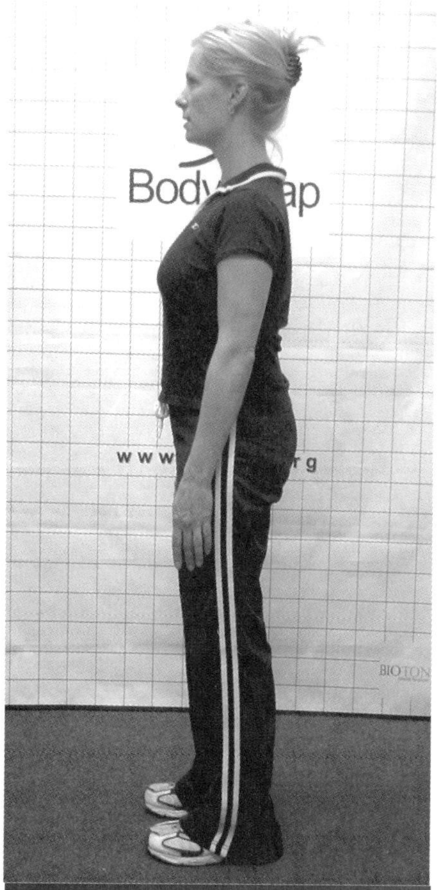

Proper postural alignment allows the kinetic chain to produce high levels of functional strength with optimal neuromuscular efficiency. **Functional strength** is the ability of the neuromuscular system to perform dynamic eccentric, isometric and con-centric muscle actions in all three planes of motion.[3,4]

Figure 5-21:
Proper Postural Alignment

NEUROMUSCULAR EFFICIENCY:
The ability of the nervous system to communicate effectively with the muscular system.

FUNCTIONAL STRENGTH:
The ability of the neuromuscular system to contract eccentrically, isometrically and concentrically in all three planes of motion.

POSTURAL DISTORTION PATTERNS:
Predictable occurrences of muscle imbalances caused by altered movement patterns.

All muscles must be activated with precise timing to work in complete synergy. Think of the muscles in the body as an orchestra. The conductor (nervous system) must bring the horn, percussion and string sections (various muscles) into the musical piece at the right time in order for the music to have a perfect melody (functional strength). The same holds true for the kinetic chain.

Without proper postural alignment, we set the body up for degeneration.[3,4,9,63,71-74] Altered movement patterns result from muscle imbalances which can place unusual stresses on the joints.[63,71] This affects other joints and muscles in the kinetic chain which can cause tissue stress throughout the body. These traumas are known as **postural distortion patterns**, which are simply predictable patterns of muscle imbalance.[3,4,7,9,63,71-74] Causes of muscle imbalances and strategies in improving these imbalances will be discussed in Chapter 6 (Flexibility Training).

How to Observe Posture

Observing Static Posture

A quick, static postural observation (done while a client is standing still) can give general structural information regarding the state of a client's muscles and joints.[74] The postural observation discussed here will be a simplified version of an ideal assessment that would be performed by a physician or physical therapist.

The brief "snapshot" looks at the client's natural appearance, much like taking a picture. The health and fitness professional should look for gross deviations in overall posture. There are five major deviations to watch for: forward head, protracted shoulders, anterior pelvic tilt, adducted and internally rotated knees and flattened feet.

These postural deviations can be grouped into three postural distortion patterns: lower-extremity, lumbo-pelvic-hip and upper-extremity.

- The lower-extremity postural distortion is characterized by flattened and externally rotated feet as well as adducted and internally rotated knees.

- The lumbo-pelvic-hip postural distortion is characterized by an anterior pelvic tilt.

- The upper-extremity postural distortion is characterized by protracted (rounded) shoulder and a forward head.

The observation itself can be performed in a couple of minutes and may be done while talking to a client or even as a client walks toward the health and fitness professional for the first workout. Table 5-6 lists each of the common postural distortions and what to look for with each.

Table 5-6: Postural Distortions and Compensations	
Postural Distortion	**Postural Compensations**
Lower-extremity postural distortion	Flat and externally rotated feet
	Adducted and internally rotated knees
Lumbo-pelvic-hip postural distortion	Anterior pelvic tilt
Upper-extremity postural distortion	Protracted shoulders
	Forward head

What to Look for When Observing Static Posture

Flattened and Externally Rotated Feet

- The feet will appear flat, or the client will say they have flat feet.

- He/she will stand/walk with their feet externally rotated.

- The inside (or medial) portion of the foot/ankle will protrude outward in the client's shoe (Figure 5-22) (Table 5-7).

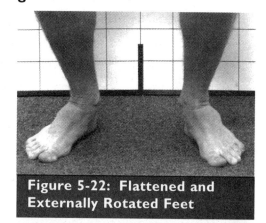

Figure 5-22: Flattened and Externally Rotated Feet

| Table 5:7: Musculature of Flattened and Externally Rotated Feet ||
Tight Musculature	Weak Musculature
Gastrocnemius	Anterior tibialis
Soleus	Posterior tibialis
Peroneals	Vastus medialis
Adductors	Gluteus medius/maximus
Iliotibial band	Hip external rotators
Psoas	
Rectus femoris	

Adducted and Internally Rotated Knees

- The knees will have a "knock-kneed" appearance where the knees converge and are not lined up over the middle of the foot (Figure 5-23) (Table 5-8).

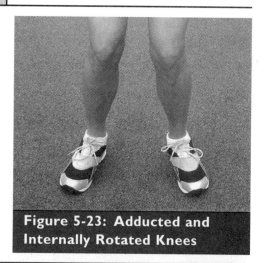

Figure 5-23: Adducted and Internally Rotated Knees

| Table 5-8: Musculature of Adducted and Internally Rotated Knees ||
Tight Musculature	Weak Musculature
Gastrocnemius	Anterior tibialis
Soleus	Posterior tibialis
Peroneals	Vastus medialis
Adductors	Gluteus medius/maximus
Iliotibial band	Hip external rotators
Psoas	
Rectus femoris	

Anterior Pelvic Tilt

- The belt line is often a good indicator. If the belt line starts higher in the back and comes down in the front, this may indicate an anterior tilt.

- A client with an anterior tilt often has fully extended or hyperextended knees (Figure 5-24) (Table 5-9).

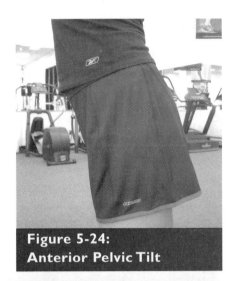

Figure 5-24:
Anterior Pelvic Tilt

Table 5-9: Musculature of Anterior Pelvic Tilt

Tight Musculature	Weak Musculature
Psoas	Gluteus medius/maximus
Rectus femoris	Bicep femoris
Adductors	Transversus abdominis
Latissimus dorsi	Internal oblique
Erector spinae	Multifidi
	Pelvic floor muscles

Protracted Shoulders

- Protracted shoulders are detectable by the roundness across the upper back and the concavity of the chest region.

- The shoulders may also appear to point in an anterior direction.

- The palm of the hand may be facing posteriorly (or away from a front view of the client) (Figure 5-25) (Table 5-10).

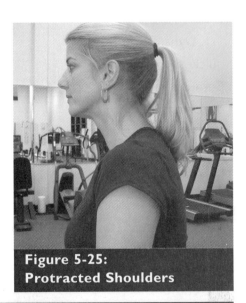

Figure 5-25:
Protracted Shoulders

Table 5-10: Musculature of Protracted Shoulders

Tight Musculature	Weak Musculature
Pectoralis major	Rhomboids
Pectoralis minor	Middle and lower trapezius
Latissimus dorsi	

Forward Head

■ A forward head sits anterior (forward) to the shoulder and often exhibit a protruding chin (Figure 5-26) (Table 5-11).

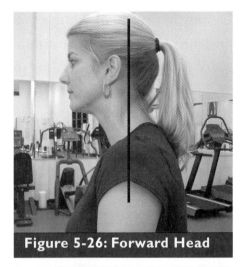

Figure 5-26: Forward Head

Table 5-11: Musculature of Forward Head	
Tight Musculature	**Weak Musculature**
Upper trapezius Levator scapulae Sternocleidomastoid	Deep cervical flexors (logus coli, longus capitus)

Chapter 6 (Flexibility Training) will provide you solutions on corrective strategies for each postural distortion.

Observing Dynamic Posture

Dynamic postural observations (looking at movements) are often the quickest way to gain an overall impression of a client's functional status. Because posture is a dynamic quality, these observations show postural distortion in its naturally dynamic setting.[3,4]

Movement observations should relate to basic functions such as squatting, pushing, pulling and balancing, in addition to providing crucial information about muscle and joint interplay. The observation process should search for any imbalances in anatomy, physiology or biomechanics that may decrease a client's results and possibly lead to injury (both in and out of the fitness environment). With the limited time that most health and fitness professionals have for observation, incorporating a systematic assessment sequence is essential. (At the end of this chapter, different assessment sequences are provided to aid in time efficiency.)

There are various assessment techniques that will be defined and described. Each assessment described also contains key kinetic chain checkpoints to observe. These assessments can also be incorporated as a first workout for your client.

Dynamic Postural Assessments

Overhead Squat Assessment

This observation is designed to assess dynamic flexibility on both sides of the body as well as integrated total body strength.

Position

1. Client stands with feet shoulder-width apart and pointed straight ahead. The foot and ankle complex should be in a neutral position.

2. Have client raise his/her arms overhead, with elbows fully extended. The upper arms should bisect the ears (Figures 5-27, 5-28 and 5-29).

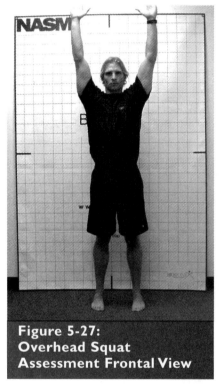

**Figure 5-27:
Overhead Squat
Assessment Frontal View**

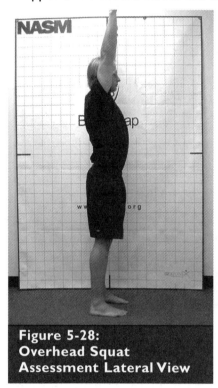

**Figure 5-28:
Overhead Squat
Assessment Lateral View**

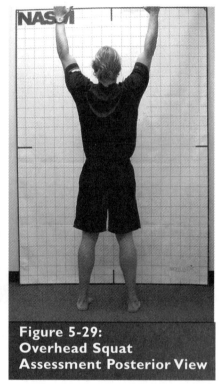

**Figure 5-29:
Overhead Squat
Assessment Posterior View**

Movement

3. Instruct client to squat to a comfortable level and return to the start position.

4. Have the client repeat the movement.

Views

5. View feet, ankles and knees from the front (Figure 5-30) (Table 5-12).

6. View the lumbo-pelvic-hip complex, shoulder and cervical complex from the side (Figure 5-31) (Table 5-12).

7. View the feet, ankles and knees, the lumbo-pelvic-hip complex and the shoulder and cervical complex from the posterior (Figure 5-32) (Table 5-12).

8. View up to five repetitions before resetting client's position.

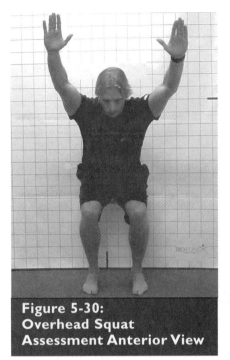

**Figure 5-30:
Overhead Squat
Assessment Anterior View**

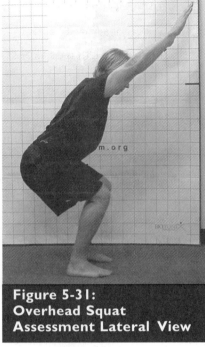

**Figure 5-31:
Overhead Squat
Assessment Lateral View**

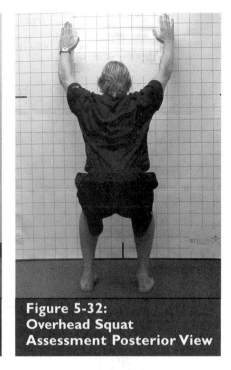

**Figure 5-32:
Overhead Squat
Assessment Posterior View**

Follow the kinetic chain checkpoints in Table 5-12 for each view. When doing an observation, record all findings, in writing.

Table 5-12: Observational Findings Overhead Squat Assessment				
View	**Kinetic Chain Checkpoints**	**Movement Observation**	**Right**	**Left**
Anterior	Feet	Turns out	☐	☐
	Knees	Moves inward	☐	☐
		Moves outward	☐	☐
Lateral	Lumbo-pelvic-hip complex	Excessive forward lean	☐	☐
		Low back arches	☐	☐
		Low back rounds	☐	☐
	Shoulder complex	Arms fall forward	☐	☐
Posterior	Feet	Heel of foot rises	☐	☐
		Foot flattens	☐	☐
	Lumbo-pelvic-hip complex	Asymmetrical weight shift	☐	☐
	Shoulder complex	Shoulder elevates	☐	☐

Single-leg Squat Assessment

The observation is designed to assess ankle proprioception, core strength and hip joint stability.

Position

1. Client should stand with hands on the hips and eyes focused on an object straight ahead.
2. Feet should be pointed straight ahead and the foot, ankle and knee and the lumbo-pelvic-hip complex should be in a neutral position (Figure 5-33).

Movement

3. Instruct client to raise one leg and place it parallel to the stance leg.
4. Have client squat to a comfortable level (Figure 5-34) and return to the start position.
5. Perform up to five repetitions before switching sides.

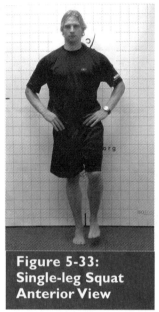

**Figure 5-33:
Single-leg Squat
Anterior View**

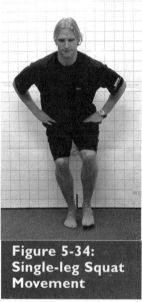

**Figure 5-34:
Single-leg Squat
Movement**

Views

6. View the foot, ankle and knee and the lumbo-pelvic-hip complex from the front.

Follow the kinetic chain checkpoints in Table 5-13. When doing an observation, record all findings, in writing.

Table 5-13: Observational Findings Single-leg Squat Assessment				
View	**Kinetic Chain Checkpoints**	**Movement Observation**	**Right**	**Left**
Anterior	Foot	Foot flattens	☐	☐
	Knee	Moves inward	☐	☐
		Moves outward	☐	☐
	Lumbo-pelvic-hip complex	Lateral hip shift	☐	☐

Pushing Assessment

Position

1. Instruct client to sit in a chest-press machine with abdomen drawn inward, feet shoulder-width apart and toes pointing forward (Figure 5-35).

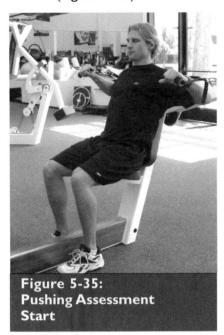

Figure 5-35:
Pushing Assessment
Start

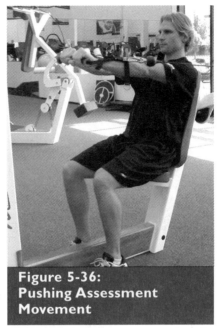

Figure 5-36:
Pushing Assessment
Movement

Movement

2. Instruct client to press handles forward and return slowly (Figure 5-36).
3. Perform up to 20 repetitions using a 2-0-2 speed (per repetition).
4. Use the checklist below to record movement faults (Table 5-14).

Table 5:14: Observational Findings Pushing Assessment			
Kinetic Chain Checkpoints	**Movement Observation**	**Right**	**Left**
Feet	Turns out	☐	☐
Knees	Moves inward	☐	☐
Lumbo-pelvic-hip complex	Low back arches	☐	☐
	Low back rounds	☐	☐
Shoulder complex	Shoulders elevate	☐	☐
Head	Head protrudes while pushing	☐	☐

Pulling Assessment

Position

1. Instruct client to sit in a rowing machine with abdomen drawn inward, feet shoulder-width apart and toes pointing forward (Figure 5-37).

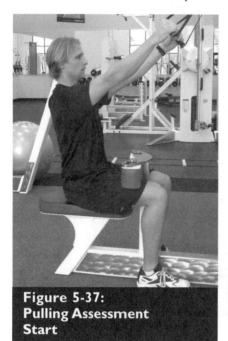

**Figure 5-37:
Pulling Assessment
Start**

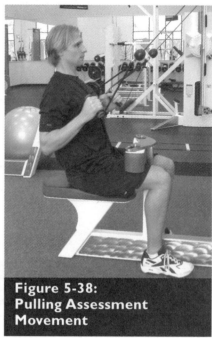

**Figure 5-38:
Pulling Assessment
Movement**

Movement:

2. Instruct client to pull handles toward their body and return slowly (Figure 5-38).
3. Perform up to 20 repetitions using a 2-0-2 speed (per repetition).
4. Use the checklist below to record movement faults (Table 5-15).

Table 5:15: Observational Findings Pulling Assessment			
Kinetic Chain Checkpoints	**Movement Observation**	**Right**	**Left**
Feet	Turns out	☐	☐
Knees	Moves inward	☐	☐
Lumbo-pelvic-hip complex	Low back arches	☐	☐
	Low back rounds	☐	☐
Shoulder complex	Shoulders elevate	☐	☐
Head	Head protrudes while pulling	☐	☐

MODULE 5-5 Summary

Posture is the alignment and function of all parts of the kinetic chain. Its main purpose is to overcome constant forces placed upon the body by maintaining structural efficiency. The kinetic chain requires constant postural equilibrium.

Proper postural alignment puts the body in a state of optimum neuromuscular efficiency allowing for proper joint mechanics and effective distribution of force throughout the kinetic chain. It lets the body produce high levels of functional strength. Without it, the body may degenerate and/or experience postural distortion patterns.

In a quick static postural observation, a health and fitness professional looks for gross deviations in overall posture, including: forward head, protracted shoulders, anterior pelvic tilt, adducted and internally rotated knees and flattened feet.

A dynamic postural observation examines basic movements and provides crucial information about how muscles and joints interact. It searches for any imbalances in anatomy, physiology or biomechanics.

There are various dynamic postural assessment techniques. Short descriptions of the purpose of each follows:

- **Overhead Squat:** Assesses dynamic flexibility and integrated total body strength.

- **Single-leg Squat:** Assesses ankle proprioception, core strength and hip joint stability.

- **Pushing:** Assesses upper extremity neuromuscular efficiency.

- **Pulling:** Assesses spinal and shoulder girdle stability.

MODULE 5-5 Quiz

1. Posture is the position from which all movement begins and ends.

   ☐ True   ☐ False

2. Proper postural alignment puts the body in a state of:

   ☐ Dynamic posture

   ☐ Optimum neuromuscular efficiency

   ☐ Uncontrolled distribution of force

3. A client with a sloping belt line and ankles that protrude inward probably has which postural deviations?

   _____

4. _____ postural observations should relate to movements such as squatting, bending, pulling, pushing and balancing.

   ☐ Static   ☐ Dynamic

5. What kind of assessment is the Single-leg Squat?

   _____

MODULE 5-6:
Performance Assessments

Performance assessments can be utilized for clients trying to improve athletic performance. These assessments will measure upper extremity stability, lower extremity agility and overall strength. Basic performance assessments include the Davies test, shark skill test, bench press strength assessment and leg press strength assessment.

Davies Test

This observation is designed to assess upper extremity agility and stabilization. This assessment may not be suitable for individuals who lack shoulder stability.

Position

1. Placing two pieces of tape on the floor, 36 inches apart.
2. Have client assume a push-up position, with one hand on each piece of tape (Figure 5-39).

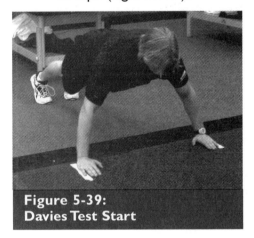

**Figure 5-39:
Davies Test Start**

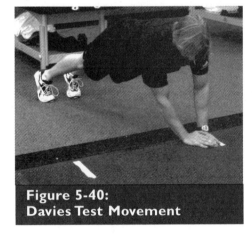

**Figure 5-40:
Davies Test Movement**

Movement

3. Instruct client to quickly move his/her right hand to touch the left hand (Figure 5-40).
4. Perform alternating touching on each side for 15 seconds.
5. Repeat for three trials.

Record the number of lines touched by both hands in Table 5-16.

Table 5-16: Observational Findings Davies Assessment			
Trial Number	**Distance of Points**	**Time**	**Repetitions Performed**
One	36 inches	15 sec.	
Two	36 inches	15 sec.	
Three	36 inches	15 sec.	

Shark Skill Test

The observation is designed to assess lower extremity agility and neuromuscular control. It should be viewed as a progression from the Single-leg Squat and, as such, may not be suitable for all individuals.

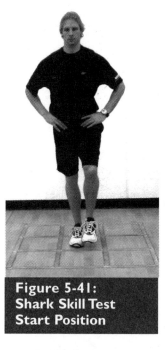

Figure 5-41:
Shark Skill Test
Start Position

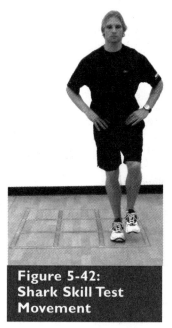

Figure 5-42:
Shark Skill Test
Movement

Position

1. Position client in the center box of a grid, with hands on hips and standing on one leg (Figure 5-41).

Movement

2. Instruct client to hop to each box in a designated pattern, always returning to the center box (Figure 5-42). Be consistent with the patterns.

3. Perform one practice run through the boxes with each foot.
4. Perform test twice with each foot (four times total). Keep track of time.
5. Record the times in Table 5-17.
6. Deduct 0.10 seconds for each of the following faults:
    i.   Non-hopping leg touches ground
    ii. Hands come off hips
    iii. Foot goes into wrong square
    iv. Foot does not return to center square

Record observations in Table 5-17.

Table 5-17: Observational Findings Shark Skill Test					
Trial	**Side**	**Time** (Seconds)	**Deduction Tally**	**Total Deducted** (# of faults x 0.1)	**Final Total** (Time - Total Deduction)
Practice	Right				
	Left				
One	Right				
	Left				
Two	Right				
	Left				

Bench Press Strength Assessment

This observation is designed to estimate the one-rep maximum, for training intensity purposes. This is considered an advanced assessment (for strength specific goals) and, as such, may not be suitable for many clients.

Position

1. Position client on a bench, lying on his/her back. Feet should be pointed straight ahead. The low back should be in a neutral position (Figure 5-43).

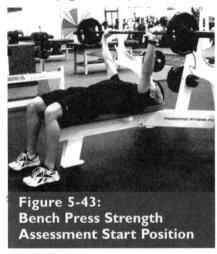

Figure 5-43: Bench Press Strength Assessment Start Position

Movement

2. Instruct the client to warm-up with a light resistance that can be easily performed 8-10 repetitions.
3. Take a one-minute rest.
4. Add 10-20 pounds (five to 10 percent of body weight) and perform 3-5 repetitions.
5. Take a two-minute rest
6. Repeat steps 4 and 5 until the individual fails at 3-5 repetitions
7. Calculate one-rep maximum (1RM) using estimation chart in the appendix.

Leg Press Strength Assessment

This observation is designed to estimate the one-rep leg press maximum, for training intensity purposes. This is considered an advanced assessment (for strength specific goals) and, as such, may not be suitable for many clients.

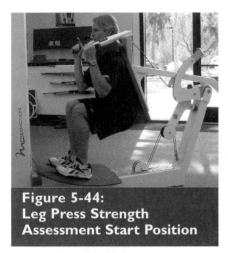

Figure 5-44: Leg Press Strength Assessment Start Position

Position

1. Position client in the leg press machine, lying on his/her back. Feet should be pointed straight ahead and knees in line with the toes. The low back should be in a neutral position (Figure 5-44).

Movement:

2. Instruct the client to warm up with a light resistance that can be easily performed 8-10 repetitions.
3. Take a one-minute rest.
4. Add 30-40 pounds (10 to 20 percent of body weight) and perform 3-5 repetitions.
5. Take a two-minute rest.
6. Repeat steps 4 and 5 until the individual fails at 3-5 repetitions
7. Calculate one-rep maximum (1RM) using estimation chart in the appendix.

MODULE 5-6 Summary

Performance assessments can be incorporated into the assessment process for clients looking to improve athletic performance. Short descriptions of the purpose of each test follows:

- **Davies:** Assesses upper extremity stability and agility
- **Shark Skill:** Assesses overall athletic ability (single-leg squat assessment progression).
- **Bench Press Strength:** Advanced assessment that estimates one-rep maximum and upper extremity strength.
- **Leg Press Strength:** Advanced assessment that estimates one-rep maximum and lower extremity strength

MODULE 5-6 Quiz

1. Which assessment tests a one-rep maximum?

   ☐ Single-leg Squat

   ☐ Davies Test

   ☐ Bench Press Strength Assessment

2. In which assessment does a client hop in a box grid?

   ☐ Single-leg Squat

   ☐ Davies Test

   ☐ Shark Skill

3. How many trials should be performed in the Davies Test?

   _____

MODULE 5-7:
Implementing the Fitness Assessment

Assessment Parameters

The fitness assessment builds the foundation for the entire template. It enables the health and fitness professional to decide the appropriate selection of flexibility, cardiorespiratory, core, balance, power and strength training exercises. Specifically, the integrated fitness assessment allows the health and fitness professional to fill in the first section of the template seen in Figure 5-45. Listed below are several example clients, along with the pertinent subjective information that would have been obtained in their first session. From this information, it will also list the appropriate objective assessments that a health and fitness professional would want to include, in order to ensure that the program is individualized to these clients' specific goals and needs.

Client 1: Lita

General Information

Age:	38
Occupation:	Secretary. She spends a lot of time sitting behind a computer and on the phone. Lita is required to wear business attire.
Lifestyle:	Has two children (ages 6 and 9). Enjoys hiking, gardening and playing sports with her kids.
Medical history:	Has had low back pain in the past (approximately 2 months ago), but does not currently experience any pain. She also, at times, experiences a feeling of "tension" through her neck when working on the computer. Lita had a C-section with her second child. She is in good overall health and is not taking any medications.
Goals:	Decrease body fat and "tone up." Become less "tense" in order to be able to continue her recreational activities and be simply "overall healthy."

Recommended Objective Assessments for Lita

- Body fat measurement
- Circumference measurement
- Resting heart rate
- Blood pressure
- Step Test or Rockport Walk Test
- Overhead Squat
- Single-leg Squat or Single-leg Balance
- Pushing Assessment (time permitting)
- Pulling Assessment (time permitting)

Client 2: Ron

General Information

Age: 72

Occupation: Retired business executive

Lifestyle: Enjoys traveling, enjoys long walks with his wife, golf, carpentry, and playing with his 7 grandkids.

Medical history: Had a triple bypass surgery (10 years ago). Takes medication for high cholesterol. Has lower back and shoulder pain after he plays golf.

Goals: Ron is 170 lbs. and is not concerned with altering his body composition. He wants to be healthy, increase some overall strength and decrease his back and shoulder pain to play golf and with his grandkids more easily.

Recommended Objective Assessments for Ron

- Obtain a medical release from Ron's physician
- Resting heart rate
- Blood pressure
- Three Minute Step Test or Rockport Walk Test

- Overhead Squat
- Single-leg Balance
- Pushing Assessment (time permitting)
- Pulling Assessment (time permitting)

Client 3: Brian

General Information

Age:	24
Occupation:	Semi-professional soccer player
Lifestyle:	He travels often, competing in various soccer tournaments. He likes to work out with weights 3-4 times per week, practices five days per week and plays in an organized game at least 2 times a week.
Medical history:	Had surgery for a torn ACL in his left knee 3 years ago and has sprained his left ankle twice since his knee surgery. Went through physical therapy for his last ankle sprain 6 months ago and was cleared to work out and play again. For the most part, his knee and ankle have not been giving him any trouble, other than some occasional soreness after games and practice. He has recently gone through a physical to begin playing again and his physician gave him a clean bill of health.
Goals:	He wants to increase his overall performance by enhancing his flexibility, speed, cardiorespiratory efficiency and leg strength. He also wants to decrease his risk of incurring other injuries. After being out of soccer due to the injury, he increased his body fat percentage and would like to lower it.

Recommended Objective Assessments for Brian

- Body fat measurement
- Three Minute Step Test or Rockport Walk Test
- Overhead Squat

- Single-leg Squat
- Davies Test
- Shark Skill Test
- Leg Press Strength Assessment

Filling in the Template

Fill in the assessment portion of the template, according to the example in Figure 5-45. The name should obviously be filled in, in order to keep proper records of the correct client. The date is necessary in order to follow a client's progression over time and keep track of what workouts occurred on what dates.

The phase signifies where in the OPT™ model the client is. This can also act as a reminder about the acute variables significant to this phase. (This will be discussed in detail later in the text.)

NASM   NATIONAL ACADEMY OF SPORTS MEDICINE

Optimum Performance Training

NAME	John Smith	DATE	March 10, 2004
TRAINER	Chere	PHASE	2: Integrated Stabilization Training
DAYS/WEEK	3	GOAL	Fat loss

CARDIO TRAINING	TIME	EQUIPMENT

WARM-UP/FLEXIBILITY	Sets	Reps	Duration	Rest	Notes
1.					
2.					
3.					
4.					

CORE and BALANCE	Sets	Reps	Tempo	Rest	Notes
1.					
2.					
3.					
4.					
5.					

REACTIVE	Sets	Reps	Tempo	Rest	Notes
1.					
2.					

SPEED, AGILITY, QUICKNESS	Sets	Reps	Tempo	Rest	Notes
1.					
2.					

STRENGTH	Exercises	Sets	Reps	Intensity	Tempo	Rest	Notes
TOTAL BODY							
CHEST							
BACK							
SHOULDERS							
BICEPS							
TRICEPS							
LEGS							

COOL-DOWN	
POST-WORKOUT FLEXIBILITY	

Figure 5-45: OPT™ Template

References

1. American College of Sports Medicine. *ACSM's guidelines for exercise testing and prescription.* 5th edition. Philadelphia: Williams & Wilkins; 1995.

2. Thomas S, Reading J, Shephard RJ. Revision of the physical activity readiness questionnaire (PAR-Q). *Can J Sports Sci* 1992;17:338-45.

3. Clark MA. *Integrated training for the new millennium.* Thousand Oaks, CA: National Academy of Sports Medicine; 2001.

4. Clark MA. *Integrated kinetic chain assessment.* Thousand Oaks, CA: National Academy of Sports Medicine; 2001.

5. Clark MA. *An integrated approach to human movement science.* Thousand Oaks, CA: National Academy of Sports Medicine; 2001.

6. Bachrach RM. The relationship of low back pain to psoas insufficiency. *J Ortho Med* 1991;13:34-40.

7. Janda V. In: Grant R (ed). *Physical therapy of the cervical and thoracic spine.* Edinburgh: Churchill Livingstone; 1988.

8. Leahy PM. Active release techniques: logical soft tissue treatment. Ch 17. In: Hammer WI (ed). *Functional soft tissue examination and treatment by manual methods.* Gaithersburg, MD: Aspen Publishers, Inc.; 1999.

9. Lewitt K. *Manipulation in rehabilitation of the locomotor system.* London: Butterworths; 1993.

10. Chaitow L. *Cranial manipulation theory and practice: osseous and soft tissue approaches.* London: Churchill Livingstone; 1999.

11. Timmons B. *Behavioral and psychological approaches to breathing disorders.* New York: Plenum Press; 1994.

12. Bullock-Saxton JE. Local sensation changes and altered hip muscle function following severe ankle sprain. *Phys Ther* 1994;74(1):17-23.

13. Freeman MAR, Wyke B. Articular reflexes at the ankle joint: an EMG study of normal and abnormal influences of ankle joint mechanoreceptors upon reflex activity in the leg muscles. *Br J Surg* 1967;54:990-1001.

14. Cornwall M, Murrell P. Postural sway following inversion sprain of the ankle. *J Am Pod Med Assoc* 1991;81:243-7.

15. Feurbach JW, Grabiner MD. Effect of the aircast on unilateral postural control: amplitude and frequency variables. *JOSPT* 1993;7:149-54.

16. Forkin DM, Koczur C, Battle R, Newton RA. Evaluation of kinesthetic deficits indicative of balance control in gymnasts with unilateral chronic ankle sprains. *JOSPT* 1996;23(4):245-50.

17. Freeman MAR, Dean MRE, Hanham IWF. The etiology and prevention of functional instability of the foot. *J Bone Joint Surg* 1965;47B:678-85.

18. Freeman MAR, Wyke B. Articular contributions to limb muscle reflexes. *Br J Surg* 1966;53:61-9.

19. Guskiewicz KM, Perrin DM. Effect of orthotics on postural sway following inversion ankle sprain. *JOSPT* 1996;23(5):326-31.

20. Nitz AJ, Dobner JJ, Kersey D. Nerve injury and grades II and III ankle sprains. *Am J Sports Med* 1985;13:177-82.

21. Wilkerson GB, Nitz AJ. Dynamic ankle stability: Mechanical and neuromuscular interrelationships. *J Sport Rehabil* 1994;3:43-57.

22. Barrack RL, Lund PJ, Skinner HB. Knee proprioception revisited. *J Sport Rehab* 1994;3:18-42.

23. Beard DJ, Kyberd PJ, O'Connor JJ, Fergusson CM. Reflex hamstring contraction latency in ACL deficiency. *J Ortho Res* 1994;12(2):219-28.

24. Boyd IA. The histological structure of the receptors in the knee joint of the cat correlated with their physiological response. *J Physiol* 1954;124:476-88.

25. Ciccotti MG, Perry J, Kerian RK, Pink M. An EMG analysis of the normal, the rehabilitated ACL deficient, and the ACL reconstructed patient during functional activities. Abstract presented at AOSSM Society's Specialty Day Meeting, San Fransisco, CA: 1993.

26. Corrigan JP, Cashman WF, Brady MP. Proprioception in the cruciate deficient knee. *J Bone Joint Surg* 1992;74B:247-50.

27. DeCarlo M, Klootwyk T, Shelbourne K. ACL surgery and accelerated rehabilitation. *J Sports Rehabil* 1997 6(2):144-56.

28. Ekholm J, Eklund G, Skoglund S. On the reflex effects from knee joint of the cat. *Acta Physiol Scand* 1960;50:167-74.

29. Feagin JA. The syndrome of a torn ACL. *Orthop Clin North Am* 1979;10:81-90.

30. Irrgang J, Whitney S, Cox E. Balance and proprioceptive training for rehabilitation of the lower extremity. *J Sport Rehabil* 1994;3:68-83.

31. Irrgang J, Harner C. Recent advances in ACL rehabilitation: clinical factors. *J Sport Rehab* 1997;6(2):111-24.

32. Johansson H, Sjolander P. Receptors in the knee joint ligaments and their role in the biomechanics of the joint. *CriticRev Biomed Engineer* 1988;18(5):341-68.

33. Johansson H. Role of knee ligaments in proprioception and regulation of muscle stiffness. *J Electomyogr Kinesiol* 1991;1(3):158-79.

34. Johansson H, Sjolander P, Sojka P. A sensory role for the cruciate ligaments. *Clin Orthop* 1991;268:161-78.

35. Noyes F, Barber S, Mangine R. Abnormal lower limb symmetry determined by functional hop test after ACL rupture. *Am J Sports Med* 1991;19(5):516-8.

36. Raunst J, Sager M, Burgner E. Proprioceptive mechanisms in the cruciate ligaments: An EMG study on reflex activity in thigh muscles. *J Traum Inj Infec Critic Car* 1996;41(3):488-93.

37. Solomonow M, Barratta R, Zhou BH. The synergistic action of the ACL and thigh muscles in maintaining joint stability. *Am J Sports Med* 1987;15:207-13.

38. Janda V. Muscle weakness and inhibition in back pain syndromes. In: Grieve GP (ed). *Modern manual therapy of the vertebral column.* New York: Churchill Livingstone; 1986.

39. Lewit K. Muscular and articular factors in movement restriction. *Man Med* 1985;1:83-5.

40. Hodges PW, Richardson CA. Neuromotor dysfunction of the trunk musculature in low back pain patients. In: Proceedings of the International Congress of the World Confederation of Physical Therapists. Washington, DC: 1995.

41. Hodges PW, Richardson CA. Inefficient muscular stabilization of the lumbar spine associated with low back pain. *Spine* 1996;21(22):2640-50.

42. Bullock-Saxton JE, Janda V, Bullock M. Reflex activation of gluteal muscles in walking: an approach to restoration of muscle function for patients with low back pain. *Spine* 1993;18(6):704-8.

43. Hodges PW, Richardson CA. Contraction of the abdominal muscles associated with movement of the lower limb. *Phys Ther* 1997;77:132-14.

44. Hodges PW, Richardson CA, Jull G. Evaluation of the relationship between laboratory and clinical tests of transverse abdominus function. *Physiother Res Int* 1996;1:30-40.

45. Richardson CA, Jull G, Toppenberg R, Comerford M. Techniques for active lumbar stabilization for spinal protection. *Aus J Physiother* 1992;38:105-12.

46. O'Sullivan PE, Twomey L, Allison G, Sinclair J, Miller K, Knox J. Altered patterns of abdominal muscle activation in patients with chronic low back pain. *Aus J Physiother* 1997;43(2):91-8.

47. Jull G, Richardson CA, Comerford M. Strategies for the initial activation of dynamic lumbar stabilization. Proceedings of manipulative physiotherapists association of australia. New South Wales; 1991.

48. Jull G, Richardson CA, Hamilton C, Hodges PW, Ng J. Towards the validation of a clinical test for the deep abdominal muscles in back pain patients. Manipulative Physiotherapists Association of Australia. Gold Coast, Queensland; 1995.

49. Glousman R, Jobe F, Tibone JE, Moynes D, Antonelli D, Perry J. Dynamic electromyographic analysis of the throwing shoulder with glenohumeral instability. *J Bone Joint Surg* 1988;70(2):220-6.

50. Broström L-Å, Kronberg M, Nemeth G. Muscle activity during shoulder dislocation. *Acta Orthop Scand* 1989;60:639-41.

51. Howell SM, Kraft TA. The role of the supraspinatus and infraspinatus muscles in glenohumeral kinematics of anterior shoulder instability. *Clin Orthop* 1991;263:128-34.

52. Kronberg M, Broström L-Å, Nemeth G. Differences in shoulder muscle activity between patients with generalized joint laxity and normal controls. *Clin Orthop* 1991;269:181-92.

53. Glousman R. Electromyographic analysis and its role in the athletic shoulder. *Clin Orthop* 1993;288:27-34.

54. Mense S, Simons DG. *Muscle pain. Understanding its nature, diagnosis, and treatment.* Philadelphia: Lippincott Williams & Wilkins; 2001.

55. Trott PH, Grant R. Manipulative physical therapy in the management of selected low lumbar syndromes. In: Twomey LT, Taylor JR (eds). *Physical therapy of the low back*. 3rd edition. New York: Churchill Livingstone; 2000.

56. Whaley MA, Kaminsky LA. Epidemiology of physical activity, physical fitness, and selected chronic diseases. Ch 2. In: American College of Sports Medicine (ed). *ACSM's resource manual for guidelines for exercise testing and prescription.* 3rd edition. Baltimore, MD: Williams & Wilkins; 1998.

57. Prate RR, Pratt MM, Blair SN, Haskell WL, Macera CA, Bouchard C, Buchner D, Ettinger W, Heath GW, King AC. Physical activity and public health: a recommendation from the centers for disease control and prevention and the american college of sports medicine. *JAMA* 1995;273:402-7.

58. Lambert EV, Bohlmann I, Cowling K. Physical activity for health: understanding the epidemiological evidence for risk benefits. *Int Sport Med J* 2001;1(5):1-15.

59. American College of Sports Medicine. *ACSM's resource manual for guidelines for exercise testing and prescription.* 3rd edition. Baltimore, MD: Williams & Wilkins; 1998.

60. Durnin JVGA, Womersley J. Body fat assessed from total body density and its estimation from skinfold thickness measurements on 481 men and women aged 16-72 years. *Br J Nutr* 1974;32:77-97.

61. Ehrman JK, Gordon PM, Visich PS, Keteyian SJ. *Clinical exercise physiology.* Champaign, IL: Human Kinetics; 2003.

62. McArdle WD, Katch FI, Katch VL. *Exercise physiology: energy, nutrition and human performance.* Philadelphia: Williams & Wilkins; 1996.

63. Kendall FP, McCreary EK, Provance PG. *Muscles testing and function.* 4th edition. Baltimore, MA: Lippincott Williams & Wilkins; 1993.

64. Norkin CC, Levangie PK. *Joint structure and function.* 2nd edition. Philadelphia, PA: F.A. Davis Company; 1992.

65. Soderberg GL. *Kinesiology.* 2nd edition. Baltimore, MD: Williams & Wilkins; 1997.

66. Rash PJ, Burke RK. *Kinesiology and applied anatomy.* Philadelphia; Lea & Febiger; 1971.

67. Gross J, Fetto J, Rosen E. *Musculoskeletal examination.* Malden, MA: Blackwell Sciences, Inc.; 1996.

68. Hansen PD, Woollacott MH, Debu B. Postural responses to changing task conditions. *Ex Brain Res* 1988;73:627-36.

69. Dietz V. Human neuronal control of automatic functional movements: interactions between central programs and afferent input. *Physiol Rev* 1992;72:33-69.

70. Liebension C. Integrating rehabilitation into chiropractic practice (blending active and passive care). Chapter 2. In: Liebenson C (ed). *Rehabilitation of the spine.* Baltimore: Williams & Wilkins; 1996.

71. Janda V. Muscle strength in relation to muscle length, pain and muscle imbalance. In: Harms-Rindahl K (ed). *Muscle strength.* New York: Churchill Livingstone; 1993.

72. Janda V. On the concept of postural muscles and posture in man. *Aus J Physiother* 1983;29(3):83-4.

73. Spring H, Illi U, Kunz H, Rothlin K, Schneider W, Tritschler T. *Stretching and strengthening exercises.* New York: Theime Medicals Publishers, Inc.; 1991.

74. Sarhmann S. Posture and muscle imbalance: Faulty lumbopelvic alignment and associated musculoskeletal pain syndromes. *Orthop Div Rev Can Phys Ther* 1992;12:13-20.

Flexibility Training Concepts

Objectives

After studying this chapter, you will be able to:

- Explain the effects of muscle imbalances on the kinetic chain.
- Provide a scientific rationale for the use of an integrated flexibility-training program.
- Differentiate between the types of flexibility techniques.
- Perform and instruct appropriate flexibility techniques for given situations.

Key Terms

- Flexibility
- Extensibility
- Dynamic range of motion
- Neuromuscular efficiency
- Dynamic functional flexibility
- Integrated flexibility training
- Postural distortion patterns
- Homeostasis
- Equilibrium
- Adaptive
- Relative flexibility

- Muscle imbalance
- Length-tension relationship
- Synergistic dominance
- Arthrokinetic dysfunction
- Neuromuscular efficiency
- Pattern overload
- Self-myofascial release
- Static stretch
- Active stretch
- Dynamic stretch

Introduction to Flexibility Training

With the completion of the assessment section, all pertinent information needed to fill out the remainder of the programming template has been gathered. The focus can now be shifted toward designing the program. The next portion of the Optimum Performance Training (OPT™) programming template that needs to be filled out is the warm-up section. In designing the warm-up program, the components of flexibility and cardiorespiratory training need to be reviewed. Most clients require flexibility training to properly perform any type of cardiorespiratory work, so that is a good place to start.

MODULE 6-1:
Current Concepts in Flexibility Training

Why is Flexibility Training Important?

Today's society is plagued by postural imbalances, primarily due to sedentary lifestyles caused by advancements in technology. More people today are spending time in office-related jobs, which require individuals to sit for long hours. More than ever before, flexibility training has become a key component in developing neuromuscular efficiency and decreasing these dysfunctions. Flexibility training may decrease the occurrences of muscle imbalances, joint dysfunctions and overuse injuries. Without optimum levels of flexibility, it may not be possible for clients to achieve their goals without getting injured.[1-6] It is critical for fitness professionals to learn about flexibility training to properly design an integrated training program.[1-5]

What is Flexibility?

Flexibility is the normal **extensibility** of all soft tissues that allow the full range of motion of a joint.[1] However, in order for soft tissue to achieve efficient extensibility, there must be optimum control throughout the entire range of motion.[4,7,8] More specifically, this optimum control can be referred to as **dynamic range of motion**. This is the combination of flexibility and the nervous system's ability to control this range of motion efficiently (or neuromuscular efficiency).

Neuromuscular efficiency is the ability of the nervous system to properly recruit the correct muscles (agonists, antagonists, synergists and stabilizers) to produce force (concentrically), reduce force (eccentrically) and dynamically stabilize (isometrically) the body's structure in all three planes of motion.[4,5]

For example when performing a lat pulldown, the latissimus dorsi (agonist) must be able to concentrically accelerate shoulder extension, adduction and internal rotation while the middle and lower trapezius and rhomboids (synergists) perform downward rotation of the scapulae. At the same time, the rotator cuff musculature (stabilizers) must dynamically stabilize the glenohumeral joint throughout the motion. If these muscles (force-couples) do not work in tandem efficiently, compensations may ensue, leading to muscle imbalances, altered joint motion and possible injury.

To allow for optimal neuromuscular efficiency, individuals must have proper flexibility in all three planes of motion. This allows for the movement needed to perform everyday activities effectively, such as bending over to tie shoes or reaching in the top cupboard for dishes (Table 6-1).[4,5]

FLEXIBILITY:
The normal extensibility of all soft tissues that allow the full range of motion of a joint.

EXTENSIBILITY:
Capability to be elongated or stretched.

DYNAMIC RANGE OF MOTION:
Controlled, accurate movement that utilizes flexibility and neuromuscular efficiency.

NEUROMUSCULAR EFFICIENCY:
The ability of the neuromuscular system to allow agonists, antagonists and stabilizers to work synergistically to produce, reduce and dynamically stabilize the entire kinetic chain in all three planes of motion.

Table 6-1: Multiplanar Flexibility		
Muscle	**Plane of Motion**	**Produces proper:**
Latissimus dorsi	Sagittal	Must have proper extensibility to allow for proper shoulder flexion
	Frontal	Must have proper extensibility to allow for proper shoulder abduction
	Transverse	Must have proper extensibility to allow for proper external humerus rotation
Biceps femoris	Sagittal	Must have proper extensibility to allow for proper hip flexion; knee extension
	Frontal	Must have proper extensibility to allow for proper hip adduction
	Transverse	Must have proper extensibility to allow for proper hip and knee internal rotation
Gastrocnemius	Sagittal	Must have proper extensibility to allow for proper dorsiflexion of ankle
	Frontal	Must have proper extensibility to allow for proper inversion of calcaneus
	Transverse	Must have proper extensibility to allow for proper internal rotation of femur

In review, flexibility requires extensibility, which requires dynamic range of motion, which requires neuromuscular efficiency. This entire chain is referred to as **dynamic functional flexibility** and is achieved by taking an integrated approach toward flexibility training.[4,5]

Flexibility training must be a multifaceted approach, which integrates various flexibility techniques in order to achieve optimum soft tissue extensibility in all planes of motion (Table 6-1).

To better understand integrated flexibility, a few important concepts must first be reviewed. These include the kinetic chain, muscle imbalances and neuromuscular control (efficiency).

Review of the Kinetic Chain

The kinetic chain is comprised of the muscular, skeletal and nervous systems. Optimum alignment and function of each component of the kinetic chain is the cornerstone of a sound training program. If one segment of the kinetic chain is misaligned and not functioning properly, predictable patterns of dysfunction develop.[4,5,7-11] These predictable patterns of dysfunction are referred to as **postural distortion patterns** and lead to decreased neuromuscular efficiency and tissue overload (Figure 6-1).[4-5,7]

DYNAMIC FUNCTIONAL FLEXIBILITY:
Multiplanar soft tissue extensibility with optimal neuromuscular efficiency throughout the full range of motion.

FLEXIBILITY TRAINING:
Physical training of the body that integrates various stretches in all three planes of motion in order to produce the maximum extensibility of tissues.

POSTURAL DISTORTION PATTERNS:
Predictable patterns of muscle imbalances.

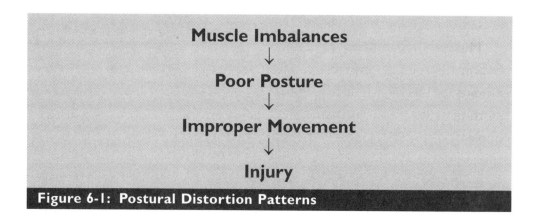

Figure 6-1: Postural Distortion Patterns

Postural distortion patterns are represented by a lack of structural integrity, resulting from decreased functioning of one (or more) components of the kinetic chain.[4,7-10] This lack of structural integrity comes in the form of altered length-tension relationships, force-couple relationships and arthrokinematics. There are several postural distortions about which the fitness professional must be aware including upper-extremity postural distortion, lumbo-pelvic-hip complex distortion and lower-extremity postural distortion, all of which are reviewed in Chapter 5.

Maximum neuromuscular efficiency of the kinetic chain can only exist if all kinetic chain components (muscular, skeletal and neural) function optimally and interdependently. The ultimate goal of the kinetic chain is to maintain **homeostasis** (or dynamic postural equilibrium).

Poor flexibility may lead to the development of **relative flexibility**, which is the process where the kinetic chain seeks the path of least resistance, during functional movement patterns.[4,8,12] A prime example of relative flexibility is seen in people who squat with their feet externally rotated (Figure 6-2). As most people today have tightness in their calf muscles, they lack the proper amount of dorsiflexion at the ankle to perform a squat with proper mechanics. By widening their stance and externally rotating their feet, they are able to decrease the amount of dorsiflexion required at the ankle to squat and, thus, compensate for this lack of flexibility. A second example is seen when people perform an overhead shoulder press with excessive lumbar extension (Figure 6-3). Individuals who possess a tight latissimus dorsi will have decreased sagittal-plane shoulder flexion. As a result, they must compensate for this lack of range of motion at the shoulder in the lumbar spine to allow for them to press the load completely above their head.

HOMEOSTASIS:
The ability or tendency of an organism or a cell to maintain internal equilibrium by adjusting its physiological processes.

RELATIVE FLEXIBILITY:
The tendency of the body to seek the path of least resistance during functional movement patterns.

Muscle Imbalance

Muscle imbalances caused by abnormal structural and functional efficiency of the kinetic chain (altered length-tension relationships, force-couple relationships and arthrokinematics) are alterations in the lengths of muscles surrounding a given joint, where some are shortened or tight and others may be lengthened, weakened and/or inhibited.[4,5,7,10] Examples of such imbalances come in the forms of the postural distortion patterns (discussed in Chapter 5): lower-extremity postural distortion, lumbo-pelvic-hip postural distortion and upper-extremity postural distortion.

Muscle imbalance can be caused by a variety of mechanisms.[1,4,5,8,12] These causes may include:

- Postural stress
- Emotional duress
- Repetitive movement
- Cumulative trauma
- Poor training technique
- Lack of core strength
- Lack of neuromuscular control (efficiency)

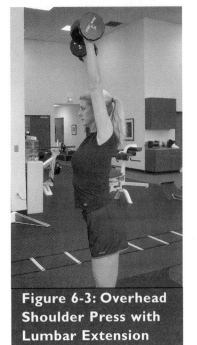

Figure 6-2: Squat with Externally Rotated Feet

Figure 6-3: Overhead Shoulder Press with Lumbar Extension

Muscle imbalances result from altered reciprocal inhibition, synergistic dominance, arthrokinetic dysfunction and overall decreased neuromuscular control. These concepts are reviewed below.

Altered Reciprocal Inhibition

Altered reciprocal inhibition is the concept of muscle inhibition caused by a tight agonist, which decreases neural drive of its functional antagonist.[1,4,7-10,13-19] For example, a tight psoas (hip flexor) would decrease neural drive the gluteus maximus (hip extensor). This results in muscle imbalances, which alter length-tension relationships and force-couple relationships, produce synergistic dominance and lead to the development of faulty movement patterns, poor neuromuscular control and arthrokinetic dysfunction.[4,5]

Synergistic Dominance

Synergistic dominance is the neuromuscular phenomenon that occurs when synergists take over function for a weak or inhibited prime mover (Table 6-2).[4,5,8,10] Think of this as your body's substitution system. When the starting player on a sports team gets tired, the coach puts in the backup player. The backup player can perform the tasks necessary to play, but not quite as well as the starter. The nervous system reacts in the same manner. For example, when the psoas is tight, it leads to reciprocal inhibition of the gluteus maximus. The result is increased force output of the synergists for hip extension (hamstrings, adductor magnus and erector spinae) to compensate for the weakened gluteus maximus. This causes faulty movement patterns, leading to arthrokinetic (joint) dysfunction and altered force-couple relationships, decreasing neuromuscular efficiency and eventually leading to injury.[4,5]

Table 6-2: Common Movement Compensations	
Body Region	**Common Movement Compensations**
Foot and ankle complex	Feet flatten Feet externally rotate
Knees	Adduct (buckle in) Abduct (bow out)
Lumbo-pelvic-hip complex	Increased lumbar extension Increased lumbar flexion
Shoulder complex	Shoulders round Shoulders elevate
Cervical spine	Head protrudes

Arthrokinetic Dysfunction

The term **arthrokinematics** refers to the motion of the joints. **Arthrokinetic dysfunction** is a biomechanical and neuromuscular dysfunction leading to altered joint motion.[4,5,7-11] Altered joint motion causes altered length-tension relationships and force-couple relationships. This affects the joint and causes poor movement efficiency. For example, externally rotating the feet when squatting forces the tibia and femur to also externally rotate. This alters length-tension relationships of the muscles at the knee and hips, putting the gluteus maximus (agonist) in a shortened position and decreasing its ability to generate force. This causes the bicep femoris and piriformis (synergists) to become synergistically dominant, altering force-couple relationships (recruitment patterns), altering arthrokinematics (joint motion) and increasing stress to the knees and low back.[4,20] Over time, this stress can lead to pain which can further alter muscle recruitment and joint mechanics.[4,5,7-10]

Neuromuscular Efficiency

As mentioned earlier, **neuromuscular efficiency** is the ability of the neuromuscular system to properly recruit muscles to produce force (concentrically), reduce force (eccentrically) and dynamically stabilize (isometrically) the entire kinetic chain in all three planes of motion.[4,5] Because the nervous system is the controlling factor behind this principle, it is important to mention that *mechanoreceptors* (or sensory receptors) located in the muscles and tendons help to determine muscle balance or imbalance. These mechanoreceptors include the muscle spindles and Golgi tendon organ.

Muscle Spindles

As mentioned in Chapter 2, muscle spindles are the major sensory organ of the muscle and are composed of microscopic fibers that lie parallel to the muscle fiber (Figure 6-4). Remember that muscle spindles are sensitive to

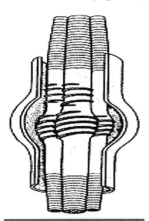

change in length and rate of length change.[5,7,21-28] When a muscle on one side of a joint is lengthened (due to a shortened muscle on the other side), the spindles of the lengthened muscle are stretched. This information is transmitted to the brain and spinal cord, exciting the muscle spindle, causing the muscle fibers to contract. This often results in muscle spasms or a feeling of tightness.[1,4,7,9]

The hamstring, in a lumbo-pelvic-hip postural distortion, is a prime example of this response, where the pelvis is rotated anteriorly (forward) (Figure 6-5).

**Figure 6-4:
Muscle Spindles**

This means that the anterior superior iliac spines (front of the pelvis) move downward (inferiorly) and the ischium (bottom posterior portion of pelvis, where the hamstrings originate) moves upward (superiorly). If the attachment of the hamstrings is moved superiorly, it increases the distance between the two attachment sites and lengthens the muscle. In this case, the hamstrings do not need to be statically stretched because they are already in a stretched position. When a lengthened muscle is stretched, it increases the excitement of the muscle spindles and further creates a contraction (spasm) response. With this scenario, the shortened hip flexors are helping to create the anterior pelvic rotation that is causing the lengthening of the hamstrings. Instead, the hip flexors need to be stretched.[20]

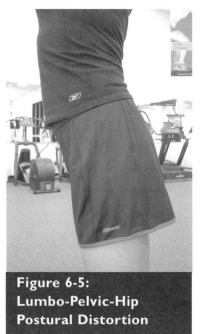

**Figure 6-5:
Lumbo-Pelvic-Hip
Postural Distortion**

(This will be reviewed later in the chapter.) Another example includes an individual whose knees adduct and internally rotate in a lower-extremity postural distortion. The lengthened muscle is the gluteus medius (hip abductor and external rotator). Thus, one would not need to stretch the gluteus medius, but instead stretch the adductor complex which pulls the femur into adduction and internal rotation. Individuals with protracted (rounded) shoulders in an upper-extremity postural distortion need not stretch the rhomboids, middle and lower trapezius (lengthened), but rather stretch the muscles pulling them into protraction (pectoralis major, pectoralis minor and latissimus dorsi).

Golgi Tendon Organs

Golgi tendon organs are located within the *musculotendinous junction* (or the point where the muscle and the tendon meet) and are sensitive to changes in muscular tension and rate of the tension change.[5,7,21-28] When excited, the Golgi tendon organ causes the muscle to relax. This prevents the muscle from being placed under excessive stress, which could result in injury.

Prolonged Golgi tendon organ stimulation provides an inhibitory action to muscle spindles (located within the same muscle). This neuromuscular phenomenon is called **autogenic inhibition** and occurs when the neural impulses sensing tension are greater than the impulses causing muscle contraction.[8,17] The phenomenon is termed "autogenic" because the contracting muscle is being inhibited by its own receptors.[4,5,8]

This is one of the main principles used in flexibility training. Proper stimulation of the Golgi tendon organ can cause relaxation in an overactive muscle.

AUTOGENIC INHIBITION:
The process when neural impulses that sense tension is greater than the impulses that cause muscles to contract, which prevents muscle spindles from contracting.

MODULE 6-1 Summary

Flexibility training may decrease the chance of muscle imbalances, joint dysfunctions and overuse injuries. It is important to have proper range of motion in all three planes. This can be achieved by implementing an integrated approach toward flexibility training.

All segments of the kinetic chain must be properly aligned to avoid postural distortion patterns, decreased neuromuscular efficiency and tissue overload. The adaptive potential of the kinetic chain is decreased by limited flexibility. This forces the body to move in an altered fashion, leading to relative flexibility.

Muscle imbalances result from altered length-tension relationships, force-couple relationships and arthrokinematics. These imbalances can be caused by poor posture, poor training technique or previous injury. These muscle imbalances result in altered reciprocal inhibition, synergistic dominance and arthrokinetic dysfunction, which in turn lead to decreased neuromuscular control.

MODULE 6-1 Quiz

1. The kinetic chain is made up of:

    ☐ Nervous system   ☐ Skeletal system

    ☐ Muscular system   ☐ All of the above

2. A prime example of relative flexibility is seen in people who squat with their feet ☐ **internally** ☐ **externally** rotated because they lack the proper amount of ankle ☐ **dorsiflexion** ☐ **plantarflexion** to perform a squat with proper mechanics.

3. Name three of the four results of muscle imbalances.

    _____

    _____

    _____

4. In autogenic inhibition, the neural impulses cause muscles to contract.

    ☐ True   ☐ False

MODULE 6-2:
Scientific Rationale for Flexibility Training

Benefits of Flexibility Training

Flexibility training is a key component for all training programs.[1,4,7,8] It is utilized for a variety of reasons, including:

- Correcting muscle imbalances
- Increasing joint range of motion
- Decreasing the excessive tension of muscles
- Relieving joint stress
- Improving the extensibility of the musculotendinous junction
- Maintaining the normal functional length of all muscles
- Improving optimum neuromuscular efficiency
- Improving function

Pattern Overload

> **PATTERN OVERLOAD:** Repetitive physical activity that moves through the same patterns of motion, placing the same stresses on the body over a period of time.

Significant numbers of people in today's society have muscular imbalances that are a result of **pattern overload**. Pattern overload is consistently repeating the same pattern of motion. There are gym members who train with the same routine repetitively. This may lead to pattern overload and place abnormal stresses on the body.

Pattern overload may not necessarily be directly related to exercise. Consider the person who has a particularly repetitive occupation such as a loading-dock employee lifting and loading packages all day. He, too, will experience a pattern overload from moving his body in repetitive ways on a daily basis. Even sitting at a computer is a repetitive stress.

Cumulative Injury Cycle

Poor posture and repetitive movements create dysfunction within the connective tissue of the kinetic chain.[1,4,5,7,29-31] This dysfunction is treated by the body as an injury and as a result, the body will initiate a repair process termed the cumulative injury cycle (Figure 6-6).[7,31]

Any trauma to the tissue of the body (such as resistance training) creates inflammation. Inflammation, in turn, activates the body's pain receptors and initiates a protective mechanism, increasing muscle tension and/or causing muscle spasm. Heightened activity of muscle spindles in particular areas of the muscle create a microspasm. As a result of the spasm, adhesions (or knots) begin to form in the soft tissue. These adhesions form a weak, inelastic matrix (unable to stretch) that decreases normal elasticity of the soft tissue.[1,4,5,7,31] The result is altered length-tension relationships (leading to altered reciprocal inhibition), altered force-couple relationships (leading to synergistic dominance) and arthrokinetic dysfunction (leading to altered joint motion).[4,5] Left unchecked, these adhesions can begin to form permanent structural changes in the soft tissue that is evident by Davis' Law.

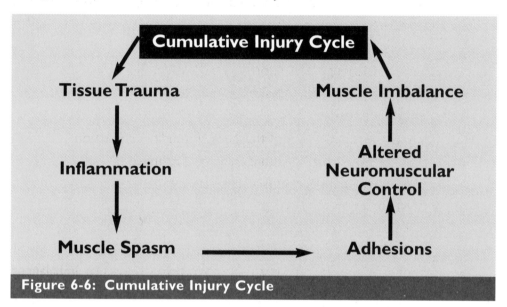

Figure 6-6: Cumulative Injury Cycle

Davis' Law states that soft tissue models along the lines of stress.[1,4,7,32] Soft tissue remodels (or rebuilds) itself with an inelastic collagen matrix that forms in a random fashion. This simply means that it usually does not run in the same direction as the muscle fibers. If the muscle fibers are lengthened, these inelastic connective tissue fibers act as roadblocks, preventing the muscle fibers from moving properly. This creates alterations in normal tissue extensibility and causes relative flexibility.[4,5,12]

For example, if a muscle is in a constant shortened state (such as the hip flexor musculature when sitting for prolonged periods every day), it will demonstrate poor neuromuscular efficiency (due to altered length-tension and force-couple relationships). In turn, this will affect joint motion (ankle, knee, hip and lumbar spine) and alter movement patterns (leading to synergistic dominance). An inelastic collagen matrix will form along the same lines of stress created by the altered muscle movements. Because the muscle is consistently short and moves in a pattern different from its intended function, the newly formed inelastic connective tissue forms along this altered pattern, reducing the ability of the muscle to extend and move in its proper manner. This is why it is imperative that a flexibility-training program be utilized to restore the normal extensibility of the entire soft tissue complex.[4,5,33,34]

It is essential for health and fitness professionals to address their clients' muscular imbalances through a fitness assessment and flexibility-training program. By neglecting these phases of programming and simply moving clients right into a resistance-training program, it will add additional loads to joints and muscles that have improper mechanics and faulty recruitment patterns.

MODULE 6-2 Summary

Flexibility training has the benefits of improving muscle imbalances, increasing joint range of motion and extensibility, relieving excessive tension of muscles and joint stress and improving neuromuscular efficiency and function.

People who physically train in a repetitive fashion (or have jobs that require moving their bodies in repetitive ways) may experience pattern overload, which places stress on the body.

Poor posture and repetitive movements may create dysfunctions in connective tissue, initiating the cumulative injury cycle. Tissue trauma creates inflammation, which leads to microspasms and decreases normal elasticity of the soft tissue.

Soft tissue rebuilds itself in a random fashion with an inelastic collagen matrix that usually does not run in the same direction as the muscle fibers. If the muscle fibers are lengthened, these inelastic connective tissue fibers act as roadblocks, creating alterations in normal tissue extensibility and causing relative flexibility. It is essential for fitness professionals to address muscular imbalances through a fitness assessment and flexibility training to restore the normal extensibility of the entire soft tissue complex.

MODULE 6-2 Quiz

1. What is one of the greatest benefits of flexibility training for today's clientele?

   _____

2. A construction worker could experience pattern overload by being bent over and hammering all day.

   ☐ True   ☐ False

3. What process does the body initiate to repair dysfunction within the connective tissue?

   _____

4. What law states that soft tissue will model along the lines of stress?

_____

MODULE 6-3:
The Flexibility Continuum

To fully appreciate the principles of flexibility training, health and fitness professionals must understand the different types. Flexibility, like any other form of training, should follow a systematic progression. This is known as the flexibility continuum.[4,5] There are three phases of flexibility training: corrective, active and functional (Figure 6-7).[1,4,13,17,35,36]

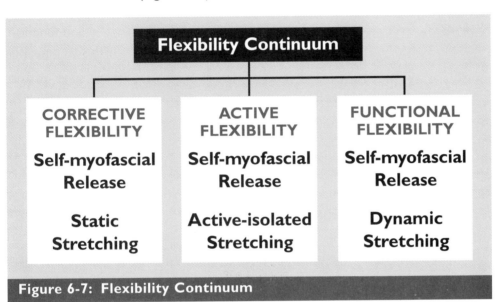

Flexibility Continuum

CORRECTIVE FLEXIBILITY	ACTIVE FLEXIBILITY	FUNCTIONAL FLEXIBILITY
Self-myofascial Release	Self-myofascial Release	Self-myofascial Release
Static Stretching	Active-isolated Stretching	Dynamic Stretching

Figure 6-7: Flexibility Continuum

Corrective Flexibility

Corrective flexibility is designed to improve muscle imbalances and altered joint motion.[4,5] It uses the principles of both reciprocal inhibition and autogenic inhibition. It includes static stretching and **self-myofascial release** (foam roll) techniques (Figure 6-8). This form of flexibility is appropriate at the stabilization level (Phases 1 and 2) of the OPT™ model.

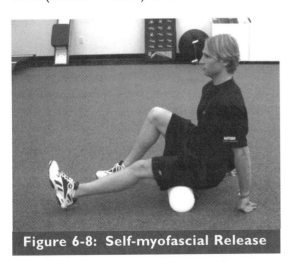

Figure 6-8: Self-myofascial Release

> **SELF-MYOFASCIAL RELEASE:**
> A flexibility technique where muscles are rolled over a cylindrical piece of foam (or foam roll), using body pressure to massage micro-adhesions in the fibrous tissue that surrounds and separates muscle tissue.

Active Flexibility

Active flexibility is designed to improve the extensibility of soft tissue and increase neuromuscular efficiency by using reciprocal inhibition.[4,5] Active flexibility allows for agonists and synergist muscles to move a limb through a full range of motion while the functional antagonists are being stretched.[4,17,37,38] For example, a supine straight-leg raise utilizes the hip flexor and quadriceps to raise the leg and hold it unsupported, while the antagonist hamstring group is stretched. Active flexibility uses active-isolated stretching and self-myofascial release techniques. This form of flexibility would be appropriate at the strength level (Phases 3, 4 and 5) of the OPT™ model.

Functional Flexibility

Functional flexibility is integrated, multiplanar soft tissue extensibility, with optimum neuromuscular control, through the full range of motion.[4,5,17] Essentially, it is movement without compensations. Therefore, if a client is compensating during training then he/she needs to be regressed to corrective and active flexibility. Functional flexibility uses dynamic flexibility and self-myofascial release techniques. This form of flexibility would be appropriate at the power level (Phases 6 and 7) of the OPT™ model.

Remember that all functional movements occur in all three planes of motion and that injuries most often occur in the transverse plane. If the appropriate soft tissue is not extensible through the full range of movement, the risk of injury dramatically increases.[2,39] Exercises that increase multiplanar soft tissue extensibility and have high levels of neuromuscular demand are preferred.

Stretching Techniques

Proper stretching is one way to enhance flexibility and can also be viewed as a continuum. The flexibility continuum consists of specific forms of stretching. For example, corrective flexibility uses self-myofascial release and static stretching; active flexibility uses self-myofascial release and active-isolated stretching; and functional flexibility uses dynamic stretching (Table 6-3). Each form of stretching manipulates the receptors and the nervous system, which in turn allows for the alteration of the muscle extensibility.[4-5]

Table 6-3: Examples of Stretching within the Flexibility Continuum		
Flexibility Type	**Type of Stretching**	**Examples**
Corrective	Self-Myofascial Release Static	Foam Roll Static Pectoral Ball Stretch
Active	Self-Myofascial Release Active-isolated	Foam Roll Active Soleus with Pronation and Supination
Functional	Self-Myofascial Release Dynamic	Foam Roll Walking Lunge with Rotation

Corrective Flexibility

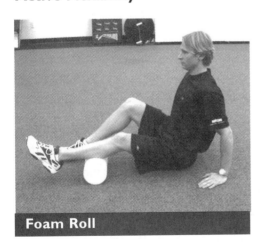

Foam Roll

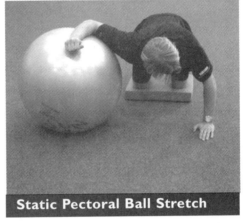

Static Pectoral Ball Stretch

Active Flexibility

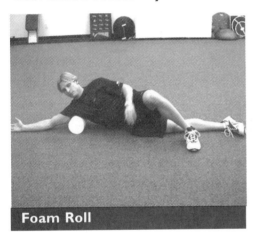

Foam Roll

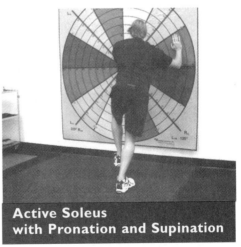

Active Soleus
with Pronation and Supination

Functional Flexibility

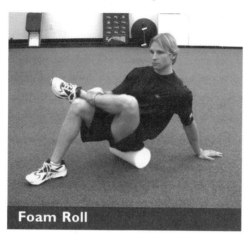

Foam Roll

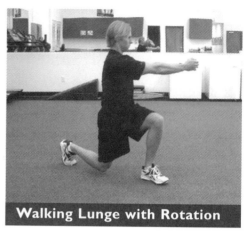

Walking Lunge with Rotation

Self-myofascial Release

Self-myofascial release is another stretching technique that focuses on the neural system and fascial system in the body (or the fibrous tissue that surrounds and separates muscle tissue). By applying gentle force to an adhesion or "knot," the elastic muscle fibers are altered from a bundled position (that causes the adhesion) into a straighter alignment with the direction of the muscle and/or fascia. The gentle pressure (applied with implements such as a foam roll) will stimulate the Golgi tendon organ and create autogenic inhibition, decreasing muscle spindle excitation and releasing the hypertonicity of the underlying musculature.[4]

It is crucial to note that when a person is using self-myofascial release he/she must find a tender spot (that indicates the presence of muscle hypertonicity) and sustain pressure on that spot for a minimum of 20-30 seconds.[4] This will increase the Golgi tendon organ activity and decrease muscle spindle activity thus the autogenic inhibition response. It may take longer, depending on the client's ability to consciously relax.

This process will help restore the body back to its optimal level of function by resetting the proprioceptive mechanisms of the soft tissue.[42] Self-myofascial release is suggested prior to static stretching for postural distortion patterns and/or prior to activity. In addition, it can be used during the cool-down process.

Gastrocnemius/Soleus

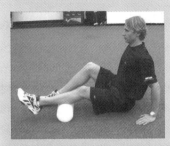

Preparation
1. Place foam roll under mid-calf.
2. Cross left leg over right leg to increase pressure (optional).

Movement
3. Draw abs in and activate glutes.
4. Slowly roll calf area to find the most tender spot.
5. Once identified, hold tender spot until the discomfort is reduced by at least 75 percent.
6. Progress to the next tender spot and hold again.
7. Repeat on opposite leg.

Peroneals

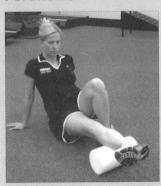

Preparation
1. Place foam roll under lateral part of calf.
2. Cross left leg over right leg to increase pressure (optional).

Movement
3. Draw abs in.
4. Slowly roll area to find the most tender spot.
5. Once identified, hold tender spot until the discomfort is reduced by at least 75 percent.
6. Progress to the next tender spot and hold again.
7. Repeat on opposite leg.

Hamstrings

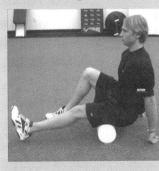

Preparation
1. Place foam roll under hamstrings with hips unsupported.
2. Cross left leg over right leg to increase pressure (optional).

Movement
3. Draw abs in.
4. Slowly roll from the back of knee toward the posterior hip to find the most tender spot, while maintaining tightness in the quadriceps.
5. Once identified, hold tender spot until the discomfort is reduced by at least 75 percent.
6. Progress to the next tender spot and hold again.
7. Repeat on opposite leg.

Iliotibial Band

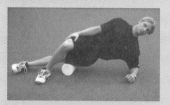

Preparation

1. Lie on one side, with legs on top of the foam roll. Cross the top leg over lower leg, with foot touching the floor and the bottom leg raised slightly off floor.
2. Maintain optimal head alignment (ears in line with shoulders).

Movement

3. Draw abs in and activate glutes.
4. Slowly roll from hip joint to lateral knee to find the most tender spot.
5. Once identified, hold tender spot until the discomfort is reduced by at least 75 percent.
6. Progress to the next tender spot and hold again.
7. Repeat on opposite leg.

Tensor Fascia Latae

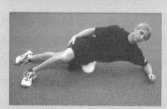

Preparation

1. Lie on one side, with the foam roll on the side and just anterior of the hip. Cross the top leg over the lower leg, with foot touching the floor and the bottom leg raised slightly off floor.
2. Maintain optimal head alignment (ears in line with shoulders).

Movement

3. Draw abs in and activate glutes.
4. Slowly roll laterally and slightly in front of the hip joint to find the most tender spot.
5. Once identified, hold tender spot until the discomfort is reduced by at least 75 percent.
6. Progress to the next tender spot and hold again.
7. Repeat on opposite leg.

Quadriceps

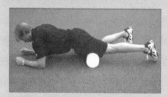

Preparation

1. Lie prone with foam roll under the anterior upper leg. Maintain proper core control.

Movement

2. Draw abs in and activate glutes.
3. Slowly roll from the pelvic bone to the knee area to find the most tender spot.
4. Once identified, hold tender spot until the discomfort is reduced by at least 75 percent.
5. Progress to the next tender spot and hold again.
6. Repeat on opposite leg.

Adductors

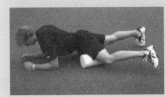

Preparation

1. Lie prone with one thigh extended and the foam roll in the groin region, under the upper thigh.

Movement

2. Draw abs in and activate glutes.
3. Slowly roll the medial thigh area to find the most tender spot.
4. Once identified, hold tender spot until the discomfort is reduced by at least 75 percent.
5. Progress to the next tender spot and hold again.
6. Repeat on opposite leg.

Piriformis

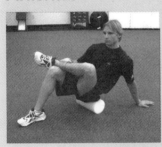

Preparation

1. Sit on top of the foam roll, positioned on the back of the hip. Cross one foot to the opposite knee.

Movement

2. Draw abs in.
3. Lean into the hip of the crossed leg. Slowly roll on the posterior hip area to find the most tender spot.
4. Once identified, hold tender spot until the discomfort is reduced by at least 75 percent.
5. Progress to the next tender spot and hold again.
6. Repeat on opposite leg.

Latissimus Dorsi

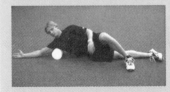

Preparation

1. Lie on the floor on one side with the arm closest to the floor outstretched and thumb facing upward.
2. Place the foam roll in the axillary area under the armpit.

Movement

3. Draw abs in and activate glutes.
4. Slowly move back and forth to find the most tender spot.
5. Once identified, hold tender spot until the discomfort is reduced by at least 75 percent.
6. Progress to the next tender spot and hold again.
7. Repeat on opposite side.

Thoracic Erector Spine

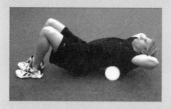

Preparation

1. Sit on the floor with foam roll placed behind the back.
2. Cross arms to the opposite shoulder to clear the shoulder blades across the mid-back. Lie back on top of the foam roll so that it is positioned under the upper back.

Movement

3. Draw abs in and activate glutes.
4. While maintaining abdominal stability, raise hips until unsupported.
5. Slowly move back and forth to find the most tender spot.
6. Once identified, hold tender spot until the discomfort is reduced by at least 75 percent.
7. Progress to the next tender spot and hold again.

Static Stretching

Static stretching is the process of passively taking a muscle to the point of tension and holding the stretch for a minimum of 20 seconds.[1,2,4,14] This is the traditional form of stretching that is most often seen in fitness today. It combines low force with longer duration.[17,40]

One of the proposed mechanisms for this type of stretching is autogenic inhibition.[5] By holding the muscle in a stretched position for a prolonged period of time, the Golgi tendon organ is stimulated and produces an inhibitory effect on the muscle spindle (autogenic inhibition). This allows the muscle to relax and provides for better elongation of the muscle.[4,5,7,41]

Static stretching should be used to decrease the muscle spindle activity of a tight muscle prior to and following activity.[5] Detailed explanations of various static stretching techniques are described below (Table 6-4).

Table 6-4: Examples of Static Stretching			
Type of Stretch	**Mechanism of Action**	**Acute Variables**	**Examples**
Static Stretch	Autogenic Inhibition	1-2 sets Hold each stretch 20-30 seconds	■ Gastrocnemius Stretch ■ 90-90 Hamstring Stretch ■ Kneeling Quadriceps Stretch ■ Standing Adductor Stretch ■ Pectoral Wall Stretch

Static Gastrocnemius Stretch

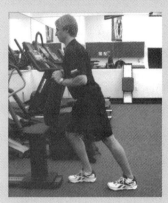

Preparation

1. Stand facing a wall or sturdy object.
2. Bring one leg forward toward the wall for support. Use upper body to lean against the wall, keeping outstretched rear leg straight.

Movement

3. Draw abs in and activate glutes.
4. Keep rear foot flat, with foot pointed straight ahead. Do not allow the rear foot to cave inward or roll outward.
5. Bend arms, move chest toward the wall and tilt pelvis forward.
6. Stop movement when slight tension is felt.
7. Hold for 20-30 seconds.
8. Switch sides and repeat.

Static Soleus Stretch

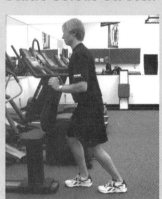

Preparation

1. Stand facing a wall or sturdy object.
2. Bring one leg forward toward the wall for support. Use upper body to lean against wall, keeping outstretched rear leg straight.

Movement

3. Draw abs in and activate glutes.
4. Keep rear foot flat, with foot pointed straight ahead. Do not allow the rear foot to cave inward or roll outward.
5. Bend rear knee until slight tension is felt.
6. Hold for 20-30 seconds.
7. Switch sides and repeat.

Static Peroneal Stretch

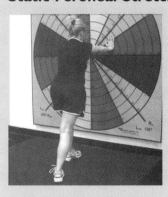

Preparation

1. Stand facing a wall or sturdy object.
2. Bring one leg forward toward the wall for support. Use upper body to lean against wall.
3. Internally rotate rear leg and invert (turn in) foot.

Movement

4. Draw abs in and activate glutes.
5. Lean forward until slight tension is felt in the lateral shin of the back leg.
6. Hold for 20-30 seconds.
7. Switch sides and repeat.

Static Straight-leg Hamstring Stretch

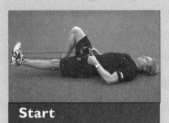
Start

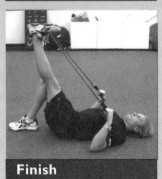
Finish

Preparation

1. Lie on floor with one leg straight.
2. Bend opposite leg and keep foot flat on the floor.

Movement

3. Draw abs in.
4. Slightly tilt pelvis anteriorly.
5. Wrap a stretch cord around the sole of the foot, near the toes, and slowly lift the straight leg until a slight stretch is felt.
6. Hold for 20-30 seconds.
7. Switch sides and repeat.

Static 90-90 Hamstring Stretch

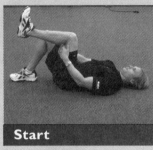
Start

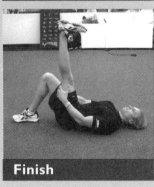
Finish

Preparation

1. Lie on floor with legs flat.
2. Flex hip and knee of one leg and create a 90-90 position.

Movement

3. Draw abs in.
4. Slightly tilt pelvis anteriorly.
5. With hands supporting leg, slowly extend the knee (without moving at the pelvis) until tension is felt.
6. Hold for 20-30 seconds.
7. Switch sides and repeat.

Static Seated Ball Hamstring Stretch

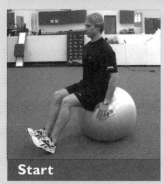

Start

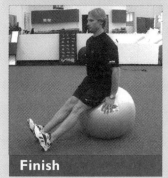

Finish

Preparation

1. Sit on ball using erect posture.
2. Extend one leg and place heel on floor.

Movement

3. Draw abs in.
4. Maintaining an extended spine, slightly roll the ball backward by leaning forward at the hips until a slight stretch is felt in the back of the extended leg.
5. Hold for 20-30 seconds.
6. Switch sides and repeat.

Static Standing Cross-leg Biceps Femoris Stretch

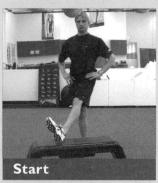

Start

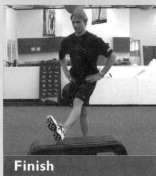

Finish

Preparation

1. Stand with erect posture and one leg straight, hip flexed, adducted and internally rotated on a bench.

Movement

2. Draw abs in.
3. Maintaining an upright posture, slightly lean forward at the hip until a slight stretch is felt in the back of the thigh.
4. Hold for 20-30 seconds.
5. Switch sides and repeat.

Static Standing Psoas Stretch

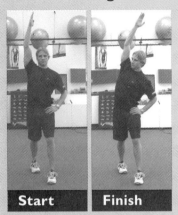

Start **Finish**

Preparation

1. Stand with one leg bent and slightly forward.
2. Internally rotate back leg.

Movement

3. Draw abs in and activate glutes.
4. Squeeze buttocks, while rotating pelvis posteriorly.
5. Slowly, move body forward until a mild tension is achieved in the front of the hip being stretched.
6. Raise the arm (on the same side as the back leg) up and over to the opposite side, while maintaining pelvis position.
7. Hold side bend position and slowly rotate backward.
8. Hold for 20-30 seconds.
9. Switch sides and repeat.

Static Kneeling Hip Flexor/Quadriceps Stretch

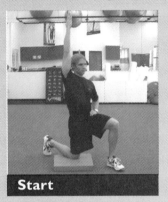

Start

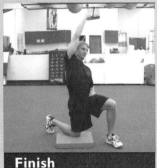

Finish

Preparation

1. Kneel with front leg bent at a 90-degree angle.
2. Internally rotate back leg.

Movement

3. Draw abs in and activate glutes.
4. Squeeze buttocks, while rotating pelvis posteriorly.
5. Slowly move body forward until a mild tension is achieved in the front of the hip being stretched.
6. Raise stretch side arm up and over to the opposite side, while maintaining pelvis position.
7. Hold side bend position and slowly rotate backward.
8. Hold for 20-30 seconds.
9. Switch sides and repeat.

Static Standing Adductor Stretch

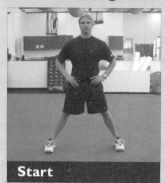

Start

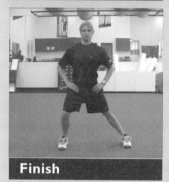

Finish

Preparation
1. Stand with one leg straight and the opposite leg bent.
2. Both feet should be pointed straight ahead.

Movement
3. Draw abs in and activate glutes.
4. Slowly move in a sideways motion toward the bent leg until a stretch in the straight leg groin area is felt.
5. Hold for 20-30 seconds.
6. Switch sides and repeat.

Seated Ball Adductor Stretch

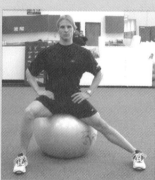

Preparation
1. Sit on ball with one leg extended and the other bent (side lunge), with weight on the bent leg.

Movement
2. Draw abs in and activate glutes.
3. Slowly shift weight toward the front foot until a slight resistance is felt on the straight leg.
4. Hold for 20-30 seconds.
5. Switch sides and repeat.

Static Adductor Magnus Stretch

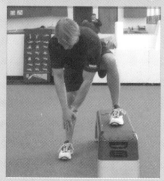

Preparation
1. Place one foot on a bench/ball/chair about waist high (or at a comfortable height).
2. The standing leg should be slightly bent at the knee and facing forward (as in proper walking position).

Movement
3. Draw abs in.
4. Slowly bend forward, reaching both arms toward the floor until a stretch is felt in the back of the raised leg.
5. Hold for 20-30 seconds.
6. Switch sides and repeat.

Static Supine Piriformis Stretch

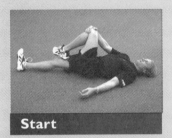

Start

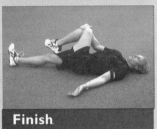

Finish

Preparation
1. Lie supine with right leg crossed over the left.

Movement
2. Draw abs in.
3. Place left hand on the lateral right knee and slowly pull to opposite shoulder, until a slight tension is felt in buttock region.
4. Hold for 20-30 seconds.
5. Switch sides and repeat.

Static Erector Spinae Cross-leg Stretch

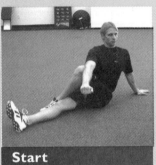

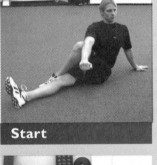

Start

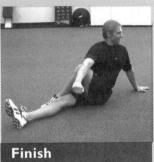

Finish

Preparation
1. Sit on ground with left leg straight and right leg bent and crossed over the left.

Movement
2. Draw abs in and activate glutes.
3. Slowly use left arm against right crossed leg to apply pressure to the point of tension.
4. Hold 20-30 seconds.
5. Switch sides and repeat.

Static Abdominal Stretch Over Ball

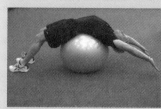

Preparation

1. Lie supine on a ball, with arms outstretched.

Movement

2. Draw abs in and activate glutes.
3. Slowly allow body to drape over the ball, extending legs and reaching with arms.
4. Hold for 20-30 seconds.

Static Latissimus Dorsi Ball Stretch

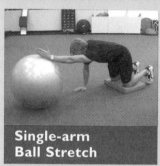

Single-arm Ball Stretch

Preparation

1. Kneel in front of a stability ball.
2. Place arm on ball, with thumb pointed straight up in the air.

Movement

3. Draw abs in and activate glutes.
4. Slowly lower body until a comfortable stretch is felt.
5. Hold for 20-30 seconds.
6. Switch sides and repeat.

Static Pectoral Ball Stretch

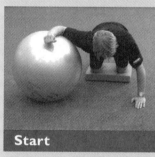

Start

Finish

Preparation

1. Kneel on the side of a stability ball with one arm supported on the ground.
2. Place one arm in a 90/90 position on ball.

Movement

3. Draw abs in and activate glutes.
4. Slowly rotate trunk forward around support arm until a slight stretch is felt in the anterior shoulder region.
5. Hold for 20-30 seconds.
6. Switch sides and repeat.
7. This stretch can also be performed standing in a doorway or against a stable object.

Static Sternocleidomastoid Stretch

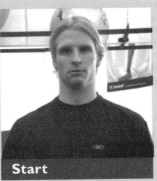

Start

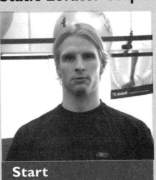

Finish

Preparation

1. Start in optimal posture and place right arm behind body, depressing shoulder.

Movement

2. Draw abs in.
3. Tuck chin and slowly draw left ear to left shoulder.
4. Continue by rotating upward toward the ceiling until a slight stretch is felt on the right side.
5. Optional: Use left hand to apply slight pressure and assist in lateral flexion and rotation.
6. Hold stretch position for 20-30 seconds.
7. Switch sides and repeat.

Static Levator Scapulae Stretch

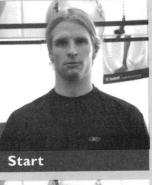

Start

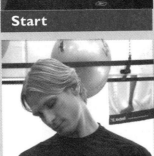

Finish

Preparation

1. Stand in optimal posture and place right arm behind body.

Movement

2. Draw abs in.
3. Tuck chin and slowly draw left ear to left shoulder.
4. Continue by rotating downward toward opposite pocket, until a slight stretch is felt on the right side
5. Optional: Use left hand to apply slight pressure and assist in lateral flexion and rotation.
6. Hold stretch position for 20-30 seconds.
7. Switch sides and repeat.

Static Scalene Stretch

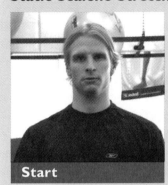

Start

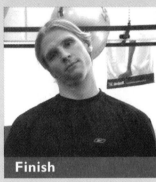

Finish

Preparation
1. Stand in optimal posture and place right arm behind body.

Movement
2. Draw abs in.
3. Tuck chin and slowly draw left ear to left shoulder.
4. Optional: Use left hand to apply slight pressure and assist in lateral flexion.
5. Hold stretch position for 20-30 seconds.
6. Switch sides and repeat.

Active-isolated Stretching

ACTIVE-ISOLATED STRETCH:
The process of using agonists and synergists to dynamically move the joint into a range of motion.

Active-isolated stretching is the process of using agonists and synergists to dynamically move the joint into a range of motion.[4,17,36] This form of stretching increases motor-neuron excitability, creating reciprocal inhibition of the muscle being stretched.

The active straight-leg hamstring stretch is a good example of active stretching.[1,4,17] The quadriceps and hip flexors contract to pull the leg up off the floor. This enhances the stretch of the hamstrings in two ways. First, it increases the length of the hamstrings. Second, the contraction of the quadriceps and hip flexors causes reciprocal inhibition (decreased neural drive and muscle spindle excitation) of the hamstrings, which allows them to elongate.

Active-isolated stretches are suggested for pre-activity warm-up, as long as no postural distortion patterns are present.[5] Typically, five to 10 repetitions of each stretch are performed and held for two to four seconds each. Detailed explanations of various active stretches are given below (Table 6-5).

Table 6-5: Examples of Active-isolated Stretching			
Type of Stretch	**Mechanism of Action**	**Acute Variables**	**Stretch Examples**
Active-isolated Stretch	Reciprocal Inhibition	1-2 sets Hold each stretch 2-4 seconds for 5-10 repetitions	■ Active Gastrocnemius ■ Active 90-90 Hamstring ■ Active Kneeling Quadriceps ■ Active Standing Adductor ■ Active Pectoral Wall

Active Gastrocnemius Stretch with Pronation and Supination

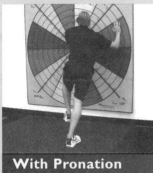

With Pronation

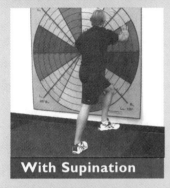

With Supination

Preparation
1. Stand near a wall or sturdy object.
2. Bring one leg forward for support. Use upper body and lean against wall.
3. The outstretched leg should form one straight line and the subtalar joint should be in a neutral position

Movement
3. Draw abs in and activate glutes.
4. Keep rear foot on the ground, with opposite hip flexed.
5. Slowly move through hips, creating controlled supination and pronation through the lower extremity.
6. Hold for 2-4 seconds and repeat for 5-10 repetitions.
7. Switch sides and repeat.

Active Soleus Stretch with Pronation and Supination

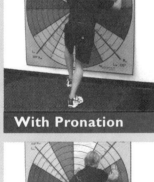

With Pronation

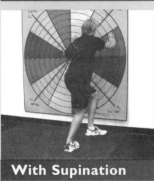

With Supination

Preparation
1. Stand near a wall or sturdy object.
2. Bring one leg forward for support. Use your upper body and lean against wall.
3. Bend back knee at a 30-degree angle and keep subtalar joint in a neutral position.

Movement
3. Draw abs in and activate glutes.
4. Keep rear foot on the ground, with opposite hip flexed.
5. Slowly move through hips, creating controlled supination and pronation through the lower extremity.
6. Hold for 2-4 seconds and repeat for 5-10 repetitions.
7. Switch sides and repeat.

Active Straight-leg Hamstring Stretch

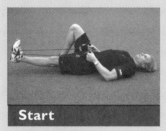

Start

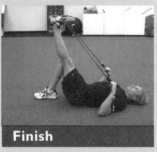

Finish

Preparation

1. Lie supine on floor with one leg straight.
2. Bend opposite leg, keeping foot flat on the floor.

Movement

3. Draw abs in and activate glutes.
4. Slightly tilt pelvis anteriorly.
5. Wrap a stretch cord around the sole of the foot, near the toes, and slowly lift the straight leg until a slight stretch is felt.
6. Hold for 2-4 seconds and repeat for 5-10 repetitions.
7. Switch sides and repeat.

Active 90-90 Hamstring Stretch

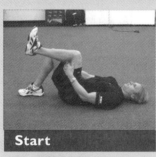

Start

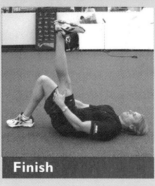

Finish

Preparation

1. Lie supine on floor with legs flat.
2. Flex hip and knee of one leg and place leg in a 90-90 position.

Movement

3. Draw abs in and activate glutes.
4. Slightly tilt pelvis anteriorly.
5. With hands supporting leg, extend and flex the knee in a controlled manner, without moving at the pelvis until tension is felt.
6. Hold for 2-4 seconds for 5-10 repetitions.
7. Switch sides and repeat.

Active Standing Psoas Stretch

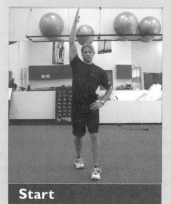

Start

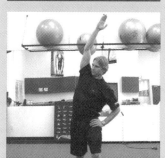

Finish

Preparation

1. Stand with one leg bent and slightly forward.
2. Position the back leg in internal rotation.

Movement

3. Draw abs in and activate glutes.
4. Squeeze buttocks, while rotating posteriorly.
5. Stride forward, in a controlled manner, until a mild tension is achieved in the front of the hip being stretched.
6. Raise stretch side arm up and over to the opposite side, while maintaining pelvic position.
7. Rotate to the back leg in a controlled manner.
8. Hold for 2-4 seconds for 5-10 repetitions.
9. Switch sides and repeat.

Active Kneeling Hip Flexor/Quadriceps Stretch

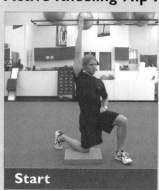

Start

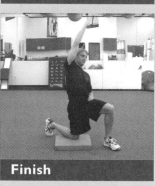

Finish

Preparation

1. Kneel with front leg at a 90-degree angle.
2. Position the back leg in internal rotation.

Movement

3. Draw abs in and activate glutes.
4. Squeeze buttocks, while rotating pelvis posteriorly.
5. Slowly move body forward until a mild tension is achieved in the front of the hip being stretched.
6. Raise arm (on the same side as the kneeling leg) up and over to the opposite side, while maintaining pelvis position.
7. Hold side bend position and slowly rotate backward.
8. Hold for 2-4 seconds for 5-10 repetitions.
9. Switch sides and repeat.

Active Standing Adductor Stretch

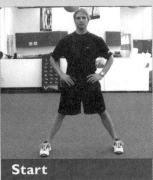

Start

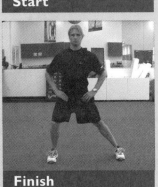

Finish

Preparation

1. Stand with both feet pointed straight ahead, with one leg straight and the opposite leg bent.
2. Place one hand superior to the greater trochanter of the straight leg.

Movement

3. Draw abs in and activate glutes.
4. Under muscular control, perform a posterior tilt of the pelvis followed by moving in a frontal/transverse direction.
5. Hold for 2-4 seconds for 5-10 repetitions.
6. Switch sides and repeat.

Active Seated Adductor Stretch

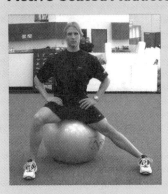

Preparation

1. Sit with both feet pointed straight ahead, with one leg straight and the opposite leg bent.
2. Place one hand superior to the greater trochanter of the straight leg.

Movement

3. Draw abs in and activate glutes.
4. Under muscular control, perform a posterior tilt of the pelvis followed by moving in a frontal/transverse direction.
5. Hold for 2-4 seconds for 5-10 repetitions.
6. Switch sides and repeat.

Pelvic Tilt on Ball

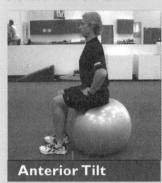

Anterior Tilt

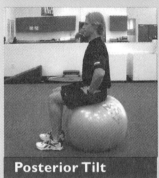

Posterior Tilt

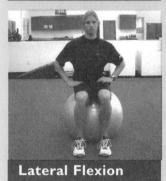

Lateral Flexion

Preparation
1. Sit on a ball with at least a 90-degree angle in the hips and knees.
2. Hands should be on hips, with feet on the floor (shoulder-width apart), pointing straight ahead.

Movement
3. Draw abs in and activate glutes.
4. Perform anterior and posterior pelvic tilts, using controlled movements.
5. Perform lateral flexion, under control, to each side.
6. Hold for 2-4 seconds for 5-10 repetitions.

Active Latissimus Dorsi Ball Stretch

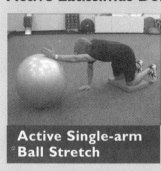

Active Single-arm Ball Stretch

Preparation
1. Kneel in front of stability ball.
2. Place arm on ball with thumb straight up in air

Movement
3. Draw abs in and activate glutes.
4. Maintaining core control, roll ball out until a comfortable stretch is felt. As ball is rolled out, posteriorly rotate pelvis.
5. Hold for 2-4 seconds for 5-10 repetitions.
6. Switch sides and repeat

Active Sternocleidomastoid Stretch

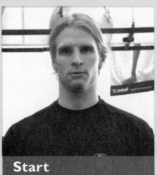

Start

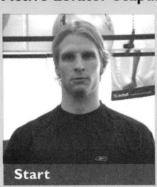

Finish

Preparation

1. Stand with optimal posture.

Movement

2. Draw abs in and activate glutes.
3. Tuck chin and, using control, draw left ear to left shoulder.
4. Continue by rotating upward toward the ceiling while retracting and depressing the right shoulder complex.
5. Hold for 2-4 seconds for 5-10 repetitions.
6. Switch sides and repeat

Active Levator Scapulae Stretch

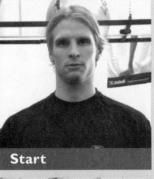

Start

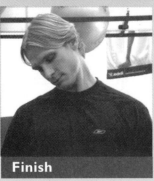

Finish

Preparation

1. Stand with optimal posture.

Movement

2. Draw abs in and activate glutes.
3. Tuck chin and rotate head to the right, in a controlled manner, while retracting and depressing shoulder complex on the left.
4. Hold for 2-4 seconds for 5-10 repetitions.
5. Switch sides and repeat.

Active Scalene Stretch

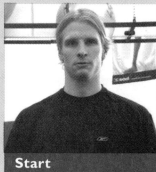

Start

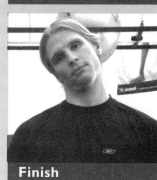

Finish

Preparation

1. Standing with optimal posture.

Movement

2. Draw abs in and activate glutes.
3. Tuck chin and laterally flex head (ear to shoulder) in a controlled manner, while retracting and depressing left shoulder complex.
4. Hold for 2-4 seconds for 5-10 repetitions.
5. Switch sides and repeat.

Dynamic Stretching

DYNAMIC STRETCH: The active extension of a muscle, using force production and momentum, in order to move the joint through the full available range of motion.

Dynamic stretching uses the force production of a muscle and the body's momentum to take a joint through the full available range of motion (Table 6-6). Dynamic stretching employs the concept of reciprocal inhibition to improve soft tissue extensibility. One can perform one set of 10 repetitions utilizing three to 10 dynamic stretches. Medicine ball rotations and walking lunges are a good example of dynamic stretching.[1,4,17] Dynamic stretching is also suggested as a pre-activity warm-up, as long as no postural distortion patterns are present.[5] It is recommended that the client have good levels of tissue extensibility, core stability and balance capabilities prior to undertaking an aggressive dynamic stretching program.

Table 6-6: Examples of Dynamic Stretching			
Type of Stretch	**Mechanism of Action**	**Acute Variables**	**Examples**
Dynamic Stretch	Reciprocal Inhibition	1 set 10-15 repetitions 3-10 exercises	■ Tube Walking ■ Push-up with Rotation ■ Prisoner Squat ■ Walking Lunge with Rotation ■ Single-leg Squat ■ Multiplanar Lunge ■ Multiplanar Hop with Stabilization

Tube Walking: Side to Side

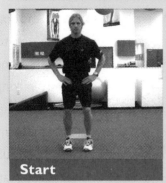

Start

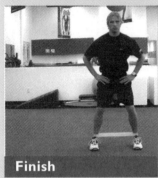

Finish

Preparation

1. Stand with feet hip-width apart, knees slightly bent and feet straight ahead.
2. Place tubing around mid-lower leg.

Movement

3. Draw abs in and activate glutes.
4. Keep feet straight ahead and take 10 small steps sideways, without allowing knees to cave inward.
5. Repeat in the opposite direction.

Tube Walking: Front to Back

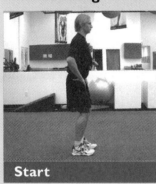

Start

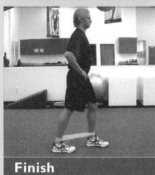

Finish

Preparation

1. Stand with feet hip-width apart, knees slightly bent and feet straight ahead.
2. Place tubing around mid-lower leg.

Movement

3. Draw abs in and activate glutes.
4. Keep feet straight ahead and take 10 small steps forward without allowing knees to cave inward.
5. Repeat moving backward.

Medicine Ball Chop and Lift

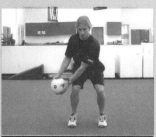

Start

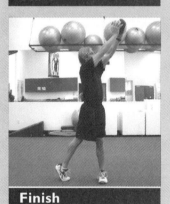

Finish

Preparation

1. Stand with feet hip-width apart, knees slightly bent and feet straight ahead.
2. Grasp a medicine ball with both hands and keep elbows fully extended.

Movement

3. Draw abs in and activate glutes.
4. Starting from optimal posture, initiate the rotational movement from the trunk outward, lifting the medicine ball from a low position to a high position.
5. Allow the hips to pivot on the back foot as the motion nears end range.
6. Perform 10 repetitions.
7. Repeat on opposite side.

Medicine Ball Rotation

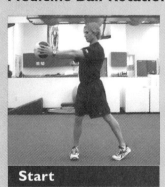

Start

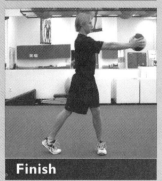

Finish

Preparation

1. Stand with feet hip-width apart, knees slightly bent and feet straight ahead.
2. Grasp a medicine ball with both hands and keep elbows fully extended.

Movement

3. Draw abs in and activate glutes.
4. Starting from optimal posture, initiate the rotational movement from the trunk, moving side to side.
5. Allow the hips to pivot on the back foot as the motion nears end range.
6. Perform 10 repetitions to each side.

Medicine Ball Extension/Flexion

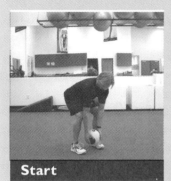

Start

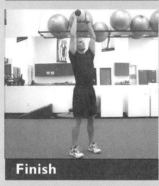

Finish

Preparation

1. Grasp a medicine ball with both hands, keeping elbows slightly bent.
2. Squat.

Movement

3. Draw abs in and activate glutes.
4. From the squat position, squeeze glutes to start extending at the ankle, knee, hip and spine.
5. Perform 10 repetitions

Russian Twist on Ball

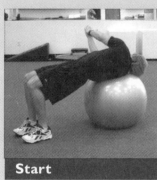

Start

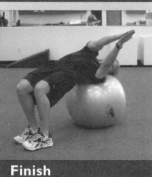

Finish

Preparation

1. Lie supine on a ball, with head and neck supported and both feet straight ahead.
2. Lift hips up until they are in line with knees and shoulders.
3. Raise arms straight up toward ceiling.

Movement

4. Draw abs in and activate glutes.
5. Maintaining core control, slowly rotate trunk to each side.
6. Perform 10 repetitions to each side.

Single-leg Squat Touchdown

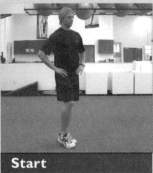

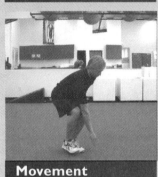

Start

Preparation

1. Stand on one leg in optimal posture, keeping raised leg parallel to the standing leg.

Movement

2. Draw abs in and activate glutes.
3. Squat, in a controlled manner, bending the ankle, knee and hip.
4. Touch toe of standing leg with the opposite hand.
5. While maintaining drawing-in maneuver and gluteal activity, return to starting position.
6. Perform 10 repetitions.
7. Repeat on opposite sides.

Movement

Single-leg Romanian Deadlift

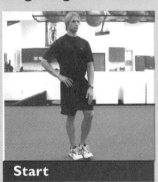

Start

Preparation

1. Stand on one leg in optimal posture, keeping raised leg parallel to the standing leg.

Movement

2. Draw abs in and activate glutes.
3. Without allowing further knee movement, bend over at the hip, touching toe of standing leg with opposite hand.
4. While maintaining abdominal drawing-in maneuver and gluteal activity, return to starting position.
5. Perform 10 repetitions.
6. Repeat on opposite side.

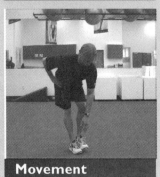

Movement

Multiplanar Lunge

Preparation

1. Stand in proper alignment with hands on hips and feet straight ahead.

Movement

2. Draw abs in and activate glutes.
3. While maintaining total body alignment, step forward (sagittal plane), descending slowly by bending at the hips, knees and ankles.
4. Use hip and thigh muscles to push up and back to the start position.
5. Perform 10 repetitions.
6. Repeat on opposite leg.
7. Progress to side lunges (frontal plane), followed by turning lunges (transverse plane).

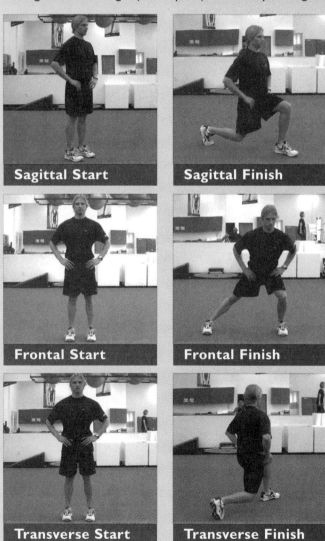

Sagittal Start — Sagittal Finish

Frontal Start — Frontal Finish

Transverse Start — Transverse Finish

Multiplanar Hop with Stabilization

Preparation

1. Stand with feet shoulder-width apart and pointed straight ahead. Hips should be in a neutral position.
2. Lift chest, retract shoulders slightly and tuck chin.

Movement

3. Draw abdominals in, activate glutes and brace.
4. Lift one leg directly beside balance leg. Dorsiflex toe, flex hip at a 90-degree angle and slightly flex knee. Maintain optimal alignment, including level hips and shoulders.
5. Hop forward (sagittal), landing on opposite foot. Stabilize and hold for two to four seconds.
6. Hop backward (sagittal), landing on opposite foot in starting position. Stabilize and hold for two to four seconds.
7. Switch legs and repeat as instructed.
8. Use the same format to move in frontal and transverse planes, hopping in a side-to-side or turning manner.

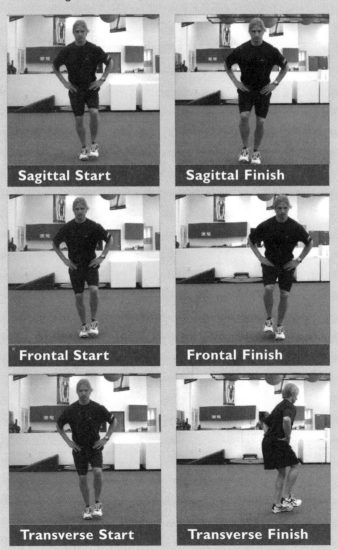

Sagittal Start   Sagittal Finish

Frontal Start   Frontal Finish

Transverse Start   Transverse Finish

Push-up with Rotation

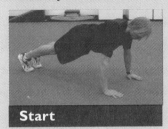

Start

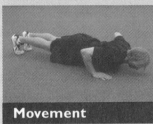

Movement

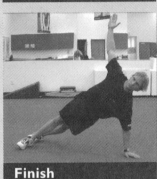

Finish

Preparation

1. Assume a push-up position with hands shoulder-width apart.

Movement

2. Draw abs in and activate glutes.
3. Slowly lower body, using control, and extend elbows, lifting body so it is perpendicular with the floor.
4. Rotate body to one side, raising arm toward ceiling. Stabilize for 2-4 seconds.
5. Return to start position.
6. Repeat on the other side.
7. Perform 10 repetitions.

Walking Lunge with Rotation

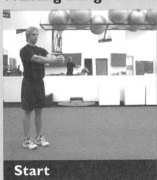

Start

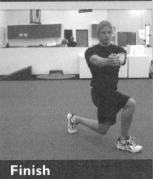

Finish

Preparation

1. Stand in proper alignment, with the hands held in front of the body.

Movement

3. Draw abs in and activate glutes.
3. While maintaining total body alignment, step forward (descending slowly) and bend at the hips, knees and ankles.
4. Slowly rotate at the spine toward the forward leg side.
5. Use hip and thigh muscles to push back up to take the next step.
6. As body is lifted, rotate spine back to the starting position.
7. Repeat on opposite side.
8. Perform 10 repetitions.

Prisoner Squat

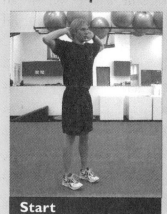

Start

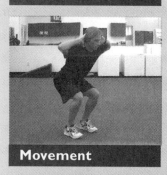

Movement

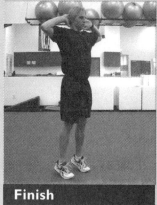

Finish

Preparation

1. Stand in proper alignment, with the hands behind the head.

Movement

2. Draw abs in and activate glutes.
3. Lower to a squat position, using control and without compensation.
4. Extend hips, knees and ankles to return to start position.
5. Raise onto toes.
6. Return to start position.
7. Perform 10 repetitions

MODULE 6-3 Summary

Flexibility training should be progressive, systematic and based on an assessment. There are three phases of flexibility training: corrective, active and functional.

Corrective flexibility improves muscle imbalances and altered joint motion by using static stretching and self-myofascial release. Active flexibility improves the extensibility of soft tissue and increases neuromuscular efficiency by using active-isolated stretching and self-myofascial release. Functional flexibility improves the extensibility of soft tissue and increases neuromuscular efficiency by using integrated, multiplanar techniques that move through the full range of motion.

Injuries most often occur in the transverse plane. If the appropriate soft tissue is not extensible through the full range of movement, the risk of injury dramatically increases. Health and fitness professionals should emphasize exercises that increase multiplanar soft tissue extensibility and have high levels of neuromuscular demand.

Each type of flexibility training consists of specific stretching techniques. Corrective flexibility uses self-myofascial release and static stretching; active flexibility uses self-myofascial release and active-isolated stretching; and functional flexibility uses self-myofascial release and dynamic stretching.

Self-myofascial release applies gentle pressure on muscle hypertonicity for 20-30 seconds. The force applied stimulates the Golgi tendon organ and creates autogenic inhibition, decreasing muscle spindle excitation and releasing the muscle hypertonicity. These techniques are suggested prior to static stretching and/or activity, as well as for cool-down.

Static stretching (the most popular form) passively takes a muscle to the point of tension and holds it there for a minimum of 20 seconds, thereby creating autogenic inhibition. These should be used prior to activity and to "reset" soft tissue following activity.

Active-isolated stretches use agonists and synergists to dynamically move joints into their ranges of motion. The reciprocal inhibition of the muscle being stretched allows for greater ranges of motion to be accessed. These are suggested for pre-activity warm-up (five to 10 repetitions, held for two to four seconds each).

Dynamic stretches use force production and momentum to take a joint through the full available range of motion. These are suggested for pre-activity warm-up as well.

MODULE 6-3 Quiz

1. Active flexibility uses the principle of:

   ☐ Reciprocal inhibition

   ☐ Autogenic inhibition

2. What tool is used in self-myofascial release?

   _____

3. Which form of flexibility utilizes self-myofascial release and active-isolated stretching?

   _____

4. Static stretches should be used for cool-down.

   ☐ True   ☐ False

5. Which type(s) of stretching stimulates the Golgi tendon organ which produces autogenic inhibition?

   _____

6. Dynamic stretching uses what to take a joint through the full available range of motion?

   ☐ Dumbbells

   ☐ Force production

   ☐ Passive motion

7. A supine straight-leg raise held for two to four seconds and repeated five to 10 times is an example of which type of stretching?

   ☐ Static

   ☐ Active-isolated

   ☐ Dynamic

8. Which type of flexibility uses dynamic stretching?

   _____

MODULE 6-4:
Practical Application of Flexibility Training

Current research has demonstrated that static stretching prior to activity decreases the rate of force production.[36,43,44] As such, static stretching is not advised prior to performing dynamic functional activities. Instead, it is more appropriate to perform a controlled dynamic functional warm-up prior to activity and save static stretching for the cool-down (Phases 3-7). If, however, an individual exhibits muscle imbalances, joint dysfunctions and postural distortions, corrective-flexibility exercises (self-myofascial release and static stretching) should be implemented prior to the controlled active/dynamic warm-up to ensure appropriate movement patterns and prevent relative flexibility (Phases 1 and 2).[4,5]

Flexibility for Postural Distortion Patterns

As previously mentioned, there are three main postural distortion patterns: lumbo-pelvic-hip complex, upper-extremity and lower-extremity. Proper flexibility is the first step to addressing these problems. Table 6-7 provides the common compensations seen during the assessment process, associated tight and weak muscles and corrective strategies for each. Chapter 8 (Core Training) and Chapter 9 (Balance Training) provide proper exercise technique for the core and balance exercises.

Table 6-7: Compensations, Muscle Imbalance and Corrective Strategies

Abnormal Movement	Tight Muscles	Weak Muscles	Corrective Strategy
Foot and Ankle Complex			
Feet Flatten	Gastrocnemius Peroneals	Gluteus Medius Anterior Tibialis Posterior Tibialis	**Foam Roll + Static/Active Stretch** Peroneals Gastrocnemius **Core Strengthening Exercises** Bridge **Balance Progression** Single-leg Balance Single-leg Balance Reach Single-leg Squat
Feet Turn Out	Soleus Biceps Femoris Piriformis	Gluteus Medius	**Foam Roll + Static/Active Stretch** Soleus Biceps Femoris Piriformis **Core Strengthening Exercises** Bridge **Balance Progression** Single-leg Balance Single-leg Balance Reach Single-leg Squat
Heels Elevate	Gastrocnemius Soleus Peroneals	Anterior Tibialis Posterior Tibialis	**Foam Roll + Static/Active Stretch** Peroneals Gastrocnemius/Soleus **Core Strengthening Exercises** Bridge **Balance Progression** Single leg Balance Single-leg Balance Reach
Knees			
Knees Adduct (Cave In)	Adductors Iliotibial Band	Gluteus Medius Gluteus Maximus	**Foam Roll + Static/Active Stretch** Adductors Iliotibial Band **Core Strengthening Exercises** Bridge **Balance Progression** Single-leg Balance Single-leg Balance Reach Single-leg Squat
Knees Abduct (Bow Out)	Biceps Femoris Iliopsoas Piriformis	Gluteus Medius Gluteus Maximus	**Foam Roll + Static/Active Stretch** Biceps Femoris Iliopsoas Piriformis **Core Strengthening Exercises** Bridge **Balance Progression** Single-leg Balance Single-leg Balance Reach Single-leg Squat

Table 6-7: Compensations, Muscle Imbalance and Corrective Strategies

Abnormal Movement	Tight Muscles	Weak Muscles	Corrective Strategy
Lumbo-pelvic-hip Complex			
Asymmetrical Weight Shifting	Gastrocnemius Soleus Biceps Femoris Adductors Iliotibial Band Iliopsoas Piriformis	Gluteus Medius Gluteus Maximus Transversus Abdominis Multifidi	**Foam Roll + Static/Active Stretch** Biceps Femoris Iliopsoas Piriformis **Core Strengthening Exercises** Bridge **Balance Progression** Single-leg Balance Single-leg Balance Reach Single-leg Squat
Low Back Arches (Anterior Tilt)	Iliopsoas Rectus Femoris Erector Spinae Latissimus Dorsi	Gluteus Maximus Gluteus Medius Lumbo-pelvic-hip Complex Stabilization Mechanism	**Foam Roll + Static/Active Stretch** Iliopsoas Rectus Femoris Erector Spinae Latissimus Dorsi **Core Strengthening Exercises** Marching Bridge **Balance Progression** Single-leg Balance Single-leg Balance Reach Single-leg Squat
Low Back Rounds (Posterior Tilt)	External Obliques Rectus Abdominis Hamstrings	Gluteus Maximus Gluteus Medius Lumbo-pelvic-hip Complex Stabilization Mechanism	**Foam Roll + Static/Active Stretch** External Obliques Rectus Abdominis Hamstrings **Core Strengthening Exercises** Bridge **Balance Progression** Single-leg Balance Single-leg Balance Reach Single-leg Squat
Abdomen Protrudes	Iliopsoas	Lumbo-pelvic-hip Complex Stabilization Mechanism	**Foam Roll + Static/Active Stretch** Iliopsoas **Core Strengthening Exercises** Marching Bridge **Balance Progression** Single-leg Balance Single-leg Balance Reach Single-leg Squat

Table 6-7: Compensations, Muscle Imbalance and Corrective Strategies

Abnormal Movement	Tight Muscles	Weak Muscles	Corrective Strategy
Shoulder Complex			
Arms Fall Forward (when overhead) or Lumbar Spine Hyperextends	Latissimus Dorsi Pectoralis Major	Middle/Lower Trapezius	**Foam Roll + Static/Active Stretch** Latissimus Dorsi Pectoralis Major **Core Strengthening Exercises** Prone Cobra Bridge **Balance** Single-leg Scaption
Elbows Flex (when arms are overhead)	Pectoralis Major	Middle/Lower Trapezius	**Foam Roll + Static/Active Stretch** Pectoralis Major **Core Strengthening Exercises** Prone Cobra **Balance** Single-leg Scaption
Shoulder Blade Protracted (Rounded Shoulders)	Pectoralis Major/Minor Latissimus Dorsi	Rhomboids Middle/Lower Trapezius Teres Minor Infraspinatus	**Foam Roll + Static/Active Stretch** Pectoralis Major/Minor Latissimus Dorsi **Core Strengthening Exercise** Prone Cobra **Balance** Single-leg Scaption
Shoulder Elevated	Upper Trapezius Levator Scapulae	Lower Trapezius	**Static/Active Stretch** Upper Trapezius Levator **Core Strengthening Exercise** Prone Cobra **Balance** Single-leg Scaption
Cervical Spine			
Forward Head	Sternocleido-mastoid Scalenes	Deep Cervical Flexors (Longus Coli/Capitus)	**Static/Active Stretch** Sternocleidomastoid Scalenes **Core Strengthening Exercise** Keep Chin Tucked

Filling in the Template

Following a fitness assessment, the flexibility portion of the template can now be filled in. On the template, select the form of flexibility your client requires. Go to the warm-up section and insert the appropriate stretches to be incorporated into the routine.

For most first-time clients and those requiring correction of postural imbalance, corrective flexibility is used prior to and following training sessions (as well as at home, on off days). Be sure to follow the flexibility guidelines for postural distortion patterns found in this chapter. Corrective flexibility will be

NASM — NATIONAL ACADEMY OF SPORTS MEDICINE

Optimum Performance Training

NAME	John Smith	**DATE**	March 10, 2004
TRAINER	Chere	**PHASE**	2: Integrated Stabilization Training
DAYS/WEEK	3	**GOAL**	Fat loss

CARDIO TRAINING	TIME		EQUIPMENT

WARM-UP/FLEXIBILITY	Sets	Reps	Duration	Rest	Notes
1. SMR: Calves, IT band, adductors	1				Hold tender spots 20-30 sec.
2.					
3. Static Stretching: Calves, hip flexors, lats	1		30 sec.		
4.					

CORE and BALANCE	Sets	Reps	Tempo	Rest	Notes
1.					
2.					
3.					
4.					
5.					

REACTIVE	Sets	Reps	Tempo	Rest	Notes
1.					
2.					

SPEED, AGILITY, QUICKNESS	Sets	Reps	Tempo	Rest	Notes
1.					
2.					

STRENGTH	Exercises	Sets	Reps	Intensity	Tempo	Rest	Notes
TOTAL BODY							
CHEST							
BACK							
SHOULDERS							
BICEPS							
TRICEPS							
LEGS							

COOL-DOWN	
POST-WORKOUT FLEXIBILITY	Static Stretching: Calves, adductors, hip flexors, pectorals

Figure 6-9: OPT™ Template

used during the first two phases of the OPT™ model.

With a proper progression through the flexibility continuum (and as the client's ability dictates), active and functional flexibility can be implemented later in strength and power levels of the OPT™ model.

The use of flexibility techniques can be a great warm-up as well as a cool-down, especially the self-myofascial release, and corrective flexibility techniques. On the template, go to the cool-down section (at the bottom) and select one or more modes: corrective flexibility, active flexibility, functional flexibility or other (which may consist of cardiovascular activity, if appropriate) (Figure 6-7).

MODULE 6-4 Summary

Current research shows that static stretching actually decreases the rate of force production, if done before activity. So, it is best to do a controlled, dynamic, functional warm-up first and cool-down with static stretching, unless an individual exhibits muscle imbalances, joint dysfunctions and postural distortions. If so, static stretching should be performed before the controlled, active/dynamic warm-up to prevent relative flexibility.

Proper flexibility is the first step to addressing three main postural distortion patterns: lumbo-pelvic-hip, upper-extremity and lower-extremity.

To fill out the warm-up flexibility portion of the template, select the form of flexibility the client requires: corrective, active or functional. First-time clients will use corrective flexibility before and after sessions. Be sure to follow the flexibility guidelines for postural distortion patterns found in this chapter. Active and functional flexibility can be implemented in the strength and power levels of the OPT™ model.

To fill out the cool-down flexibility portion of the template, select one or more modes: corrective flexibility, active flexibility, functional flexibility or other.

MODULE 6-4 Quiz

1. An athlete should do static stretching as a warm-up prior to dynamic activity?

    ☐ True   ☐ False

2. A pectoral ball stretch is a good static stretch for which kind of postural distortion(s)?

    ☐ Lumbo-pelvic-hip   ☐ Upper-extremity   ☐ Lower-extremity

3. The kneeling hip flexor/quadriceps stretch is appropriate for which postural distortion(s)?

    ☐ Lumbo-pelvic-hip   ☐ Upper-extremity   ☐ Lower-extremity

References

1   Alter MJ. *Science of flexibility.* 2nd edition. Champaign, IL: Human Kinetics; 1996.

2. Bandy WD, Irion JM, Briggler M. The effect of time and frequency of static stretching on flexibility of the hamstring muscles. *Phys Ther Abstract* Oct 1997;77(10):1090-6.

3. Clanton TO, Coupe KJ. Hamstring strains in athletes: diagnosis and treatment. *J Am Acad Orthop Surg* Jul-Aug 1998;6(4):237-48.

4. Clark MA. *Integrated flexibility training.* Thousand Oaks, CA: National Academy of Sports Medicine; 2001.

5. Clark MA. *Integrated training for the new millennium.* Thousand Oaks, CA: National Academy of Sports Medicine; 2000.

6. Condon SA. Soleus muscle electromyographic activity and ankle dorsiflexion range of motion during four stretching procedures. *Phys Ther* 1987;67:24-30.

7. Chaitow L. *Muscle energy techniques.* New York: Churchill Livingstone; 1997.

8. Clark MA. *Integrated neuromuscular stabilization training.* Thousand Oaks, CA: National Academy of Sports Medicine; 2001.

9. Janda V. Muscle spasm — a proposed procedure for differential diagnosis. *Man Med* 199;6136-9.

10. Liebension C. Integrating rehabilitation into chiropractic practice (blending active and passive care). Chapter 2. In: Liebenson C (ed). *Rehabilitation of the spine.* Baltimore: Williams and Wilkins; 1996.

11. Poterfield J, DeRosa C. *Mechanical low back pain; perspectives in functional anatomy.* Philadelphia: WB Saunders; 1991.

12. Gossman MR, Sahrman SA, Rose SJ. Review of length-associated changes in muscle: experimental evidence and clinical implications. *Phys Ther* 1982;62:1799-1808.

13. Halbertsma JPK, Van Bulhuis AI, Goeken LNH. Sport stretching: effect on passive muscle stiffness of short hamstrings. *Arch Phys Med Rehabil* 1996;77(7):688-92.

14. Holcomb WR. Improved stretching with proprioceptive neuromuscular facilitation. *J NSCA* 2000;22(1):59-61.

15. Moore MA, Kukulka CG. Depression of hoffmann reflexes following voluntary contraction and implications for proprioceptive neuromuscular facilitation therapy. *Phys Ther* Apr 1991;71(4):321-9.

16. Moore MA. Electromyographic investigation of muscle stretching techniques. *Med Sci Sports Exerc* 1980;12:322-9.

17. Sady SP, Wortman M, Blanke D. Flexibility training: ballistic, static, or proprioceptive neuromuscular facilitation? *Arch Phys Med Rehabil* Jun 1982;63(6):261-3.

18. Sherrington C. *The integrative action of the nervous system.* New Haven, CT: Yale University Press; 1947.

19. Wang RY. Effect of proprioceptive neuromuscular facilitation on the gait of patients with hemiplegia of long and short duration. *Phys Ther* Dec 1994;74(12):1108-15.

20. Bachrach RM. Psoas: dysfunction/insufficiency, sacroiliac dysfunction and low back pain. Chapter 25. In Vleeming A, Mooney V, Dorman T, Snijders C, Stoeckart R (eds). *Movement, stability and low back pain.* London: Churchill Livingstone; 1997.

21. Cohen H. *Neuroscience for rehabilitation.* 2nd edition. Philadelphia: Lippincott Williams & Wilkins; 1999.

22. Liebension C. Active rehabilitation protocols. Chapter 18. In: Liebension C (ed). *Rehabilitation of the spine.* Baltimore: Williams & Wilkins; 1996.

23. Milner-Brown A. *Neuromuscular physiology.* Thousand Oaks, CA: National Academy of Sports Medicine; 2001.

24. Fox SI. *Human physiology.* 5th edition. Dubuque, IA: Wm. C. Brown Publishers; 1996.

25. Vander A, Sherman J, Luciano D. *Human physiology: the mechanisms of body function.* 8th edition. New York: McGraw-Hill; 2001.

26. Enoka RM. *Neuromechanical basis of kinesiology.* 2nd edition. Champaign, IL: Human Kinetics; 1994.

27. McClosky DJ. Kinesthetic sensibility. *Physiol Rev* 1978; 58:763-820.

28. Grigg P. Peripheral neural mechanisms in proprioception. *J Sports Rehab* 1994;3:2-17.

29. Janda V. In: Grant R (ed). *Physical therapy of the cervical and thoracic spine.* Edinburgh: Churchill Livingstone; 1988.

30. Lewitt K. *Manipulation in rehabilitation of the locomotor system.* London: Butterworths; 1993.

31. Leahy PM. Active release techniques: Logical soft tissue treatment. Chapter 17. In: Hammer WI (ed). *Functional soft tissue examination and treatment by manual methods.* Gaithersburg, MD: Aspen Publishers, Inc.; 1999.

32. Spencer AM. *Practical podiatric orthopedic procedures.* Cleveland: Ohio College of Podiatric Medicine; 1978.

33. Woo SLY, Buckwalter JA. *Injury and repair of the musculoskeletal soft tissues.* American Academy of Orthopedic Surgeons; 1987.

34. Zairns B. Soft tissue injury and repair-biomechanical aspects. *Int Journal Sports Med* 1982;3:9-11.

35. Beaulieu JA. Developing a stretching program. *Physic Sports Med* 1981;9:59.

36. Evjenth O, Hamburg J. *Muscle stretching in manual therapy — a clinical manual.* Alfta, Sweden: Alfta Rehab; 1984.

37. Tannigawa M. Comparison of the hold-relax procedure and passive mobilization on increasing muscle length. *Phys Ther* 1972;52:725.

38. Voss DE, Ionla MK, Meyers BJ. *Proprioceptive neuromuscular facilitation.* 3rd edition. Philadelphia: Harper and Row Publishers; 1985.

39. Akeson WH, Woo SLY. The connective tissue response to immobility: biochemical changes in periarticular connective tissue of the immobilized rabbit knee. *Clin Orthoped Rel Res* 1973;93:356-62.

40. Sapega A, Quedenfeld T, Moyer R. Biophysical factors in range of motion exercises. *Phys Sports Med* 1981;9:57.

41. Etnyre BR, Abraham LD. Gains in range of ankle dorsiflexion using three popular stretching techniques. *Am J Phys Med* 1986;65:189.

42. Barnes JF. Myofascial release. In: Hammer WI (ed). *Functional soft tissue examination and treatment by manual methods.* 2nd edition. Chapter 16. Gaithersburg, MD: Aspen Publishers, Inc; 1999.

43. Brieg A, Troup JDG. Biomechanical considerations in the straight leg raising test. *Spine* 1974;4:243-50.

44. Donatelli R, Owens-Burkhart H. Effects of immobilization on the extensibility of periarticular connective tissue. *JOSPT* 1981;3:67.

CHAPTER SEVEN

Cardiorespiratory Training Concepts

Objectives

After studying this chapter, you will be able to:

- Define cardiorespiratory training.
- Describe how cardiorespiratory training is used within an integrated training program.
- Provide the guidelines for proper cardiorespiratory training.
- Design cardiorespiratory training programs for a variety of clients.
- Perform and instruct appropriate cardiorespiratory techniques.

Key Terms

- Cardiorespiratory training
- General warm-up
- Specific warm-up
- Frequency
- Intensity
- Time
- Type
- Enjoyment
- Excess post-exercise oxygen consumption (EPOC)

MODULE 7-1: Current Concepts in Cardiorespiratory Training

The flexibility portion of the OPT™ model has been completed. The next component to be filled out is the second portion of the warm-up section: cardiovascular activity (often referred to as cardio). Within this text, we will also refer to this as **cardiorespiratory training**.

Cardiorespiratory training is simply training that involves and places a stress on the cardiorespiratory system. This means that any form of activity (walking on a treadmill, playing basketball, weight training, etc.) can be used as a form of cardiorespiratory training.[1] This is a major concept that can be used to the health and fitness professional's advantage, allowing him/her to maximize the efficiency of the time spent with a client.

> **CARDIO-RESPIRATORY TRAINING:** Any physical activity that involves and places stress on the cardiorespiratory system.

Why is Cardiorespiratory Training Important?

All exercise, regardless of the duration and/or intensity, must utilize the cardiorespiratory system to either sustain the activity and/or recuperate from it.[2,3] Cardiorespiratory exercise in the fitness industry is traditionally viewed as requiring a certain piece of equipment (such as the treadmill, stationary bicycle or even "aerobics" classes). In this case, cardiorespiratory training becomes a separate component of an overall workout program that is used in a few distinct ways. These include:

- Warm-up
- Cool-down
- Workout

The following sections will review each of these forms of cardiorespiratory training, their importance and examples of traditional as well as integrated approaches.

Forms of Cardiorespiratory Training
Warm-up

A warm-up is generally described as a preparing of the body for physical activity. It can be either general in nature or more specific to the activity.[4,5] A **general warm-up** consists of movements that do not necessarily have any movement specificity to the actual activity to be performed. (Examples include warming up by walking on a treadmill or riding a stationary bicycle prior to weight training.) A **specific warm-up** consists of movements that more closely mimic those of the actual activity. (Examples include performing body-weight squats and push-ups prior to weight training.)

The proposed benefits of a warm-up are outlined in Table 7-1.[2,4-6]

There is speculation as to whether a warm-up is helpful in the prevention of musculoskeletal injury. While some researchers claim benefits to a warm-up, others show no change between the use of a warm-up prior to exercise and no warm-up.[7-9] It is proposed, however, that while a warm-up may not be directly associated to injury prevention, it may be beneficial for enhancing overall performance, as indicated by the benefits listed above. In this case, better overall function of the kinetic chain may allow for more efficient and effective movement patterns and thus decrease the chance of future injuries.

Warm-ups have been shown to have a possible inhibitory effect on the accumulation of intercellular acidosis during subsequent exercise bouts.[10] Acidosis is the accumulation of excessive hydrogen (H+) that causes increased acidity (pH) of the blood and muscle that is related to (but, not caused by)

GENERAL WARM-UP: Low-intensity exercise consisting of movements that do not necessarily relate to the more intense exercise that is to follow.

SPECIFIC WARM-UP: Low-intensity exercise consisting of movements that mimic those that will be included in the more intense exercise that is to follow.

Table 7-1: Benefits and Effects of a Warm-up

Benefits	Effects
Increased heart and respiratory rate	Increases cardiorespiratory system's capacity to perform work
	Increases blood flow to active muscle tissue
	Increases the oxygen exchange capacity
Increased tissue temperature	Increases rate of muscle contraction
	Increases efficiency of opposing muscle contraction and relaxation
	Increases metabolic rate
	Increases the soft tissue extensibility
Increased psychological preparation for bouts of exercise	Increases the mental readiness of an individual

lactic acid.[2] Increased acidic levels have been associated with neuromuscular fatigue.[2,11] In turn, neuromuscular fatigue can lead to a decrease in the ability of a muscle to produce sufficient amounts of force.[12,13] The inability of muscles to produce proper levels of force can lead to altered recruitment patterns.[14-17] This can further lead to synergistic dominance and potential injury.[18-24] Thus, a warm-up may provide protection from an injury and should be viewed as an important component of a complete workout.

Practical Application for a Warm-up

NASM suggests that the cardiorespiratory portion of a warm-up should last five to 10 minutes at a low-to-moderate intensity. However, depending on the client's goals and objectives, this can be altered. Furthermore, the cardiorespiratory portion of a warm-up is usually considered a general warm-up. A complete warm-up should include a general and a specific warm-up. A first-time client, with excessive postural distortion patterns, may initially (the first one to three workouts) spend half of the workout time on the warm-up. Table 7-2 provides examples of suggested warm-ups utilizing flexibility and cardiorespiratory exercise for a client in the stabilization level (Phases 1 and 2) of the OPT™ model.

Once a client has demonstrated an understanding of the techniques necessary for self-myofascial release (foam rolling) and static stretching and operation of the cardiorespiratory equipment, he/she should begin performing this warm-up prior to time spent with the health and fitness professional. This should take place after the first one to three sessions (or as the health and fitness professional deems appropriate). This will then allow for increased

Table 7-2: Warm-up for the Stabilization Level Client

Components	Examples	Time
Self-myofascial Release (pre-warm-up flexibility)	Gastrocnemius/Soleus Iliotibial Band Glutes/Piriformis Latissimus Dorsi	5-10 minutes
Cardiorespiratory	Elliptical Trainers Steppers Treadmills Bicycles	5-10 minutes
Static Stretching	Gastrocnemius/Soleus Adductors Iliopsoas Latissimus Dorsi Pectoralis Major/Minor	10-15 minutes

training time in which to focus on other aspects of the training program.

It is very important that the health and fitness professional have a full understanding of the proper cardiorespiratory and flexibility techniques, as his/her demonstration will determine the success of the client. It is imperative to provide clear and concise instructions to the client to allow for proper assimilation of the information

Table 7-3 provides an example warm-up for the client who has progressed to the strength level (Phases 3, 4 and 5) of the OPT™ model.

Table 7-4 provides a sample warm-up for the client who has progressed to the power level (Phases 6 and 7) of the OPT™ model. Bear in mind that traditional

Table 7-3: Warm-up for the Strength Level Client

Components	Examples	Time
Self-myofascial Release (pre-warm-up flexibility)	Gastrocnemius/Soleus Iliotibial Band Glutes/Piriformis Latissimus Dorsi	5-10 minutes
Cardiorespiratory	Elliptical Trainers Steppers Treadmills Bicycles	5-10 minutes
Active-isolated Stretching	Gastrocnemius/Soleus Adductors Iliopsoas Latissimus Dorsi Pectoralis Major/Minor	3-5 minutes

Table 7-4: Warm-up for the Power Level Client (Dynamic, Functional Warm-up)		
Components	**Examples**	**Time**
Self-myofascial Release (pre-warm-up flexibility)	Gastrocnemius/Soleus Iliotibial Band Glutes/Piriformis Latissimus Dorsi	5-10 minutes
Dynamic Stretching (10 repetitions of each)	Prisoner Squat Walking Lunge with Twist Push-up with Rotation Tube Walking Medicine Ball Rotation: PNF Single-leg Squat Multiplanar Hop	10 minutes

cardiorespiratory exercises may not be necessary in this form of a warm-up because the listed dynamic stretches can be performed in a circuit (performing one exercise after the other), providing an ample cardiorespiratory warm-up.

It should be reemphasized that a warm-up should prepare the body for an activity, not fatigue the body before the activity begins. Again, this can lead to altered muscle recruitment and detract from the purpose of proper training. Keeping the activity to a moderate duration and intensity level will help ensure a proper warm-up.

Cool-down

A cool-down provides the body with a smooth transition from exercise back to a steady state of rest. In essence, a cool-down is the opposite of the warm-up. This portion of a workout is often overlooked and viewed as less important than the other components.[2] However, proper use of a cool-down can have a significant impact on a client's overall health. Sufficient time for a cool-down period is approximately five to 10 minutes.[25] The proposed benefits of a cool-down are shown in Figure 7-1.[2,4,6,25,26]

Practical Application for a Cool-down

If an individual is performing cardiorespiratory exercise for an extended period of time, it will be vital that he/she slowly decrease the intensity of the exercise (40-50 percent of maximum heart rate) and work at this lowered intensity for five to 10 minutes. This will help in gradually decreasing the heart rate back down to a resting state. It will also ensure that blood does not pool to the lower extremities, leading to dizziness and/or possible fainting.

- **May improve flexibility**
- **Removes waste by-products, via the blood**
- **Minimizes muscle soreness**
- **Allows cardiorespiratory system to respond to lower demand**
- **Avoids dizziness and or possible fainting**
- **Provides an emotional balance following exercise stress**

Figure 7-1: Benefits of a Cool-down

Flexibility is also an important component to be utilized in the cool-down. Because one of the goals of a cool-down is to relax muscles and bring them back to their original resting length after a workout, corrective stretching (self-myofascial release and static stretching) would be the appropriate form of stretching during a cool-down.

The first one to three workouts (or more, if deemed appropriate by the health and fitness professional) should be monitored for completeness and technique with a first-time client. Once the client and the health and fitness professional feel confident that the proper techniques are being employed, the cool-down can be performed on the client's own time.

It is important for the client to understand the importance of both the warm-up and the cool-down. This helps to alleviate any anxiety on the part of the client and/or health and fitness professional that not enough time is being dedicated to the "workout." As the client is capable of a greater workload and requires more time for the "workout," the warm-up and cool-down can be performed before and after the workout by the client independently.

Decreases
- **Daily fatigue**
- **Anxiety**
- **Depression**
- **Coronary artery disease (CAD)**
- **Hypertension**
- **Noninsulin dependent diabetes mellitus**
- **Cancer**
- **Osteoporosis**
- **Obesity**

Increases
- **Flexibility (potentially)**
- **Work, recreational and sports performance**
- **Sense of well-being**
- **Blood lipid profile**
- **Insulin sensitivity**
- **Glucose tolerance**
- **Immunity**

Figure 7-2: Benefits of Cardiorespiratory Activities and/or Exercise

Cardiorespiratory Training as a Workout

Most people who perform cardiorespiratory exercise are looking for improvements in their health and/or fitness levels. However, it has been suggested that there is a difference between the level of activity required for health versus that necessary for increased fitness.[27-32] It is viewed that activity levels that may not necessarily produce significant improvements in fitness may have marked effects on health.[30] In either scenario, cardiorespiratory activities and/or exercise have a profound effect on the overall physical and mental health of a participant summarized in Table 7-2.[1,27-35]

These benefits accrue as the result of many physiological adaptations to cardiorespiratory training. The adaptations are summarized in Table 7-5.

Table 7-5: Adaptations to Cardiorespiratory Training	
Variable	**Response**
VO$_2$ max	Increase
Stroke volume	Increase
Cardiac output	Increase
Oxidative capacity of muscle	Increase
Resting heart rate	Decrease
Exercising heart rate	Decrease

MODULE 7-1 Summary

In the fitness industry, cardiorespiratory exercise is typically associated with certain pieces of equipment. However, the cardiorespiratory system is used to either sustain or recover from all physical activity. Integrated cardiorespiratory training is simply training that involves and places a stress on the cardiorespiratory system. Thus, any form of activity can be used as a form of cardiorespiratory training.

Cardiorespiratory training can be used as the warm-up, cool-down or as the workout itself. Regardless of a client's goals, cardiorespiratory training should be incorporated into the program.

A warm-up prepares the body for physical activity and can be either general in nature or more specific to the activity. Typically, the cardiorespiratory portion of a warm-up should last five to 10 minutes at a low-to-moderate intensity.

A cool-down of five to 10 minutes provides the body with an essential transition from exercise back to a steady state of rest. Flexibility (corrective stretching) is also an important component of the cool-down to bring muscles back to their original resting length after a workout.

Once a client has demonstrated an understanding of proper technique, he/she can begin performing the warm-up and cool-down alone, prior to and after time spent with the health and fitness professional.

By using a variety of methods to incorporate cardiorespiratory training into one's exercise routine, the health and fitness professional can effectively ensure optimum health in clients, maximize results by minimizing the body's ability to adapt, increase enjoyment of each training session, maximize the personalized aspect of program design and increase retention and referrals.

MODULE 7-1 Quiz

1. All exercise, regardless of the duration and/or intensity, must utilize the cardiorespiratory system to either sustain the activity and/or recuperate from it.

   ☐ True   ☐ False

2. Why aren't traditional cardiorespiratory exercises necessary in the warm-up of the power level?

   _____

   _____

   _____

3. A cool-down ensures that blood does not pool in the _____ extremities, leading to dizziness and/or possible fainting.

   ☐ upper
   ☐ lower

4. One adaptive benefit of cardiorespiratory exercise is that it
   ☐ **increases** ☐ **decreases** resting heart rate and
   ☐ **increases** ☐ **decreases** exercising heart rate.

MODULE 7-2: General Guidelines for Cardiorespiratory Training

Any form of training must have certain guidelines to allow for the development of a proper program. These guidelines also serve to quantify activity.[1,33] For these purposes, NASM uses the F.I.T.T.E. factors (Figure 7-3).[1,33,36]

F	Frequency
I	Intensity
T	Time
T	Type
E	Enjoyment

Figure 7-3: The F.I.T.T.E. Factors

Frequency

Frequency refers to the number of training sessions or activity sessions for a given timeframe. The timeframe usually consists of a week. But, depending on the client and his/her goals, it may be one workout, a day, a month or a year. For general health requirements (Table 7-6), the recommended frequency of activity is preferably every day of the week, for small quantities of time.[27] For improved fitness levels, the frequency is three to five days per week (Table 7-7).[1,33]

FREQUENCY:
The number of training sessions in a given timeframe.

Intensity

Intensity refers to the level of demand the activity places on the body. This is usually measured by heart rate and/or maximal oxygen consumption (VO_2 max).[1,33] For general health requirements (Table 7-6), moderate intensity is preferred.[27] This would be perceived as enough demand to increase heart and respiratory rates, but not cause exhaustion or breathlessness.[1,33] For improved fitness levels (Table 7-7), the intensity recommended is 40-85 percent of heart rate reserve (HRR) or 60-90 percent of maximal heart rate (HR max).[1,33]

INTENSITY:
The level of demand that a given activity places on the body.

Time

Time refers to the length of time engaged in the activity. This is usually measured in minutes. For general health requirements (Table 7-6), approximately 30 total minutes a day is recommended.[27] This could be six five-minute bouts, three 10-minute bouts or two 15-minute bouts (or any other combination equaling 30 minutes). For improved fitness levels (Table 7-7), the time recommended is approximately 20-60 minutes.[1,33] This will vary, depending on the goal.

TIME:
The length of time an individual is engaged in a given activity.

Type

Type refers to the mode or activity utilized. This can be virtually any activity. For general health requirements, this may consist of:

- Using stairs (versus elevators)
- Parking farther from the desired location and walking a longer distance
- Mowing the yard with a push mower
- Raking leaves by hand
- Gardening
- Dancing

For improved fitness levels, this may consist of:

- Treadmill, stationary bike, stepper, etc.
- Aerobic classes
- Sports
- Weight training

Enjoyment

Enjoyment refers to the amount of pleasure derived from the activity by the client. This is often an overlooked component of program design by the health and fitness professional. One of the most important aspects of creating a program is that it fits with a client's personality and interests. This does not mean that the client dictates what it is that a health and fitness professional does.

One of the most important components of a properly designed training program is that it must be enjoyable. This means that the program and its activities must coincide with the personality, likes and dislikes of the client. This translates into compliance, and that will equal results. A client is much more apt to continue with a program that is fun and challenging. By complying with a structured program, the client will achieve the desired results. This ultimately allows for higher level of retention, results and referrals. For the health and fitness professional, this means having a drastic impact on the life of another human being.

Recommendations

Exercise parameters used for improved health have been shown to differ from those that are recommended for improved fitness levels (Tables 7-6 and 7-7).[27-33] The benefits from exercise (listed earlier in Figure 7-2), however, can be derived from the general health guidelines listed in Table 7-6. This is important for the health and fitness professional to realize, especially for first time and/or deconditioned clients. Any activity above what the client is currently involved in will produce some benefit.

Table 7-6: General Health Activity Recommendations				
Frequency	**Intensity**	**Time**	**Type**	**Enjoyment**
5-7 days per week	Moderate (enough to increase heart and respiration rates)	30 minutes total per day	General activities: Walking Using stairs Dancing Mowing the yard	The higher, the better

Table 7-7: Improved Fitness Recommendations				
Frequency	**Intensity**	**Time**	**Type**	**Enjoyment**
5-7 days per week	40-85% VO_2 max or 60-90% HR max	20-60 minutes per day	Any activity	The higher, the better

The fitness guidelines shown in Table 7-7 may be too extreme for the beginning client. Many clients will not be able to perform the fitness level guidelines for integrated cardiorespiratory training of 20 minutes at 60 percent of HR max for three to five days per week. However, accumulating a total 30 minutes of exercise per day over a five-to-seven-day period may be more attainable. It has been shown that performing three 10-minute bouts of exercise is just as effective as one 30-minute continuous bout of the same exercise.[37-39] Also, exercising at lower intensities (40 percent of VO_2 max) has been shown to be beneficial for sedentary people, when compared to higher intensities (80 percent of VO_2 max) for general health and fitness purposes.[40]

MODULE 7-2 Summary

The F.I.T.T.E. guidelines allow for the development of a proper program and quantify its variables. Recommendations are listed below.

Frequency: Almost every day of the week for short quantities of time.

Intensity: Moderate enough to increase heart and respiratory rates.

Time: 20-60 total minutes a day, depending on goals.

Type: Any kind of activity from gardening to weight training.

Enjoyment: The program and its activities should coincide with the personality, likes and dislikes of the client.

MODULE 7-2 Quiz

1. A timeframe can consist of a day, month or year, depending on the client's goals.

    ☐ True   ☐ False

2. How is intensity usually measured?

    _____

3. It has been shown that performing three 10-minute bouts of exercise is just as effective as one 30-minute continuous bout of the same exercise.

    ☐ True   ☐ False

4. For the general health and fitness of sedentary individuals, exercising at ☐ **lower** ☐ **higher** intensities has been shown to be more beneficial than ☐ **lower** ☐ **higher** intensities.

MODULE 7-3:

Cardiorespiratory Training and its Relation to Appearance

The Myth of the "Fat Burning" Zone

While many clients and health and fitness professionals realize the overall benefits of cardiorespiratory exercise, the primary manner in which it is utilized is as a workout, to reduce body fat. It is generally assumed that body fat reduction can only result from extended periods of time on a piece of cardio equipment (or in an aerobic classes). There is still a popular trend of thinking that suggests there is a magical "fat burning" zone for exercise. However, body fat reduction can only take place when there is more energy being burned than consumed. This is known as the *Law of Thermodynamics*.[2] To gain a better insight into effectively using cardiorespiratory training and its role in fat loss, the mystique of the "fat burning" zone must be eliminated.

Cardiorespiratory training, as with any other form of training, falls under the principle of specificity. Typically, the "fat burning" zone is thought of as the time when body is mainly using fat as fuel. However, to design appropriate cardiorespiratory training programs, the energy systems used at different generalized heart rate zones must be examined.

Fat and glucose are major sources of fuel for exercise. In order for them to be used more efficiently, the body must be able to receive enough oxygen (O_2). Oxygen allows fat and glucose to be "burned" as fuel. This, in turn, produces the waste products of carbon dioxide (CO_2) and water. (Think of this like a car burning gasoline, with the body's "exhaust" being CO_2 and water.)

The amount of O_2 and CO_2 exchanged in the lungs normally equals that used and released by body tissues. This allows the body to use these respiratory gasses to estimate caloric expenditure. The method is called indirect calorimetry. It can be measured with a metabolic analyzer to detect an individual's respiratory exchange ratio (RER). RER is the ratio of CO_2 produced to the volume of O_2 consumed.[2]

Table 7-8 gives a guide for determining how many of the calories burned come from carbohydrates and fats.[41] To estimate the amount of energy used by the body, first determine the type of energy sources (carbohydrate, fat or protein) that are being oxidized (or burned for energy). The fact that fat and carbohydrates differ in the amount of oxygen used (in addition to the fact that carbon dioxide is produced during oxidization) can help to determine what kind of fuel is being used.

Table 7-8: Respiratory Exchange Ratio (RER) and the Percentage of Calories Derived from Fats and CHO		
RER	**% from Carbohydrates**	**% from Fats**
0.71	0.0	100.0
0.75	15.6	84.4
0.80	33.4	66.6
0.85	50.7	49.3
0.90	67.5	32.5
0.95	84.0	16.0
1.00	100.0	0.0

RER = VCO_2 / VO_2 measured at a steady state of exercise

The body uses the highest percent of its fuel from fat when the body has a RER of 0.71 (Table 7-8). If the body uses a maximal percent of its fuel from fat at 0.71 RER, then why shouldn't an individual exercise at this level all the time? The answer lies in the fact that the only time the body can be at 0.71 RER is when it is at complete rest. This is how the fat burning zone originated. Though the percentage of fat being burned is maximal, the amount of energy used (and calories burned) is minimal and, therefore, not very productive for the goal of weight/fat loss. Remember, it is not how much fat an individual burns that ultimately dictates body fat reduction. Instead, it is how many calories are burned.

Excess Post-exercise Oxygen Consumption (EPOC)

One of the main objectives of the human body is to expend as little energy as possible. In order to do so, it must readily adapt to the demands placed upon it. Fortunately, the human body is a highly adaptable organism, with the capability to streamline physical and mental demands over time, using minimal energy.[42-46] A health and fitness professional must understand this principle and be able to utilize it in order to produce desirable results in the client.

One way a health and fitness professional can combat this is by maximizing the caloric expenditure of a training session. This is made easier by maximizing the O_2 consumption needed for the duration of (as well as the recovery from) the training session. This recovery oxygen consumption is known as **excess post-exercise oxygen consumption (EPOC)**.

EPOC is simply the state where the body's metabolism is elevated following exercise.[2,47] This means that the body is burning more calories following exercise than before the exercise was initiated. Think of EPOC as a caloric afterburner that is caused by exercise (much like a car engine stays warm for a period of time after it has been driven). Following exercise, the body must utilize increased amounts of oxygen to replenish energy supplies, lower tissue temperature and return the body to a resting state.[2,47]

EXCESS POST-EXERCISE OXYGEN CONSUMPTION (EPOC): Elevation of the body's metabolism following exercise.

Research has indicated that the higher the intensity (percentage of VO_2 max and/or percentage of HR max) of the training session, the greater the magnitude of EPOC.[48-50] Furthermore, it has been shown that splitting the training session into multiple sessions (usually two) of equal time has the greatest effect on EPOC.[49-52]

MODULE 7-3 Summary

When the goal is body fat reduction, the key is to focus on burning calories, not burning fat. To do this, it must be determined what percentage of calories being burned come from carbohydrates and fats.

Oxygen allows fat and glucose to be "burned" as fuel. A metabolic analyzer can be used to detect an individual's respiratory exchange ratio (RER). RER is the ratio of carbon dioxide produced to the volume of oxygen consumed. Once RER is determined, the caloric percentages can be figured out.

The body is designed to expend as little energy as possible. This can be avoided by maximizing the caloric expenditure of a training session and thus, the excess post-exercise oxygen consumption (EPOC). The body will continue to burn more calories following exercise than before exercise was initiated. Increased intensity and splitting training sessions into multiple sessions will both result in higher EPOC.

MODULE 7-3 Quiz

1. The Law of Thermodynamics states that body fat reduction can only take place when there is more _____ being burned than consumed.

2. The amount of O_2 and CO_2 exchanged in the lungs is normally _____ that used and released by body tissues?
    - ☐ Less than
    - ☐ Equal to
    - ☐ Greater than

3. When is the only time that the body can be at 0.71 RER?

    _____

4. Following exercise, the body must utilize increased amounts of oxygen to replenish energy supplies, raise tissue temperature and return the body to a resting state.
    - ☐ True   ☐ False

MODULE 7-4:
Cardiorespiratory Training Modalities

Cardiorespiratory training, as with any other form of training, falls under the General Adaptation Syndrome and the Principle of Specificity. This means that the body will adapt to the level of stressed placed upon it and will then require more or varied amounts of stress to produce a higher level of adaptation carryover. A cardiorespiratory training program for a client who may desire adaptations for weekend sports will probably be different than a client who desires general conditioning. The variance of the cardiorespiratory training program will place a different demand on the bioenergetic continuum and will ultimately affect the client's adaptations and goals. There are several methods of incorporating cardiorespiratory exercise into a client's program. As such, stage training and circuit training will be discussed below.

Stage Training

In order to ensure continual adaptation, cardiorespiratory training programs must be designed to progress in an organized fashion and to minimize the risk of over-training and injury.[53] This is the basis behind the stage training system.

Stage training is a three-stage programming system that uses different heart rate training zones based on one's RER. Those zones are organized to maximize cardiorespiratory training benefits. The three different stages of cardiorespiratory training mimic the three stages of training seen in the OPT™ model. Each stage will help to create a strong cardiorespiratory base to build on in subsequent stages.

Table 7-9: Respiratory Exchange Ratio (RER) and Heart Rate Zones					
Heart Rate Zone	**RER**	**Heart Rate Percentage**	**Energy System**	**Energy Source**	**Activity**
Zone One	0.80-0.90	65-75%	Aerobic	Muscle glycogen and fatty acids	Walking or jogging
Zone Two	0.95-1.0	80-85%	Aerobic/ Anaerobic	Muscle glycogen and lactic acid	Group exercise classes
Zone Three	1.1	86-90%	Anaerobic	ATP/CP and muscle glycogen	Sprinting

Translating RER into Heart Rate Zones

Before discussing each stage, it is essential to know how to translate RER into heart rate zones. The RER numbers seen in Table 7-8 correspond easily with heart rate zones. Table 7-9 demonstrates estimated heart rate numbers that coincide with the RER to give a predictable and usable number to work with. Also shown are the energy system, energy source and example activity. The heart rates are broken up into three heart rate zones that are easily used for program design.

Zone One

Zone One consists of a heart rate of approximately 65-75 percent of a predicted heart rate maximum (calculated as 220 - client's age). While this equation is not accurate for everyone, it is a good general tool. This zone is a "recovery zone." It is a great zone to start in and is consistently used for beginners to improve the blood's ability to deliver oxygen throughout the body and remove waste. Regular exercise increases blood volume, which allows more blood to get to the cells. The result is a greater flow of oxygen to a greater number of cells throughout the body, thus helping the cells work to their capacity and allowing the heart to become stronger. This form of training fits very well with the beginning phases of the OPT™ model (stabilization level) where the goal is to increase blood supply to tissue for recovery. There may be times, however, that even this zone will be too high for some clients. In this case, the general health activity recommendations (Table 7-6) will become very important guidelines to follow.

Zone Two

Zone Two consists of a heart rate of approximately 80-85 percent of a predicted heart rate maximum. This is near the anaerobic threshold. Anaerobic threshold is the point when the body can no longer produce enough energy for the muscles with normal oxygen intake (aerobic energy system in Zone One). As a result, it begins to produce higher levels of lactic acid than can be removed from the body. Training and staying at an aerobic level will result in more calories burned with a higher percent of those calories coming from fat. Thus, one of the main goals of cardiorespiratory training is to increase the anaerobic threshold. Many people who perform high-intensity workouts every time they use a piece of fitness equipment or attend a group exercise class are usually in this zone, and not truly performing high-intensity training. Zone Two would be appropriate for individuals who have progressed to the strength level of the OPT™ model.

Zone Three

Zone Three consists of a heart rate of approximately 86-90 percent of a predicted heart rate maximum. This is a true high-intensity workout and cannot be sustained for long periods of time (more than 10-60 seconds). Zone Three training should be used in a workout with zones one and two. Staying in Zone One or Two all the time will also cause clients to hit a plateau. The reason is simple: to improve fitness level or increase metabolism, the body must be overloaded. Based on the General Adaptation Syndrome, the same high-intensity level of exercise performed during every workout will exhaust the body and not allow recovery enough to do an overload workout. This will not allow for adaptation and realization of the client's goal. Similarly, doing the same low-intensity level of exercise during every workout will not place enough stress on the body to force an adaptation. The solution is to progress a client to the point that he/she can use all three heart rate zones of training, over the course of each week, varying the intensity for each workout.[54-55] For most clients, going to Zone Three once a week is enough. Caution must be exercised to not spend too much time in Zone Three, which can lead to over-training.[53] Zone Three training would be appropriate for the individual who has progressed to the power level of the OPT™ model.

Translating Heart Rate Zones into Stages

After understanding the different zones and their function, each of these zones can be applied in a systematic fashion utilizing stage training.

Stage I (Stabilization Level)

This stage is for the beginner who has not been working out and only uses heart rate training Zone One (Table 7-9). Just like in weight training, a base needs to be established first. In this stage, clients should start slow and work up to 30-60 minutes in Zone One. Sixty-five to 75 percent of maximum heart rate should be low enough to ensure the client is in an aerobic state. If the client has never worked out before, he/she might start in Zone One for only five minutes and/or reduce the heart rate percentage to the General Health Activity Recommendations (Table 7-6). Stage I training also helps a client to better meet the muscular endurance demands of the stabilization level of training in the OPT™ model.

Clients who can maintain Zone One heart rate for at least 30 minutes two to three times per week, will be ready for Stage II. A beginner, however, might take two to three months to meet this demand. An example might be walking on a treadmill at a speed of three miles per hour. The speed may change for each session in order to stay in Zone One. During this stage, it will be apparent if the heart rate zones created are good for the client. The progression for this stage of cardiorespiratory training is to slowly add time to the client's light workout.

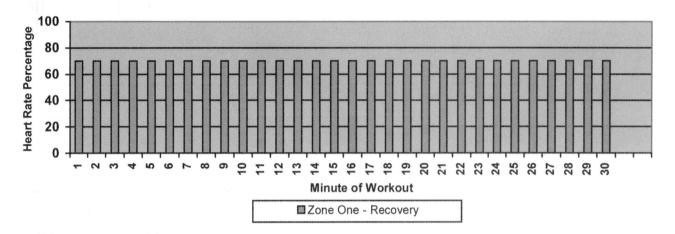

Figure 7-4: Stage I (Stabilization Level) Training Parameters

Stage II (Strength Level)

This stage is for the intermediate client who has built a good cardiorespiratory base and will use heart rate Zones One and Two (Figure 7-5). The focus in this stage is on increasing the workload (speed, incline, level, etc.) in a way that will help the client alter heart rate in and out of each zone. Remember, it doesn't matter how hard the equipment is working; what matters is how hard the client is working. This will be determined by heart rate. Some clients can start in this zone if they have been working out for a while with a low intensity and have created the aerobic base. Stage II training helps increase the cardiorespiratory capacity needed for the workout styles in the strength level of the OPT™ model.

Stage II is the introduction to interval training in which intensities are varied throughout the workout. The workout will proceed as follows:

1. Start by warming up in Zone One for five to 10 minutes.

2. Move into a one-minute interval in Zone Two (Figure 7-5). Gradually increase the workload to raise the heart rate up to the Zone Two within that minute. Once the heart rate reaches 80-85 percent of maximum heart rate, maintain it for the rest of that minute. It might take 45 seconds to reach that heart rate, which means the client will only be at the top end for 15 seconds before reducing the workload (speed, incline or level), and returning to Zone One.

3. After the one-minute interval, return to Zone One for five minutes.

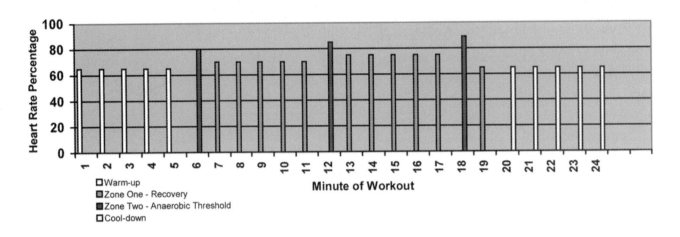

Figure 7-5: Stage II (Strength Level) Training Parameters

4. Repeat this if the client has time and can recover back into the Zone One range. The most important part of the interval is to recover back to Zone One between the intervals.

During the first workout, adjustments may need to be made. The first thing to look at is the one-minute push. Did the client get to the Zone Two heart rate? Was it easy? Could he/she hold that heart rate? (Also, make sure the client was pushing hard enough and didn't progress the workload too slowly.) Based on the answers to these questions, start to create a more accurate, modified training zone for the client.

1. If the client wasn't able to reach the predicted Zone Two in one minute, then use the heart rate he/she was able to reach as their "85 percent."

2. Take five percent off this number to get the lower end of the client's readjusted zone (85 - 5 = 80 percent).

   a. For example, if 150 beats per minute (bpm) was the predicted 85 percent of HR max, but the client was only able to work up to 145 bpm during the one-minute push, 145 bpm should now be considered that client's 85 percent HR max.

   b. Take five percent off 145 (5 percent of 145 is 7 beats; 145 - 7 = 138). So, 138 bpm is the individual's 80 percent of HR max.

3. If the client got into the readjusted Zone Two, and then reaching the zones was fine, work slowly to increase the client's time in this zone.

4. If the client's heart rate goes above the predicted zone and he/she still can recover back to Zone One at the end, add a couple of bpms to the zone and then work on increasing the time.

It is very important to point out that in Stage II, it will be important to alternate days of the week with Stage I training (Figure 7-6). This means alternating sessions every workout.

Figure 7-6 displays a monthly plan for a three-days-per-week schedule. Start with Stage I on Monday. Then, move to Stage II on Wednesday and go back to Stage I on Friday. The next week, start with Stage II and so on. Rotate the stages to keep workouts balanced. This will become very important in Stage III. The monthly plan is only a general guide and may changed, based upon the workout (if any) being performed on that day.

Week	1							2							3							4						
Day	M	T	W	T	F	S	S	M	T	W	T	F	S	S	M	T	W	T	F	S	S	M	T	W	T	F	S	S
CET																												
IST																												
SET																												
MDT																												
MST																												
EET																												
MPT																												
Cardio	S1		S2		S1			S2		S1		S2			S1		S2		S1			S2		S1		S2		
Flexibility																												
KCA																												

S1 = Stage I   S2 = Stage II

Figure 7-6: The Monthly Plan

Stage III (Power Level)

This stage is for the advanced client who has built a very good cardiorespiratory base and will use heart rate Zones One, Two and Three. It should not be used by beginning or intermediate clients. Failure to comply with these standards could result in a critical health-related injury to a client. It is imperative that health and fitness professionals follow the proper assessment procedures to avoid legal issues regarding client care.

The focus in this stage is on further increasing the workload (speed, incline, level, etc.) in a way that will help the client alter heart rate in and out of each zone (Figure 7-7). Stage III training increases the capacity of the energy systems needed at the power level of the OPT™ model.

The workout will proceed as follows:

1. Warm up in Zone One for up to 10 minutes.

2. Then, increase the workload every 60 seconds until reaching Zone Three. This will require a slow climb through Zone Two for at least two minutes.

3. After pushing for another minute in Zone Three, decrease the workload. This one-minute break is an important minute to help gauge improvement.

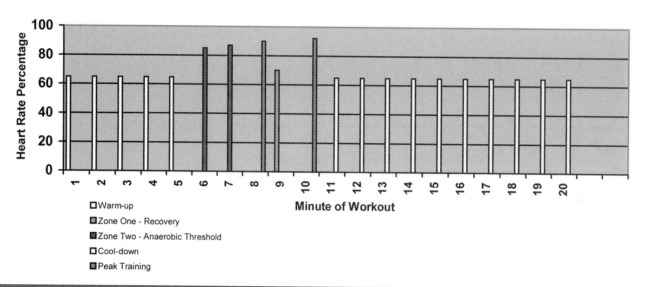

☐ Warm-up
◼ Zone One - Recovery
◼ Zone Two - Anaerobic Threshold
☐ Cool-down
◼ Peak Training

Figure 7-7: Stage III (Power Level) Training Parameters

4. Drop the client's workload down to the level he/she was just working in, prior to starting the Zone Three interval. During this minute, the heart rate will drop.

   a. As improvements are made over several weeks of training, the heart rate will drop more quickly. The faster the heart rate drops, the stronger the heart is getting.

   b. If the client is not able to drop to the appropriate heart rate during the one-minute break, assume that he/she is tired and about to over-train. The solution is to stay in Zone One or Two for the rest of the workout. The bottom line is that the client is not rested enough to do that type of exercise on that day (which may be due to a hard workout the day before, not enough sleep or poor nutrition). Monitoring heart rate is an excellent tool in avoiding over-training.

5. If the heart rate does drop to a normal rate, then overload the body again and go to the next zone, Zone Three, for one minute.

6. After this minute, go back to Zone One for 10 minutes before starting over.

It is vital when training at this level to rotate all three stages. There will be a low (Stage I), medium (Stage II) and high intensity day (Stage III) to help minimize the risk of over-training. The monthly plan, shown in Figure 7-8, is only a general guide and may change based upon the workout (if any) that is being performed on that day.

Week		1							2							3							4					
Day	M	T	W	T	F	S	S	M	T	W	T	F	S	S	M	T	W	T	F	S	S	M	T	W	T	F	S	S
CET																												
IST																												
SET																												
MDT																												
MST																												
EET																												
MPT																												
Cardio	S1		S2		S3			S1		S2		S3			S1		S2		S3			S1		S2		S3		
Flexibility																												
KCA																												

S1 = Stage I   S2 = Stage II   S3 = Stage III

Figure 7-8: The Monthly Plan

The importance of understanding the three stages of cardiorespiratory training (and using them in an alternating manner) is that EPOC, in and of itself, does not ensure weight loss or increased total caloric expenditure for a given exercise session or its recovery. Rather, it can be a large contributor to the total caloric expenditure, depending on the intensity and duration of the exercise, by increasing the amount of oxygen consumed following exercise.[48-52] Simply increasing the intensity for the same type of training will not produce consistent increases in fitness levels and weight control, as the body will soon adapt.[44] For the intermediate and advanced client, this information becomes crucial to obtaining optimal results. Many clients fail to push themselves to force a new level of fitness and results. That is the purpose of a health and fitness professional. By increasing a client's intensity through the three heart rate zones seen in Stage III training, the client can take greater advantage of EPOC and help ensure greater results.

Circuit Training

One of the most beneficial forms of cardiorespiratory training is **circuit training**. Circuit training allows for comparable fitness results without spending extended periods of time to achieve them. It is a very time-efficient manner in which to train a client and will be thoroughly described, as it pertains to cardiorespiratory training.

Circuit training programs consist of a series of resistance training exercises that an individual performs, one after the other, with minimal rest. An example would include:

1. Ball Dumbbell Chest Press
2. Standing Cable Row
3. Standing Overhead Dumbbell Press
4. Standing Dumbbell Curl

5. Ball Dumbbell Tricep Extension
6. Step-up
7. Rest

Several recent studies have compared the effects of circuit weight training to traditional endurance forms of exercise (such as treadmills, cross-country skiing, jogging and/or bicycling), in relation to energy expenditure, strength and improving physical fitness.[56-59] It was demonstrated that circuit weight training:

- Was just as beneficial as traditional forms of cardiorespiratory exercise for improving and/or contributing to improved fitness levels.[56,55]

- Produced greater levels of excess post-exercise energy expenditure (EPOC) and strength.[57,58]

- Produced near-identical caloric expenditure for the same given time span, when compared to walking at a fast pace.[55]

With the assumption that circuit weight training is an effective form of cardiorespiratory training, research has looked at various alterations within a circuit weight-training program. When circuit weight training was compared to circuit weight training with a combined 30 seconds of running between each exercise station, no statistical difference was found between the two protocols.[60] Circuit weight training has also been looked at comparing two different rest protocols: 20 seconds and 60 seconds between each exercise.[61] It was found that while 20 seconds of rest produced a higher EPOC, 60 seconds of rest produced higher total caloric expenditure. This was attributed to the fact that in the 60-second rest group, the total workout time was greater and utilized more total energy.[61] However, this is not to be interpreted as advice to take long rest periods and slow a workout down. Much of the benefit derived from shorter rest periods may be lost after three minutes of rest.[62]

A prime example of how circuit training can be implemented into one's program (and still utilize the F.I.T.T.E. principle) can been seen in a client who dislikes traditional cardiorespiratory activity, but loves to weight train. By structuring the client's weight-training program in a specific manner (circuit training), a health and fitness professional can accomplish cardiorespiratory work and weight training while keeping the client happy. Circuit training can also incorporate traditional cardiorespiratory exercise into the routine. Some examples may include:

Beginning Client (Stabilization Level)

- 5-10 minutes   Flexibility (self-myofascial release and static stretching)
- 5-10 minutes   Stage I cardiorespiratory training
- 15-20 minutes   Circuit weight training
- 5-10 minutes   Stage I cardiorespiratory training
- 5-10 minutes   Flexibility (self-myofascial release and/or static stretching)

Intermediate Client (Strength Level)

- 5-10 minutes   Warm-up: Flexibility (self-myofascial release and active-isolated stretching)
- 5-10 minutes   Stage II cardiorespiratory training
- 15-20 minutes   Circuit weight training
- 5-10 minutes   Stage II cardiorespiratory training
- 5-10 minutes   Cool-down: Flexibility (self-myofascial release and/or static stretching)

At this level, the warm-up and cool-down may be performed separately by the client, prior to or after meeting with the health and fitness professional. This will allow for more time to be spent on the cardiorespiratory and circuit training components.

Advanced Client (Power Level)

- 5-10 minutes   Flexibility (self-myofascial release and dynamic stretching)
- 5-10 minutes   Stage III cardiorespiratory training
- 15-20 minutes   Circuit weight training
- 5-10 minutes   Stage II cardiorespiratory training
- 5-10 minutes   Flexibility (self-myofascial release and/or static stretching)

Again, at this level, the warm-up and cool-down may be performed prior to or after meeting with the health and fitness professional.

Filling in the Template

The information in this chapter allows the warm-up and/or the Cardio Training section of the OPT™ template to be completed (Figure 7-9) section. Here, enter the desired form of cardio that will be used for the warm-up or cardio workout. Note the amount of time and stage in the Cardio Training section.

NASM
NATIONAL ACADEMY OF SPORTS MEDICINE

Optimum Performance Training

NAME	John Smith	**DATE**	March 10, 2004
TRAINER	Chere	**PHASE**	2: Integrated Stabilization Training
DAYS/WEEK	3	**GOAL**	Fat loss

CARDIO TRAINING: Stage I	TIME: 20 min.	EQUIPMENT: Elliptical Trainer

WARM-UP/FLEXIBILITY	Sets	Reps	Duration	Rest	Notes
1. SMR: Calves, IT band, adductors	1				Hold tender spots 20-30 sec.
2. Cardio: Elliptical Trainer			5 min.		
3. Static Stretching: Calves, hip flexors, lats	1		30 sec.		
4.					

CORE and BALANCE	Sets	Reps	Tempo	Rest	Notes
1.					
2.					
3.					
4.					
5.					

REACTIVE	Sets	Reps	Tempo	Rest	Notes
1.					
2.					

SPEED, AGILITY, QUICKNESS	Sets	Reps	Tempo	Rest	Notes
1.					
2.					

STRENGTH	Exercises	Sets	Reps	Intensity	Tempo	Rest	Notes
TOTAL BODY							
CHEST							
BACK							
SHOULDERS							
BICEPS							
TRICEPS							
LEGS							

COOL-DOWN	
POST-WORKOUT FLEXIBILITY	Static Stretching: Calves, adductors, hip flexors, pectorals

Figure 7-9: OPT™ Template

MODULE 7-4 Summary

Different cardiorespiratory training programs place different demands on the bioenergetic continuum and ultimately affect a client's adaptations and goals. Stage training is a three-stage programming system that uses different heart rate training zones, based on the respiratory exchange ratio (RER). Zone One consists of a heart rate of approximately 65-75 percent of a predicted heart rate maximum and is intended for beginners and used as a recovery zone for more advanced clients. Zone Two is near the anaerobic threshold, at 80-85 percent of heart rate maximum, and is intended for individuals who have progressed to the strength level of the OPT™ model. Zone Three is at 86-90 percent of heart rate maximum, and is intended for short bouts for individuals who have progressed to the power level of the OPT™ model. These zones can be translated into three stages, which dictate in which zone and for what length of time cardiorespiratory activity should be performed.

Circuit training programs consist of a series of resistance training exercises that an individual performs, one after the other, with minimal rest. Thus, they allow for comparable fitness results in shorter periods of time. It is also a good way to accomplish cardiorespiratory work during weight training.

MODULE 7-4 Quiz

1. The three different stages of cardiorespiratory training can mimic the three stages of training seen in the OPT™ model.

   ☐ True   ☐ False

2. One of the main goals of cardiorespiratory training is to increase the _____ threshold.

3. Why won't continuing to increase the intensity for a type of training produce consistent increases in fitness levels and weight control?

   _____

4. Which of the following is/are true about circuit weight training?

   ☐ It is not as beneficial as traditional forms of cardiorespiratory exercise for improving fitness levels.

   ☐ It produces greater levels of EPOC.

   ☐ It produces near-identical caloric expenditure for the same given time span, when compared to walking at a fast pace.

MODULE 7-5: Postural Considerations in Cardiorespiratory Training

As any form of cardiorespiratory training involves movement, it must follow the same kinetic chain technique parameters as flexibility and resistance training exercises. Selecting the appropriate form of cardiorespiratory training is also important for the beginner and should be approached as follows:

Clients Who Possess an Upper-extremity Postural Distortion

It is important to note that clients with an upper-extremity postural distortion pattern will have a tendency to elevate and protract their shoulders and extend the cervical spine (protract the head). The health and fitness professional must watch closely for the following kinetic chain deviations:

■ During use of stationary bicycles, treadmills and elliptical trainers, watch for rounding of shoulders and protruding head.

■ On steppers and treadmills, watch for the grasping of the handles (with an over-supinated or over-pronated hand position), which will cause elevated and protracted shoulders and a protracted head. If possible, this equipment should be used without the assistance of the hands to increase the stabilization component, elevating the caloric expenditure and balance requirements.

■ In settings where a television is present, watch for excessive cervical extension or rotation of the head to view the television.

Clients Who Possess a Lumbo-pelvic-hip Postural Distortion

It is important to note that clients with a lumbo-pelvic-hip postural distortion will have a tendency to hyperextend the low back and minimize hip extension. The health and fitness professional must watch closely for the following kinetic chain deviations:

■ Initial use of bicycles and/or steppers may not be warranted, as the hips are placed in a constant state of flexion, adding to a shortened hip flexor complex. If they are used, emphasize hip flexor stretches prior to and after use.

■ Treadmill speed should be kept to a controllable pace, to avoid over-striding. The hips will not be able to properly extend and will cause the low back to overextend, placing increased stress on the low back. Hip flexor stretches should be emphasized prior to and after use.

Clients Who Possess a Lower-extremity Postural Distortion

It is important to note that clients with a lower-extremity postural distortion will have a tendency to flatten the foot, internally rotate and adduct at the knees and hips. The health and fitness professional must watch closely for the following kinetic chain deviations:

■ Use of all cardio equipment that involves the lower extremities will require proper flexibility of the ankle joint (gastrocnemius and soleus muscles). Clients lacking this proper range of motion will over-pronate (feet flatten, evert and externally rotate), regardless of whether they are on the bicycle, treadmill, steppers and/or in an aerobics classes. This will only perpetuate their problem. Emphasize foam rolling for calves, adductors, iliotibial (IT) band, tensor fascia latae (TFL) and latissimus dorsi as well as hip flexor stretches.

■ Clients with a lower-extremity postural distortion will initially have a decreased ability to decelerate (to perform proper eccentric muscle actions of the lower extremity). Using the treadmill and steppers that require climbing (and/or aerobics classes) may initially be too extreme for constant repetition, especially if clients are allowed to hold on and speed up the pace. If these modalities are used, emphasize the foam roll protocol and keep the pace at a controllable speed.

MODULE 7-5 Summary

Because movement is involved, it is vital to monitor kinetic chain checkpoints with clients who are performing cardiorespiratory activity. For clients who have upper-extremity postural distortion, watch for elevated and protracted shoulders and extended cervical spine, particularly on cardio machinery. Individuals with a lumbo-pelvic-hip postural distortion may hyperextend the low back and minimize hip extension. It may be best to avoid bicycles and steppers for these clients and emphasize hip flexor stretches. Clients with a lower-extremity postural distortion will have a tendency to flatten feet and/or internally rotate and adduct at the knees and hips. With these clients stress foam rolling techniques to the calves and adductors.

MODULE 7-5 Quiz

1. Clients with lumbo-pelvic-hip postural distortion should use bicycles and steppers to place the hips into flexion.

   ☐ True   ☐ False

2. Clients who lack a proper dorsiflexion range of motion will typically do what on cardio machinery?

   _____

3. With which postural distortion is it important to watch for excessive cervical extension in clients who are watching television?

   ☐ Lower-extremity

   ☐ Upper-extremity

   ☐ Lumbo-pelvic-hip complex

References

1. Holly RG, Shaffrath JD. Cardiorespiratory endurance. Chapter 52. In: American College of Sports Medicine (ed). *ACSM's resource manual for guidelines for exercise testing and prescription.* 3rd edition. Baltimore, MD: Williams & Wilkins; 1998.

2. Brooks GA, Fahey TD, White TP. *Exercise physiology: human bioenergetics and its application.* 2nd edition. Mountain View, CA: Mayfield Publishing Company; 1996.

3. Greenhaff PL, Timmons JA. Interaction between aerobic and anaerobic metabolism during intense muscle contraction. In: Holsey JO (ed). *Exercise and sport science reviews.* Vol 26. Baltimore: Williams & Wilkins; 1998. pp. 1-30.

4. Alter MJ. *Science of flexibility.* 2nd edition. Champaign, IL: Human Kinetics; 1996.

5. Kovaleski JE, Gurchiek LR, Spriggs DH. Musculoskeletal injuries: risks, prevention and care. Ch 57. In: American College of Sports Medicine (ed). *ACSM's resource manual for guidelines for exercise testing and prescription.* 3rd edition. Baltimore, MD: Williams & Wilkins; 1998.

6. Karvonen J. Importance of warm-up and cool-down on exercise performance. *Med Sports Sci* 1992;35:182-214.

7. Wilford HN, East JB, Smith FH, Burry LA. Evaluation of warm-up for improved flexibility. *Am J Sports Med* 1986;14(4):316-9.

8. Walter SD, Hart LE, McIntosh JM, Sutton JR. The ontario cohort study of running related injuries. *Arch Intern Med* 1989;149(11):2561-4.

9. van Mechelen W, Hlobil H, Kemper HCG, Voorn WJ, de Jongh R. Prevention of running injuries by warm-up, cool-down, and stretching exercises. *Am J Sports Med* 1993;21(5):711-9.

10. Kato Y, Ikata T, Takai H, Takata S, Sairyo K, Iwanaga K. Effects of specific warm-up at various intensities on energy metabolism during subsequent exercise. *J Sports Med Phys Fitn* 2000;40(2):126-30.

11. Fitts RH. Cellular mechanisms of muscle fatigue. *Physiol Rev* 1994;74:49.

12. Andrews MA, Godt RE, Nosek TM. Influence of physiological L(+)-lactate concentrations on contractility of skinned striated muscle fibers of rabbit. *J Appl Physiol* 1996;80(6):2060-5.

13. Metzger JM, Moss RL. Effects of tension and stiffness due to reduced pH in mammalian fast- and slow-twitch skinned skeletal muscle fibres. *J Physiol* 1990;428:737-50.

14. Dorfman LJ, Howard JE, McGill KC. Triphasic behavioral response of motor units to submaximal fatiguing exercise. *Muscl Nerv* 1990;13:621-8.

15. Garland SJ, Enoka RM, Serrano LP, Robinson GA. Behavior of motor units in human biceps brachii during submaximal fatiguing contraction. *J Appl Physiol* 1994;76(6):2411-9.

16. Grimby L. Single motor unit discharge during voluntary contraction and locomotion. In: Jones NL, McCartney N, McComas AJ (eds). *Human muscle power*. Champaign, IL: Human Kinetics; 1986.

17. Moritani T, Muro M, Nagata A. Intramuscular and surface electromyogram changes during muscle fatigue. *J Appl Physiol* 1986;60:1179-85.

18. Edgerton VR, Wolf S, Roy RR. Theoretical basis for patterning EMG amplitudes to assess muscle dysfunction. *Med Sci Sports Exerc* 1996;28(6):744-51.

19. Clark MA. *Integrated training for the new millennium*. Thousand Oaks, CA: National Academy of Sports Medicine; 2001.

20. Clark MA. *Integrated kinetic chain assessment*. Thousand Oaks, CA: National Academy of Sports Medicine; 2001.

21. Janda V. In: Grant R (ed). *Physical therapy of the cervical and thoracic spine*. Edinburgh: Churchill Livingstone; 1988.

22. Janda V. *Muscle function testing*. London: Butterworths; 1983.

23. Liebension C. Integrating rehabilitation into chiropractic practice (blending active and passive care). Ch 2. In: Liebenson C (ed). *Rehabilitation of the spine*. Baltimore: Williams & Wilkins; 1996.

24. Hammer WI. Muscle imbalance and postfacilitation stretch. Ch 12. In: Hammer WI (ed). *Functional soft tissue examination and treatment by manual methods*. 2nd edition. Gaithsburg, MD: Aspen Publishers, Inc.; 1999.

25. Carter R III, Watenpaugh DE, Wasmund WL, Wasmund SL, Smith ML. Muscle pump and central command during recovery from exercise in humans. *J Appl Physiol* 1999;87(4):1463-9.

26. Raine NM, Cable NT, George KP, Campbell IG. The influence of recovery posture on post-exercise hypotension in normotensive men. *Med Sci Sports Exerc* 2001;33(3):404-12.

27. Pate RR, Pratt MM, Blair SN, Haskell WL, Macera CA, Bouchard C, Buchner D, Ettinger W, Heath GW, King AC. Physical activity and public health: a recommendation from the centers for disease control and prevention and the american college of sports medicine. *JAMA* 1995;273:402-7.

28. Lambert EV, Bohlmann I, Cowling K. Physical activity for health: understanding the epidemiological evidence for risk benefits. *Int Sport Med J* 2001;1(5):1-15.

29. Blair SN, Wei M. Sedentary habits, health, and function in older women and men. *Am J Health Promot* 2000;15(1):1-8.

30. Blair SN, Kohl HW, Barlow CE, Paffenbarger RS Jr, Gibbons LW, Macera CA. Changes in physical fitness and all-cause mortality. A prospective study of healthy and unhealthy men. *JAMA* 1995;273(14):1093-8.

31. Blair SN. Physical inactivity and cardiovascular disease risk in women. *Med Sci Sports Exerc* 1996;28(1):9-10.

32. Smolander J, Blair SN, Kohl HW III. Work ability, physical activity, and cardiorespiratory fitness: 2-year results from Project Active. *J Occup Environ Med* 2000;42(9):906-10.

33. American College of Sports Medicine. *ACSM's guidelines for exercise testing and prescription.* 5th edition. Philadelphia: Williams & Wilkins; 1995.

34. Wei M, Schwertner HA, Blair SN. The association between physical activity, physical fitness, and type 2 diabetes mellitus. *Compr Ther* 2000;26(3):176-82.

35. Andreoli A, Monteleone M, Van Loan M, Promenzio L, Tarantino U, De Lorenzo A. Effects of different sports on bone density and muscle mass in highly trained athletes. *Med Sci Sports Exerc* 2001;33(4):507-11.

36. American College of Sports Medicine American College of Sports Medicine position stand. The recommended quantity and quality of exercise for developing and maintaining CR and muscular fitness in healthy adults. *Med Sci Sports Exerc* 1990;22(2):265-74.

37. Murphy MH, Hardman AE. Training effects of short and long bouts of brisk walking in sedentary women. *Med Sci Sports Exerc* 1998;30(1):152-7.

38. Snyder KA, Donnelly JE, Jabobsen DJ, Hertner G, Jakicic JM. The effects of long-term, moderate intensity, intermittent exercise on aerobic capacity, body composition, blood lipids, insulin, and glucose in overweight females. *Int J Obes Relat Metab Disord* 1997;21(12):1180-9.

39. Thomas DQ, Lewis HL, McCaw ST, Adams MJ. The effects of continuous and discontinuous walking on physiological response in college-age subjects. *J Strength Cond Res* 2001;15(2):264-5.

40. Branch JD, Pate RR, Bourque SP. Moderate intensity exercise training improves cardiorespiratory fitness in women. *J Wom Health Gend Bas Med* 2000;9(1):65-73.

41. Wilmore JH, Costill DL. *Physiology of sport and exercise.* Champaign, IL: Human Kinetics; 1994.

42. Sale DG. Neural adaptation to resistance training. *Med Sci Sports Exerc* 1988;20(5):S135-S145.

43. Enoka RM. Muscle strength and its development. New perspectives. *Sport Med* 1988;6:146-68.

44. Westerterp KR, Meijer GAL, Janssen GME, Saris WHM, Hoor F. Long-term effect of physical activity on energy balance and body composition. *Br J Nutr* 1992;68(1):21-30.

45. Conley DL, Krahenbuhl GS. Running economy and distance running performance of highly trained athletes. *Med Sci Sports Exerc* 1980;12:357.

46. Enoka RM. *Neuromechanical basis of kinesiology.* 2nd edition. Champaign, IL: Human Kinetics; 1994.

47. Gaesser GA, Brooks GA. Metabolic bases of excess post-exercise oxygen consumption: a review. *Med Sci Sports Exerc* 1984;16:29-43.

48. Bahr R, Ingnes I, Vaage O, Sejersted O, Newsholme E. Effect of duration of exercise on excess post-exercise O_2 consumption. *J Appl Physiol* 1987;62:485-90.

49. Bahr R, Gronnerod O, Sejersted O. Effect of supramaximal exercise on excess post-exercise O_2 consumption. *Med Sci Sports Exerc* 1992;24:66-71.

50. Gore C, Whithers R. Effect of exercise intensity and duration on post-exercise metabolism. *J Appl Physiol* 1990;68:2362-8.

51. Laforgia J, Whithers RT, Shipp NJ, Gore CJ. Comparison of energy expenditure elevations after submaximal and supramaximal running. *J Appl Physiol* 1997;82:661-6.

52. Almuzaini KS, Potteiger JA, Green SB. Effects of split exercise sessions on excess postexercise oxygen consumption and resting metabolic rate. *Can J Appl Physiol* 1998;23(5):433-43.

53. Gerald S, Zavorsky DL, Montgomery DP. Effect of intensity interval workouts on running economy using three recovery durations. *Eur J Appl Physiol* 1998;77:224-30.

54. Henritze J, Weltman A, Schurrer RL, Barlow K. Effects of training at and above the lactate threshold on the lactate threshold and maximal oxygen uptake. *Eur J Appl Physiol* 1985;54:84-8.

55. Weltman A, Seip RL, Snead D, Weltman JY, Haskvitz EM, Evans WS, Veldhuis JD, Rogol AD. Exercise training at and above the lactate threshold in previously untrained women. *Int J Sport Med* 1992;13:257-63.

56. Kaikkonen H, Yrlama M, Siljander E, Byman P, Laukkanen R. The effect of heart rate controlled low resistance circuit weight training and endurance training on maximal aerobic power in sedentary adults. *Scand J Med Sci Sports* 2000;10(4):211-5.

57. Jurimae T, Jurimae J, Pihl E. Circulatory response to single circuit weight and walking training sessions of similar energy cost in middle-aged overweight females. *Clin Physiol* 2000;20(2):143-9.

58. Burleson MA, O'Bryant HS, Stone MH, Collins MA, Triplett-McBride T. Effect of weight training exercise and treadmill exercise on post-exercise oxygen consumption. *Med Sci Sports Exerc* 1998;30(4):518-22.

59. Gillette CA, Bullough RC, Melby CL. Postexercise energy expenditure in response to acute aerobic or resistive exercise. *Int J Sport Nutr* 1994;4(4):347-60.

60. Gettman LR, Ward P, Hagan RD. A comparison of combined running and weight training with circuit weight training. *Med Sci Sports Exerc* 1982;14(3):229-34.

61. Haltom RW, Kraemer R, Sloan R, Hebert EP, Frank K, Tryniecki JL. Circuit weight training and its effects on postexercise oxygen consumption. *Med Sci Sports Exerc* 1999;31(11):1613-8.

62. Dudley GA, Tesch PA, Harris RT, et al. Influence of eccentric action on the metabolic cost of resistance exercise. *Aviat Space Environ Med* 1991;62:543-50.

CHAPTER EIGHT

Core Training Concepts

Objectives

After studying this chapter, you will be able to:

- Understand the importance of the core musculature.
- Differentiate between the stabilization system and the movement system.
- Rationalize the importance of core training.
- Design a core-training program for clients at any level of training.
- Perform, describe and instruct various core-training exercises.

Key Terms

- Core
- Drawing-in maneuver
- Intramuscular coordination
- Intermuscular coordination

MODULE 8-1:
Concepts in Core Training

This chapter discusses the importance of core training and how to implement this component into a client's program. Successive chapters discuss balance training and reactive training and how these additional components can be incorporated into a training program that will enhance overall functional efficiency.

Core Musculature

The **core** has been defined as the lumbo-pelvic-hip complex, thoracic and cervical spine.[1,2] The core is where the body's center of gravity is located and where all movement begins.[3-7] An efficient core is necessary for maintaining proper muscle balance throughout the entire kinetic chain (Figure 8-1).

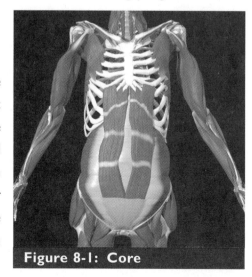

Figure 8-1: Core

There are 29 muscles that attach to the lumbo-pelvic hip complex. Optimum lengths (or length-tension relationships), recruitment patterns (or force-couple relationships) and joint motions (or arthrokinematics) in the muscles of the lumbo-pelvic-hip complex establish neuromuscular efficiency throughout the entire kinetic chain.[7] This allows for efficient acceleration, deceleration and stabilization during dynamic movements, as well as the prevention of possible injuries.[3-13]

The musculature of the core is divided into two categories: the stabilization system and the movement system (Table 8-1). The stabilization system is primarily responsible for stability of the lumbo-pelvic-hip complex, whereas the movement system is responsible for movement of the core.

The core operates as an integrated functional unit, whereby the stabilization system must work in concert with the movement system. When working optimally, each structural component distributes weight, absorbs force and transfers ground-reaction forces.[1,7,14] As such, these interdependent systems must be trained appropriately to allow the kinetic chain to function efficiently during dynamic activities. This means that we must work from the inside (stabilization system) out (movement system). Training the muscles of the movement system prior to the muscles of the stabilization system would not make structural, biomechanical or logical sense. This would be analogous to building a house without a foundation. The foundation must be developed first to provide a stable platform for the remaining components of the house to be built upon. One must be stable first in order to move efficiently.

Table 8-1: Muscles of the Core	
Stabilization System	**Movement System**
Transversus Abdominis	Latissimus Dorsi
Internal Oblique	Erector Spinae
Lumbar Multifidus	Iliopsoas
Pelvic Floor Muscles	Hamstrings
Diaphragm	Hip Adductors
Transversospinalis	■ Adductor Magnus
	■ Adductor Longus
	■ Adductor Brevis
	■ Gracilis
	■ Pectineus
	Hip Abductors
	■ Gluteus Minimus
	■ Gluteus Medius
	■ Tensor Fascia Latae
	Rectus Abdominis
	External Oblique

Importance of Properly Training the Stabilization System

Many individuals have developed strength, power, neuromuscular control and muscular endurance in the movement system which enables them to perform functional activities.[1,7,10,12,14] Few people, however, have properly developed the

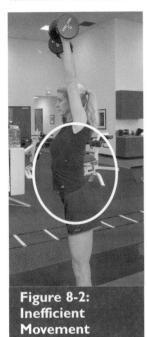

deep stabilization muscles required for lumbo-pelvic-hip complex stabilization.[11-13] The body's stabilization system (core) has to be operating with maximal efficiency to effectively utilize the strength, power, neuromuscular control and muscular endurance that has been developed in the prime movers. If the movement system musculature of the core is strong and the stabilization system is weak, the kinetic chain senses imbalance and forces are not being transferred and/or utilized properly. This leads to compensation, synergistic dominance and inefficient movements.[1,7,11-13,14] Examples include performing a lunge, squat or overhead press with excessive spinal extension (Figure 8-2).

Figure 8-2: Inefficient Movement

A weak core is a fundamental problem that causes inefficient movement and can lead to predictable patterns of injury.[7,11-13,14,15] Many people have a strong rectus abdominis, external obliques and erector spinae, but weak stabilizing muscles. This results in lack of stabilization and unwanted motion of the individual vertebrae, thus increasing forces throughout the lumbo-pelvic-hip complex that may result in low back pain and injury.[7,14,16]

MODULE 8-1: Summary

The core is the beginning point for movement and the center of gravity for the body. It consists of the lumbo-pelvic-hip complex, thoracic and cervical spine. If the core is unstable during movement, it does not allow optimum stabilization force reduction, production and transference to occur throughout the kinetic chain.

An efficient core is necessary for maintaining proper muscle balance throughout the entire kinetic chain. Optimum lengths (length-tension relationships), recruitment patterns (force-couple relationships) and joint motions (arthrokinematics) in the muscles of the lumbo-pelvic-hip complex establish neuromuscular efficiency throughout the entire kinetic chain. This allows for efficient acceleration, deceleration and stabilization during dynamic movements, as well as the prevention of possible injuries.

The musculature of the core is divided into two categories: stabilization and movement systems. The stabilization system is primarily responsible for stability of the lumbo-pelvic-hip complex. The movement system is responsible for movement, force production and force reduction of the core. Training should begin from the inside (stabilization system) out (movement system). If the core's movement-system musculature is strong and the stabilization system is weak, the kinetic chain senses imbalance and forces are not being transferred and/or utilized properly. This all may result in compensation, synergistic dominance and inefficient movements.

MODULE 8-1: Quiz

1. The core is which of the following?

   ☐ The lumbo-pelvic-hip complex, thoracic and cervical spine

   ☐ Where the body's center of gravity is located

   ☐ Where all movement begins

   ☐ All of the above

2. What are the two categories of core musculature?

   _____ and _____

3. Which muscle is part of the movement system?

   ☐ Transversus abdominis

   ☐ Iliopsoas

4. The movement system should be trained before the stabilization system.

   ☐ True   ☐ False

MODULE 8-2: Scientific Rationale for Core Stabilization Training

Similarities in Individuals with Chronic Back Pain

Researchers have found that in individuals with chronic low back pain (85 percent of U.S. adults) have decreased activation of certain muscles: transversus abdominis, internal obliques, pelvic floor muscles, multifidus, diaphragm and deep erector spinae.[11-13,17-19] These individuals also have decreased stabilization endurance.[3,4,20,21]

Performing traditional abdominal exercises without proper lumbo-pelvic-hip stabilization has been shown to increase pressure on the discs and compressive forces in the lumbar spine.[11-13,17,21-24] Furthermore, performing traditional low back hyperextension exercises without proper lumbo-pelvic-hip stabilization has been shown to increase pressure on the discs to dangerous levels. These unsupported exercises can cause damage to the ligaments supporting the vertebrae, which may lead to a narrowing of openings in the vertebrae that spinal nerves pass through.[20,22,24]

Therefore, it is crucial for fitness professionals to incorporate a systematic, progressive approach when training the core, ensuring the muscles that stabilize the spine (stabilization system) are strengthened prior to the musculature that moves the spine (movement system).

Solutions for Stabilization

Fortunately, additional research has demonstrated increased electromyogram (EMG) activity and pelvic stabilization when an abdominal **drawing-in maneuver** is performed before core training (Figure 8-3).[20,22,25-32] This maneuver involves:

1. Pull in the region just below the naval toward the spine (drawing-in maneuver).

Also, maintaining the cervical spine in a neutral position during core training improves posture, muscle balance and stabilization. If a forward protruding head is noticed during movement, the sternocleidomastoid is preferentially recruited. This increases the compressive forces in the cervical spine. It can also lead to pelvic instability and muscle imbalances as a result of the pelvo-occular reflex. This reflex is important to maintain the eyes level during movement.[33,34] If the sternocleidomastoid muscle is hyperactive and extends the upper cervical spine, the pelvis rotates anteriorly to realign the eyes. This can lead to muscle imbalances and decreased pelvic stabilization.[33,34]

> **DRAWING-IN MANEUVER:** The action of pulling the belly button in toward the spine.

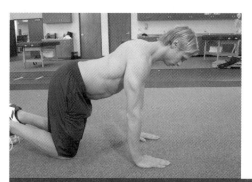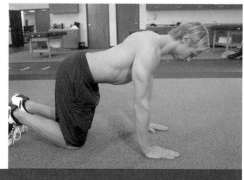

Figure 8-3: Drawing-in Maneuver

Requirements for Core Training

The core-stabilization system (transversus abdominis, internal obliques, pelvic floor musculature, diaphragm, transversospinalis and multifidus) consists primarily of slow-twitch, Type I muscle fibers, which respond best to time under tension.[3-6] This means that these muscles need sustained contractions (six to 20 seconds) to improve **intramuscular coordination**, and motor-unit recruitment within a muscle. This enhances static and dynamic stabilization of the lumbo-pelvic-hip complex.

The core-movement system (rectus abdominis, erector spinae, external obliques, latissimus dorsi, adductors, hamstrings and iliopsoas) is primarily geared toward movement of the lumbo-pelvic-hip complex. These muscles must work synergistically with the stabilization system to ensure optimal **intermuscular coordination** of the lumbo-pelvic-hip complex.

INTRAMUSCULAR COORDINATION: The ability of the neuromuscular system to allow optimal levels of motor unit recruitment and synchronization within a muscle.

INTERMUSCULAR COORDINATION: The ability of the neuromuscular system to allow all muscles to work together with proper activation and timing between them.

MODULE 8-2: Summary

Individuals who have chronic low back pain activate their core muscles less and have a lower endurance for stabilization. Performing traditional abdominal and/or low back exercises without proper pelvic stabilization may cause abnormal forces throughout the lumbo-pelvic-hip complex. These exercises may lead to tissue overload cause damage. However, the pelvis can be stabilized by using the drawing-in maneuver before core training. In addition, keeping the cervical spine in a neutral position during core training improves posture, muscle balance and stabilization.

The stabilization system of the core requires sustained contractions of between six and 20 seconds to properly stimulate the motor units. These muscles must be trained over prolonged periods of time to increase endurance and allow for dynamic postural control.

The movement system of the core is primarily geared toward movement of the lumbo-pelvic-hip complex. These muscles must work synergistically with the stabilization system to ensure optimal force production, force reduction and dynamic stabilization of the lumbo-pelvic-hip complex.

MODULE 8-2: Quiz

1. Research shows that individuals who have chronic low back pain display an increased activation of the transversus abdominis, internal oblique, pelvic floor muscles, multifidus, diaphragm and deep erector spinae.

    ☐ True   ☐ False

2. The drawing-in maneuver involves pulling in the region just below the _____ toward the _____.

3. A forward protruding head during movement is a sign that the sternocleidomastoid is preferentially recruited. This causes:

    ☐ Decreased compressive forces in the cervical spine

    ☐ The pelvis to rotate posteriorly

    ☐ The pelvo-occular reflex and muscle imbalances

4. The stabilization system of the core requires sustained contractions of what length?

    _____

MODULE 8-3:
Designing a Core-training Program

CORE-TRAINING DESIGN PARAMETERS

The core musculature is an integral component of the protective mechanism that relieves the spine of harmful forces that occur during functional activities.[35] A core-training program is designed to help an individual develop stabilization, strength, power, muscle endurance and neuromuscular efficiency in the lumbo-pelvic-hip complex. This integrated approach facilitates balanced muscular functioning of the entire kinetic chain.[1,7,14]

Greater neuromuscular control and stabilization strength offers a more biomechanically efficient position for the entire kinetic chain, thereby allowing optimum neuromuscular efficiency.[7,14]

Thus, a core-training program must be systematic and progressive.[7,14] Fitness professionals must follow specific program guidelines, proper exercise-selection criteria and detailed program variables to achieve consistent success with clients (Figure 8-4).[7,14]

Exercise Selection

Progressive
- Easy to hard
- Simple to complex
- Known to unknown
- Stable to unstable

Systematic
- Stabilization
- Strength
- Power

Activity/Goal-specific

Integrated

Proprioceptively challenging
- Stability ball
- BOSU
- Reebok Core Board
- Half foam roll
- Airex pad
- Dyna Disc
- Bodyblade

Based in current science

Variables

Plane of motion
- Sagittal
- Frontal
- Transverse

Range of motion
- Full
- Partial
- End-range

Type of resistance
- Stability ball
- Cable
- Tubing
- Medicine ball
- Power ball
- Dumbbells
- Other

Body position
- Supine
- Prone
- Side-lying
- Kneeling
- Half-kneeling
- Standing
- Staggered-stance
- Single-leg
- Standing progression on unstable surface

Speed of motion
- Stabilization
- Strength
- Power

Duration

Frequency

Amount of feedback
- Fitness-professional cues
- Kinesthetic awareness

Figure 8-4: Program Design Parameters for Core Training

Levels of Core Training

There are three levels of training within the OPT™ model: stabilization, strength and power (Figure 8-5). A proper core-training program follows the same systematic progression.

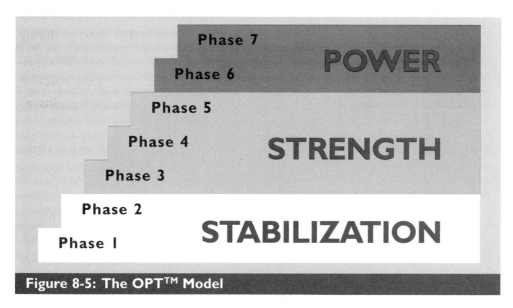

Phase 7	
Phase 6	**POWER**
Phase 5	
Phase 4	**STRENGTH**
Phase 3	
Phase 2	
Phase 1	**STABILIZATION**

Figure 8-5: The OPT™ Model

Stabilization

In core-stabilization training (Phases 1 and 2), exercises involve little motion through the spine and pelvis. These exercises are designed to improve the functional capacity of the stabilization system.[7,14] Exercises in this level include:

- Marching
- Floor Bridge
- Ball Bridge
- Floor Prone Cobra
- Quadruped Opposite Arm/Leg Raise

- Prone Iso-ab
- Prone Iso-ab with Hip Extension
- Prone Iso-ab with Hip Abduction
- Side-lying Iso-ab
- Two-leg Reverse Hyper

Marching

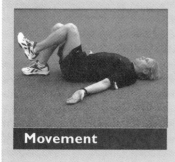

Movement

Preparation
1. Lie supine on floor with knees bent, feet flat, toes pointing straight ahead and arms by sides.

Movement
2. Draw abs in, activate the glutes.
3. Lift one foot off the floor only as high as can be controlled. Maintain the drawing-in maneuver.
4. Hold for one to two seconds.
5. Slowly lower.
6. Repeat on the opposite leg.

Floor Bridge

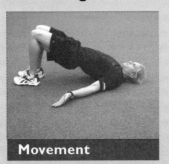

Movement

Preparation

1. Lie supine on the floor with knees bent, feet flat on floor and toes shoulder-width apart and pointing straight ahead.
2. Place arms to the side, palms up.

Movement

3. Draw abs in, activate glutes.
4. Lift pelvis off the floor until the knees, hips and shoulders are in line.
5. Slowly lower pelvis to the floor.
6. Repeat as instructed.
7. To progress, perform as a single-leg exercise.

Ball Bridge

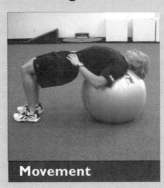

Movement

Preparation

1. Lie supine on a stability ball (ball between shoulder blades) with hands on hips. Place feet flat on floor with toes shoulder-width apart and pointing straight ahead. Allow the back to curve over the ball so that glutes are near the floor.

Movement

2. Draw abs in, activate glutes.
3. Lift pelvis until knees are bent at a 90-degree angle and the body forms a straight line from shoulders to knees.
4. Slowly lower pelvis toward the floor.
5. Repeat as instructed.

Floor Prone Cobra

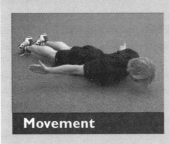

Movement

Preparation

1. Lie prone on the floor with arms in front of body, palms facing toward ground.

Movement

2. Draw abs in, activate glutes, and pinch shoulder blades together.
3. Lift chest off the floor.
4. Hold for one to two seconds.
5. Slowly return body to the ground, keeping chin tucked.
6. Repeat as instructed.

Quadruped Opposite Arm/Leg Raise

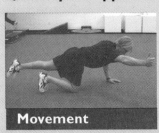

Preparation

1. Start on all fours, with the spine in a neutral position.

Movement

2. Draw abs in and tuck chin.
3. Slowly raise the right arm (thumb up) and the left leg with toes pointed away from the body (triple extension). Keep both arm and leg straight while lifting them to body height.
4. Hold for one to two seconds
5. Slowly return both arm and leg to the ground, maintaining optimal alignment.
6. Repeat alternating sides, as instructed.
7. Regress by raising one arm or leg independently.

Prone Iso-ab

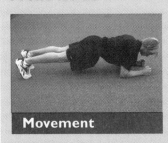

Preparation

1. Lie prone on the floor with feet together and forearms on ground. Clench hands into fists and place at shoulder level.

Movement

2. Draw abs in, activate glutes.
3. Lift entire body off the ground until it forms a straight line from head to toe, resting on forearms and toes.
4. Hold for one to two seconds.
5. Slowly return body to the ground, keeping chin tucked and back flat.
6. Repeat as instructed.
7. To regress, perform with the knees on the floor or with hands on a bench and feet on the floor.

Prone Iso-ab with Hip Extension

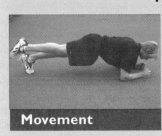

Preparation

1. Lie prone on the floor with feet together and forearms on ground. Clench hands into fists and place at shoulder level.

Movement

2. Draw abs in and activate glutes.
3. Lift entire body off the ground until it forms a straight line from head to toe, resting on forearms and toes.
4. Extend right hip by activating glutes and lifting right leg off the ground, putting leg in triple extension (hip and knee extension, ankle dorsiflexion).
5. Hold for one to two seconds.
6. Slowly return body to the ground, keeping chin tucked and back flat.
7. Switch sides and repeat as instructed.

Prone Iso-ab with Hip Abduction

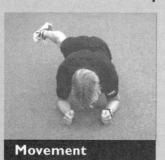

Movement

Preparation

1. Lie prone on the floor with feet together and forearms on ground. Clench hands into fists and place at shoulder level.

Movement

2. Draw abs in and activate glutes.
3. Lift entire body off the ground until it forms a straight line from head to toe, resting on forearms and toes.
4. Extend right hip by activating glutes and lifting right leg off the ground, putting leg in triple extension (hip and knee extension, ankle dorsiflexion).
5. Abduct hip.
6. Hold for one to two seconds.
7. Slowly adduct hip and return body to the ground, keeping chin tucked and back flat.
8. Switch sides and repeat as instructed.

Side-lying Iso-ab

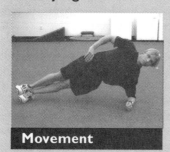

Movement

Preparation

1. Lie on one side with feet and legs stacked on top of each other and forearm on ground.

Movement

2. Draw abs in and activate glutes.
3. Lift hips and legs off the ground until the body forms a straight line from head to toe, resting on forearm and feet.
4. Hold for one to two seconds.
5. Slowly lower body to the ground
6. Switch sides and repeat as instructed.

Two-leg Reverse Hyper

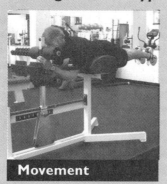

Movement

Preparation

1. Lie prone on a bench with the upper body supported by the bench and the lower body suspended in air.

Movement

2. Draw abs in and activate glutes.
3. Extend legs directly behind the body into triple extension (hips, knees, ankles).
4. Slowly return legs to start position.
5. Repeat as instructed.
6. Progress by performing as a single-leg (alternating) exercise.

Strength

In core-strength training (Phases 3, 4 and 5), the exercises involve more dynamic eccentric and concentric movements of the spine throughout a full range of motion. The specificity, speed and neural demand are also progressed in this level. These exercises are designed to improve dynamic stabilization, concentric strength (force production), eccentric strength (force reduction) and neuromuscular efficiency of the entire kinetic chain.[7,14] Exercises in this level include:

Floor
- Short-lever Crunch
- Long-lever Crunch

Ball
- Crunch
- Crunch with Rotation
- Cobra

Bench
- Knee-up
- Reverse Crunch
- Reverse Crunch with Rotation
- Back Extension

Cable/Tubing
- Rotation
- Lift
- Chop

Floor Exercises

Short-lever Floor Crunch

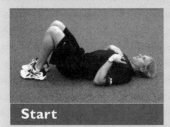
Start

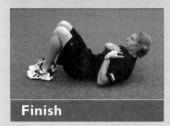
Finish

Preparation
1. Lie supine on the floor with knees bent, feet flat on floor and toes shoulder-width apart and pointing straight ahead.
2. Place arms across the chest.

Movement
3. Draw abs in and tuck chin.
4. Slowly crunch upper body forward, bringing the lower rib cage toward hips.
5. Slowly lower upper body to the floor, maintaining a drawn-in and chin-tucked position.
6. Repeat as instructed.

Long-lever Floor Crunch

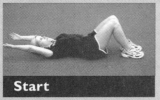
Start

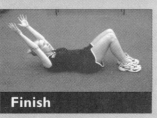
Finish

Preparation

1. Lie supine on the floor with knees bent, feet flat on floor and toes shoulder-width apart and pointing straight ahead.
2. Place arms straight overhead.

Movement

3. Draw abs in and tuck chin.
4. Slowly crunch upper body forward, bringing the lower rib cage toward hips and keeping arms directly overhead.
5. Slowly lower upper body to the floor, maintaining a drawn-in and chin-tucked position.
6. Repeat as instructed.

Ball Exercises
Short-lever Ball Crunch

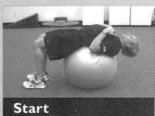

Start

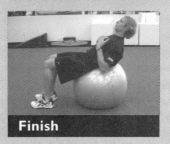
Finish

Preparation

1. Lie supine on a stability ball (ball under low back) with knees bent at a 90-degree angle. Place feet flat on floor with toes shoulder-width apart and pointing straight ahead. Allow back to extend over curve of ball. Cross arms across chest.

Movement

2. Draw abs in and activate glutes.
3. Slowly crunch upper body forward, raising shoulder blades off the ball and tucking chin to chest.
4. Slowly lower upper body over the ball, maintaining a drawn-in position.
5. Repeat as instructed.
6. To progress, perform as a long-lever exercise.

Short-lever Ball Crunch with Rotation

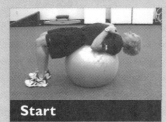
Start

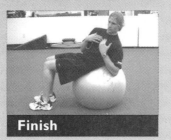
Finish

Preparation

1. Lie supine on a stability ball (ball under low back) with knees bent at a 90-degree angle. Place feet flat on floor with toes shoulder-width apart and pointing straight ahead. Allow back to extend over curve of ball. Cross arms across chest.

Movement

2. Draw abs in and activate glutes.
3. Slowly crunch upper body forward, raising shoulder blades off the ball and tucking chin to chest.
4. At the top position, rotate trunk to one side.
5. Return trunk to neutral position and slowly lower upper body over the ball, maintaining a drawn-in position.
6. Repeat as instructed.
7. To progress, perform as a long-lever exercise.

Ball Cobra

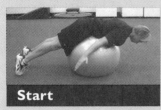

Start

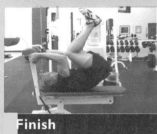

Finish

Preparation

1. Lie prone on a stability ball (ball under abdomen). Keep feet pointed toward floor with legs straight.
2. Extend arms in front of body.

Movement

3. Draw abs in and activate glutes.
4. Bring arms around to the side of the body by pinching shoulder blades back and down.
5. Lift chest off ball, keeping back and neck in proper alignment.
6. Lower chest to ball and return arms to front of body.
7. Repeat as instructed.

Bench Exercises
Reverse Crunch

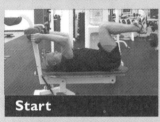

Start

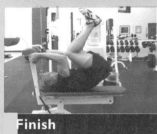

Finish

Preparation

1. Lie supine on a bench with hips and knees bent at a 90-degree angle, feet in the air and hands gripping a stable object for support.

Movement

2. Draw abs in and activate glutes.
3. Lift hips off the bench while bringing the knees toward the chest.
4. Slowly lower the hips to the bench.
5. Repeat as instructed.

Reverse Crunch with Rotation

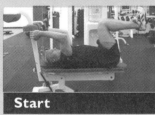

Start

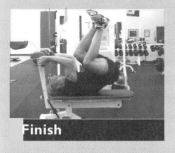

Finish

Preparation

1. Lie supine on a bench with hips and knees bent at a 90-degree angle, feet in the air and hands gripping a stable object for support.

Movement

2. Draw abs in and activate glutes.
3. Lift hips off the bench while bringing the knees toward the chest.
4. At the end range, rotate hips to one side.
5. Return hips to a neutral position and slowly lower the hips to the bench.
6. Repeat as instructed.

Knee-up

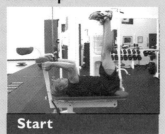

Start

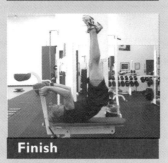

Finish

Preparation

1. Lie supine on a bench with hips bent at a 90-degree angle, legs pointing straight up in the air and hands gripping a stable object for support.

Movement

2. Draw abs in and activate glutes.
3. Lift hips off the bench (use abs, not arms) while pressing toes toward the ceiling.
4. Slowly lower the hips to the bench.
5. Repeat as instructed.

Back Extension

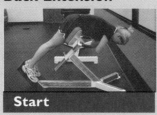

Start

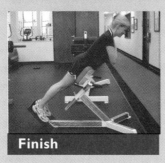

Finish

Preparation

1. Lie prone on a back-extension bench with legs straight and toes shoulder-width apart and pointing straight ahead.
2. Place pads on thighs and cross arms over the chest.

Movement

3. Bend forward at waist to end range.
4. Draw abs in, activate glutes, tuck chin and retract shoulder blades.
5. Raise upper body to a neutral position, keeping chin tucked and shoulder blades retracted and depressed.
6. Slowly lower upper body toward the ground to end range.
7. Repeat as instructed.

Cable/Tubing Exercises
Cable Rotation

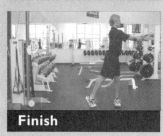

Start

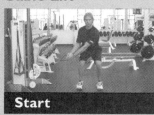

Finish

Preparation
1. Stand with feet shoulder width apart, knees slightly flexed and toes pointing straight ahead.
2. Hold a cable with both hands directly in front of chest, with arms extended and shoulder blades retracted and depressed.

Movement
3. Draw abs in, activate glutes and tuck chin.
4. Rotate body away from the weight stack using abdominals and glutes. Allow back foot to pivot and put back leg into triple extension (hips, knee, ankle).
5. Slowly return to start position.
6. Repeat as instructed.

Cable Lift

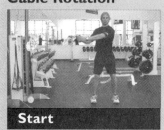

Start

Finish

Preparation
1. Stand in a semi-squat position with feet shoulder width apart and pointed straight ahead. Lift chest.
2. Hold a cable with both hands at the level of the knee closest to the weight stack with arms fully extended.

Movement
3. Draw abs in, activate glutes and tuck chin.
4. Keeping arms extended, lift the cable diagonally and rotate the body using hips, abs and glutes and allowing the back foot to pivot.
5. Lift until the hands reach eye level and the back leg achieves triple extension (hips, knee, ankle).
6. Slowly return to start position.
7. Repeat as instructed.

Cable Chop

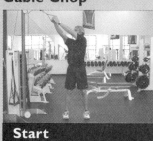

Start

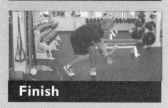

Finish

Preparation
1. Stand with feet shoulder width apart, pointed straight ahead and arms extended.
2. Hold a cable with both hands at shoulder level.

Movement
3. Draw abs in, activate glutes and tuck chin.
4. Keeping arms extended, lower the cable diagonally and rotate the body using hips, abs and glutes and allowing the back foot to pivot.
5. Lower until the hands reach knee level and the back leg achieves triple extension (hips, knee, ankle).
6. Slowly return to start position.
7. Repeat as instructed.

Power

In core-power training (Phases 6 and 7), exercises are designed to improve the rate of force production of the core musculature.[7,14] These forms of exercise prepare an individual to dynamically stabilize and generate force at more functionally applicable speeds. Although these exercises are traditionally performed with a medicine ball, tubing can be an option if a medicine ball is not available or applicable. Exercises in this level include:

- Rotation Chest Pass
- Ball Medicine Ball Pullover
- Back Extension Throw
- Soccer Throw
- Overhead Medicine Ball Throw
- Medicine Ball Squat Jump

Rotation Chest Pass

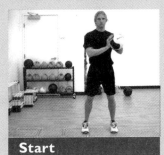
Start

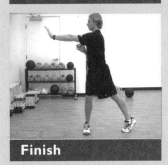
Finish

Preparation

1. Stand upright, with body turned at a 90-degree angle to a wall, with feet shoulder width apart and toes pointing straight ahead.
2. Hold a medicine ball (between five and 10 percent of body weight) in hands at chest level.

Movement

3. Draw abs in and activate glutes.
4. Use abs, hips and glutes to rotate body quickly and explosively to face the wall. As body turns, pivot back leg and allow it to go into triple extension (hips, knee, ankle).
5. Throw medicine ball at wall with the rear arm extending and applying force.
6. Catch and repeat as quickly as can be controlled.

Ball Medicine Ball Pullover

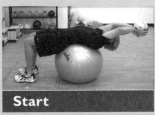
Start

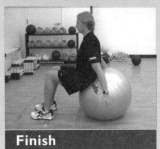
Finish

Preparation

1. Lie on a stability ball (ball under low back) with knees bent at a 90-degree angle, feet flat on floor and toes pointing straight ahead.
2. Hold a medicine ball (between five and 10 percent of body weight) overhead with arms extended.

Movement

3. Draw abs in, activate glutes and tuck chin.
4. Quickly crunch forward, throwing medicine ball against the wall.
5. As the ball releases, continue pulling the arms through to the sides of the body.
6. At the end of the follow-through, shoulder blades should be retracted and depressed.
7. Catch ball and repeat.

Back Extension Throw

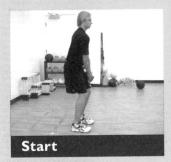

Start

Finish

Preparation
1. Stand with back toward a wall with feet shoulder-width apart, knees slightly bent and toes pointing straight ahead.
2. Hold a medicine ball (between five and 10 percent of body weight) at waist level.

Movement
3. Draw abs in and activate glutes.
4. Use abs, hips and glutes to quickly rotate body, allowing rear leg to pivot and ready triple extension (hips, knee, ankle). Avoid arching the back and keep abdominals drawn in at all times.
5. Throw the ball against the wall as body rotates.
6. Use a scooping motion to catch ball.
7. Repeat as quickly as can be controlled.
8. This exercise can be performed continuously to one side or by alternating sides.

Soccer Throw

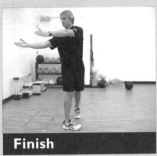

Start   **Finish**

Preparation
1. Stand facing a wall with feet shoulder-width apart and pointing straight ahead.
2. Hold a medicine ball (between five and 10 percent of body weight) overhead.

Movement
3. Draw abs in, activate glutes and tuck chin.
4. While stepping forward, throw the medicine ball against the wall by pulling arms down to the side and retracting and depressing shoulder blades. Keep abdomen drawn in and chin tucked as the ball is thrown. Do not arch back.
5. Repeat exercise by alternating legs.

Medicine Ball Jump Squat

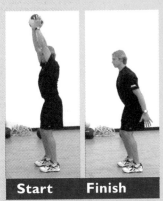

Movement   Finish

Preparation
1. Stand with feet shoulder-width apart, toes pointing straight ahead and knees aligned over toes.
2. Hold a medicine ball (between five and 10 percent of body weight) at chest level.

Movement
3. Draw abs in and activate glutes.
4. Squat down slightly and jump up into the air, extending arms overhead.
5. Land softly on the balls of the feet in a controlled manner, with feet straight ahead, knees over mid-foot.
6. Return the medicine ball back to chest level.
7. Repeat as instructed, spending as little time on the ground as possible.

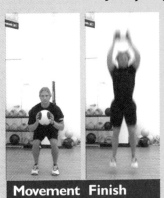

MODULE 8-3: Summary

The core musculature helps protect the spine from harmful forces that occur during functional activities. A core-training program is designed to increase stabilization strength, power, muscle endurance and neuromuscular control in the lumbo-pelvic-hip complex. Core-training programs must be systematic, progressive, activity-/goal-specific, integrated and proprioceptively challenging.

A proper core-training program follows the same systematic progression as the OPT™ model: stabilization, strength and power. In core-stabilization training (Phases 1 and 2), the emphasis is on stabilization of the lumbo-pelvic-hip complex. It improves the function of the stabilization system. In core-strength training (Phases 3, 4 and 5), the spine moves dynamically through a full range of motion, with exercises that require greater specificity, speed and neural demand. These exercises improve neuromuscular efficiency of the entire kinetic chain. Exercises of core-power training (Phases 6 and 7) improve the rate of force production of in the musculature of the lumbo-pelvic-hip complex (movement system).

MODULE 8-3: Quiz

1. An integrated core-training program creates greater _____ and _____ and, in turn, a more _____ position for the entire kinetic chain, thereby allowing optimum _____.

   a. Neuromuscular efficiency
   b. Stabilization strength
   c. Biomechanically efficient
   d. Neuromuscular control

2. Name four of the eight variables that must be taken into consideration when designing a core-training program.

   _____

   _____

   _____

   _____

3. In core-stabilization training, exercises involve little motion through the spine and pelvis.

   ☐ True   ☐ False

4. Indicate whether the following exercises are *stabilization*, *strength* or *power* exercises.

   Back Extension: _____

   Rotation Chest Pass: _____

   Ball Bridge: _____

   Back Extension Throw: _____

MODULE 8-4:
Implementing a Core Training Program

Core Training Design Parameters

Implementing a core-training program requires that fitness professionals follow the progression of the OPT™ model (Figure 8-5). For example, if a client is in the stabilization level of training (Phase 1 or 2), select core-stabilization exercises. For a different client in the strength level of training (Phase 3, 4 or 5), the fitness professional should select core-strength exercises. For an advanced client in the power level of training (Phase 6 or 7), select core-power exercises (Table 8-2).

Core Systems	OPT™ Level	Phase(s)	Exercise	Number of Exercises	Sets	Reps	Tempo	Rest
Stabilization	Stabilization	1 2	Core Stabilization	1-4	1-3	10-20	3-10 sec hold	0-90 sec.
Movement	Strength	3 4 5	Core Strength	0-4	2-4	8-12	3/2/1 - 1/1/1	0-60 sec.
Movement	Power	6	Core Power	0-2	2-4	8-12	As fast as can be controlled	0-90 sec.
		7	Included in resistance-training portion of workout.					

Table 8-2: Integrated Core Training Program Design

Filling in the Template

To fill in the program template (Figure 8-6), go to the section labeled Core and Balance. You will then refer to Table 8-2 for the appropriate type of core exercise (stabilization, strength or power), the appropriate number of core exercises and the appropriate acute variables specific to the phase of training your client will be working in (1-7).

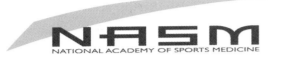

Optimum Performance Training™

NAME: JOHN SMITH

TRAINER: CHERE

DAYS/WEEK: 3

DATE: March 10, 2004

PHASE: 2: Integrated Stabilization Training

GOAL: Fat Loss

CARDIO TRAINING: Stage 1	TIME: 20 min	EQUIPMENT: Elliptical Trainer

WARMUP/FLEXIBILITY	Sets	Reps	Duration	Rest	Notes
1. SMR: Calves, IT band, adductors	1				Hold tender spots 20-30 sec.
2. Cardio: Elliptical trainer			5 min.		
3. Static Stretching: Calves, hip flexors, lats	1		30 sec.		
4.					

CORE & BALANCE	Sets	Reps	Tempo	Rest	Notes
1. Quadruped Arm Opposite Leg Raise	1-3	12-20	3-10 sec. hold	0	Circuit training
2. Floor bridge	1-3	12-20	3-10 sec. hold	0	

REACTIVE	Sets	Reps	Tempo	Rest	Notes
1.					
2.					

SPEED, AGILITY, QUICKNESS	Sets	Reps	Time	Rest	Notes
1.					
2.					

STRENGTH	Exercise	Sets	Reps	Intensity	Tempo	Rest	Notes
TOTAL BODY							
CHEST							
BACK							
SHOULDERS							
BICEPS							
TRICEPS							
LEGS							

COOL-DOWN	
POST-WORKOUT FLEXIBILITY	Static Stretching: Calves, adductors, hip flexors, pectorals

Figure 8-6: OPT™ Template

MODULE 8-4: Summary

To choose the proper exercises when designing a program, follow the progression of the OPT™ model. In the stabilization level, choose one to four core stabilization exercises. In the strength level, select zero to four core strength exercises. In the power level, pick zero to two core power exercises.

MODULE 8-4: Quiz

1. What kind of core exercises would you choose for a client in Phase 4 of the OPT™ model?

   ☐ Core stabilization

   ☐ Core strength

   ☐ Flexibility

   ☐ All of the above

2. How many repetitions of each core power exercise should a client perform?

   _____

3. A client in Phase 7 of the OPT™ model should do how many sets of each core exercise?

   _____

References

1. Aaron G. The use of stabilization training in the rehabilitation of the athlete. Sports Physical Therapy Home Study Course. 1996.

2. Dominguez RH. *Total body training*. East Dundee, IL: Moving Force Systems; 1982.

3. Gracovetsky S, Farfan H. The optimum spine. *Spine* 1986;11:543-73.

4. Gracovetsky S, Farfan H, Heuller C. The abdominal mechanism. *Spine* 1985;10:317-24.

5. Panjabi MM. The stabilizing system of the spine. Part I: Function, dysfunction, adaptation, and enhancement. *J Spinal Disord* 1992;5:383-9.

6. Panjabi MM, Tech D, White AA. Basic biomechanics of the spine. *Neurosurg* 1980; 7:76-93.

7. Clark MA. *Integrated training for the new millennium*. Thousand Oaks, CA: National Academy of Sports Medicine; 2001.

8. Sahrmann S. Posture and muscle imbalance: faulty lumbo-pelvic alignment and associated musculoskeletal pain syndromes: *Orthop Div Rev Can Phys Ther* 1992;12:13-20.

9. Sahrmann S. Diagnosis and treatment of muscle imbalances and musculoskeletal pain syndrome. Continuing Education Course. St. Louis; 1997.

10. Dominguez RH. *Total body training*. East Dundee, IL: Moving Force Systems; 1982.

11. Hodges PW, Richardson CA. Neuromotor dysfunction of the trunk musculature in low back pain patients. In: Proceedings of the international congress of the world confederation of physical therapists. Washington, DC; 1995.

12. Hodges PW, Richardson CA. Inefficient muscular stabilization of the lumbar spine associated with low back pain. *Spine* 1996;21(22):2640-50.

13. Hodges PW, Richardson CA. Contraction of the abdominal muscles associated with movement of the lower limb. *Phys Ther* 1997;77:132-4.

14. Clark MA. *Integrated core stabilzation training*. Thousand Oaks, CA: National Academy of Sports Medicine; 2001.

15. Jesse J. *Hidden causes of injury, prevention, and correction for running athletes*. Pasadena, CA: The Athletic Press; 1977.

16. Janda V. Muscle weakness and inhibition in back pain syndromes. In: Grieve GP. *Modern manual therapy of the vertebral column*. New York: Churchill Livingstone; 1986.

17. Hodges PW, Richardson CA, Jull G. Evaluation of the relationship between laboratory and clinical tests of transverse abdominus function. *Physiother Res Int* 1996;1:30-40.

18. O'Sullivan PE, Twomey L, Allison G, Sinclair J, Miller K, Knox J. Altered patterns of abdominal muscle activation in patients with chronic low back pain. *Aus J Physiother* 1997;43(2):91-8.

19. Richardson CA, Jull G. Muscle control-pain control. What exercises would you prescribe? *Man Med*;1:2-10,195.

20. Beim G, Giraldo JL, Pincivero DM, Borror MJ, Fu FH. Abdominal strengthening exercises: a comparative EMG study. *J Sports Rehab* 1997;6:11-20.

21. Calliet R. *Low back pain syndrome.* Oxford, England: Blackwell; 1962.

22. Ashmen KJ, Swanik CB, Lephart SM. Strength and flexibility characteristics of athletes with chronic low back pain. *J Sports Rehab* 1996;5:275-86.

23. Nachemson A. The load on the lumbar discs in different positions of the body. *Clin Orthoped* 1966;122.

24. Norris CM. Abdominal muscle training in sports. *Br J Sports Med* 1993;7(1):19-27.

25. Liebenson CL. Active muscle relaxation techniques. Part I. Basic principles and methods. *J Manip Physiol Ther* 1989;12(6):446-54.

26. Chek P. Scientific abdominal training. Correspondence Course. La Jolla, CA: Paul Chek Seminars; 1992.

27. Bittenham D, Brittenham G. *Stronger abs and back.* Champaign, IL: Human Kinetics; 1997.

28. Gustavsen R, Streeck R. *Training therapy; prophylaxis and rehabilitation.* New York: Thieme Medical Publishers; 1993.

29. Hall T, David A, Geere J, Salvenson K. *Relative recruitment of the abdominal muscles during three levels of exertion during abdominal hollowing.* Gold Coast, Queensland: Manipulative Physiotherapists Association of Australia; 1995.

30. Miller MI, Medeiros JM. Recruitment of the internal oblique and transverse abdominus muscles on the eccentric phase of the curl-up. *Phys Ther* 1987;67(8):1213-7.

31. O'Sullivan PE, Twomey L, Allison G. *Evaluation of specific stabilizing exercises in the treatment of chronic low back pain with radiological diagnosis of spondylolisthesis.* Gold Coast, Queensland: Manipulative Physiotherapists Association of Australia; 1995.

32. Richardson CA, Jull G, Toppenberg R, Comerford M. Techniques for active lumbar stabilization for spinal protection. *Aus J Physiother* 1992;38:105-12.

33. Lewit K. Muscular and articular factors in movement restriction. *Man Med* 1985;1:83-5.

34. Lewit K. *Manipulative therapy in the rehabilitation of the locomotor system.* London: Butterworths; 1985.

35. Bullock-Saxton JE. Muscles and joint: inter-relationships with pain and movement dysfunction. Course Manual. Nov 1997.

CHAPTER NINE

Balance Training Concepts

Objectives

After studying this chapter, you will be able to:

- Describe balance and its purpose.
- Rationalize the importance of balance training.
- Design a balance-training program for clients in any level of training.
- Perform, describe and instruct various balance-training exercises.

Key Terms

- Dynamic joint stabilization
- Multisensory condition
- Controlled instability

MODULE 9-1: Concepts in Balance Training

The Importance of Balance

Whether on a basketball court, stability ball or walking down stairs, maintaining balance is key to all functional movements. In functional activities, balance does not work in isolation. Therefore, it should not be thought of as an isolated component of function. Balance is a component of all movements, regardless of whether strength, speed, flexibility or endurance dominates the movement.[1,2]

Balance is often thought of as a static process. However, functional balance is a dynamic process involving multiple neurological pathways. Maintenance of postural equilibrium (or balance) is an integrated process requiring optimal muscular balance (or length-tension relationships and force-couple relationships), joint dynamics (or arthrokinematics) and neuromuscular efficiency.[1,2]

The integrated performance paradigm (Figure 9-1) shows that adequate force reduction and stabilization are required for optimum force production. The ability to reduce force at the right joint, at the right time and in the right plane of motion requires optimum levels of functional dynamic balance and neuromuscular efficiency.[1,2]

Importance of Properly Training the Balance Mechanism

Balance training should constantly stress an individual's limits of stability (or balance threshold). An individual's limit of stability is the distance outside of the base of support that he/she can go without losing control of his/her center of gravity. This threshold must be constantly stressed in a multiplanar, proprioceptively enriched environment, utilizing functional movement patterns to improve dynamic balance and neuromuscular efficiency.[1,2]

Training functional movements in a proprioceptively enriched environment (unstable, yet controllable) with appropriate progressions (floor, balance beam, half foam roll, Airex pad, Dyna Disc), correct technique and at varying speeds, facilitates maximal sensory input to the central nervous system, resulting in the selection of the proper movement pattern.[1,2]

Fitness professionals must implement progressive, systematic training programs in order to develop consistent, long-term changes in each client. Traditional program design often results in an incomplete training program, which does not challenge the proprioceptive mechanisms of the kinetic chain.

Balance training fills the gap left by traditional training. It focuses on functional movement patterns in a multisensory, unstable environment.[3,4] The design and implementation of balance into a program is critical for developing, improving and restoring the synergy and synchronicity of muscle-firing patterns required for dynamic joint stabilization and optimal neural muscular control.[3-6]

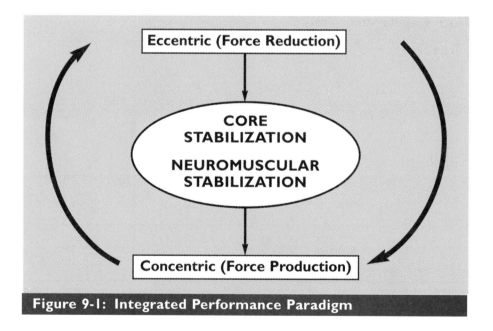

Eccentric (Force Reduction)

CORE STABILIZATION

NEUROMUSCULAR STABILIZATION

Concentric (Force Production)

Figure 9-1: Integrated Performance Paradigm

MODULE 9-1: Summary

Balance is key to all functional movement. However, it does not work in isolation and is not static. Maintenance of postural equilibrium is an integrated, dynamic process requiring optimal muscular balance, joint dynamics and neuromuscular efficiency. Balance training should challenge an individual's ability to stabilize outside their normal base of support. By training in a multisensory environment, there will be more of a demand on the nervous system's ability to activate the right muscles at the right time in the right plane of motion.

MODULE 9-1: Quiz

1. The limit of stability is the distance a person can go outside of his base of support, without losing control of his _____.

2. The integrated performance paradigm demonstrates that adequate force reduction and stabilization are required for optimum force production.

    ☐ True   ☐ False

3. What type of environment is created by training with any of the following implements: floor, balance beam, half foam roll, Airex pad, Dyna Disc?

    _____

4. Balance is an isolated activity.

    ☐ True   ☐ False

MODULE 9-2:
Scientific Rationale for Balance Training

Benefits of Balance Training

Balance training has been shown to be particularly beneficial to improve **dynamic joint stabilization**.[7-14] Dynamic joint stabilization refers to the ability of the kinetic chain to stabilize a joint during movement. Some examples of this include:

- The rotator cuff stabilizing the head of the humerus on the glenoid fossa while performing a push-up
- The gluteus medius and adductor complex stabilizing the hip when performing a squat
- The posterior tibialis and peroneus longus stabilizing the foot and ankle complex when performing a calf raise.

Balance and neuromuscular efficiency are improved through repetitive exposure to a variety of **multisensory conditions**.[5,6] An example of this would be having a client balance on one foot on a half foam roll, while squatting down and reaching across the body, toward the floor. This helps facilitate the nervous system to achieve maximal sensorimotor integration, resulting in the selection of the proper movement pattern.

The main goal of balance training is to continually increase the client's awareness of his/her limit of stability (or kinesthetic awareness) by creating **controlled instability**.[1] An example of this could range from having a 65-year-old client balance on one foot, to having a 25-year-old client balance on one foot on a half foam roll or Dyna Disc.

Balance and Joint Dysfunctions

Research has demonstrated that specific kinetic chain imbalances (such as altered length-tension relationships, force-couple relationships and arthrokinematics) in individuals leads to altered balance and neuromuscular efficiency.[15-24]

Alterations in the kinetic chain before, during or after exercises further affect the quality of movement and perpetuate faulty movement patterns. The faulty movement patterns alter the firing order of the muscles involved, disturbing specific functional movement patterns and decreasing neuromuscular efficiency.[15,25,26] Prime movers may be slow to activate, while synergists, stabilizers and neutralizers substitute and become overactive (synergistic dominance). This leads to abnormal joint stress, which affects the structural integrity of the kinetic chain. This may lead to pain, joint dysfunction and further decrease neuromuscular efficiency.[17]

Research has demonstrated that joint dysfunction creates muscle inhibition.[17,27,28] Joint injury results in joint swelling, which results in the interruption of sensory input from articular, ligamentous and muscular mechanoreceptors to the central nervous system (Figure 9-2).[29] This results in a clinically evident disturbance in proprioception. It has been demonstrated that sensory feedback to the central nervous system is altered, following ankle sprains, ligamentous injuries to the knee and low back pain.[17,19,20,30-34] This is critical for the fitness professional to understand because 85 percent of the adult U.S. population experiences low back pain and an estimated 80,000 to 100,000 anterior cruciate ligament (ACL) injuries and two million ankle sprains occur annually.

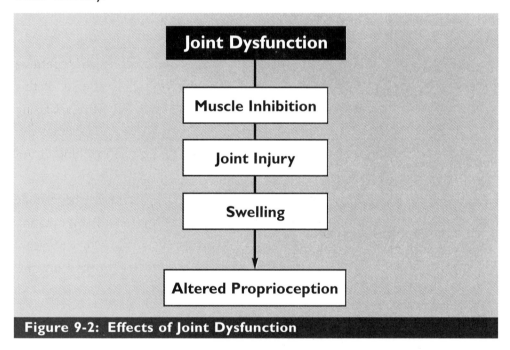

Figure 9-2: Effects of Joint Dysfunction

Thus, muscle imbalances, joint dysfunctions, pain and swelling can lead to altered balance. Therefore, the majority of the clients that fitness professionals work with may have decreased neuromuscular efficiency. It is imperative to understand balance and how to design a balance routine that caters to the needs of today's client.

MODULE 9-2 Summary

Balance training benefits dynamic joint stabilization. Its main goal is to continually increase awareness of limits of stability. Repetitive exposure to varied multisensory conditions can improve balance and neuromuscular efficiency. Training should occur in an unstable environment in which an individual can still safely control movements.

Individuals with altered neuromuscular control likely have specific kinetic chain imbalances. These affect the quality of movement, create faulty movement patterns and lead to lowered neuromuscular efficiency. This may contribute to synergistic dominance, which can cause joint dysfunction and pain elsewhere. Joint dysfunction creates muscle inhibition, which alters balance and leads to tissue overload and injury.

The majority of fitness clients have decreased neuromuscular efficiency and problems with balance.

MODULE 9-2 Quiz

1. Joint dysfunctions, pain and swelling can lead to altered balance.

    ☐ True   ☐ False

2. When the body stabilizes a joint during movement, it is known as what?

    _____

3. Joint dysfunction may lead to:

    ☐ Synergistic dominance

    ☐ Muscle inhibition

    ☐ Decreased neuromuscular control

    ☐ All of the above

4. A training environment should be as unstable as possible.

    ☐ True   ☐ False

MODULE 9-3:
Designing a Balance Training Program

Balance Training Design Parameters

A balance-training program is a vital component of any integrated training program. It ensures optimum neuromuscular efficiency of the entire kinetic chain. The program must be systematic and progressive.[1,2] Fitness professionals must follow specific program guidelines, proper exercise selection criteria and detailed program variables (Figure 9-3).[1,2]

Exercise Selection	Variables	Type of resistance
Safe	**Plane of motion**	**Body position**
Progressive	■ Sagittal	■ Two-leg
■ Easy to hard	■ Frontal	■ Staggered-stance
■ Simple to complex	■ Transverse	■ Single-leg
■ Known to unknown	**Range of motion**	■ Multiposition
■ Stable to unstable	■ Full	— Upright
■ Static to dynamic	■ Partial	— 30°
■ Slow to fast	■ End-range	— 45°
■ Two-arm/leg to single-arm/leg	**Multisensory**	— 75°
■ Stable to unstable	■ Half foam roll	— 90°
■ Eyes open to eyes closed	■ Reebok Core Board	**Speed of motion**
Systematic	■ Airex pad	**Duration**
■ Stabilization	■ Dyna Disc	**Frequency**
■ Strength	■ BOSU	**Amount of feedback**
■ Power		
Proprioceptively challenging		
■ Floor		
■ Balance beam		
■ Half foam roll		
■ Airex pad		
■ Dyna Disc		

Figure 9-3: Program Design Parameters for Balance Training

Levels of Balance Training

There are three levels of training within the OPT™ model: stabilization, strength and power (Figure 9-5). A proper balance-training program follows the same systematic progression.

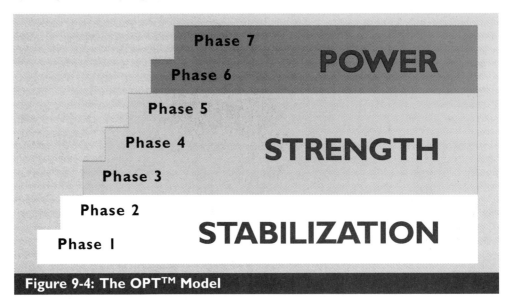

Figure 9-4: The OPT™ Model

Stabilization Level

In balance-stabilization training, exercises involve little joint motion. They are designed to improve reflexive joint stabilization contractions to increase joint stability.[1,2] This means that when the body is placed in unstable environments, it must react by contracting the right muscles at the right time to maintain balance. Exercises in this level include:

- Single-leg Balance
- Single-leg Hip Internal and External Rotation
- Single-leg Hip Flexion and Extension
- Single-leg Balance Reach
- Single-leg Rotation
- Single-leg Lift and Chop

Single-leg Balance

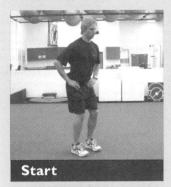

Start

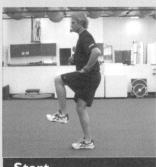

Finish

Preparation

1. Stand with feet shoulder-width apart and pointed straight ahead. Hips should be in a neutral position.
2. Lift chest, retract shoulders slightly and tuck chin.

Movement

3. Draw abs in and activate glutes.
4. Lift one leg directly beside balance leg. Dorsiflex toe, flex hip at a 90-degree angle and slightly flex knee. Maintain optimal alignment, including level hips and shoulders.
5. Hold for five to 20 seconds.
6. Slowly return to original position.
7. Switch legs and repeat as instructed.

Single-leg Hip Flexion and Extension

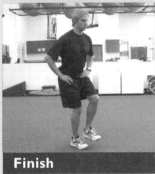

Start

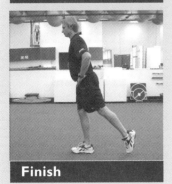

Finish

Preparation

1. Stand with feet shoulder-width apart and pointed straight ahead. Hips should be in a neutral position.
2. Lift chest, retract shoulders slightly and tuck chin.

Movement

3. Draw abs in and activate glutes.
4. Lift one leg directly beside balance leg. Dorsiflex toe, flex hip at a 90-degree angle and slightly flex knee. Maintain optimal alignment, including level hips and shoulders.
5. Slowly flex and extend hip of lifted leg, holding each end position for two seconds.
6. Slowly return to original position.
7. Switch legs and repeat as instructed.

Single-leg Balance Reach (Sagittal, Frontal and Transverse)

Preparation
1. Stand with feet shoulder-width apart and pointed straight ahead. Hips should be in a neutral position.
2. Lift chest, retract shoulders slightly and tuck chin.

Movement
3. Draw abs in and activate glutes.
4. Lift one leg directly beside balance leg. Dorsiflex toe, flex hip at a 90-degree angle and slightly flex knee. Maintain optimal alignment, including level hips and shoulders.
5. Move lifted leg to the front of the body (sagittal). Hold for two seconds.
6. Slowly return to original position.
7. Move lifted leg to the side of the body (frontal). Hold for two seconds.
8. Slowly return to original position.
9. Externally rotate balance hip and move lifted leg to the rear of the body (transverse). Hold for two seconds.
10. Slowly return to original position.
11. Switch legs and repeat as instructed.

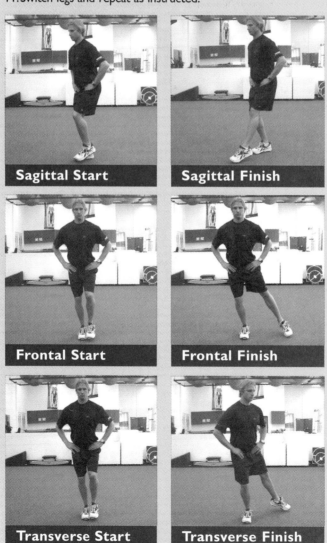

Sagittal Start   Sagittal Finish

Frontal Start   Frontal Finish

Transverse Start   Transverse Finish

Single-leg Lift and Chop

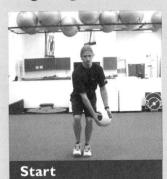

Start

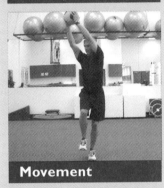

Movement

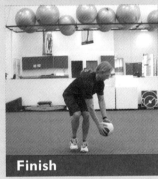

Finish

Preparation

1. Stand with feet shoulder-width apart and pointed straight ahead. Hips should be in a neutral position.
2. Hold medicine ball (between five and 10 percent of body weight) in extended hands.
3. Lift chest, retract shoulders slightly and tuck chin.

Movement

4. Draw abs in and activate glutes.
5. Lift one leg directly beside balance leg. Dorsiflex toe, flex hip at a 90-degree angle and slightly flex knee. Maintain optimal alignment, including level hips and shoulders.
6. Extend arms so that hands are at the outside of the balance leg.
7. Lift medicine ball in a diagonal pattern, rotating the body using hips, abs and glutes until medicine ball is overhead. Hold for two seconds.
8. Slowly return to original position.
9. Switch legs and repeat as instructed.

Strength Level

In balance-strength training, exercises involve more dynamic eccentric and concentric movement of the balance leg, through a full range of motion. Movements require dynamic control in mid-range of motion, with isometric stabilization at the end-range of motion. The specificity, speed and neural demand are progressed in this level. These exercises are designed to improve the neuromuscular efficiency of the entire kinetic chain.[1,2] Exercises in this level include:

- Single-leg Squat
- Single-leg Squat Touchdown
- Single-leg Romanian Deadlift
- Lunge to Balance
- Step-up to Balance

Single-leg Squat

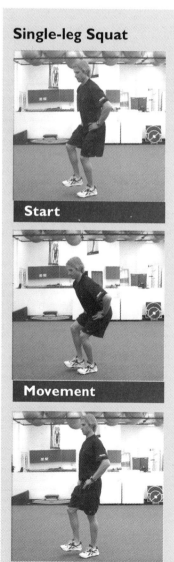

Start

Movement

Finish

Preparation

1. Stand with feet shoulder-width apart and pointed straight ahead. Hips should be in a neutral position.
2. Lift chest, retract shoulders slightly, tuck chin and place hands on hips.

Movement

3. Draw abs in and activate glutes.
4. Lift one leg directly beside balance leg. Dorsiflex toe, flex hip at a 90-degree angle and slightly flex knee. Maintain optimal alignment, including level hips and shoulders.
5. Slowly squat as if sitting in a chair. Lower to first point of compensation. Hold for two seconds.
6. Slowly stand upright but pushing through heel, using abs and glutes.
7. Switch legs and repeat as instructed.

Single-leg Squat Touchdown

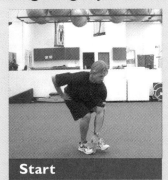

Start

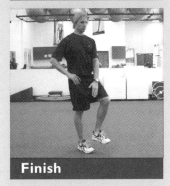

Finish

Preparation

1. Stand with feet shoulder-width apart and pointed straight ahead. Hips should be in a neutral position.
2. Lift chest, retract shoulders slightly, tuck chin and place hands on hips.

Movement

3. Draw abs in and activate glutes.
4. Lift one leg directly beside balance leg. Dorsiflex toe, flex hip at a 90-degree angle and slightly flex knee. Maintain optimal alignment, including level hips and shoulders.
5. Slowly squat as if sitting in a chair, reaching hand opposite of balance leg toward lower foot and keeping chest lifted.
6. Lower to first point of compensation. Hold for two seconds.
7. Slowly stand upright but pushing through heel, using abs and glutes.
8. Switch legs and repeat as instructed.

Single-leg Romanian Deadlift

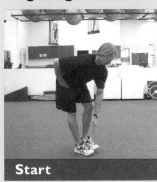

Start

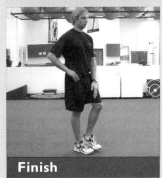

Finish

Preparation

1. Stand with feet shoulder-width apart and pointed straight ahead. Hips should be in a neutral position.
2. Lift chest, retract shoulders slightly, tuck chin and place hands on hips.

Movement

3. Draw abs in and activate glutes.
4. Lift one leg directly beside balance leg. Dorsiflex toe, flex hip at a 90-degree angle and slightly flex knee. Maintain optimal alignment, including level hips and shoulders.
5. Slowly reach hand toward stabilizing foot.
6. Lower to first point of compensation. Hold for two seconds.
7. Slowly stand upright, using abs and glutes.
8. Switch legs and repeat as instructed.

Lunge to Balance

Preparation

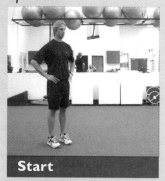

Start

1. Stand with feet shoulder-width apart and pointed straight ahead. Hips should be in a neutral position.
2. Lift chest, retract shoulders slightly, tuck chin and place hands on hips.

Movement

3. Draw abs in and activate glutes.
4. Lunge forward, landing on the heel of lunge foot with toes pointed straight ahead and knee directly over the toes. Both knees should be bent at 90-degree angles. The front foot should be flat and the back heel should be lifted.
5. Stabilize.
6. Push off of front foot through heel onto back leg, straightening balance leg and lifting opposite leg so that hip and knee are flexed at 90-degree angles with foot dorsiflexed.
7. Switch sides and repeat as instructed.

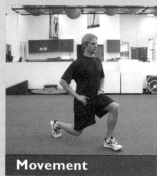

Movement

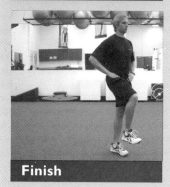

Finish

Step-up to Balance

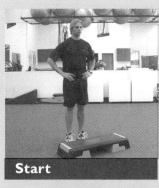

Start

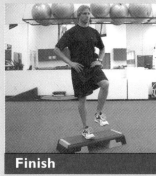

Finish

Preparation

1. Stand in front of a box or platform (between six and 18 inches) with feet shoulder-width apart and pointed straight ahead. Hips should be in a neutral position.
2. Lift chest, retract shoulders slightly and tuck chin.

Movement

3. Draw abs in and activate glutes.
4. Step onto box with one leg, keeping toes pointed straight ahead and knee directly over the toes.
5. Push through front heel and stand upright, balancing on one leg, lifting opposite leg so that hip and knee are flexed at 90-degree angles with foot dorsiflexed.
6. Stabilize.
7. Return lifted leg to the ground, keeping toes and knees aligned.
8. Switch sides and repeat as instructed.

Power Level

In balance-power training, exercises are designed to develop high levels of eccentric strength, dynamic neuromuscular efficiency and reactive joint stabilization.[1,2] Exercises in this level include:

- Multiplanar Hop with Stabilization
    — Sagittal Plane Hop with Stabilization
    — Frontal Plane Hop with Stabilization
    — Transverse Plane Hop with Stabilization
- Single-leg Box Hop-up with Stabilization
- Single-leg Box Hop-down with Stabilization
- Single-leg Hop with Stabilization

Multiplanar Hop with Stabilization
(Sagittal, Frontal and Transverse)

Preparation

1. Stand with feet shoulder-width apart and pointed straight ahead. Hips should be in a neutral position.
2. Lift chest, retract shoulders slightly and tuck chin.

Movement

3. Draw abs in and activate glutes.
4. Lift one leg directly beside balance leg. Dorsiflex toe, flex hip at a 90-degree angle and slightly flex knee. Maintain optimal alignment, including level hips and shoulders.
5. Hop forward (sagittal), landing on opposite foot. Stabilize and hold for two to four seconds.
6. Hop backward (sagittal), landing on opposite foot in starting position. Stabilize and hold for two to four seconds.
7. Switch legs and repeat as instructed.
8. Use the same format to move in frontal and transverse planes, hopping in a side-to-side or turning manner.

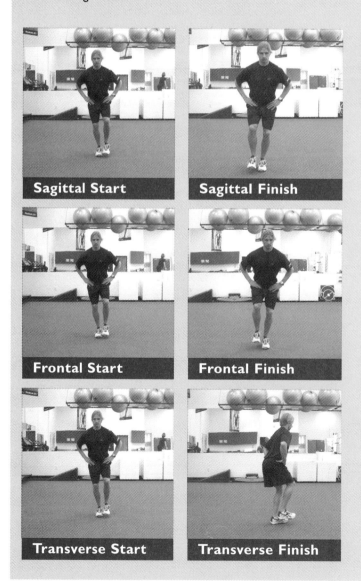

Sagittal Start | Sagittal Finish

Frontal Start | Frontal Finish

Transverse Start | Transverse Finish

Single-leg Box Hop-up with Stabilization

Preparation

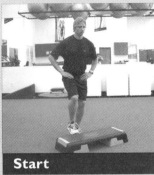

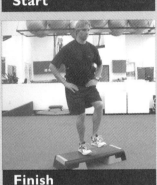

1. Stand in front of a box or platform (between six and 18 inches) with feet shoulder-width apart and pointed straight ahead. Hips should be in a neutral position.
2. Lift chest, retract shoulders slightly and tuck chin.

Movement

3. Draw abs in and activate glutes.
4. Lift one leg directly beside balance leg. Dorsiflex toe, flex hip at a 90-degree angle and slightly flex knee. Maintain optimal alignment, including level hips and shoulders.
5. Using arms, jump up and land on top of box, keeping toes pointed straight ahead and knee directly over the toes. Stablize. Hold for two to four seconds.
6. Step off box, keeping toes and knees aligned.
7. Switch sides and repeat as instructed.
8. Use the same format to hop in the frontal and transverse planes.

Single-leg Box Hop-down with Stabilization

Preparation

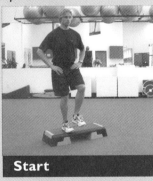

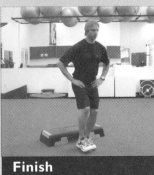

1. Stand on a box or platform (between six and 18 inches) with feet shoulder-width apart and pointed straight ahead. Hips should be in a neutral position.
2. Lift chest, retract shoulders slightly and tuck chin.

Movement

3. Draw abs in and activate glutes.
4. Lift one leg directly beside balance leg. Dorsiflex toe, flex hip at a 90-degree angle and slightly flex knee. Maintain optimal alignment, including level hips and shoulders.
5. Using arms, jump off box and land on ground, keeping toes pointed straight ahead and knee directly over the toes. Stablize. Hold for two to four seconds.
6. Step onto box, keeping toes and knees aligned.
7. Switch sides and repeat as instructed.
8. Use the same format to hop in the frontal and transverse planes.

Single-leg Hop with Stabilization

Preparation

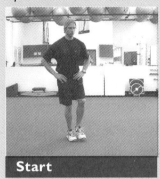

Start

1. Stand with feet shoulder-width apart and pointed straight ahead. Hips should be in a neutral position.
2. Lift chest, retract shoulders slightly and tuck chin.

Movement

3. Draw abs in and activate glutes.
4. Lift one leg directly beside balance leg. Dorsiflex toe, flex hip at a 90-degree angle and slightly flex knee. Maintain optimal alignment, including level hips and shoulders.
5. Squat slightly as if sitting in a chair.
6. Jump up, extending arms overhead.
7. Land softly, maintaining optimal alignment and returning arms to sides. Stabilize and hold for two to four seconds.
8. Switch legs and repeat as instructed.

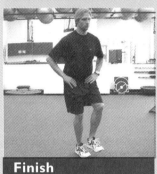

Finish

MODULE 9-3 Summary

A balance-training program is designed to ensure optimum neuromuscular efficiency of the entire kinetic chain. Balance training programs must be systematic and progressive, following specific program guidelines, proper exercise selection criteria and detailed program variables.

A proper balance-training program follows the same systematic progression as the OPT™ model: stabilization, strength and power levels of training. Exercises in the stabilization level of balance training do not involve much joint motion and improve joint stability. In the strength level of balance training, the balancing leg moves dynamically through a full range of motion, with exercises that require greater specificity, speed and neural demand. These movements require isometric stabilization at the end-range of motion. They improve neuromuscular efficiency of the entire kinetic chain. Exercises in the power level of balance training improve high levels of eccentric strength, dynamic neuromuscular efficiency and reactive joint stabilization.

MODULE 9-3 Quiz

1. Which guidelines must be taken into consideration when designing a balance training program?

    ☐ Proprioceptively challenging

    ☐ Isolated

    ☐ Systematic

    ☐ Unrelated to activities

    ☐ Creative

    ☐ Progressive

2. In the stabilization level of balance training, exercises involve little joint motion to _____ joint stability.

    ☐ Increase

    ☐ Decrease

3. Match the exercises to either stabilization, strength or power levels of training:

    Single-leg Balance:_____

    Single-leg Hop with Stabilization:_____

    Single-leg Squat:_____

    Lunge to Balance:_____

MODULE 9-4:
Implementing a Balance Training Program

Balance Training Design Parameters

Implementing a balance-training program requires that fitness professionals follow the progression of the OPT™ model. For example, if a client is in the stabilization level of training (Phase 1 or 2), select balance-stabilization exercises. For a client in the strength level of training (Phase 3, 4 or 5), the fitness professional should select balance-strength exercises. For an advanced client in the power level of training (Phase 6 or 7), select balance-power exercises (Table 9-2).

Table 9-2: Balance Training Program Design

OPT™ Level	Phase(s)	Exercise	Number of Exercises	Sets	Reps	Tempo	Rest
Stabilization	1 2	Balance Stabilization	1-4	1-3	10-20 (or single-leg 6-10 each)	3-10 sec hold	0-90 sec.
Strength	3 4 5	Balance Strength	0-4	2-4	8-12	3/2/1 - 1/1/1	0-60 sec.
Power	6	Balance Power	0-3	2-4	8-12	Controlled. Hold stabilization position for 3-5 seconds.	0-90 sec.
	7	*Included in resistance-training portion of workout.*					

Filling in the Template

To fill in the program template, go to the section labeled Core and Balance. You will then refer to Table 9-2 for the appropriate type of balance exercise (stabilization, strength or power), the appropriate number of balance exercises and the appropriate acute variables specific to the phase of training your client will be working in (1-7).

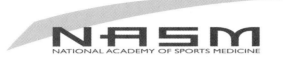

Optimum Performance Training™

NAME:	JOHN SMITH	**DATE:**	March 10, 2004
TRAINER:	CHERE	**PHASE:**	2: Integrated Stabilization Training
DAYS/WEEK:	3	**GOAL:**	Fat Loss

CARDIO TRAINING: Stage 1	TIME: 20 min	EQUIPMENT: Elliptical Trainer

WARMUP/FLEXIBILITY	Sets	Reps	Duration	Rest	Notes
1. SMR: Calves, IT band, adductors	1				Hold tender spots 20-30 sec.
2. Cardio: Elliptical trainer			5 min.		
3. Static Stretching: Calves, hip flexors, lats	1		30 sec.		

CORE & BALANCE	Sets	Reps	Tempo	Rest	Notes
1. Quadruped Arm Opposite Leg Raise	1-3	12-20	3-10 sec. hold	0	Circuit training
2. Floor bridge	1-3	12-20	3-10 sec. hold	0	
3. Single-leg Hip Flexion/Extension	**1-3**	**6-10/leg**	**3-10 sec. hold**	**60 sec.**	

REACTIVE	Sets	Reps	Tempo	Rest	Notes
1.					
2.					

SPEED, AGILITY, QUICKNESS	Sets	Reps	Time	Rest	Notes
1.					
2.					

STRENGTH	Exercise	Sets	Reps	Intensity	Tempo	Rest	Notes
TOTAL BODY							
CHEST							
BACK							
SHOULDERS							
BICEPS							
TRICEPS							
LEGS							

COOL-DOWN	
POST-WORKOUT FLEXIBILITY	Static Stretching: Calves, adductors, hip flexors, pectorals

Figure 9-5: OPT™ Template

MODULE 9-4 Summary

To choose the right exercises when designing a program, follow the progression of the OPT™ model. In the stabilization level, choose one to four balance-stabilization exercises. In the strength level, select zero to four balance-strength exercises (optional in Phases 4 and 5). In the power level, pick from zero to three balance-power exercises.

MODULE 9-4 Quiz

1. What kind of exercises would you choose for a client in Phase 3 of the OPT™ model?

   _____

2. What is the optimal tempo for a single-leg balance reach?

   _____

References

1. Clark MA. *Integrated training for the new millennium.* Thousand Oaks, CA: National Academy of Sports Medicine; 2001.

2. Clark MA. *Integrated neuromuscular stabilization training.* Thousand Oaks, CA: National Academy of Sports Medicine; 2001.

3. Tippet S, Voight M. *Functional progressions for sports rehabilitation.* Champaign, IL: Human Kinetics; 1995.

4. Voight M, Cook G. Clinical application of closed kinetic chain exercise. *J Sport Rehab* 1996;5(1):25-44.

5. Lephart SM. *Re-establishing proprioception, kinesthesia, joint position sense, and neuromuscular control in rehabilitation.* In: Rehabilitation techniques in sports. Prentice WE (Second Edition). St. Louis, MO: Mosby Publishing; 1993.

6. Guskiewicz KM, Perrin DM. Research and clinical applications of assessing balance. *J Sport Rehab* 1996;5:45-63.

7. Balogun JA, Adesinasi CO, Marzouk DK. The effects of wobble board exercise training program on static balance performance and strength of the lower extremity muscles. *Physiother Can* 1992;44:23-30.

8. Barrack RL, Skinner HB. Proprioception in the ACL deficient knee. *Am J Sports Med* 1989;17:1-6.

9. Barret D. Proprioception and function after ACL reconstruction. *J Bone Joint Surg* 1991;73:833-7.

10. Blackburn TA. Rehabilitation of ACL injuries. *Orthop Clin North Am* 1985;16(2):241-69.

11. Freeman MAR, Wyke B. Articular reflexes at the ankle joint: an EMG study of normal and abnormal influences of ankle joint mechanoreceptors upon reflex activity in the leg muscles. *Br Journal of Surg* 1967;54:990-1001.

12. Freeman MAR. Coordination exercises in the treatment of functional instability of the foot. *Phys Ther* 1964;44:393-5.

13. Hirokawa S, Solomonow M. Muscular co-contraction and control of knee stability. *J Electromyogr Kinesiol* 1991;1(3):199-208.

14. Ihara H, Nakayama A. Dynamic joint control training for knee ligament injuries. *Am J Sports Med* 1986;14:309-14.

15. Edgerton VR, Wolf S, Roy RR. Theoretical basis for patterning EMG amplitudes to assess muscle dysfunction. *Med Sci Sports Exerc* 1996;28(6):744-51.

16. Janda V. *Muscle weakness and inhibition in back pain syndromes.* In: Grieve GP. Modern manual therapy of the vertebral column. New York: Churchill Livingstone; 1986.

17. Lewit K. Muscular and articular factors in movement restriction. *Man Med* 1985;1:83-85.

18. Janda V, Vavrova M. Sensory motor stimulation video. Brisbane, Australia: Body Control Systems; 1990.

19. Hodges PW, Richardson CA. *Neuromotor dysfunction of the trunk musculature in low back pain patients.* In: Proceedings of the international congress of the world confederation of physical therapists. Washington, DC; 1995.

20. Hodges PW, Richardson CA. Inefficient muscular stabilization of the lumbar spine associated with low back pain. *Spine* 1996;21(22):2640-50.

21. O'Sullivan PE, Twomey L, Allison G, Sinclair J, Miller K, Knox J. Altered patterns of abdominal muscle activation in patients with chronic low back pain. *Aus J Physiother* 1997;43(2):91-8.

22. Borsa PA, Lephart SM, Kocher MS, Lephart SP. Functional assessment and rehabilitation of shoulder proprioception for glenohumeral instability. *J Sports Rehab* 1994;3:84-104.

23. Janda V. *Muscle function testing.* London: Butterworth; 1983.

24. Janda V. *Muscles, central nervous system regulation, and back problems.* In: Korr IM (ed). Neurobiologic mechanisms in manipulative therapy. New York: Plennum Press; 1978.

25. Liebension C. Integrating rehabilitation into chiropractic practice (blending active and passive care). Chapter 2. In Liebenson C (ed.). *Rehabilitation of the spine.* Baltimore: Williams and Wilkins; 1996.

26. Sahrmann S. Diagnosis and treatment of muscle imbalances and musculoskeletal pain syndrome. Continuing Education Course. St. Louis; 1997.

27. Rowinski MJ. Afferent neurobiology of the joint. In: Gould JA (ed). *Orthopedic and sports physical therapy.* St. Louis: Mosby; 1990..

28. Warmerdam ALA. *Arthrokinetic therapy; manual therapy to improve muscle and joint function.* Course manual. Marshfield, WI; 1996.

29. Fahrer H, Rentsch HU, Gerber NJ, Beyler C, Hess CW. Knee effusion and reflex inhibition of the quadriceps. A bar to effective retraining. *J Bone Joint Surg* 1988;70B:635-9.

30. Solomonow M, Barratta R, Zhou BH. The synergistic action of the ACL and thigh muscles in maintaining joint stability. *Am J Sports Med* 1987;15:207-13.

31. Bullock-Saxton JE, Janda V, Bullock M. Reflex activation of gluteal muscles in walking: an approach to restoration of muscle function for patients with low back pain. *Spine* 1993;18(6):704-8.

32. Janda V. *Physical therapy of the cervical and thoracic spine.* In: Grant R (ed). New York: Churchill Livingstone; 1988.

33. Jull G, Richardson CA, Comerford M. Strategies for the initial activation of dynamic lumbar stabilization. Proceedings of Manipulative Physiotherapists Association of Australia. New South Wales; 1991.

34. Jull G, Richardson CA, Hamilton C, Hodges PW, Ng J. *Towards the validation of a clinical test for the deep abdominal muscles in back pain patients.* Gold Coast, Queensland: Manipulative Physiotherapists Association of Australia; 1995.

CHAPTER TEN

Reactive (Power) Training Concepts

Objectives

After studying this chapter, you will be able to:

- Describe reactive training and its purpose.
- Rationalize the importance of integrated reactive training.
- Design a reactive-training program for clients in any level of training.
- Perform, describe and instruct various reactive-training exercises.

Key Terms

- Power
- Reactive training
- Plyometric
- Rate of force production

MODULE 10-1:
Concepts in Reactive Training

The final component necessary in enhancing stability is reactive training. It is separate from core and balance training section on the program template because an individual must possess proper core strength and have an ability to balance efficiently prior to performing reactive exercises. This chapter reviews the importance of reactive training and how to design and incorporate a reactive routine into your client's program regimen.

The Importance of Reactive Training

Enhanced performance during functional activities emphasizes the ability of muscles to exert maximal force output in a minimal amount of time (also known as *rate of force production*). Success in most functional activities depends on the speed at which muscular force is generated. Power and reactive neuromuscular control represents a component of function. It is perhaps the best measure of success in activities that require rapid force production.

Power is defined as the ability to exert maximal force in the shortest period of time. **Reactive training** is defined as a quick, powerful movement involving an eccentric contraction, followed immediately by an explosive concentric contraction.[1] This is accomplished through the use of **plyometric**

> **POWER:**
> Ability of muscles to exert maximal force in the shortest period of time.

337

REACTIVE TRAINING:
Exercises that utilize quick, powerful movements involving an eccentric contraction immediately followed by an explosive concentric contraction.

PLYOMETRIC:
Exercise that enhances muscular power through quick, repetitive expanding and contracting of muscles.

INTEGRATED PERFORMANCE PARADIGM:
in order to move with precision, forces must be reduced (eccentrically), stabilized (isometrically) and then produced (concentrically).

exercise and defines the stretch shortening cycle of the integrated performance paradigm (Figure 10-1), which states that in order to move with precision, forces must be reduced (eccentrically), stabilized (isometrically) and then produced (concentrically).[2] These exercises enhance the excitability, sensitivity and reactivity of the neuromuscular system, increase rate of force production, motor-unit recruitment, firing frequency (rate coding) and synchronization.

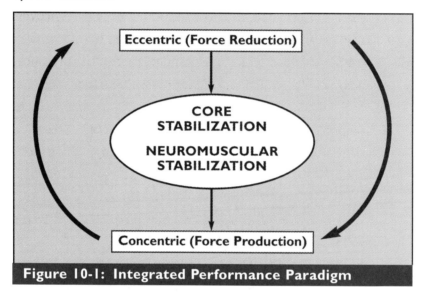

Figure 10-1: Integrated Performance Paradigm

These training exercises are a progression that can be incorporated once a client has achieved proper core and balance stabilization capabilities. Ample isometric stabilization strength (developed through core and balance stabilization exercise) decreases the time between the eccentric contraction and concentric contraction, resulting in decreased tissue overload and potential injury when performing reactive training. Reactive exercises also employ the stimulation of the body's proprioceptive mechanism and elastic properties to generate maximal force output in the minimal amount of time.[2,3]

All movement patterns that occur during functional activities involve a series of repetitive stretch-shortening cycles (eccentric and concentric contractions). The neuromuscular system must react quickly and efficiently following an eccentric muscle action to produce a concentric contraction and impart the necessary force (or acceleration) in the appropriate direction. Muscles produce the necessary force to change the direction of an object's center of mass.[4] Therefore, specific functional exercises that emphasize a rapid change in direction must be utilized to prepare each client for the functional demands of a specific activity.[2,3]

Reactive training provides the ability to train specific movement patterns in a biomechanically correct manner at a more functionally appropriate speed.

This provides better functional strengthening of the muscle, tendon and ligaments to meet the demands of everyday activities and sports.[2,3] The ultimate goal of reactive training is to increase the reaction time of the muscle action spectrum (eccentric deceleration, isometric stabilization and concentric acceleration).[5] This is also known as **rate of force production**.

The speed of muscular exertion is limited by neuromuscular coordination. This means that the body will only move within a range of speed that the nervous system has been programmed to allow.[4] Reactive training improves neuromuscular efficiency and improves the range of speed set by the central nervous system (or rate of force production). Optimum reactive performance of any activity depends on the speed at which muscular forces can be generated.[2,3]

This is another component of program design that is often overlooked in traditional training programs. It is often perceived by many to be too dangerous, potentially increasing the risk of injury. However, reactive training has a systematic progression sequence that allows a client to begin with less demanding exercises and progress to more demanding exercises as he/she adapts. This is no different than any other form of training. If too-advanced exercises are assigned to a client, he/she will not have the ability to perform them correctly and will compensate. This leads to synergistic dominance and faulty movement patterns. When placed within the proper programming scheme with proper progression, reactive training can be a vital component to achieving optimal performance of any activity at any level of ability.

For example, a 60-year-old woman and a 25-year-old male professional athlete may not both need to train for maximal strength. However, they both need stabilization strength and endurance as well as the ability to produce force quickly to perform daily activities efficiently. Therefore, the ability to react and produce sufficient force to avoid a fall or an opponent is paramount. The specificity of training concept dictates that both clients are trained in a more velocity-specific environment.[6] The speed of the repetition or movement is at a faster tempo, similar to movements seen in daily activities.

> **RATE OF FORCE PRODUCTION:** Ability of muscles to exert maximal force output in a minimal amount of time.

MODULE 10-1 Summary

The ability to react and generate force quickly is crucial to overall function and safety during movement. Reactive training is defined as a quick, powerful movement involving an eccentric contraction, followed immediately by an explosive concentric contraction. Reactive training can enhance one's ability to dynamically stabilize, reduce and produce forces at speeds that are functionally applicable to the tasks at hand.

The nervous system only recruits muscles at speeds at which it has been trained. If it is not trained to recruit muscles quickly, when met with a demand for fast reaction, the nervous system will not be able to respond appropriately. The ultimate goal of integrated reactive training is to increase the reaction time of muscle action spectrum (or rate of force production).

It is important to note, however, that reactive/power training should only be incorporated into an individual's exercise program once they have obtained proper flexibility, core strength and balance capabilities. This reiterates the importance of utilizing a progressive and systematic approach when designing the reactive component of your client's training regimen.

MODULE 10-1 Quiz

1. Reactive training aims to generate ☐ **minimal** ☐ **maximal** force output in the ☐ **minimal** ☐ **maximal** amount of time.

2. Why might a 60-year old woman need reactive training?

   _____

3. Increasing the reaction time of the muscle action spectrum is also known as _____.

4. All movement patterns that occur during functional activities involve a series of repetitive stretch-shortening cycles.

   ☐ True   ☐ False

MODULE 10-2:
Designing a Reactive-training Program

Reactive Training Design Parameters

A reactive-training program is a vital component of any integrated training program. The program must be systematic and progressive.[2,3] A client must exhibit proper levels of core strength and balance before progressing into reactive training. Fitness professionals must follow specific program guidelines, proper exercise selection criteria and detailed program variables (Figure 10-2).[2,3]

Exercise Selection	Variables
Safe	**Plane of motion**
Done with supportive shoes	■ Sagittal
Performed on a proper training surface	■ Frontal
■ Grass field	■ Transverse
■ Basketball court	**Range of motion**
■ Tartan track surface	■ Full
■ Rubber track surface	■ Partial
Performed with proper supervision	**Type of resistance**
Progressive	■ Medicine ball
■ Easy to hard	■ Power ball
■ Simple to complex	**Type of implements**
■ Known to unknown	■ Tape
■ Stable to unstable	■ Cones
■ Body weight to loaded	■ Boxes
Activity-specific	**Muscle action**
	■ Eccentric
	■ Isometric
	■ Concentric
	Speed of motion
	Duration
	Frequency
	Amplitude of movement

Figure 10-2: Program Design Parameters for Reactive-training

Levels of Reactive Training

There are three levels of training within NASM's OPT™ model: stabilization, strength and power (Figure 10-3).

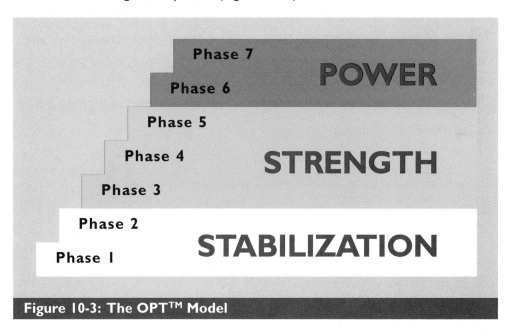

Figure 10-3: The OPT™ Model

Stabilization

In reactive-stabilization training, exercises involve little joint motion. They are designed to establish optimum landing mechanics, postural alignment and reactive neuromuscular efficiency.[2,3] When an individual lands during these exercises, he/she should hold the landing position (or stabilize) for three to five seconds before repeating. Exercises in this level include:

- Squat Jump with Stabilization
- Box Jump-up with Stabilization
- Box Jump-down with Stabilization
- Horizontal Jump with Stabilization

Squat Jump with Stabilization

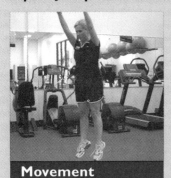

Movement

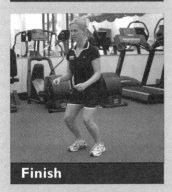

Finish

Preparation

1. Stand with feet shoulder-width apart and pointed straight ahead. Hips should be in a neutral position and knees should be aligned over mid-foot with arms held at sides.

Movement

2. Draw abs in and activate glutes.
3. Squat slightly as if sitting in a chair.
4. Jump up, extending arms overhead.
5. Land softly, maintaining optimal alignment and returning arms to sides. Stabilize and hold for two to four seconds.
6. Repeat as instructed.

Box Jump-up with Stabilization

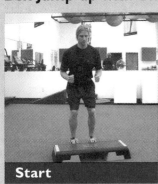

Start

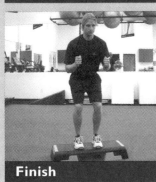

Finish

Preparation

1. Stand in front of a box or platform (between six and 18 inches) with feet shoulder-width apart and pointed straight ahead. Hips should be in a neutral position.
2. Lift chest, retract shoulders slightly and tuck chin.

Movement

3. Draw abs in and activate glutes.
4. Using arms, jump up and land on top of box, keeping toes pointed straight ahead and knees directly over the toes. Stabilize. Hold for two to four seconds.
5. Step off box, keeping toes and knees aligned.
6. Repeat as instructed.
7. As a progression, perform in the frontal the transverse plane

Box Jump-down with Stabilization

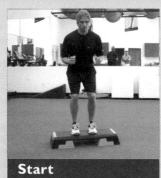

Start

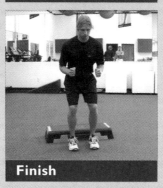

Finish

Preparation

1. Stand on a box or platform (between six and 18 inches) with feet shoulder-width apart and pointed straight ahead. Hips should be in a neutral position.
2. Lift chest, retract shoulders slightly and tuck chin.

Movement

3. Draw abs in and activate glutes.
4. Using arms, jump up and land on floor, keeping toes pointed straight ahead and knees directly over the toes. Stablize. Hold for two to four seconds.
5. Step onto box, keeping toes and knees aligned.
6. Repeat as instructed.
7. As a progression, perform in the frontal the transverse plane

Horizontal Jump with Stabilization

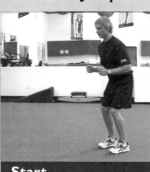

Start

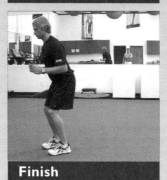

Finish

Preparation

1. Stand with feet shoulder-width apart and pointed straight ahead. Hips should be in a neutral position.
2. Lift chest, retract shoulders slightly and tuck chin.

Movement

3. Draw abs in and activate glutes.
4. Swinging arms forward, jump forward (long jump) as far as can be controlled.
5. Land softly, maintaining optimal alignment and returning arms to sides. Stabilize and hold for two to four seconds.
6. Repeat as instructed.
7. As a progression, perform in the frontal the transverse plane

Strength Level

In reactive-strength training, exercises involve more dynamic eccentric and concentric movement through a full range of motion. The specificity, speed and neural demand are also progressed in this level. These exercises are designed to improve dynamic joint stabilization, improve eccentric strength, rate of force production and neuromuscular efficiency of the entire kinetic chain.[2,3] These exercises are performed in a more repetitive fashion (spending a short amount of time on the ground). Exercises in this level include:

- Squat Jump
- Tuck Jump
- Butt Kick
- Power Step-up

Squat Jump

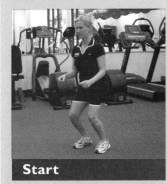

Start

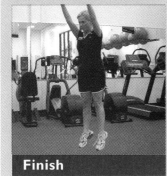

Finish

Preparation
1. Stand with feet shoulder-width apart and pointed straight ahead. Hips should be in a neutral position and knees should be aligned over mid-foot with arms held at sides.

Movement
2. Draw abs in and activate glutes.
3. Squat slightly as if sitting in a chair.
4. Jump up, extending arms overhead.
5. Land softly, maintaining optimal alignment and returning arms to sides.
6. Repeat as instructed.

Tuck Jump

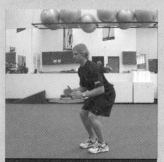

Start

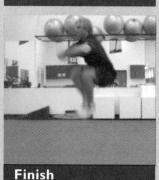

Finish

Preparation

1. Stand with feet shoulder-width apart and pointed straight ahead. Hips should be in a neutral position and knees should be aligned over mid-foot with arms held at sides.

Movement

2. Draw abs in and activate glutes.
3. Jump up, bringing knees to chest.
4. Land softly, maintaining optimal alignment and returning arms to sides.
5. Repeat as instructed.

Butt Kick

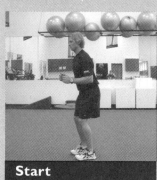

Start

Finish

Preparation

1. Stand with feet shoulder-width apart and pointed straight ahead. Hips should be in a neutral position and knees should be aligned over mid-foot with arms held at sides.

Movement

2. Draw abs in and activate glutes.
3. Jump up, bringing heels to glutes and avoiding arching of the lower back.
4. Land softly, maintaining optimal alignment and returning arms to sides.
5. Repeat as instructed.

Power Step-up

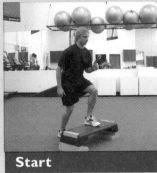

Start

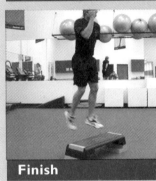

Finish

Preparation

1. Stand in front of a box or platform (between six and 18 inches) with feet shoulder-width apart and pointed straight ahead. Hips should be in a neutral position.
2. Lift chest, retract shoulders slightly and tuck chin.

Movement

3. Draw abs in and activate glutes.
4. Place one foot on top of box.
5. Forcefully push off leg on top of box, putting leg into full extension.
6. Switch legs, keeping weight on the upper leg and maintaining optimal alignment.
7. Repeat as instructed.

Power Level

In the power level of reactive training, exercises involve the entire muscle action spectrum and contraction velocity spectrum used during integrated, functional movements. These exercises are designed to improve the rate of force production, eccentric strength, reactive strength, reactive joint stabilization, dynamic neuromuscular efficiency and optimum force production.[2,3] These exercises are performed as fast and as explosively as possible. Exercises in this level include:

- Squat Jump
- Box Jump
- Ice Skater
- Single-leg Power Step-up
- Proprioceptive Plyometrics: Cones or Hurdles

Box Jump-up

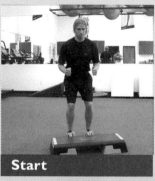

Start

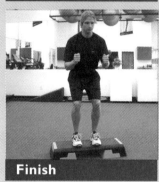

Finish

Preparation

1. Stand in front of a box or platform (between six and 18 inches) with feet shoulder-width apart and pointed straight ahead. Hips should be in a neutral position.
2. Lift chest, retract shoulders slightly and tuck chin.

Movement

3. Draw abs in and activate glutes.
4. Using arms, jump up and land on top of box, keeping toes pointed straight ahead and knees directly over the toes.
5. Step off box, keeping toes and knees aligned.
6. Repeat as instructed, spending as little time on the box as possible.

Ice Skater

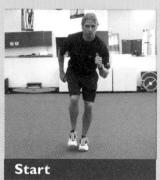

Start

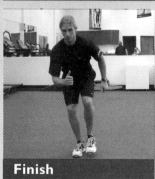

Finish

Preparation

1. Stand with feet shoulder-width apart and pointed straight ahead. Hips should be in a neutral position.
2. Lift chest, retract shoulders slightly, tuck chin and place hands on hips.

Movement

3. Draw abs in and activate glutes.
4. Quickly hop from side to side, switching legs and maintaining optimum alignment.
5. Repeat as instructed, as quickly as can be controlled.

Single-leg Power Step-up

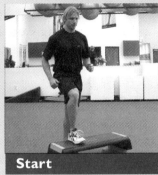

Start

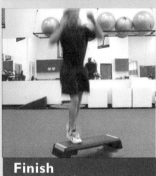

Finish

Preparation

1. Stand in front of a box or platform (between six and 18 inches) with feet shoulder-width apart and pointed straight ahead. Hips should be in a neutral position.
2. Lift chest, retract shoulders slightly and tuck chin.

Movement

3. Draw abs in and activate glutes.
4. Place one foot on top of box.
5. Forcefully push off leg on top of box, putting leg into full extension.
6. Land on same leg, keeping weight on the upper leg and maintaining optimal alignment.
7. Repeat as instructed, as quickly as can be controlled.

Proprioceptive Plyometrics

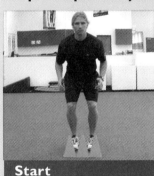

Start

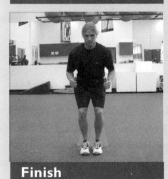

Finish

Preparation

1. Stand with feet shoulder-width apart and pointed straight ahead. Hips should be in a neutral position.
2. Lift chest, retract shoulders slightly, tuck chin and place hands on hips.

Movement

3. Draw abs in and activate glutes.
4. Jump (two legs) or hop (one leg) front to back, side to side or in a diagonal pattern over cones, hurdles or other implements.
5. Land softly and maintaining optimal alignment.
6. Repeat as instructed, as quickly as can be controlled.

MODULE 10-2 Summary

A reactive-training program is designed to enhance neuromuscular efficiency, increase rate of force production, and improve functional eccentric strength. The program must:

- Be systematic
- Be progressive
- Follow specific program guidelines
- Follow proper exercise selection criteria
- Incorporate proper program variables.

A client must exhibit proper levels of core strength and balance before progressing into reactive training.

A proper reactive training program follows the same systematic progression as the OPT™ model: stabilization, strength and power levels of training. Exercises in the stabilization level of reactive training do not involve much joint motion. They improve landing mechanics, postural alignment and reactive neuromuscular efficiency. In the strength level of reactive training, exercises involve more movement through a full range of motion, requiring greater specificity, speed and neural demand. These movements improve dynamic joint stabilization, the rate of force production and eccentric neuromuscular efficiency. Exercises in the power level of reactive training are performed as fast and explosively as possible. They improve rate of force production, reactive strength, dynamic neuromuscular efficiency and optimum force production.

MODULE 10-2 Quiz

1. Which safety guideline is most appropriate to take consideration of when designing a reactive-training program?

☐ Progressive

☐ Performed alone

☐ Performed on extremely hard surfaces

☐ Performed with unsupportive shoes

☐ Start in unstable environments

2. In which level of reactive training should clients hold the landing position?

_____

3. Match the exercises to either stabilization, strength or power levels of training:

Ice Skater:_____

Box Jump-up with Stabilization:_____

Tuck Jump:_____

Squat Jump with Stabilization:_____

MODULE 10-3:
Implementing a Reactive Training Program

Reactive Training Design Parameters

Implementing a reactive-training program requires that health and fitness professionals follow the progression of the OPT™ model. For example, if a client is in the stabilization level of training (Phases 1 and 2), select reactive-stabilization exercises. For a different client in the strength level of training (Phases 3, 4 and 5), a fitness professional should select strength-reactive exercises. For an advanced client in the power level (Phases 6 and 7), select reactive-power exercises (Table 10-1). At this level, however, it may not be necessary to include reactive exercises into the routine as reactive/power exercises will be included in the resistance-training portion of the program.

Table 10-1: Integrated Reactive Training Program Design							
OPT™ Level	Phase(s)	Exercise	Number of Exercises	Sets	Reps	Tempo	Rest
Stabilization	1 2	Reactive Stabilization	0-2	0-3	3-8	Controlled. Hold stabilization position for 3-5 seconds.	0-90 sec.
Strength	3 4 5	Reactive Strength	0-4	2-4	8-12	Repeating	0-60 sec.
Power	6	Reactive Power	0-2	2-4	8-12	Explosive	0-90 sec.
	7	*Included in resistance-training portion of workout.*					

Filling in the Template

To fill in the program template (Figure 10-4), go to the section labeled Reactive. You will then refer to Table 10-1 for the appropriate type of reactive exercise (stabilization, strength or power), the appropriate number of reactive exercises and the appropriate acute variables specific to the phase of training your client will be working in (1-7).

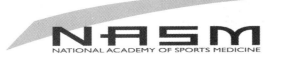

Optimum Performance Training™

NAME:	JOHN SMITH		**DATE:**	March 10, 2004
TRAINER:	CHERE		**PHASE:**	2: Integrated Stabilization Training
DAYS/WEEK:	3		**GOAL:**	Fat Loss

CARDIO TRAINING: Stage 1	**TIME:** 20 min	**EQUIPMENT:** Elliptical Trainer

WARMUP/FLEXIBILITY	Sets	Reps	Duration	Rest	Notes
1. SMR: Calves, IT band, adductors	1				Hold tender spots 20-30 sec.
2. Cardio: Elliptical trainer			5 min.		
3. Static Stretching: Calves, hip flexors, lats	1		30 sec.		

CORE & BALANCE	Sets	Reps	Tempo	Rest	Notes
1. Quadruped Arm Opposite Leg Raise	1-3	12-20	3-10 sec. hold	0	Circuit training
2. Floor bridge	1-3	12-20	3-10 sec. hold	0	
3. Single-leg Hip Flexion/Extension	1-3	6-10/leg	3-10 sec. hold	60 sec.	

REACTIVE	Sets	Reps	Tempo	Rest	Notes
1. Jump with Stabilization	**1-3**	**5-8**	**3 sec. hold**	**60 sec.**	
2.					

SPEED, AGILITY, QUICKNESS	Sets	Reps	Time	Rest	Notes
1.					
2.					

STRENGTH	Exercise	Sets	Reps	Intensity	Tempo	Rest	Notes
TOTAL BODY							
CHEST							
BACK							
SHOULDERS							
BICEPS							
TRICEPS							
LEGS							

COOL-DOWN	
POST-WORKOUT FLEXIBILITY	Static Stretching: Calves, adductors, hip flexors, pectorals

Figure 10-4: Template

MODULE 10-3 Summary

To choose the right exercises when designing a program, follow the progression of the OPT™ model. In the stabilization level, choose zero to two reactive-stabilization exercises. In the strength level, select zero (optional in Phases 4 and 5) to four reactive-strength exercises. There is no need to include power level exercises as they are included in the resistance training portion of the workout.

MODULE 10-3 Quiz

1. What kind of exercises would you choose for a client in Phase 2 of the OPT™ model?

_____

2. What should the tempo for a tuck jump be?

_____

References

1. Wilk KE, Voight M. Plyometrics for the overhead athlete. In: Andrews JR, Wilk KE (eds). *The athletic shoulder.* New York: Churchill Livingstone; 1993.

2. Clark MA. *Integrated reactive neuromuscular training.* Thousand Oaks, CA: National Academy of Sports Medicine; 2001.

3. Clark MA. *Integrated training for the new millennium.* Thousand Oaks, CA: National Academy of Sports Medicine; 2001.

4. Voight M, Draovitch P. Plyometrics. In: Albert M (ed). *Eccentric muscle training in sports and orthopedics.* New York: Churchill Livingstone; 1991.

5. Voight M, Brady D. Plyometrics. In: Devies GL (eds). 4th edition. *A compendium of isokenitics in clinical usage.* Onalaska: S&S Publishers; 1992.

6. Allman FL. *Sports medicine.* New York: Academic Press; 1974.

CHAPTER ELEVEN

Speed, Agility and Quickness Training Concepts

Objectives

After studying this chapter, you will be able to:

- Describe speed, agility and quickness training and its purpose.
- Rationalize the importance of speed, agility and quickness training.
- Design a speed, agility and quickness-training program for clients at any level of training.
- Perform, describe and instruct various speed, agility and quickness training exercises.

Key Terms

- Speed
- Agility
- Quickness

MODULE 11-1: Concepts in Speed, Agility and Quickness (SAQ) Training

The programming component of speed, agility and quickness (SAQ) training is similar to reactive training and follows the same concepts of the integrated performance paradigm. *Speed* in this text essentially refers to straight-ahead speed. *Agility* refers to short bursts of movement that involve change of direction. *Quickness* refers to the ability to react to a stimulus and change the motion of the body.

This form of training is often viewed as being beneficial only for the athlete. However, by using the proper progression as seen in the OPT™ model, the health and fitness professional can effectively use SAQ training to add intensity and complexity, increase the cardiorespiratory demand and provide a simple and exciting variety to a routine workout.

SAQ training allows a client to enhance his/her ability to accelerate, decelerate and dynamically stabilize the entire body during higher velocity, acceleration and deceleration movements, in all planes of motion (such as running, cutting and changing direction). It may further help the nervous system to respond or react more efficiently to demands placed upon it and enhance muscular recruitment and coordination, when performed with correct mechanics.[1]

Speed

Speed is the ability to move the body in one intended direction as fast as possible. It is the product of stride rate and stride length.[2,3] *Stride rate* is the number of strides taken in a given amount of time (or distance). It may be improved with proper core strength, reactive training and technique. *Stride length* is the distance covered in one stride, during running. Research has found that optimum stride length at maximum velocity has a high correlation to leg length. It is approximately 2.1 to 2.5 times leg length.[1,3,4] Speed is an ability that can be learned and trained for by following in integrated training program seen in the OPT™ model.[5]

Proper Sprint Mechanics

Proper running mechanics allow the client to maximize forces generated by muscles, so that maximum velocity can be achieved in the shortest possible time.

This includes frontside and backside mechanics. *Frontside mechanics* is the emphasis on triple flexion of the front leg. Triple flexion includes the actions of:

- Ankle dorsiflexion,
- Knee flexion,
- Hip flexion and
- Keeping the lumbar spine neutral.

Backside mechanics is the emphasis on triple extension of the back leg. Triple extension includes the actions of:

- Ankle plantarflexion,
- Knee extension,
- Hip extension and
- Keeping the lumbar spine neutral.

Agility

Agility is the ability to start (or accelerate), stop (or decelerate and stabilize) and change direction quickly, while maintaining proper posture.[6] This requires high levels of neuromuscular efficiency because the client is constantly regaining a center of gravity over his/her base of support, while changing directions, at various speeds.

Agility training can enhance eccentric neuromuscular control, dynamic flexibility, dynamic postural control, functional core strength and proprioception. Proper agility training can also help to prevent injury by enhancing the body's ability to effectively control eccentric forces in all planes of motion as well as by improving the structural integrity of the connective tissue. Proper technique for agility drills should follow the guidelines seen in Table 11-1.

Quickness

Quickness (or reaction time) is the ability to react and change body position with maximum rate of force production, in all planes of motion and from all body positions, during functional activities. Quickness involves the ability to react to visual, auditory, and kinesthetic feedback during functional activities with minimal hesitation. Proper technique for quickness drills should follow the guidelines seen in Table 11-1.

AGILITY:
The ability to accelerate, decelerate, stabilize and change direction quickly, while maintaining proper posture.

QUICKNESS:
The ability to react and change body position with maximum rate of force production, in all planes of motion, from all body positions, during functional activities.

Table 11-1: Kinetic Chain Checkpoints during Running Movements	
Body Position	**Comments**
Foot/Ankle Complex	The foot/ankle should be pointing straight ahead in a dorsiflexed position when it hits the ground.
	Excessive flattening or external rotation of the foot will create abnormal stress throughout the rest of the kinetic chain and decrease overall performance.
Knee Complex	The knees must remain straight ahead. If the athlete demonstrates excessive adduction and internal rotation of the femur during the stance phase, it decreases force production and lead to overuse injuries.
Lumbo-pelvic-hip Complex	The body should have a slight lean during acceleration. During maximum velocity, the lumbo-pelvic-hip complex should be fairly neutral, without excessive extension or flexion, unless to reach for an object.
Head	The head should remain in line with the lumbo-pelvic-hip complex and the lumbo-pelvic-hip complex should be in line with the legs. The head/neck should not compensate and move into extension, unless necessary to track an object (such as a ball) as this can affect the position of the lumbo-pelvic-hip complex (pelvo-occular reflex).

MODULE 11-1 Summary

Similar to reactive training, the programming component of speed, agility and quickness (SAQ) training follows the same concepts of the integrated performance paradigm. It can add intensity, complexity, cardiorespiratory demand and variety to a routine workout for regular clients as well as athletes. It enhances proprioceptive acceleration, deceleration and dynamic stabilization of the entire body, during higher velocity movements.

Speed is the ability to move the body in one intended direction as fast as possible. It is the product of stride rate and stride length. It can be learned and trained for. Proper running mechanics (including frontside and backside mechanics) allow an athlete to maximize forces generated by muscles, so that maximum velocity can be achieved in the shortest possible time.

Agility refers to short bursts of movement that involve change of direction. It is the ability to start, stop and change direction quickly, while maintaining proper posture. High levels of neuromuscular efficiency are required. It can help to prevent injury by enhancing control of eccentric forces in all planes of motion.

Quickness is the ability to react to a stimulus and change the motion of the body, with maximum rate of force production, in all planes of motion and from all body positions, during functional activities. Reactions are based on visual, auditory and kinesthetic feedback and require minimal hesitation.

MODULE 11-1 Quiz

1. Research has found that optimum stride length at maximum velocity is approximately how many times leg length?

   ☐ 1.1 - 1.5

   ☐ 2.1 - 2.5

   ☐ 3.1 - 3.5

   ☐ 4.1 - 4.5

2. Proper agility training can help to prevent injury by improving the structural integrity of connective tissue.

   ☐ True   ☐ False

3. _____ include the actions of ankle plantarflexion, knee extension, hip extension and keeping the lumbar spine neutral.

   ☐ Frontside mechanics

   ☐ Backside mechanics

MODULE 11-2:
SAQ Drills and Programming Strategies

It must be stressed that the programming guidelines presented in Table 11-2 are only suggestions and should be gauged on the total volume of training for all components (core, balance, reactive and resistance) in a workout. The success of a SAQ program is also dependent upon the client's core, balance and reactive capabilities. The higher these capabilities, the better and safer results a client will enjoy from his/her program. All exercises should be performed with precise technique and kinetic chain control, to minimize risk of injury.

SAQ Speed Ladder Drills

- One-ins
- Two-ins
- Side shuffle
- In-in/Out-out
- Side In-in/Out-out
- In-in-out (Zigzag)
- Ali Shuffle
- Ali Crossover
- W Weave

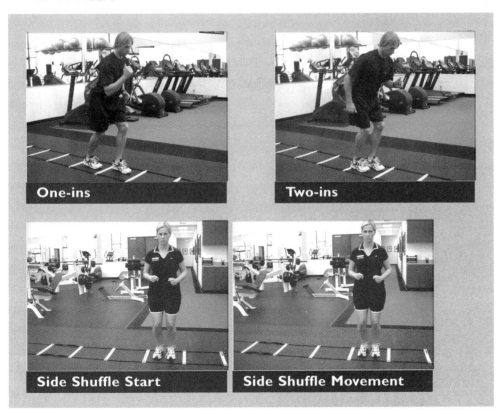

One-ins

Two-ins

Side Shuffle Start

Side Shuffle Movement

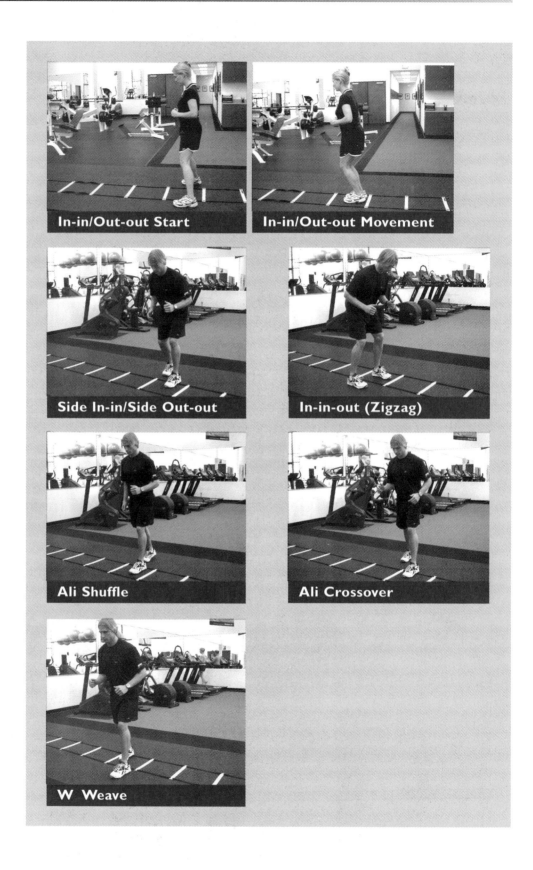

In-in/Out-out Start

In-in/Out-out Movement

Side In-in/Side Out-out

In-in-out (Zigzag)

Ali Shuffle

Ali Crossover

W Weave

SAQ Cone Drills

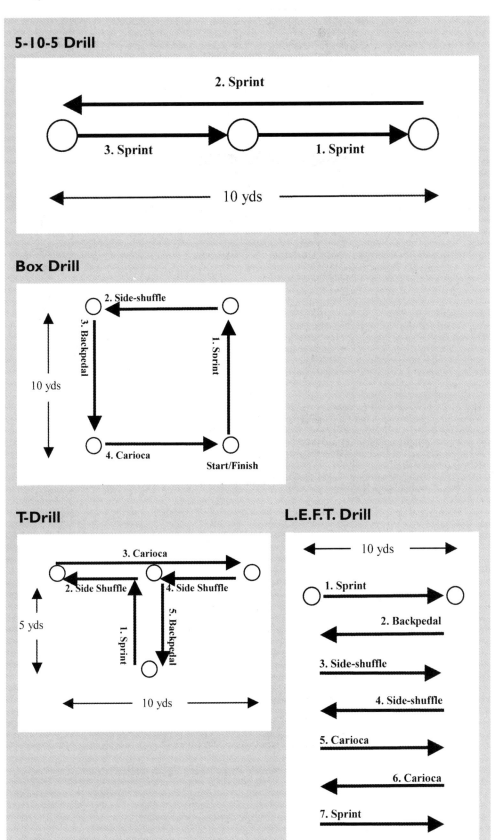

5-10-5 Drill

2. Sprint

3. Sprint   1. Sprint

10 yds

Box Drill

2. Side-shuffle

3. Backpedal   1. Sprint

10 yds

4. Carioca

Start/Finish

T-Drill

3. Carioca

2. Side Shuffle   4. Side Shuffle

1. Sprint   5. Backpedal

5 yds

10 yds

L.E.F.T. Drill

10 yds

1. Sprint

2. Backpedal

3. Side-shuffle

4. Side-shuffle

5. Carioca

6. Carioca

7. Sprint

Table 11-2: SAQ Program Design					
OPT™ Level	Phase(s)	Exercise	Sets	Reps	Rest
Stabilization	I	None	n/a	n/a	n/a
	2	4-6 Speed ladder drills	1-2	Half ladder*	0-60 sec.
		1-2 cone drills	1-2		0-90 sec.
Strength	3	6-9 Speed ladder drills	3-4	Half ladder*	0-60 sec.
	4				
	5	1-2 cone drills	2-3		0-90 sec.
Power	6	6-9 Speed ladder drills	3-6	Half ladder*	0-60 sec.
	7	2-4 cone drills	3-6		0-90 sec.

* *Most speed ladders come in two sections that snap together. Half of a speed ladder consists of using only one section.*

Filling in the Template

To fill in the program template (Figure 11-1), go to the section labeled Speed, Agility and Quickness. You will then refer to Table 11-2 for the appropriate type of exercises (ladder and/or cones), the appropriate number of exercises and the appropriate acute variables specific to the phase of training your client will be working in (1-7).

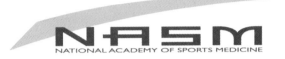

Optimum Performance Training™

NAME:	JOHN SMITH	DATE:	March 10, 2004
TRAINER:	CHERE	PHASE:	2: Integrated Stabilization Training
DAYS/WEEK:	3	GOAL:	Fat Loss

CARDIO TRAINING: Stage 1	TIME: 20 min	EQUIPMENT: Elliptical Trainer

WARMUP/FLEXIBILITY	Sets	Reps	Duration	Rest	Notes
1. SMR: Calves, IT band, adductors	1				Hold tender spots 20-30 sec.
2. Cardio: Elliptical trainer			5 min.		
3. Static Stretching: Calves, hip flexors, lats	1		30 sec.		

CORE & BALANCE	Sets	Reps	Tempo	Rest	Notes
1. Quadruped Arm Opposite Leg Raise	1-3	12-20	3-10 sec. hold	0	Circuit training
2. Floor bridge	1-3	12-20	3-10 sec. hold	0	
3. Single-leg Hip Flexion/Extension	1-3	6-10/leg	3-10 sec. hold	60 sec.	

REACTIVE	Sets	Reps	Tempo	Rest	Notes
1. Jump with Stabilization	1-3	5-8	3 sec. hold	60 sec.	
2.					

SPEED, AGILITY, QUICKNESS	Sets	Reps	Time	Rest	Notes
1. Speed Ladder	1-2			60 sec.	4 exercises
2. Box Drill	1-2			60 sec.	1-2 drills

STRENGTH	Exercise	Sets	Reps	Intensity	Tempo	Rest	Notes
TOTAL BODY							
CHEST							
BACK							
SHOULDERS							
BICEPS							
TRICEPS							
LEGS							

COOL-DOWN	
POST-WORKOUT FLEXIBILITY	Static Stretching: Calves, adductors, hip flexors, pectorals

Figure 11-1: OPT™ Template

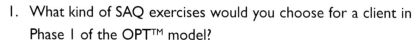
MODULE 11-2 Summary

Programming guidelines must be gauged on the total volume of training for all components in a workout. A client's core, balance and reactive capabilities will determine the success and safety of the program. Precise technique and kinetic chain control are required to minimize risk of injury. Various speed ladder and cone drills may be used in programming.

MODULE 11-2 Quiz

1. What kind of SAQ exercises would you choose for a client in Phase 1 of the OPT™ model?

_____

2. What is the recommended rest period for ladder drills?

_____

References

1. Brown LE, Ferrigno VA, Santana JC. *Training for speed, agility, and quickness.* Champaign, IL: Human Kinetics; 2000.

2. Luhtanen P, Komi PV. Mechanical factors influencing running speed. *Biomechanics VI-B.* In: Asmussen E, Jorgensen K (ed). Baltimore: University Park Press; 1978. pp. 23-29.

3. Mero A, Komi PV, Gregor RJ. Biomechanics of sprint running. *Sports Med* 1992;13(6):376-92.

4. Leierer S. A guide for sprint training. *Athl J* 1979;59(6):105-6.

5. McFarlane B. Developing maximal running speed. *Track Field Q Rev* 1985;83(2):4-9.

6. Parsons LS, Jones MT. Development of speed, quickness and agility for tennis athletes. *Strength Cond J* 1998;20:14-9.

CHAPTER TWELVE

Resistance Training Concepts

Objectives

After studying this chapter, you will be able to:

- Describe the stages of the General Adaptation Syndrome.
- Define and describe the Principle of Specificity.
- List and define the various stages of strength and training systems.

Key Terms

- General Adaptation Syndrome
- Alarm Reaction
- Resistance Development
- Exhaustion
- Periodization
- Principle of Specificity
- Specific Adaptation to Imposed Demands (SAID Principle)
- Mechanical Specificity

- Neuromuscular Specificity
- Metabolic Specificity
- Strength
- Muscular endurance
- Stability
- Strength endurance
- Hypertrophy
- Maximal strength
- Power

Introduction to Resistance Training

The final component of the OPT™ template that must be addressed is the resistance training portion. This section of the template is traditionally considered the "workout" portion of a session. It consists of filling in the exercise for each body part (chest, back, shoulders, etc.), the sets, repetitions, intensity (or weight), tempo (or speed of repetition) and the rest interval (or amount of rest given between each exercise). The resistance component of training or programming is generally seen as the most important. However, it should be very evident by now that without a proper assessment and flexibility protocol and attention to the client's goals, resistance training can become more of a hindrance than help.

There is quite a bit of information that a health and fitness professional needs to review in order to create and understand an effective resistance training program. The following modules will explore many concepts in resistance training, as well as address many misconceptions. They will focus on adaptations, progressive strength adaptations derived from resistance training, training systems used to acquire strength and specific resistance training exercise progressions.

ADAPTATION

is a function of

General Adaptation Syndrome

+

Principle of Specificity

Figure 12-1: Resistance Training Principle of Adaptation

MODULE 12-1: Adaptation

Resistance Training Principle of Adaptation

There are many important resistance training principles that a health and fitness professional must understand. The most important, perhaps, is that of adaptation (Figure 12-1).[1-7]

Adaptation

One of the many unique qualities that the human body displays is its ability to adapt or adjust its functional capacity to meet the desired needs. This is perhaps the root of all training and conditioning. The desire to seek an adaptation is the driving force behind most clients and training programs. Whether the goal is cosmetic in nature, health or performance-related, resistance training has been shown to produce many desirable effects (Figure 12-2). A good understanding of this phenomenon is important for the health and fitness professional.

General Adaptation Syndrome

GENERAL ADAPTATION SYNDROME: The kinetic chain's ability to adapt to stresses placed upon it.

The kinetic chain seeks to maintain a state of physiological balance (or homeostasis).[5] In order to do this, it must be able to adapt to stresses placed upon it. This ability to adapt to stress is known as the **General Adaptation Syndrome**. This general pattern of adaptation was brought forth by Hans Selye who showed that the kinetic chain responds and adapts to the stresses placed upon it. In order to respond, however, the body must be confronted

Physiological
- ■ Improved cardiovascular efficiency
- ■ Beneficial endocrine and serum lipid adaptations

Physical
- ■ Increased lean body mass
- ■ Decreased body fat

Performance
- ■ Increased metabolic efficiency
- ■ Increased tissue tensile strength
- ■ Increased bone density

Figure 12-2: Adaptive Benefits from Resistance Training

with a stressor or some form of stress that creates the need for a response (Table 11-1).[6] Selye outlined three stages of response to stress:[6]

- ■ Alarm Reaction
- ■ Resistance Development
- ■ Exhaustion

Alarm Reaction

The alarm reaction is the initial reaction to a stressor (Table 12-1). It allows for the activation of protective processes within the body. For example, a person who decides to begin resistance training places his body under the stress of increased amounts of force on his/her bones, joints, muscles, connective tissues and nervous system. This creates a need for increased oxygen and blood supply to the right areas in his/her body, as well as an increased neural recruitment to the muscles. Initially, the individual's body is very inefficient at responding to the demands placed upon it. Thus, the body must increase its ability to meet these new demands.[5,6]

> **ALARM
> REACTION:**
> The initial reaction
> to a stressor.

Resistance Development

During the **resistance development** stage, the body increases its functional capacity to adapt to the stressor (Table 12-1). After repeated training sessions, the kinetic chain will increase its capability to efficiently recruit muscle fibers and distribute oxygen and blood to the proper areas in the body. However, once adapted, the body will require increased stress to produce a new response.[5,6]

Health and fitness professionals often understand this adaptation response, but use it with improper application. In this scenario, many professionals only

> **RESISTANCE
> DEVELOPMENT:**
> The body increases
> its functional
> capacity to adapt
> to the stressor.

manipulate or adjust the amount of weight the client uses, when, in fact, this is only one of many ways that increased stress can be placed on the body. The next chapter will discuss the importance of manipulating many acute variables to properly enhance the kinetic chain to avoid breakdown or exhaustion.

Exhaustion

Prolonged stress or stress that is intolerable to a client will produce **exhaustion** or distress (Table 12-1). When the stressor is too much for the system to handle, it causes a breakdown or injury such as:[5,6]

- Stress fractures
- Muscle strains
- Joint pain
- Emotional fatigue

In turn, many of these will lead to the initiation of the Cumulative Injury Cycle.

This is the prime rationale for utilizing the OPT™ model (a systematic, progressive training program) that is based on science and proven through application. Resistance training (and any other form of training) must be cycled through different stages that increase stress placed on the kinetic chain and also allow for sufficient rest and recuperation. More information about the **periodization** of training (OPT™ model) will be detailed in the next chapter.

In the above example, if the resistance is continually increased with the intention of stressing the muscles of the body to produce a size and/or strength change, it can lead to injury of the muscle, joint or connective tissue. This is a result of the fact that connective tissues (such as ligaments and tendons) do not adapt as quickly as muscles, due to their lack of blood supply.[8-11] It is important to have a complete understanding of how the kinetic chain functions in order to properly manipulate it for optimum adaptation with minimal risk of injury.

There are many different tissues in the body (muscle fibers, connective tissue, etc.) and each have a different adaptive potential to stresses. This means that training programs should provide a variety of intensities and stresses to optimize the adaptation of each tissue to ensure the best possible results. Adaptation can be more specifically applied to certain aspects of the kinetic chain depending on the training technique(s) employed. This is evident by the Principle of Specificity.

EXHAUSTION:
Prolonged stress or stress that is intolerable and will produce exhaustion or distress to the system.

PERIODIZATION:
Division of a training program into smaller, progressive stages.

Table 12-1: The General Adaptation Syndrome	
Stage	**Reaction**
Alarm Reaction	Initial reaction to stressor such as increased oxygen and blood supply to the necessary areas of the body.
Resistance Development	Increased functional capacity to adapt to stressor such as increasing motor unit recruitment.
Exhaustion	A prolonged intolerable stressor produces fatigue and leads to a breakdown in the system or injury.

The Principle of Specificity: The SAID Principle

The **Principle of Specificity** is often referred to as the SAID Principle, which stands for **Specific Adaptation to Imposed Demands**. Essentially, this means that the body will specifically adapt to the type of demand placed upon it. For example, if someone repeatedly lifts heavy weights, that person will produce higher levels of maximal strength. If a person repeatedly lifts lighter weights for many repetitions, that person will develop higher levels of endurance.

This is a fairly simple concept to understand and implies that, in essence, you get what you train for. However, the Principle of Specificity is often used out of context and can become misleading to the health and fitness professional who does not remember the basic sciences previously discussed. That is, there are different tissues in the body that each respond to a different stimulus. In order to make the Principle of Specificity a safe and effective tool, it must be used appropriately.

The body must progress through different stages of adaptation to ensure that all of the necessary tissues are developed to properly meet the desired goal. Connective tissue recovers slower to training than muscle, but also must be strong in order for muscles to generate high levels of force. If emphasis is placed on training muscles to get big and/or strong, prior to training for connective tissue strength and endurance, there is risk of increased injury.

Remember that Type I muscle fibers function differently than Type II muscle fibers and are vitally important for postural stabilization. In order to train with higher intensities, proper postural stabilization is required. Therefore, tissues need to be trained differently to prepare them for higher levels of training, which are necessary to achieve many of the goals in a planned, organized manner. This is the specific purpose behind the three main adaptations of training within the OPT™ model that will be discussed in the next module.

PRINCIPLE OF SPECIFICITY OR SPECIFIC ADAPTATION TO IMPOSED DEMANDS (SAID PRINCIPLE): Principle that states the body will adapt to the specific demands that are placed upon it.

The degree of adaptation that occurs during training is directly related to the mechanical, neuromuscular and metabolic specificity of the training program.[4,12-57] In other words, the more specifically a health and fitness professional manipulates the exercise routine to meet the actual goal, the greater the carryover the training program will have on that goal. It is important to remember that if a specific adaptation is required or desired, it must be trained for. The body can only adapt if it has a reason to adapt.

- **Mechanical specificity** refers to the weight and movements placed on the body.[52-58] To develop endurance in the legs, light weights must be used over many repetitions with leg exercises. To develop maximal strength in the chest, heavy weights must be used during chest related exercises.

- **Neuromuscular specificity** refers to the speed of contraction and exercise selection.[20,59-63] To develop higher levels of power in the legs, low weight, high velocity contractions must be performed in a plyometric manner (such as those seen in reactive training power level exercises). To develop higher levels of stability while pushing, chest exercises will need to be performed, with controlled, unstable exercises, at slower speeds. (An example would be a dumbbell chest press performed on a stability ball.)

- **Metabolic specificity** refers to the energy demand placed upon the body.[64-69] To develop endurance, training will require prolonged bouts of exercise, with minimal rest periods between sets. To develop maximal strength or power, training will require longer rest periods, so the intensity of each bout of exercise remains high.

This is a very important concept for the health and fitness professional to understand and implement in their training program. A client must be trained to meet the specific demands of his/her daily life and goal(s).

As an example, imagine this concept were being applied to a client with the goal of body fat reduction. It is understood that: [70-72]

1. Mechanically, the body burns more calories when movements are performed in the standing position (versus a seated or lying position) with moderate weights.

2. Neuromuscularly, the body burns more calories when more muscles are being used over longer periods of time in controlled, unstable environments.

3. Metabolically, the body burns more calories when rest periods are controlled in order to minimize full recuperation.

MECHANICAL SPECIFICITY:
The specific muscular exercises using different weights and movements that are performed to increase strength or endurance in certain body parts.

NEUROMUSCULAR SPECIFICITY:
The specific muscular exercises using different speeds and styles that are performed to increase neuromuscular efficiency.

METABOLIC SPECIFICITY:
The specific muscular exercises using different levels of energy that are performed to increase endurance, strength or power.

Following these specificity guidelines, this client should perform more of the exercises in a standing position with moderate weight. The client should also recruit and use more muscles on each exercise, while metabolically monitoring rest periods. This method will get the client to effectively burn more calories and achieve the goal of body fat reduction.

MODULE 12-1 Summary

A well-designed, integrated training program produces optimum levels of:

- Strength,
- Neuromuscular control,
- Power,
- Flexibility,
- Endurance and
- Alterations in body composition.

To achieve this, the body is required to adapt to specifically imposed demands and stresses. The ability to adapt to stress is known as the General Adaptation Syndrome. There are three stages of response to stress: 1. Alarm Reaction (or initial activation of protective processes within the body), 2. Resistance Development (or an increase in the functional capacity to adapt to a stressor) and 3. Exhaustion (or stress that is too much for the system and causes an injury). To avoid injury, adaptive programs must use a planned training methodology (periodization) that cycles through different stages and allows for sufficient rest and recuperation. Adaptive programs have several benefits, including:

Physiological
- Improved cardiovascular efficiency

Physical
- Decreased body fat
- Increased lean body mass

Performance
- Metabolic efficiency
- Tissue tensile strength
- Bone density

Adaptation must relate to a client's goals and the design of the program. There are different types of strength and different systems of strength training that may be employed in order to create a more individualized and systematic program for the client. There are also many different tissues in the body and each respond to different stresses as seen in the Principle of Specificity/Specific

Adaptation to Imposed Demands (or SAID Principle). Training programs should provide a variety of intensities and stresses to optimize the adaptation of each tissue to ensure the best possible results. The degree of adaptation that occurs during training is directly related to the mechanical, neuromuscular and metabolic specificity of the training program.

MODULE 12-1 Quiz

1. In order for the kinetic chain to respond and adapt to stresses, it must be confronted with what?

   _____

   _____

2. The Principle of Specificity is also known as what?

   _____

3. After repeated training sessions, the kinetic chain will _____ its capability to efficiently recruit muscle fibers and distribute oxygen and blood to the proper areas in the body?

   ☐ Increase

   ☐ Decrease

4. Connective tissues (such as ligaments and tendons) adapt just as quickly as muscles.

   ☐ True   ☐ False

MODULE 12-2:
Progressive Strength Adaptations from Resistance Training

The concept of adaptation makes it clear that some type of change will occur based upon the stresses placed on the body. Resistance training programs are designed to produce changes that result in various strength adaptations. Whether the goal is to increase muscle mass, develop better athletic performance or reduce body fat, the use of resistance training is an important component of any program. This will help ensure optimal health and longevity for the client. The healthier a client remains, the longer they can train. The longer they can train without entering the exhaustion stage (General Adaptation Syndrome) and developing tissue breakdown or injury, the greater amount of change or adaptation they will realize.

Following the concepts of the General Adaptation Syndrome and the Principle of Specificity, a health and fitness professional can plan the appropriate fitness, wellness and/or performance program for their client.

Definition of Strength

Strength is the ability of the neuromuscular system to produce internal tension (in the muscles and connective tissue that pull on the bones) to overcome an external force.[73,74] Whether the external force demands the neuromuscular system to produce stability, endurance, maximal strength or power, it still requires a form of internal tension. This internal tension produced is *strength adaptation*. The specific form of strength or internal tension that is produced from training is based upon the style of training used by the client (Principle of Specificity).

Traditionally, resistance training programs have focused on developing maximal strength in individual muscles, emphasizing one plane of motion. Since all muscles function eccentrically, isometrically and concentrically in all three planes of motion at different speeds, a training program should utilize a progressive approach that emphasizes the appropriate exercise selection, all muscle actions and repetition tempos (see Chapter 13).[1,4,13,51,75]

Strength adaptations obtained from resistance training can be divided into three main categories of stabilization, strength and power as seen in the OPT™ model. Each adaptation can be defined by the emphasis that is placed on the neuromuscular system (Principle of Specificity) and all occur in a progressive sequence: stabilization before strength; strength before power. Each adaptation

> **STRENGTH:**
> **The ability of the neuromuscular system to produce internal tension in order to overcome an external force.**

category can be further divided into more specific adaptations, summarized in Table 12-2, that are a result of resistance training.[1,60]

Table 12-2: Specific Adaptations in the OPT™ Model	
Category	**Specific Adaptations**
Stabilization	Muscular Endurance
	Stability
Strength	Strength Endurance
	Hypertrophy
	Maximal Strength
Power	Power

Stabilization

Stabilization adaptations build the foundation for optimum human movement and should be the beginning point for all first time clients. Stabilization adaptation should also be revisited periodically by advanced clients. Stabilization must be established prior to training for other adaptations because it specifically focuses on the recruitment of tissues in the body responsible for postural stability. This includes tissue such as Type I muscle fibers and connective tissue. The General Adaptation Syndrome and Principle of Specificity both dictate that in order to maximize training for these tissues, a program must use high repetition schemes with low to moderate volume and intensity in a postural position that challenges the stability of the body. This means, more simply, training for muscular endurance in unstable positions that can be safely controlled. This challenges the body's ability to structurally stabilize itself.

The emphasis is placed on the nervous system in this adaptation category. Initial gains that are noted in strength originate from within the nervous system.[40,55,76-78] For muscles to function properly, they must be appropriately linked to the nervous system by motor units.

Recruitment of motor units is generally determined by their size (Size Principle).[79] Smaller motor units (Type I) are recruited before larger motor units (Type II). It has been noted that many clients who are new to resistance training have not established the ability to recruit a high percentage of motor units.[55,76] By focusing on high repetitions with low intensities at slow velocities, a beginning client can be taught precise exercise technique and establish the right connection between the brain and muscles, without placing improper stresses on the body.

The two primary adaptations that are achieved in this level of training are muscular endurance and stability. Both of these adaptations increase the ability of the body to produce internal tension and, as a result, increase specific forms of strength for each client.

Muscular Endurance

Muscular endurance is the ability to produce and maintain relatively low levels of force over prolonged periods of time. The ability to overcome gravity, ground reaction forces and momentum, on a continual basis, is vital in the prevention of injury and allows proper kinetic chain alignment and performance.[1,13,57] This is most important for maintaining proper length-tension relationships in the muscles to minimize unwanted stress on the joints and reduce the risk of entering the exhaustion phase of General Adaptation Syndrome and eventual injury. It promotes proper stabilization during training, as well as maintenance of better posture throughout the day, increasing a client's sense of well-being.

> **MUSCULAR ENDURANCE:**
> The ability of the body to produce low levels of force and maintain them for extended periods of time.

Stability

Stability is the ability of the kinetic chain's stabilizing muscles to provide optimal dynamic joint stabilization and maintain correct posture during all movements. This requires high levels of muscular endurance to allow for optimal recruitment of prime movers, increasing force production and force reduction.[73,74]

Research has repeatedly demonstrated that training with controlled, unstable exercises increases the body's ability to stabilize and/or balance itself.[80,82] Conversely, if training is not performed with controlled unstable exercises, clients will not gain the same level of stability and may even worsen.[82,83]

Stability is arguably the most important adaptation because it increases the ability of the kinetic chain to stabilize the lumbo-pelvic-hip complex and joints during movement, to allow the arms and legs to work more efficiently.

> **STABILITY:**
> The ability of the body to maintain postural equilibrium and support joints during movement.

Strength

Strength adaptations provide the necessary progression from the stabilization adaptations of training to increase the stress placed upon the body, allowing for new adaptations to be achieved. Type II muscle fibers are more predominantly recruited to increase the body's capacity to produce internal tension. The General Adaptation Syndrome and Principle of Specificity both dictate that in order to maximize training for these tissues, a program must use low to moderate repetition schemes with moderate to high volume and intensity.

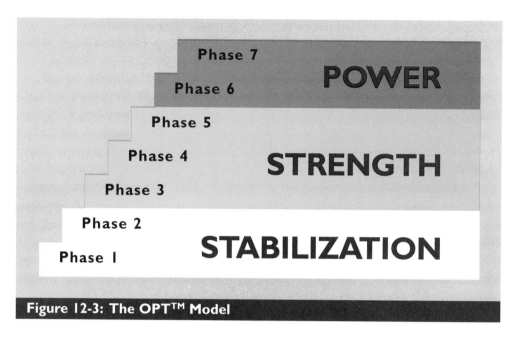

Figure 12-3: The OPT™ Model

The emphasis in this adaptation category is on both the nervous and muscular systems. Heavier weights and higher volumes of training are used to increase the recruitment, synchronization and the firing rate of motor units, while placing necessary mechanical stress on the muscles to increase their size and/or strength.[40,55,76-78] Strength endurance, hypertrophy and maximal strength are the primary adaptations seen in this level of training.

Strength Endurance

STRENGTH ENDURANCE: The ability of the body to repeatedly produce high levels of force, over prolonged periods of time.

Strength endurance is the ability to repeatedly produce higher levels of force for prolonged periods of time. Whereas muscular endurance involves lower intensities of force being used with higher repetitions (12-25) and minimal rest between sets, strength endurance allows the body to use higher levels of force with lower repetitions (six to 12) and more sets, repeatedly, with minimal rest. This adaptation is often trained with the use of supersets (Chapter 13 — Program Design,).[57,74,75]

Hypertrophy

HYPERTROPHY: Enlargement of skeletal muscle fibers in response to overcoming force from high volumes of tension.

Hypertrophy is the enlargement of skeletal muscle fibers in response to increased volumes of tension, as seen in resistance training.[84,85] Muscle hypertrophy is characterized by the increase in the cross-sectional area of individual muscle fibers and is believed to result from an increase in the myofibril proteins (myofilaments).[86,89] While hypertrophy is not externally visible for many weeks (four to eight weeks) in a beginning client, the process begins in the early stages of training, regardless of the intensity.[21,58,90-100] However, muscle fibers must be recruited in order to induce hypertrophy.[7,101] The nervous system must establish the proper connection to effectively communicate with each muscle fiber. This provides the necessary information as to why clients should start and revisit the stabilization level of training before entering into the strength level.

Maximal Strength

Maximal strength is the maximum force that a muscle can produce in a single, voluntary effort, regardless of how fast the load moves. In order for a muscle to produce maximal force, all of the muscle's motor units must be recruited.[40,55,76-78] This is to ensure that as many possible muscle fibers are involved in the contraction. One means of increasing strength lies in the ability to recruit a maximal amount of motor units.

Maximum strength can be improved through stabilization training. This type of training improves the ability of the neuromuscular system to better recruit motor units within a muscle (intramuscular coordination) and in synergy with many other muscles (intermuscular coordination). This allows the nervous system to appropriately use muscles to stabilize a joint while other muscles are lifting maximal loads.[1,4,13,51,57,75]

> **MAXIMAL STRENGTH:**
> The maximum force that a muscle can produce in a single, voluntary effort, regardless of velocity.

Power

The adaptation of power uses the stabilization and strength adaptations and applies them at more realistic speeds and forces, seen in everyday and sporting activities. The focus is now on getting the neuromuscular system to generate force as quickly as possible (rate of force production).

Power is the ability of the neuromuscular system to produce the greatest possible force in the shortest possible time. This is represented by the simple equation of force multiplied by velocity.[102]

An increase in either force and/or velocity will produce an increase in power. This can be achieved by increasing the weight (force), as seen in the strength adaptations and/or increasing the speed with which weight is moved (velocity). Power training allows for increased rate of force production by increasing the number of motor units activated, the synchronization between them and the speed at which they are activated.[76,77,103] The General Adaptation Syndrome and Principle of Specificity both dictate that in order to maximize training for this adaptation, both heavy and light loads must be moved as fast and as controlled as possible.

> **POWER:**
> Ability of the neuromuscular system to produce the greatest force in the shortest time.

MODULE 12-2 Summary

Resistance training programs produce changes that result in various strength adaptations. Strength is the ability of the neuromuscular system to produce internal tension to overcome an external force. Traditionally, resistance training programs have focused on developing maximal strength in individual muscles. However, today's training program should emphasize appropriate exercise selection, all muscle actions and repetition tempos. Training adaptations can be divided into three main categories: stabilization, strength and power.

Stabilization adaptations should be the beginning point for all first time clients. Use high repetitions with low/moderate volume and low/moderate intensity, in a postural position that challenges the stability of the body. The two primary adaptations that are achieved are muscular endurance and stability.

Strength adaptations should utilize low/moderate repetition schemes with moderate/high volume and moderate/high intensity. Heavier weights and higher volumes of training are used to improve the function of motor units, while placing stress on the muscles to increase size and/or strength. Strength endurance, hypertrophy and maximal strength are the primary adaptations seen in this period of training. Strength endurance uses higher levels of force with lower repetitions (six to 12) and more sets, repeatedly, with minimal rest. It is often trained with the use of supersets.

Power is the ability of the neuromuscular system to produce the greatest possible force in the shortest possible time. An increase in either force (weight) and/or velocity (speed with which weight is moved) will produce an increase in power. In order to maximize training for this adaptation, both heavy and light loads must be moved as fast and as controlled as possible.

MODULE 12-2 Quiz

1. In which category does the specific adaptation of muscular endurance fall?

    ☐ Power ☐ Strength ☐ Stabilization

2. An increase in either force and/or velocity will produce an ☐ **increase** ☐ **decrease** in power.

3. Strength endurance allows the body to use lower levels of force with lower repetitions and fewer sets.

    ☐ True ☐ False

MODULE 12-3:
Resistance Training Systems

Originally, power lifters, Olympic lifters and bodybuilders were the ones who designed most resistance training programs. Many of these styles of resistance training programs remain popular today because of marketing or gym science, not because they scientifically demonstrate superiority over other programs in bringing about increases in stabilization, strength and/or power.

Following a systematic, integrated training program and manipulating key training variables is necessary to achieve optimal gains in specific forms of strength.[1,13,35,52,57,104] The OPT™ model follows a progressive, systematic approach that enables the health and fitness professional to make consistent gains with all clients. It can be manipulated in many ways to achieve various goals. There are many training systems that can be utilized to structure a resistance training program for different effects. We will review several of the most common training systems that are currently used in the fitness industry. These systems are summarized in Table 12-5 at the end of the module and are explained below.

Resistance Training Systems Explained

The Single-set System

The single-set system is one of the oldest training methods.[25] The single-set system entails performance of one set of each exercise. Each set usually consists of eight to 12 repetitions of each exercise at a controlled tempo. It is usually recommended that this system be performed two times per week in order to promote sufficient development and maintenance of muscle mass.[104] Although multiple-set training is promoted as being more beneficial for strength and hypertrophy gains in advanced clients, the single-set system has been shown to be as beneficial for a beginning level client.[25,105-108]

This system of training should be explored by the health and fitness professional to help customize program design. Often in the training industry, single-set training is negatively perceived as not providing enough stimuli for adaptation. However, when reviewing the physiology of how the kinetic chain operates and current research, this may not be true.[25,106] In fact, most first-time clients *should* follow a single-set program to allow for proper adaptive responses of the connective tissue and nervous system, prior to engaging in more rigorous training systems. By not giving a client more than they can handle, synergistic dominance and injury can be avoided. Applying variation to rest periods, repetitions and intensity, single-set training can make a program very demanding for even the advanced client.

The Multiple-set System

This resistance training system has been popular since the 1940s.[75] The multiple-set system of training consists of performing a multiple number of sets for each exercise. The resistance, sets and repetitions that are performed can be selected according to the goals and needs of the client (see Chapter 13).[75,110,111] Multiple-set training can be appropriate for both novice and advanced clients, but has specifically been shown to be superior to single-set training for the advanced client.[104,112-116] It appears that the increased volume (sets, reps and/or intensity) is necessary for further improvement, but must be administered appropriately to avoid over-training.[7,117,118]

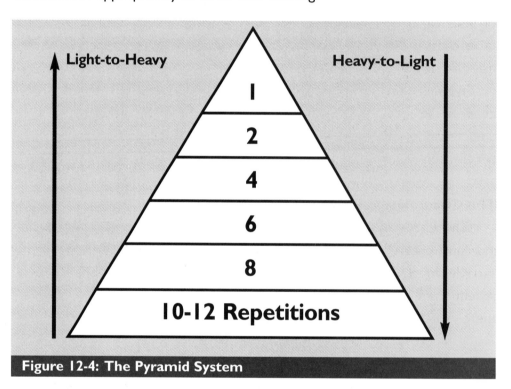

Light-to-Heavy   **Heavy-to-Light**

1
2
4
6
8
10-12 Repetitions

Figure 12-4: The Pyramid System

The Pyramid System

The pyramid system involves a progressive or regressive step approach that either increases weight with each set, or decreases weight with each set (Figure 12-4).[104]

In the *light-to-heavy system*, the individual performs 10-12 repetitions with a light load and increases the resistance for each following set, until the individual can perform one to two repetitions, usually in four to six sets. This system can easily be used for workouts that involve only two to four sets or higher repetition schemes (12-20 repetitions).

The *heavy-to-light system* works in the opposite direction. The individual begins with a heavy load (following a warm-up) for one to two repetitions then decreases the load and increases the repetitions for four to six sets.[104]

The Superset System

The superset system utilizes a couple of exercises performed in rapid succession of one another. This system features the use of independent subsystems with similar principles (namely, compound-set and tri-set systems).[104]

Compound-sets involve the performance of two exercises for antagonistic muscles. For example, an individual may perform a set of bench presses followed by cable rows (chest/back). Working opposing musculature allows for better recovery before the start of another set. In addition, it is more time efficient.[104]

Tri-sets use three exercises in rapid succession for the same muscle group or body part. For example, an individual may perform dumbbell incline press, cable chest press and ball push-ups all in succession (chest superset).[104] This may also be performed with two exercises.

Typically, supersetting involves sets of eight to 12 repetitions with no rest between sets or exercises. However, any number of repetitions can be employed. The superset system is popular among bodybuilders and may be beneficial for muscular hypertrophy and muscular endurance.[104,114]

The Circuit Training System

The circuit training system consists of a series of exercises that an individual performs one after the other, with minimal rest. The typical acute variables for a circuit-training program include one to three sets of eight to 15 repetitions with 15-60 seconds of rest between exercises.[104,119,120] However, these variables can be manipulated to enhance the desired effect.

---

1. **Ball Two-arm Dumbbell Chest Press**
2. **Single-leg Cable Pulldown**
3. **Ball Combo I**
4. **Single-leg Dumbbell Curl**
5. **Supine Ball Dumbbell Tricep Extension**
6. **Step-up**
7. **Rest**

**Figure 12-5:
The OPT™ Circuit for Phase 2: Integrated Stabilization Training**

These exercises should be performed immediately after each other for two to three sets of 12-20 repetitions each (in Phase 2 of the OPT™ model).

Circuit training is a great training system for those individuals with limited time and for those who want to alter body composition.[13,104,119-121]

The Peripheral Heart Action System

The Peripheral Heart Action System is another variation of circuit training that alternates upper body and lower body exercises throughout the circuit. The number of exercises per sequence varies with the program's goal. The individual performs eight to 20 repetitions per exercise, depending on the desired adaptation and phase of training they are using in the OPT™ model. This system is very beneficial for incorporating an integrated, multidimensional program and for altering body composition.[104,121] An example for each of the three main adaptations are shown in Table 12-3.

Table 12-3: Peripheral Heart Action System — Sample Workout		
Stabilization	**Strength**	**Power**
Ball Dumbbell Chest Press	Bench Press	Medicine Ball Chest Pass
Ball Squat	Barbell Squat	Squat Jump
Standing Cable Row	Seated Row	Soccer Throw
Step-up to balance	Lunge	Power Step Ups
Standing Alternating-arm Dumbbell Shoulder Press	Seated Dumbbell Shoulder Press	Side Oblique Throw

The Split-routine System

A split-routine system involves breaking the body up into parts to be trained on separate days. Many bodybuilders, mass dominant and strength athletes (football, shot put, etc.) use the split-routine system. Bodybuilders typically perform many exercises for the same body part to bring about optimal muscular hypertrophy. By breaking up the body into parts that can be trained on different days, more work can be performed for the allotted time per workout. Split-routines come in all sizes and shapes. A few typical split-routines are shown in Table 12-4.

Any derivative of these outlined routines can be (and have been) used. The important issue with some of these routines is recovery time. When training each body part more than once a week, volume and intensity should be accounted for.

Vertical Loading and Horizontal Loading

Vertical loading is a resistance training system used by NASM and follows the OPT™ model. It progresses a workout vertically down the template, by alternating body parts trained from set to set. Looking at the OPT™ template, it is seen that the resistance training section involves the following exercises:

- Total body
- Chest

- Back
- Shoulders
- Biceps
- Triceps
- Legs

Table 12-4: Split-Routine System — Sample Workouts		
Routine	**Day(s) Performed**	**Body Parts Trained**
2 Day	Monday	Chest/Shoulders/Triceps
	Thursday	Back/Biceps/Legs
3 Day	Monday	Chest/Shoulders/Triceps
	Wednesday	Legs
	Friday	Back/Biceps
4 Day	Monday and Thursday	Chest/Shoulders/Triceps
	Tuesday and Friday	Back/Biceps/Legs
5 Day	Monday	Chest
	Tuesday	Legs
	Wednesday	Back
	Thursday	Shoulders
	Friday	Arms
6 Day	Monday and Friday	Chest/Shoulders/Triceps
	Tuesday and Saturday	Legs
	Wednesday and Sunday	Back/Biceps

In a vertically loaded workout, the client would perform the first exercise (total body) for the required repetitions and then move to the chest exercise for the next set of repetitions. After the chest exercise, the client would move on to the back exercise and so forth, until all exercises have been completed. Once completed, the client would then start back at the first exercise (total body) and run through the exercises again for the desired amount of sets. This can also be done in a circuit style, by minimizing the rest periods in between exercises.

This system of training can be very beneficial for allowing maximal recovery to each body part while minimizing the amount of time wasted on rest. For example, if it takes one minute to perform each exercise, by the time the client returns to the chest exercise, seven to 10 minutes could have passed, which is far more than necessary for full ATP/CP recovery. Even though seven to 10 minutes have passed, the client has been constantly moving and has performed one set of every exercise in their workout.

Horizontal loading refers to performing all sets of an exercise or body part before moving on to the next exercise or body part. For example, if performing three sets of a chest exercise and three sets of a back exercise, the client would perform all three sets of the chest exercise before moving on to the back exercise. The progression of exercises is therefore said to be horizontal across the template. This is the method most commonly used in the fitness environment.

The drawback to the horizontal loading system is the amount of time typically spent resting, which can often add up to more time then the actual workout itself. Horizontal loading can be a metabolic progression if rest periods are monitored and limited to 30-90 seconds between sets. It forces the same muscle group to work with minimal recovery. This can cause metabolic and hypertrophy related adaptations to occur in the muscle.[65,69,104]

Table 12-5: Resistance Training Systems	
Type	**Definition**
Single-set	Performing one set of each exercise.
Multiple-set	Performing a multiple number of sets for each exercise.
Pyramid	Increasing (or decreasing) weight with each set.
Superset	Performing a couple of exercises in rapid succession.
Circuit Training	Performing a series of exercises, one after the other, with minimal rest.
Peripheral Heart Action	A variation of circuit training that uses different exercises for each set through the circuit.
Split-routine	A routine that trains different body parts on separate days.
Vertical Loading	Performing exercises on the OPT™ template one after the other, in a vertical manner down the template.
Horizontal Loading	Performing all sets of an exercise (or body part) before moving on to the next exercise (or body part).

Filling in the Template

To fill in the program template (Figure 12-6), go to the section labeled strength. You will then refer to the following section for the appropriate type of resistance training exercise (stabilization, strength or power), the appropriate number of exercises depending on the phase. The appropriate acute variables can be found in the next chapter, Program Design, specific to the phase of training your client will be working in.

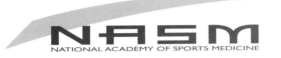

Optimum Performance Training™

NAME: JOHN SMITH

TRAINER: CHERE

DAYS/WEEK: 3

DATE: March 10, 2004

PHASE: 2: Integrated Stabilization Training

GOAL: Fat Loss

CARDIO TRAINING: Stage 1	TIME: 20 min	EQUIPMENT: Elliptical Trainer

WARMUP/FLEXIBILITY	Sets	Reps	Duration	Rest	Notes
1. SMR: Calves, IT band, adductors	1				Hold tender spots 20-30 sec.
2. Cardio: Elliptical trainer			5 min.		
3. Static Stretching: Calves, hip flexors, lats	1		30 sec.		

CORE & BALANCE	Sets	Reps	Tempo	Rest	Notes
1. Quadruped Arm Opposite Leg Raise	1-3	12-20	3-10 sec. hold	0	Circuit training
2. Floor bridge	1-3	12-20	3-10 sec. hold	0	
3. Single-leg Hip Flexion/Extension	1-3	6-10/leg	3-10 sec. hold	60 sec.	

REACTIVE	Sets	Reps	Tempo	Rest	Notes
1. Jump with Stabilization	1-3	5-8	3 sec hold	60 sec	
2.					

SPEED, AGILITY, QUICKNESS	Sets	Reps	Time	Rest	Notes
1. Speed Ladder	1-2			60 sec.	4 exercises
2. Box Drill	1-2			60 sec.	1-2 drills

STRENGTH	Exercise	Sets	Reps	Intensity	Tempo	Rest	Notes
TOTAL BODY							
CHEST	Standing Cable Chest Press	1-3	12-20	60-70%	4-2-1	0	Circuit training
BACK	Standing Cable Row	1-3	12-20	60-70%	4-2-1	0	
SHOULDERS	Standing Dumbbell Shoulder Press	1-3	12-20	60-70%	4-2-1	0	
BICEPS							
TRICEPS							
LEGS	Step-up to Balance	1-3	12-20	60-70%	4-2-1	90 sec	

COOL-DOWN	
POST-WORKOUT FLEXIBILITY	Static Stretching: Calves, adductors, hip flexors, pectorals

Figure 12-6: OPT™ Template

MODULE 12-3 Summary

The OPT™ method follows a progressive, systematic approach that enables the health and fitness professional to make consistent gains with all clients through training manipulations to achieve various goals. There are many training systems that can be utilized to structure a resistance training program for different effects.

The single-set system entails performance of one set of each exercise, usually of eight to 12 repetitions. This system has been shown to be beneficial for strength and hypertrophy gains in the beginning level client.

The multiple-set system of training consists of performing a multiple number of sets for each exercise, with resistance, sets and repetitions adjusted according to the goals/needs of the client. This system is superior to single-set training for the advanced client.

The pyramid system involves a progressive or regressive step approach that either increases weight with each set, or decreases weight with each set.

The superset system utilizes a couple of exercises performed in rapid succession of one another, usually eight to 12 repetitions with no rest between sets or exercises. This system can be performed as compound-sets or tri-sets. It is popular among bodybuilders for muscular hypertrophy and muscular endurance.

The circuit training system programs consist of a series of exercises that an individual performs one immediately after the other, with minimal rest. It is a good system for clients with limited time and those who want to alter body composition.

The Peripheral Heart Action System is another variation of circuit training that alternates upper body and lower body exercises (of varied numbers) throughout the circuit.

A split-routine system involves breaking the body up into parts to be trained on separate days so that more work can be performed for the allotted time per workout. When training each body part more than once a week, recovery period, volume and intensity should be accounted for.

Vertical loading and horizontal loading progress a workout vertically or horizontally down the OPT™ template, by alternating body parts trained from set to set. In a vertically loaded workout, the client would perform the each exercise until all exercises have been completed and then run through the exercises again for the desired amount of sets. This can also be done in a circuit style, by minimizing the rest periods in between exercises to allow maximal recovery to each body part and minimize the amount of time wasted on rest. In a horizontally loaded workout, the client would perform all sets of an exercise or body part before moving on to the next exercise or body part.

MODULE 12-3 Quiz

1. _____ training is promoted as being more beneficial for strength and hypertrophy gains in advanced clients.

   ☐ Single-set

   ☐ Multiple-set

2. Compound-sets involve the performance of exercises in rapid succession for the same muscle group or body part.

   ☐ True   ☐ False

3. Which system is good for clients with limited time as well as for those who want to alter body composition?

   _____

4. _____ loading refers to performing all sets of an exercise or body part before moving on to the next exercise or body part.

   ☐ Vertical

   ☐ Horizontal

5. How is Peripheral Heart Training System different from circuit training?

   _____

   _____

   _____

   _____

   _____

6. What is the important thing to remember for split-routine system workouts?

   _____

MODULE 12-4: Exercises

Total Body Exercise Descriptions

TOTAL BODY STABILIZATION EXERCISES

Squat to Row Progression

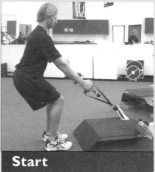

Start

Finish

Preparation

1. Face a cable machine with both feet shoulder-width apart, with feet pointing straight ahead and knees over second and third toes.
2. Hold cables with arms extended at chest level.

Movement

3. Draw abs in and activate glutes.
4. Perform a three-quarter squat, keeping lower extremity in proper alignment.
5. Before any compensation occurs, activate glutes and stand to a fully upright position.
6. While standing, begin to row, by pulling the cable, squeezing shoulder blades and pulling thumbs to your armpits.
7. The row should be complete by the time the legs are fully extended.
8. Repeat by extending the arms and squatting
9. Progressions
   a. Two-leg, alternating-arm
   b. Two-leg, single-arm
   c. Single-leg, two-arm
   d. Single-leg, alternating-arm
   e. Single-leg, single-arm

Squat, Curl to Press Progression

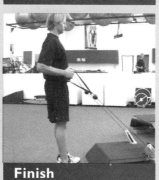

Start

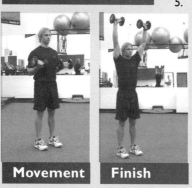

Movement   **Finish**

Preparation

1. Begin with both feet shoulder-width apart, with feet pointing straight ahead and knees over second and third toes.
2. Hold two dumbbells in hands at chest level (palms facing body).

Movement

3. Draw abs in and activate glutes.
4. Perform a three-quarter squat, keeping lower extremity in proper alignment.
5. Before any compensation occurs, activate glutes and stand to a fully upright position.
6. Once stabilized, press the dumbbells overhead until both arms are fully extended, with palms facing away.
7. Slowly return the dumbbells back to chest and repeat.
8. Regressions
   a. Ball Squat, Curl to Press
9. Progression:
   a. Alternating-arm
   b. Single-arm

Single-leg Squat, Curl to Press

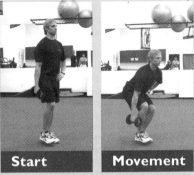

Start | Movement

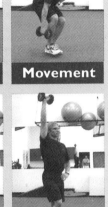

Movement | Finish

Preparation

1. Place one hand on hip and a dumbbell in the other.
2. Balance on one leg, with knee flexed slightly and aligned over second and third toes.

Movement

3. Draw abs in and activate glutes.
4. Keeping opposite leg directly beside stance leg, slowly squat down.
5. Lower down to the first point of compensation.
6. Then, push through heel, activate glutes and stand back upright until the hip and knee are extended.
7. Hold this balance position and press the dumbbells overhead.
8. Lower weight back to chest and repeat.
9. Regression
   a. Squat, Curl to Press
10. Progression
   a. Single-leg Squat Touchdown, Curl to Press

Single-leg Squat Touchdown to Overhead Press

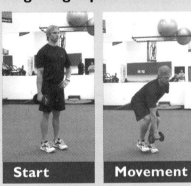

Start | Movement

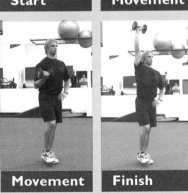

Movement | Finish

Preparation

1. Place one hand on hip and a dumbbell in the other.
2. Balance on one leg, with knee flexed slightly and aligned over second and third toes.

Movement

3. Draw abs in and activate glutes.
4. Keeping opposite leg directly beside stance leg, slowly squat down.
5. Reach with the dumbbell toward stabilizing foot. Keep chest up while lowering and maintain optimal alignment of lower extremity.
6. Lower down to the first point of compensation.
7. Then, push through heel, activate glutes and stand back upright until the hip and knee are extended.
8. Hold this balance position and press the dumbbell overhead.
9. Lower weight back to chest and repeat.
10. Regression
   a. Single-leg Squat, Curl to Press
11. Progression
   a. Unstable surface

Single-leg Romanian Deadlift to Overhead Press

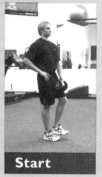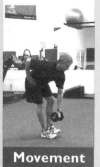

Start — Movement

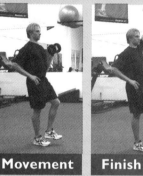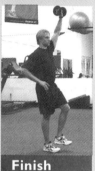

Movement — Finish

Preparation
1. Place one hand on hip and a dumbbell in the other.
2. Balance on one leg, with knee flexed at a five-degree angle and aligned over second and third toes.

Movement
3. Draw abs in and activate glutes.
4. Keep "floating" leg directly beside stance leg and slowly bend over at the waist, maintaining five degrees of knee flexion.
5. Reach with the dumbbell toward stabilizing foot. While lowering, maintain optimal alignment of lower extremity.
6. Lower to the first point of compensation.
7. Then, activate glutes and stand back upright until hip is extended.
8. Hold a balanced position and press the dumbbell overhead.
9. Lower weight back to chest and repeat.
10. Regression
    a. Decrease range of motion
11. Progression
    a. Balance beam
    b. Reebok Core Board
    c. Half foam roll
    d. Airex pad
    e. Dyna Disc

Multiplanar Step-up, Balance to Overhead Press

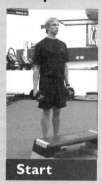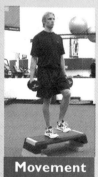

Start — Movement

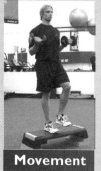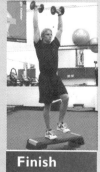

Movement — Finish

Preparation
1. Stand in front of a box (six to 18 inches high) with feet shoulder-width apart.
2. Hold dumbbells in both hands at chest level.

Movement
3. Draw abs in and activate glutes.
4. Step onto a box with one leg, keeping foot pointed straight ahead and knee lined up over mid-foot.
5. Push through heel and stand up straight, balancing on one leg.
6. Flex the other leg at the hip and knee.
7. Once balance has been established, press the dumbbells overhead until both arms are fully extended.
8. Slowly return the dumbbells to chest.
9. Return opposite leg to the ground and step off the box.
10. Repeat on other leg.
11. Regression
    a. Omit balance
12. Progression
    a. Frontal plane
    b. Transverse plane

TOTAL BODY STRENGTH EXERCISES

Lunge to Two-arm Dumbbell Press

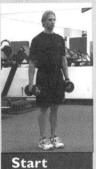
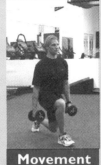

Start **Movement**

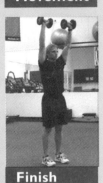

Movement **Finish**

Preparation

1. Begin with both feet shoulder-width apart.
2. Hold two dumbbells in hands at chest level (palms facing body).

Movement

3. Draw abs in and activate glutes.
4. Lunge forward, landing on the heel of lunge foot.
5. Then, come to a stabilized position with front foot pointing straight ahead and knee directly over second and third toes.
6. Both knees should now be bent at a 90-degree angle, front foot should be flat on the ground and back foot should have the heel lifted off the ground.
7. From this position, drive off of front foot (heel first) and back into a standing position.
8. In this stable position, press the dumbbells overhead until arms are fully extended.
9. Lower weight to chest and repeat.

Step-up to Two-arm Press

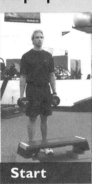
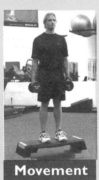

Start **Movement**

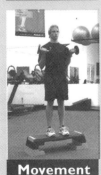
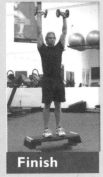

Movement **Finish**

Preparation

1. Stand in front of a box (six to 18 inches high) with feet shoulder-width apart.
2. Hold two dumbbells in both hands at chest level (palms facing body).

Movement

3. Draw abs in and activate glutes.
4. Step onto box with one leg, keeping foot pointed straight ahead and knee lined up over mid-foot.
5. Push through heel and stand up straight with both legs on top of box.
6. Once stabilization has been established, press the dumbbells overhead until both arms are fully extended.
7. Slowly return the dumbbells back to chest.
8. Step off the box and return to the ground, maintaining alignment of the lower extremity.
9. Repeat on other leg.

Squat to Two-arm Press

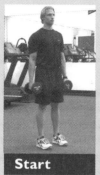
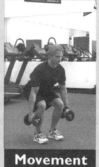

Start   **Movement**

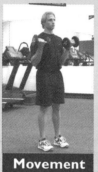
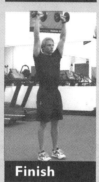

Movement   **Finish**

Preparation

1. Begin with both feet shoulder-width apart and pointing straight ahead, and knees over second and third toes.
2. Hold two dumbbells in hands at chest level (palms facing body).

Movement

3. Draw abs in and activate glutes.
4. Perform a three-quarter squat, keeping lower extremity in proper alignment.
5. Before any compensation occurs, activate glutes and stand to a fully upright position.
6. Once stabilized, press the dumbbells overhead until both arms are fully extended, with palms facing away.
7. Slowly return the dumbbells to chest and repeat.

Squat to Two-arm Row

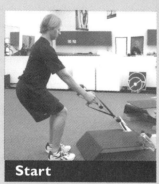

Start

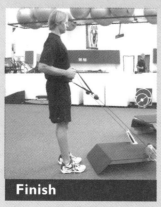

Finish

Preparation

1. Begin facing a cable machine with both feet shoulder-width apart and pointing straight ahead, and knees over second and third toes.
2. Hold cables with arms extended at chest level.

Movement

3. Draw abs in and activate glutes.
4. Perform a three-quarter squat, keeping lower extremity in proper alignment.
5. Before any compensation occurs, activate glutes and stand to a fully upright position.
6. While standing, begin to row, by pulling the cable, squeezing shoulder blades and pulling thumbs to armpits.
7. The row should be complete by the time the legs are fully extended.
8. Repeat by extending the arms and squatting.

Barbell Romanian Deadlift, Shrug, Calf Raise

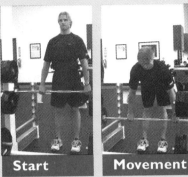

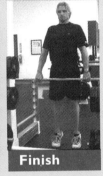

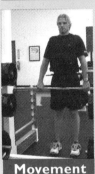

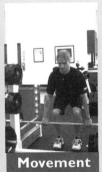

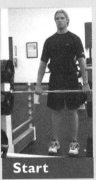

Start | Movement | Movement | Finish

Preparation

1. Barbell should be on the ground.
2. Begin with both feet shoulder-width apart, with toes pointing forward and knees bent at a five-degree angle.

Movement

3. Draw abs in and activate glutes.
4. Grab the barbell with both hands (grip slightly wider than shoulder-width).
5. Maintaining a drawn-in position, contract the glutes and lift the barbell until in a fully upright position.
6. Retract shoulder blades and shrug shoulders up toward ears.
7. Hold the shrug and perform a calf raise by putting pressure over the big toe.
8. Return to original position by reversing the order of the exercise.

Barbell Russian Deadlift, Shrug, Calf Raise

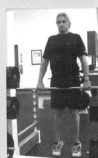

Start | Movement | Movement | Finish

Preparation

1. Barbell should be on the ground.
2. Begin with both feet shoulder-width apart and pointing forward, and knees in line with toes.

Movement

3. Draw abs in and activate glutes.
4. Squat down and grab the barbell with both hands (grip slightly wider than shoulder-width).
5. Maintaining a drawn-in position, drive through the heels, contract the glutes and lift the barbell until in a fully upright position.
6. Retract shoulder blades and shrug shoulders toward ears.
7. Hold the shrug and perform a calf raise by putting pressure over the big toe.
8. Return to original position by reversing the order of the exercise.

TOTAL BODY POWER EXERCISES

Two-arm Push Press

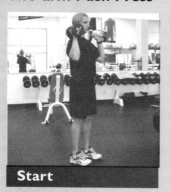

Start

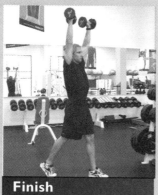

Finish

Preparation
1. Stand with feet shoulder-width apart.
2. Hold two dumbbells in hands at chest.

Movement
3. Draw abs in and activate glutes.
4. Quickly drive dumbbells up, as if doing a shoulder press.
5. At the same time, drive the legs into a stagger stance position. Back leg should be in triple extension with the front leg bent slightly.
6. Maintain optimal alignment on the return to the starting position.
7. Bring feet to shoulder-width distance and dumbbells to chest level.

Single-arm Dumbbell Snatch

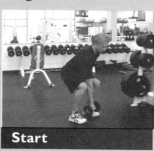

Start

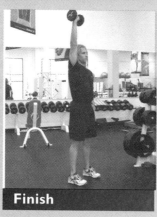

Finish

Preparation
1. Stand with feet shoulder-width apart, toes pointing forward and knees slightly flexed.
2. Hold one dumbbell held in one hand in front of the knees.
3. Keep the chest up.

Movement
4. Draw abs in and activate glutes.
5. Quickly snatch the dumbbell by keeping arm straight, bending the knees and using the shoulder and legs to get the dumbbell to an overhead position.
6. Establish a balanced position, with the dumbbell slightly in front of the ear and the arm fully extended.
7. To return to a starting position, bend the elbow, lower the dumbbell back to shoulder level and then to knee level.

Barbell Clean

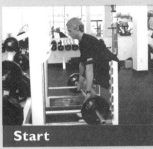

Start

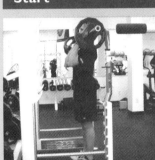

Finish

Preparation
1. Stand with feet shoulder-width apart, toes pointing forward.
2. Bend the knees slightly.
3. Bend over at the waist, grasping the barbell with both hands slightly farther than shoulder-width apart (palms facing body).

Movement
4. Draw abs in and activate glutes.
5. Keeping a drawn-in position, rapidly lift the barbell up to shoulder level.
6. Bend knees to a semi-squat position.
7. Contract glutes to stand into a full upright position, with bar resting on the chest.
8. Carefully lower the barbell back to the ground.

Chest Exercise Descriptions
CHEST STABILIZATION EXERCISES
Dumbbell Chest Press Progression

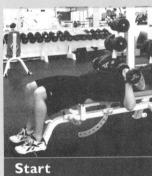

Start

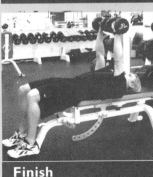

Finish

Preparation
1. Lie on flat bench with knees bent.
2. Feet should be flat on the bench, shoulder-width apart with toes pointing straight ahead.
3. Hold one dumbbell in each hand, at chest level, slightly outside of body line, with elbows flexed.

Movement
4. Draw abs in and activate glutes.
5. Press both dumbbells straight up and then together, by extending elbows and contracting chest.
6. Hold.
7. Slowly return dumbbells toward body, by flexing elbows and allowing shoulders to retract and depress.
8. Regression
   a. Chest Press Machine
9. Progression
   a. Alternating-arm
   b. Single-arm

Ball Dumbbell Chest Press Progression

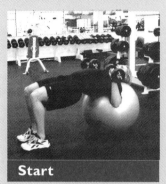

Start

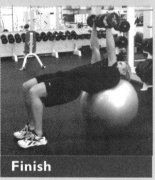

Finish

Preparation

1. Lie on stability ball, with ball placed between shoulder blades.
2. Maintain a bridge position by contracting glutes and keeping shoulders, hips and knees at the same level.
3. Feet should be shoulder-width apart with toes pointing straight ahead.
4. Hold one dumbbell in each hand, at chest level, slightly outside of body line, with elbows flexed.

Movement

5. Draw abs in and activate glutes.
6. Press both dumbbells straight up and then together, by extending elbows and contracting chest.
7. Hold.
8. Slowly return dumbbells toward body, by flexing elbows and allowing shoulders to retract and depress.
9. Regression
   a. Dumbbell Chest Press on Bench
10. Progression
    a. Alternating-arm
    b. Single-arm

Push-up Progression

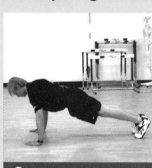

Start

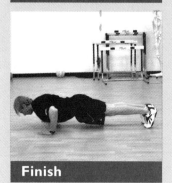

Finish

Preparation

1. Begin in a push-up position with feet and hands on the floor slightly wider than shoulder-width apart.

Movement

2. Draw abs in and activate glutes.
3. Keeping back flat, slowly lower body toward ground, by flexing elbows and retracting and depressing shoulder blades.
4. Stop at first point of compensation.
5. Push back up to starting position, by extending elbows and contracting chest. Do not allow head to jut forward.
6. Regression
   a. On knees
   b. Hands on bench, feet on floor
   c. Wall Push-up
7. Progression
   a. Hands on Reebok Core Board
   b. Hands on medicine balls
   c. Hands on stability ball

Standing Cable Chest Press Progression

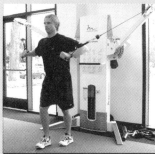

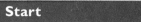
Start

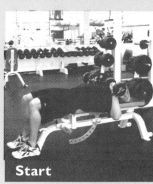
Finish

Preparation

1. Stand, back to the weight stack, with feet shoulder-width apart and pointing straight ahead, and knees slightly flexed.
2. Maintain a stable position with knees over second and third toes.
3. Hold a cable in each hand at chest height (palms facing ground), with elbows flexed and slightly below shoulder level.

Movement

4. Draw abs in and activate glutes.
5. Press cables forward and together, by extending elbows and contracting chest. Do not allow head to jut forward.
6. Slowly return hands to original position, by flexing elbows and retracting shoulder blades.
7. Regression
   a. Seated
   b. Staggered stance
8. Progression
   a. Alternating-arm
   b. Single-arm
   c. Single-leg, two-arm
   d. Single-leg, alternating-arm
   e. Single-leg, single-arm

CHEST STRENGTH EXERCISES

Flat Dumbbell Chest Press

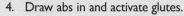

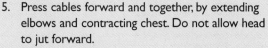
Start

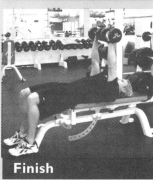
Finish

Preparation

1. Lie on flat bench with knees bent.
2. Feet should be flat on the bench, shoulder-width apart with toes pointing straight ahead.
3. Hold one dumbbell in each hand, at chest level, slightly outside of body line, with elbows flexed.

Movement

4. Draw abs in and activate glutes.
5. Press both dumbbells straight up and then together, by extending elbows and contracting chest.
6. Hold.
7. Slowly return dumbbells toward body, by flexing elbows and allowing shoulders to retract and depress.

Incline Dumbbell Chest Press

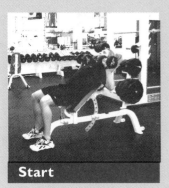

Start

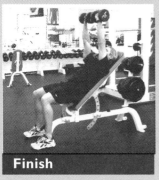

Finish

Preparation

1. Lie with back flat on incline bench, feet flat on floor and toes pointing straight ahead.
2. Hold one dumbbell in each hand, at chest level, slightly outside of body line, with elbows flexed.

Movement

3. Draw abs in and activate glutes.
4. Press both dumbbells straight up and then together, by extending elbows and contracting chest.
5. Hold.
6. Slowly return dumbbells toward body, by flexing elbows and allowing shoulders to retract and depress.

Barbell Bench Press

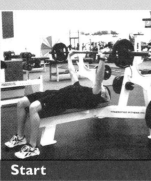

Start

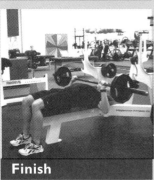

Finish

Preparation

1. Lie on flat bench, feet flat on floor and toes pointing straight ahead.
2. Hold a barbell and grasp the bar, with hands slightly wider than shoulder-width apart.

Movement

3. Draw abs in and activate glutes.
4. Slowly lower the bar toward the chest, by flexing elbows and retracting and depressing shoulder blades. Avoid letting the back arch or the head jut forward.
5. Press the bar back up, extending arms and contracting chest, until elbows are fully extended.

Incline Barbell Bench Press

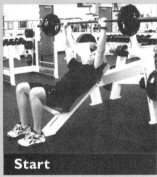

Start

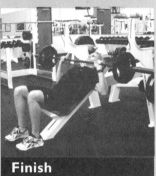

Finish

Preparation
1. Lie flat an incline bench, feet flat on floor and toes pointing straight ahead.
2. Hold a barbell and grasp the bar, with hands slightly wider than shoulder-width apart.

Movement
3. Draw abs in and activate glutes.
4. Slowly lower the bar toward the top of the chest, by flexing elbows and retracting and depressing shoulder blades. Avoid letting the back arch or the head jut forward.
5. Press the bar back up, extending arms and contracting chest, until elbows are fully extended.

Chest Press Machine

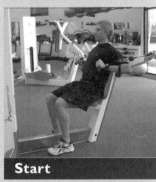

Start

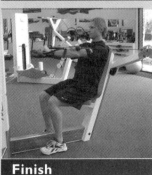

Finish

Preparation
1. Sit at machine.
2. Make any adjustments necessary to fit body.
3. Select desired weight.
4. Keep the chin tucked.

Movement
5. Draw abs in and activate glutes.
6. Press weight forward, until arms are fully extended.
7. Hold.
8. Slowly return weight to original position, by flexing elbows and allowing shoulder blades to retract and depress.

CHEST POWER EXERCISES

Two-arm Medicine Ball Chest Pass

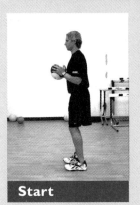

Start

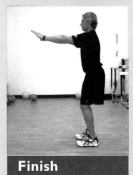

Finish

Preparation

1. Stand, facing wall or partner.
2. Hold a medicine ball (five to 10 percent of body weight) with both hands, elbows flexed, at chest level.

Movement

3. Draw abs in and activate glutes.
4. Push and release the ball toward the wall as hard as possible, by extending the elbows and contracting the chest. Do not allow the shoulders to elevate.
5. Catch the ball.
6. Repeat as quickly as possible, under control.

Staggered-stance Two-arm Medicine Ball Chest Pass

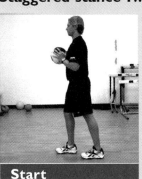

Start

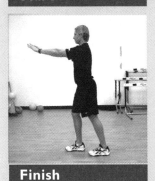

Finish

Preparation

1. Stand with a staggered stance, facing wall, with feet pointing straight ahead and knee slightly flexed.
2. Maintain a stable position with knees over second and third toes.
3. Hold a medicine ball (five to 10 percent of body weight) with both hands, elbows flexed, at chest level.

Movement

4. Draw abs in and activate glutes.
5. Push and release the ball toward the wall as hard as possible, by extending the elbows and contracting the chest. Do not allow the shoulders to elevate.
6. Catch the ball.
7. Repeat as quickly as possible, under control.

Rotation Chest Pass

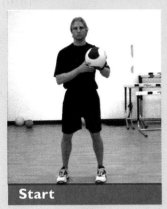

Start

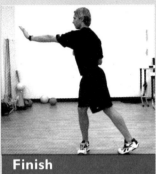

Finish

Preparation

1. Stand, with body turned at a 90-degree angle from a wall.
2. Feet should be shoulder-width apart, toes pointing straight ahead.
3. Hold a medicine ball (five to 10 percent of body weight) with both hands, elbows flexed, at chest level.

Movement

4. Draw abs in and activate glutes.
5. Use abs, hips, and glutes to rotate body quickly and explosively toward the wall.
6. As body turns, pivot back leg and allow it to go into triple extension.
7. With the upper body, push the medicine ball (as if doing a chest pass). Use the arm farthest from the wall to extend and apply force.
8. Catch the ball.
9. Repeat as quickly as possible, under control.

Plyometric Push-up

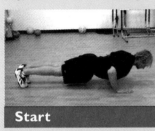

Start

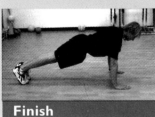

Finish

Preparation

1. Begin in a push-up position with feet and hands on the floor slightly wider than shoulder-width apart.

Movement

2. Draw abs in and activate glutes.
3. Draw in abdomen and contract glutes.
4. Keeping back flat, slowly lower body toward ground, by flexing elbows and retracting and depressing shoulder blades.
5. Stop at first point of compensation.
6. In one explosive motion, push back up away from the ground as quickly as possible, allowing for the hands to come off the floor. Do not allow head to jut forward.
7. Allow for hands to land back on the floor, control yourself back toward the ground and repeat.

Speed Bench Press

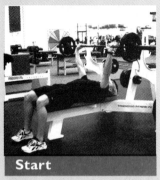
Start

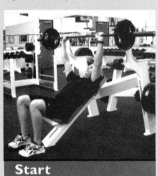
Finish

Preparation
1. Lie on flat bench, feet flat on floor and toes pointing straight ahead.
2. Hold a barbell and grasp the bar, with hands slightly wider than shoulder-width apart.

Movement
3. Draw abs in and activate glutes.
4. Lower the bar toward the chest in a controlled fashion, by flexing elbows and retracting and depressing shoulder blades. Avoid letting the back arch or the head jut forward.
5. In one explosive motion, press the bar up away from the chest, extending arms and contracting chest, until elbows are fully extended.
6. Repeat in a quick, yet controlled, fashion.

Speed Incline Bench Press

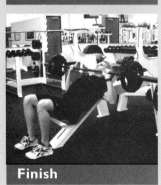
Start

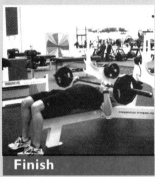
Finish

Preparation
1. Lie flat on an incline bench, feet flat on floor and toes pointing straight ahead.
2. Hold a barbell and grasp the bar, with hands slightly wider than shoulder-width apart.

Movement
3. Draw abs in and activate glutes.
4. Lower the bar toward the top of the chest in a controlled fashion, by flexing elbows and retracting and depressing shoulder blades. Avoid letting the back arch or the head to jut forward.
5. In one explosive motion, press the bar up away from the chest, extending arms and contracting chest, until elbows are fully extended.
6. Repeat in a quick, yet controlled, fashion.

Back Exercise Descriptions
BACK STABILIZATION EXERCISES
Standing Cable Row Progression

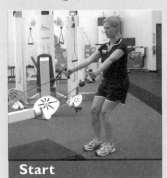

Start

Finish

Preparation
1. Stand facing a cable machine, with feet shoulder-width apart and pointing straight ahead, and knees over second and third toes.
2. Hold cables, with arms extended at chest level.

Movement
3. Draw abs in and activate glutes.
4. With knees slightly flexed, row cable by flexing elbows.
5. Bring thumbs toward the armpits, keeping the shoulder blades retracted and depressed.
6. Maintain a drawn-in position. Do not allow the head to jut forward.
7. Hold.
8. Slowly return arms to original position, by extending the elbows
9. Regression
   a. Seated
10. Progression
   a. Alternating-arm
   b. Single-arm
   c. Single-leg, two-arm
   d. Single-leg, alternating-arm
   e. Single-leg, single-arm

Standing Cable Pulldown Progression

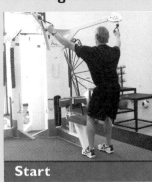

Start

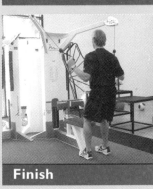

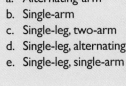

Finish

Preparation
1. Stand on both feet with feet pointing straight ahead and knees slightly flexed over second and third toes.
2. Grasp a cable in each hand (arms extended) with palms facing sides of the body.
3. Keep the hips level.

Movement
4. Draw abs in and activate glutes.
5. Perform a pulldown by retracting and depressing the shoulder blades and flexing the elbows.
6. Hold.
7. Slowly extend arms to return to original position.
8. Regression
   a. Seated
9. Progression
   a. Alternating-arm
   b. Single-arm
   c. Single-leg, two-arm
   d. Single-leg, alternating-arm
   e. Single-leg, single-arm

Standing Cable Extension Progression

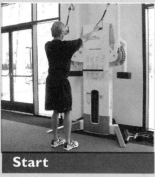

Start

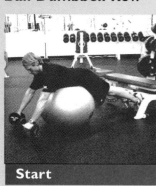

Finish

Preparation

1. Stand on both feet with feet pointing straight ahead, and knees slightly flexed and over second and third toes.
2. Grasp a cable in each hand (arms extended in front of body at eye level).
3. Keep the hips level.

Movement

4. Draw abs in and activate glutes.
5. Extend the shoulders, by retracting and depressing the shoulder blades.
6. While keeping arms fully extended, bring them to the sides of body.
7. Hold.
8. Return arms (in their flexed position) to the front of the body at eye level.
9. Regression
   a. Seated
10. Progression
    a. Alternating-arm
    b. Single-arm
    c. Single-leg, two-arm
    d. Single-leg, alternating-arm
    e. Single-leg, single-arm

Ball Dumbbell Row

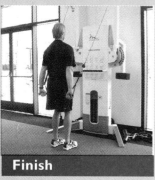

Start

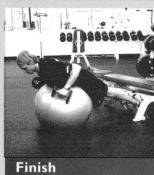

Finish

Preparation

1. Begin in a prone position, with stability ball under abdomen.
2. Keep feet pointed down, legs completely straight.
3. Hold dumbbells in each hand and extend arms in front of body.

Movement

4. Draw abs in and activate glutes.
5. Lift chest off the ball.
6. Row the dumbbells by retracting and depressing shoulder blades.
7. Flex elbows, bringing thumbs toward armpits.
8. Hold.
9. Return dumbbells slowly to ground, by extending elbows and allowing shoulders to protract at end-range.
10. Regression
    a. Kneeling over ball
11. Progression
    a. Alternating-arm
    b. Single-am

Ball Dumbbell Cobra

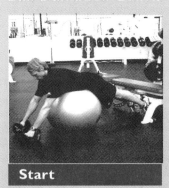

Start

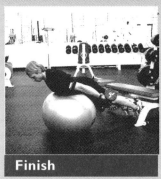

Finish

Preparation

1. Begin in a prone position, with stability ball under abdomen.
2. Keep feet pointed down, legs completely straight.
3. Hold dumbbells in each hand and extend arms in front of body.

Movement

4. Draw abs in and activate glutes.
5. Squeeze glutes and bring arms around to the side of body, by pinching shoulder blades back and down.
6. Lift chest off the ball and keep back and neck in proper alignment.
7. Hold.
8. Slowly lower chest to ball, simultaneously returning arms in front of body to the ground.
9. Regression
   a. Kneeling over ball
10. Progression
    a. Alternating-arm
    b. Single-arm

Dumbbell Row Progression

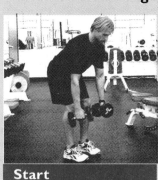

Start

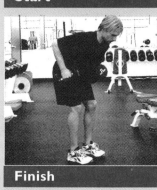

Finish

Preparation

1. Stand on both feet.
2. Bend at the waist until chest is at a 45-degree angle to the ground.
3. Feet should be straight ahead with knees over second and third toes.
4. Allow arms to extend and hang in front of body with a dumbbell in each hand.

Movement

5. Draw abs in and activate glutes.
6. Row the dumbbells, by retracting and depressing shoulder blades.
7. Flex elbows, while bringing thumbs toward armpits. Do not allow back to arch.
8. Slowly return dumbbells to their original position, by extending at the elbow.
9. Regression
   a. Decrease flexion at waist
   b. Standing Cable Row
10. Progression
    a. Alternating-arm
    b. Single-arm
    c. Single-leg, two-arm
    d. Single-leg, alternating-arm
    e. Single-leg, single-arm

Dumbbell Cobra Progression

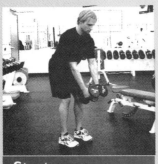

Start

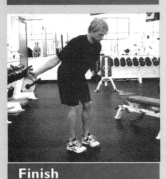

Finish

Preparation
1. Stand on both feet.
2. Bend at the waist until chest is at a 45-degree angle to the ground.
3. Feet should be straight ahead with knees over second and third toes.
4. Allow arms to extend and hang in front of body with a dumbbell in each hand.

Movement
5. Draw abs in and activate glutes.
6. Slowly move arms in a circular pattern until they are by the sides of the body.
7. Externally rotate shoulders so that the palms are supinated and shoulder blades retracted and depressed.
8. Hold.
9. Keep chin tucked and abdomen drawn in.
10. Return to start position.
11. Regression
    a. Decrease flexion at waist
    b. Standing using cables or light tubing
12. Progression
    a. Alternating-arm
    b. Single-arm
    c. Single-leg, two-arm
    d. Single-leg, alternating-arm
    e. Single-leg, single-arm

BACK STRENGTH EXERCISES

Seated Cable Row

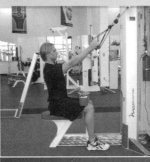

Start

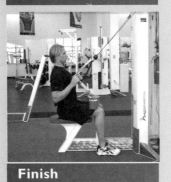

Finish

Preparation
1. Sit facing a cable machine, with feet shoulder-width apart and pointing straight ahead, and knees over second and third toes.
2. Hold cables, with arms extended at chest level.

Movement
3. Draw abs in and activate glutes.
4. Row cable by flexing elbows and pulling the handles toward the trunk.
5. Bring thumbs toward the armpits, keeping the shoulder blades retracted and depressed.
6. Maintain a drawn-in position. Do not allow the head to jut forward.
7. Hold.
8. Slowly return arms to original position, by extending the elbows.

Pull-up

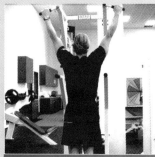

Start

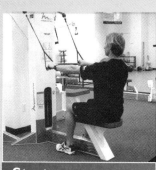

Finish

Preparation

1. Begin by grasping a pull-up bar with palms either facing body or away from body and hands slightly wider than shoulder-width apart.
2. Keep trunk straight and bend knees at a 90-degree angle.

Movement

3. Draw abs in and activate glutes.
4. While performing a drawing-in maneuver, pull chest up to bar, by flexing at elbows and retracting and depressing shoulder blades.
5. Keep head in a neutral position throughout exercise.
6. Hold.
7. Slowly lower body back toward ground, by extending the arms.

Seated Cable Extension

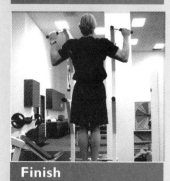

Start

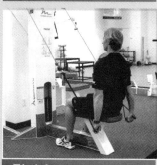

Finish

Preparation

1. Stand facing a cable machine, with feet shoulder-width apart and pointing straight ahead, and knees over second and third toes. Knees should be slightly flexed.
2. Hold cables, with arms extended at chest level.

Movement

3. Draw abs in and activate glutes.
4. Perform extension of the shoulders, by bringing arms to the side of the body, while retracting and depressing the shoulder blades.
5. Keep arms fully extended during exercise.
6. Hold.
7. Slowly return arms to original position, at eye level, in front of body.

Seated Lat Pulldown

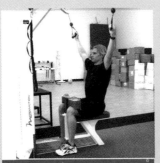

Start

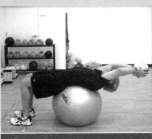

Finish

Preparation

1. Sit at machine.
2. Make any adjustments necessary to fit body.
3. Select desired weight.
4. Grasp both handles.
5. Sit upright with shoulders retracted and depressed.

Movement

6. Draw abs in and activate glutes.
7. Pull handles toward the body, by flexing elbows. Do not arch back or allow head to jut forward.
8. Hold at end range.
9. Slowly return weight to original position, by extending elbows.

BACK POWER EXERCISES

Ball Medicine Ball Pullover Throw

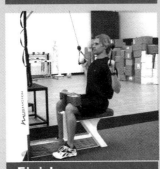

Start

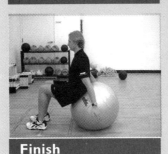

Finish

Preparation

1. Facing a wall, place stability ball under low back, bend knees at a 90-degree angle, keep feet flat and toes pointing straight ahead.
2. Hold a medicine ball (five to 10 percent of body weight) overhead with both hands, with arms extended.

Movement

3. Draw abs in and activate glutes.
4. Using abdominals, quickly crunch forward.
5. Throw the medicine ball off the wall.
6. As the ball releases, continue pulling the arms through all the way to the sides of the body.
7. Keep chin tucked throughout the exercise.
8. Repeat as quickly as possible, under control.

Soccer Throw

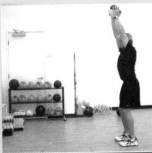

Start

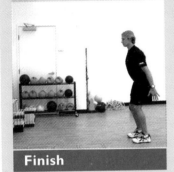

Finish

Preparation

1. Stand facing a wall, with feet pointing straight ahead and shoulder-width apart.
2. Hold a medicine ball (five to 10 percent of body weight) overhead, with both hands.

Movement

3. Draw abs in and activate glutes.
4. Take a step forward.
5. At the same time, throw the medicine ball off the wall, by pulling arms down to side and retracting and depressing shoulder blades.
6. Keep abdomen drawn in. Do not arch back and keep chin tucked as the ball is thrown.
7. Repeat exercise by alternating step legs.

Woodchop Throw

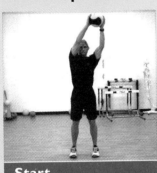

Start

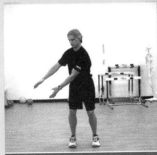

Finish

Preparation

1. Stand facing a wall, with feet pointing straight ahead, shoulder-width apart.
2. Hold a medicine ball (five to 10 percent of body weight) at one shoulder.
3. Keep knees slightly flexed.

Movement

4. Draw abs in and activate glutes.
5. Quickly pull the medicine ball toward the floor, throwing the ball toward the opposite foot (in a woodchop motion).
6. While throwing, extend elbows, pull with lats and draw in abdomen.
7. Catch ball off the floor.
8. Repeat.

Shoulder Exercise Descriptions
SHOULDER STABILIZATION EXERCISES
Seated Ball Dumbbell Flexion

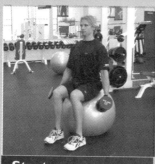

Start

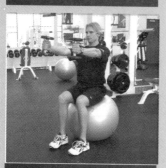

Finish

Preparation
1. Sit on a stability ball.
2. Keep feet pointed straight ahead.
3. Hold dumbbells in each hand and keep arms to the side of body.

Movement
4. Draw abs in and activate glutes.
5. Keeping the arms straight, raise the arms in front of the body to shoulder level.
6. Hold, then slowly lower arms back to the side of the body and repeat
7. Regression
   a. Seated on bench
8. Progression
   a. Alternating-arm
   b. Single-arm

Seated Ball Dumbbell Scaption

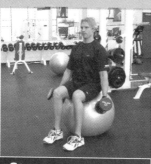

Start

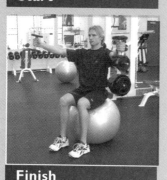

Finish

Preparation
1. Sit on a stability ball.
2. Keep feet pointed straight ahead.
3. Hold dumbbells in each hand and keep arms to the side of body.

Movement
4. Draw abs in and activate glutes.
5. Raise both arms, thumbs up, at a 45-degree angle in front of the body to eye level.
6. Keep shoulder blades retracted and depressed throughout the exercise. Do not allow the back to arch.
7. Hold.
8. Return arms slowly back to the side of the body.
9. Regression
   a. Seated on bench
10. Progression
    a. Alternating-arm
    b. Single-arm

Seated Ball Dumbbell Abduction

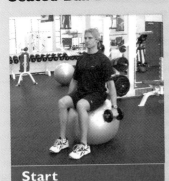

Start

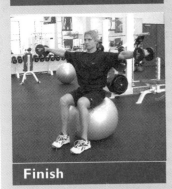

Finish

Preparation
1. Sit on a stability ball.
2. Keep feet pointed straight ahead.
3. Hold dumbbells in each hand and keep arms to the side of body.

Movement
4. Draw abs in and activate glutes.
5. Raise both arms, thumbs up, to the side of the body to shoulder level.
6. Keep shoulder blades retracted and depressed throughout the exercise. Do not allow the back to arch.
7. Hold.
8. Return arms slowly back to the side of the body.
9. Regression
   a. Seated on bench
10. Progression
    b. Alternating-arm
    c. Single-arm

Prone Dumbbell Scaption

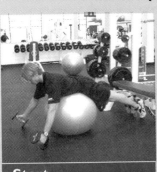

Start

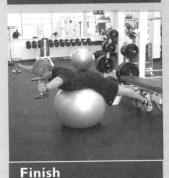

Finish

Preparation
1. Lie prone on a stability ball.
2. Keep feet, knees and hips extended.
3. Hold dumbbells in each hand with arms in front of the stability ball.

Movement
4. Draw abs in and activate glutes.
5. Raise both arms, thumbs up, at a 45-degree angle in front of the body to eye level.
6. Keep shoulder blades retracted and depressed throughout the exercise. Do not allow the back to arch.
7. Hold.
8. Return arms slowly back to the floor and repeat.
9. Regression
   a. Kneeling over the ball
10. Progression
    a. Alternating-arm
    b. Single-arm

Prone Dumbbell Abduction

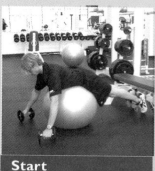

Start

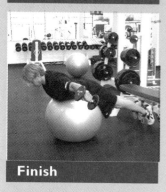

Finish

Preparation

1. Lie prone on a stability ball with abdomen on ball.
2. Keep feet, knees and hips extended.
3. Hold dumbbell in each hand with arms in front of the stability ball.

Movement

4. Draw abs in and activate glutes.
5. Raise both arms, thumbs up, into a "T" position.
6. Keep shoulder blades retracted and depressed throughout the exercise. Do not allow the back to arch.
7. Hold.
8. Return arms slowly back to the floor and repeat.
9. Regression
   a. Kneeling over the ball
10. Progression
    a. Alternating-arm
    b. Single-arm

Prone Dumbbell Cobra

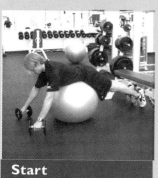

Start

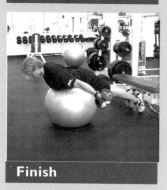

Finish

Preparation

1. Lie prone on a stability ball with abdomen on ball.
2. Keep feet pointed down and legs completely straight.
3. Hold dumbbells in each hand and extend arms in front of body.

Movement

4. Draw abs in and activate glutes.
5. Bring arms around to the side of body, by pinching shoulder blades back and down.
6. Lift chest off the ball and keep back and neck in proper alignment.
7. Hold.
8. Slowly lower chest to ball, simultaneously returning arms in front of body to the ground.
9. Regression
   a. Kneeling over ball
10. Progression
    a. Alternating-arm
    b. Single-arm

Ball Combo I

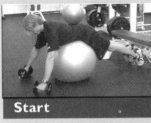
Start

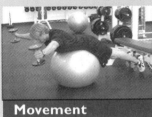
Movement

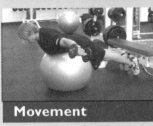
Movement

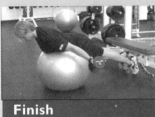
Finish

Preparation

1. Lie prone on a stability ball with abdomen on ball.
2. Keep feet pointed down and legs completely straight.
3. Hold dumbbell in each hand.

Movement

4. Draw abs in and activate glutes.
5. Lift chest off the ball and keep back and neck in proper alignment. Extend arms in front of body
6. Lift arms to body height at a 45-degree angle keeping thumbs up and pinching shoulder blades back and down (scaption).
7. Move arms straight out to side with thumbs up (abduction).
8. Move arms to the side of the body with thumbs up, retract and depress shoulder blades (cobra).
9. Hold at each location and then return arms to extended position in front of body and repeat.
10. Regression
    a. Kneeling over ball
11. Progression
    a. Alternating-arm
    b. Single-arm

Prone Rear Delt Row

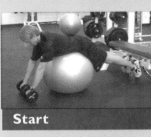
Start

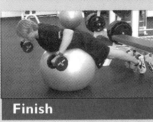
Finish

Preparation

1. Lie prone on a stability ball with abdomen on ball.
2. Keep feet pointed down and legs completely straight.
3. Hold dumbbell in each hand and extend arms in front of ball.

Movement

4. Draw abs in and activate glutes.
5. Lift chest off the ball.
6. Row the dumbbells by retracting and depressing shoulder blades keeping the elbows up toward the shoulders.
7. Hold.
8. Return dumbbells slowly to ground, by extending elbows and allowing shoulders to protract at end-range.
9. Regression
    a. Kneeling over ball
10. Progression
    b. Alternating-arm
    c. Single-arm

413

Prone External Rotation

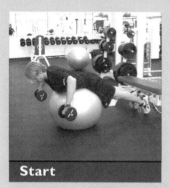

Start

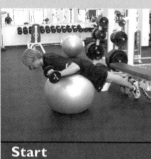

Finish

Preparation

1. Lie prone on a stability ball with abdomen on ball.
2. Keep feet pointed down and legs completely straight.
3. Hold dumbbell in each hand and extend arms in front of ball.

Movement

4. Draw abs in and activate glutes.
5. Life chest off the ball.
6. Row the dumbbells by retracting and depressing shoulder blades keeping the elbows up toward the shoulders.
7. Externally rotate the shoulders so the hands come up toward ear level
8. Hold.
9. Slowly internally rotate hands so they are point toward the ground, then slowly lower hands back to the ground by extending elbows and allowing shoulders to protract at end-range.
10. Regression
    a. Kneeling over ball
11. Progression
    b. Alternating-arm
    c. Single-arm

Prone Military Press

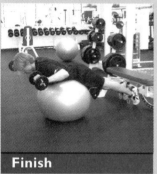

Start

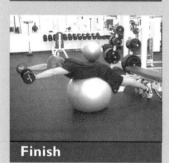

Finish

Preparation

1. Lie prone on a stability ball with abdomen on ball.
2. Keep feet pointed down and legs completely straight.
3. Hold dumbbell in each hand and begin with elbows and shoulders at 90-degree angles. Shoulders should be externally rotated as far as possible with scapula in a retracted and depressed position.

Movement

4. Draw abs in and activate glutes.
5. Press both arms directly overhead by extending elbow. Slowly return it to starting position and repeat.
6. Regression
    a. Kneeling over ball
7. Progression
    b. Alternating-arm
    c. Single-arm

Ball Combo II

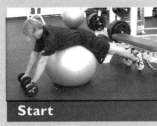
Start

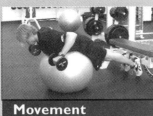
Movement

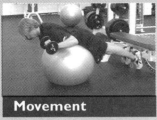
Movement

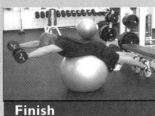
Finish

Preparation

1. Lie prone on the ball and position with ball underneath your hips and abs.
2. Put hips in a neutral position.
3. Keep head neutral with chin drawn in.
4. Extend hip, knees, and ankles (triple extension).
5. Hold dumbbell in each hand and extend arms in front of ball.

Movement

6. Draw abs in and activate glutes.
7. With arms extended in front of you row them in by pinching shoulder blades together (rear delt row)
8. Externally rotate shoulders so hands are at ear level (external rotation)
9. Press the arms overhead (prone military press)
10. Bring hands back down to ear level
11. Internally rotate shoulders so hands are pointing down to the floor and finally bring the arms to start position in front of the ball.
12. Regression
    a. Kneeling over ball
13. Progression
    a. Alternating-arm
    b. Single-arm

Standing Cable External Rotation

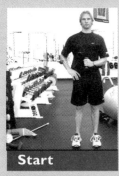
Start

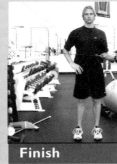
Finish

Preparation

1. Stand on both feet, hip-width apart and pointing straight ahead, and knees over second and third toes.

Movement

2. Draw abs in and activate glutes.
3. Begin by placing a towel under the arm with the upper arm at the side of the body.
4. Externally rotate the shoulder in the opposite direction of the pull of the cable.
5. Hold.
6. Slowly internally rotate shoulder to the starting position and repeat.
7. Regression
    a. Seated
8. Progression
    a. Different shoulder position
    b. Single-leg

Standing Cable Internal Rotation

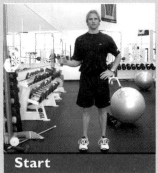

Start

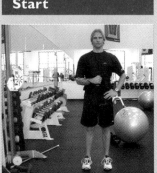

Finish

Preparation

1. Stand on both feet, hip-width apart and pointing straight ahead, and knees over second and third toes.

Movement

2. Draw abs in and activate glutes.
3. Begin by placing a towel under the arm with the upper arm at the side of the body.
4. Internally rotate the shoulder in the opposite direction of the pull of the cable.
5. Hold.
6. Slowly externally rotate shoulder to the starting position and repeat.
7. Regression
   a. Seated
8. Progression
   a. Different shoulder position
   b. Single-leg

Standing Dumbbell Scaption Progression

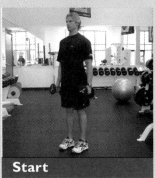

Start

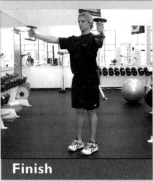

Finish

Preparation

1. Stand with feet shoulder-width apart, pointing straight ahead, knees over second and third toes and slightly flexed.
2. Hold dumbbells at side, with palms facing side of body.

Movement

3. Draw abs in and activate glutes.
4. Raise both arms, thumbs up, at a 45-degree angle in front of the body, until hands reach eye level.
5. Keep shoulder blades retracted and depressed throughout the exercise. Do not allow the back to arch.
6. Hold.
7. Slowly return arms back to sides of body and repeat.
8. Regression
   a. Seated
9. Progression
   a. Two-leg, alternating-arm
   b. Two-leg, single-arm
   c. Single-leg, two-arm
   d. Single-leg, alternating-arm
   e. Single-leg, single-arm

Standing Dumbbell PNF

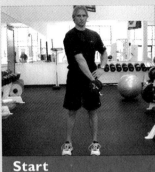

Start

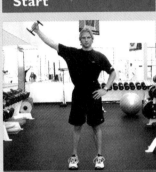

Finish

Preparation

1. Stand with feet shoulder-width apart, pointing straight ahead knees over second and third toes slightly flexed.

Movement

2. Draw abs in and activate glutes.
3. Begin with free arm extended across body, with thumb facing front pocket on opposite side.
4. Raise arm in extended position on a diagonal pattern, across the body (as if drawing a sword out of its sheath).
5. Lift arm, supinate forearm and externally rotate shoulder until hand is at eye level and at a 45-degree angle to the body.
6. Hold.
7. Slowly return arm across the body and thumb to pocket (as if placing the sword back into its sheath).
8. Regression
   a. Seated
9. Progression
   a. Single-leg

Standing Dumbbell Military Press Progression

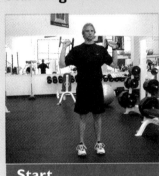

Start

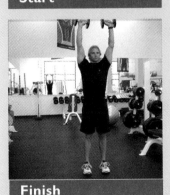

Finish

Preparation

1. Stand with feet shoulder-width apart, pointing straight ahead, and knees over second and third toes.
2. Hold dumbbells at shoulder level, with palms away.

Movement

3. Draw abs in and activate glutes.
4. Press the dumbbells overhead until both arms are fully extended, with palms facing away.
5. Arms should be slightly in front of ears.
6. Hold.
7. Slowly return dumbbells back to chest and repeat.
8. Regression
   a. Seated
9. Progression
   a. Two-leg, alternating-arm
   b. Two-leg, single-arm
   c. Single-leg, two-arm
   d. Single-leg, alternating-am
   e. Single-leg, single-arm

SHOULDER STRENGTH EXERCISES

Seated Dumbbell Shoulder Press

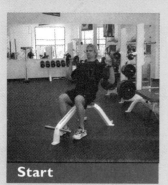

Start

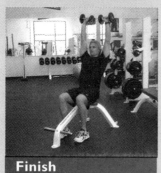

Finish

Preparation

1. Sit on a bench, feet flat on floor, shoulder-width apart, and toes pointing straight ahead.
2. Hold one dumbbell in each hand, with palms facing away from body.
3. Begin with elbows near sides of body and hands at chest level. Shoulders should be externally rotated as far as possible with scapulae in a retracted and depressed position.

Movement

4. Draw abs in and activate glutes.
5. Press arms directly overhead by extending elbow. Do not allow head to jut forward or back to arch.
6. Slowly return to starting position and repeat.

Standing Dumbbell Military Press

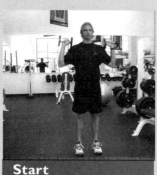

Start

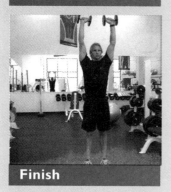

Finish

Preparation

1. Stand with feet shoulder-width apart, pointing straight ahead, and knees over second and third toes.
2. Hold dumbbells at shoulder level, with palms away.

Movement

3. Draw abs in and activate glutes.
4. Press the dumbbells overhead until both arms are fully extended, with palms facing away.
5. Arms should be slightly in front of ears.
6. Hold.
7. Slowly return dumbbells back to chest and repeat.

Seated Shoulder Press Machine

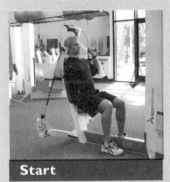

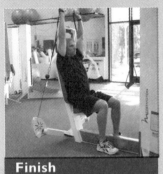

Preparation
1. Sit at machine.
2. Make any adjustments necessary to fit body.
3. Select desired weight.
4. Keep the chin tucked.

Movement
5. Draw abs in and activate glutes.
6. Press weight overhead, until arms are fully extended.
7. Hold.
8. Slowly return weight to original position, by flexing elbows and allowing shoulder blades to retract and depress.

SHOULDER POWER EXERCISES

Medicine Ball Scoop Toss

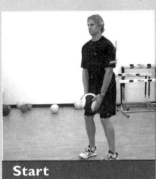

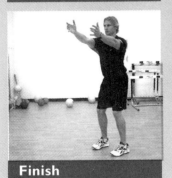

Preparation
1. Stand with feet straight ahead, hip-width apart, knees slightly bent and lined up over second and third toes, hip neutral, shoulders slightly retracted, and chin tucked.
2. Have a partner stand in front of yourself to receive and toss back the medicine ball.
3. Hold a medicine ball at the opposite side hip.

Movement
4. Draw abs in and activate glutes.
5. Maintaining body alignment, rotate the body using the glutes and abs, allowing the trailing leg to pivot.
6. Toss the medicine ball to a partner as body rotates.
7. Use a scooping motion to catch ball as the partner tosses it back and repeat in a quick, yet controlled, fashion.
8. Repeat on both sides.

Medicine Ball Side Oblique Throw

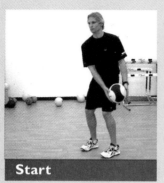

Start

Preparation

1. Stand with a partner positioned behind, but to the side.
2. Feet should be shoulder-width apart, toes pointing straight ahead, and knees flexed slightly over second and third toes.
3. Hold a medicine ball at the opposite side hip of the partner.

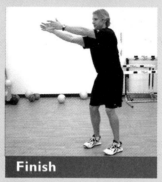

Finish

Movement

4. Draw abs in and activate glutes.
5. Maintaining body alignment, rotate the body using the glutes and abs, allowing the trailing leg to pivot.
6. Toss the medicine ball to a partner as body rotates.
7. Use a scooping motion to catch ball as the partner tosses it back and repeat in a quick, yet controlled, fashion.
8. Repeat on both sides.

Overhead Medicine Ball Throw

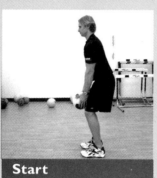

Start

Preparation

1. Stand with back to a wall.
2. Feet should be shoulder-width apart, toes pointing straight ahead.
3. Hold a medicine ball with both hands, at knee level.
4. Keep chest up.

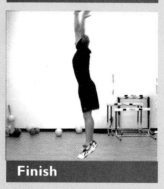

Finish

Movement

5. Draw abs in and activate glutes.
6. Begin to lower into a semi-squat position.
7. Then, jump off the ground explosively, extending arms overhead.
8. Throw the medicine ball off the wall.
9. Release the ball before arms pass ears. Do not allow the back to go into hyperextension.
10. Land in a controlled and stable manner, avoiding all compensation.

Bicep Exercise Descriptions
BICEP STABILIZATION EXERCISES
Single-leg Dumbbell Curl

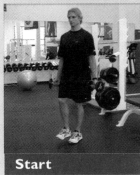
Start

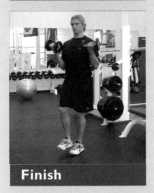

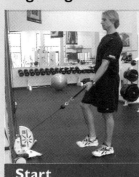
Finish

Preparation
1. Stand on one foot with foot pointed straight ahead, and knee slightly flexed over second and third toes.
2. Allow arms to extend and hang to the sides of the body with a dumbbell in each hand.
3. Keep hips level.

Movement
4. Draw abs in and activate glutes.
5. Perform a bicep curl by flexing the elbow.
6. Slowly return dumbbells to their original position, by extending at the elbow.
7. Regression
   a. Two-leg
8. Progression
   a. Alternating-arm
   b. Single-arm

Single-leg Cable Curl

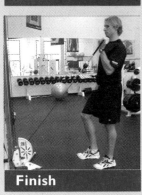
Start

Finish

Preparation
1. Stand on one foot with foot pointed straight ahead, and knee slightly flexed over second and third toes.
2. Allow arms to extend and hang to the sides of the body with a dumbbell in each hand.
3. Keep hips level.

Movement
4. Draw abs in and activate glutes.
5. Perform a bicep curl, by flexing the elbow.
6. Slowly lower the cable back to the side of the body, by extending the elbow.
7. Regression
   a. Two-leg
8. Progression
   a. Single-leg, alternating-arm
   b. Single-leg, single-arm

Single-leg Barbell Curl

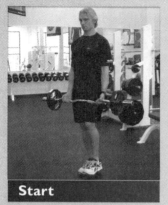

Start

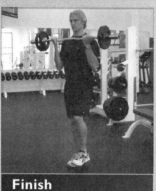

Finish

Preparation
1. Stand on one foot with foot pointed straight ahead, and knee slightly flexed over second and third toes.
2. Hold a barbell in both hands (palms facing up) with arms extended in front of body.
3. Keep hips level.

Movement
4. Draw abs in and activate glutes.
5. Perform a barbell curl by flexing both elbows, keeping the shoulder blades retracted.
6. Curl bar up to chest level.
7. Slowly lower the bar back to original position, by extending the elbows.
8. Regression
   a. Two-leg

BICEP STRENGTH EXERCISES

Standing Two-arm Dumbbell Bicep Curl

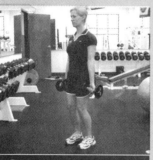

Start

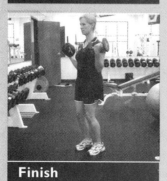

Finish

Preparation
1. Stand with feet shoulder-width apart, pointing straight ahead, and knees over second and third toes.
2. Hold dumbbell in each hand with arms at sides.
3. Keep hips level.

Movement
4. Draw abs in and activate glutes.
5. Perform a bicep curl by flexing the elbow.
6. Keep shoulder blades retracted throughout the exercise.
7. Slowly return dumbbells to their original position, by extending at the elbow.

Standing Barbell Bicep Curl

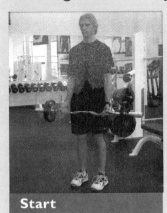

Start

Preparation
1. Stand with feet shoulder-width apart and pointed straight ahead, and knees slightly flexed over second and third toes.
2. Hold a barbell in both hands (palms facing up) with arms extended in front of body.
3. Keep hips level.

Movement
4. Draw abs in and activate glutes.
5. Perform a barbell curl, by flexing both elbows, while keeping the shoulder blades retracted.
6. Curl bar up to chest level.
7. Slowly lower the bar back to original position, by extending the elbows.

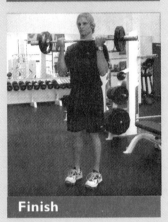

Finish

Seated Hammer Curl

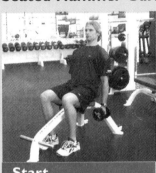

Start

Preparation
1. Sit on a bench with feet shoulder-width apart and pointed straight ahead, and knees over second and third toes.
2. Hold a dumbbell in each hand with arms extended at sides.

Movement
3. Draw abs in and activate glutes.
4. Perform a bicep curl by flexing the elbow, while keeping the palms facing the side of the body, at chest level.
5. Keep shoulder blades retracted throughout the exercise.
6. Slowly return dumbbells to their original position, by extending at the elbow.

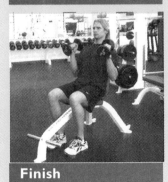

Finish

Bicep Curl Machine

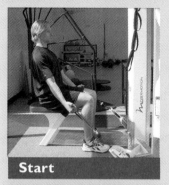

Start

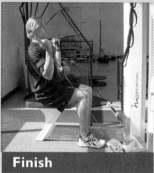

Finish

Preparation
1. Sit at machine.
2. Make any adjustments necessary to fit body.
3. Select desired weight.

Movement
4. Draw abs in and activate glutes.
5. Perform a curl by flexing elbows, while keeping shoulder blades retracted. Do not allow head to jut forward.
6. Curl until end-range.
7. Slowly return weight to original position, by extending elbows.

Tricep Exercise Descriptions

Tricep Stabilization Exercises

Supine Ball Dumbbell Tricep Extensions

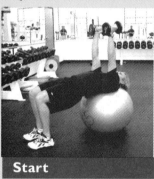

Start

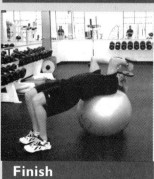

Finish

Preparation
1. Lie on a stability ball, with ball between shoulder blades.
2. Maintain a bridge position by contracting glutes and keeping shoulders, hips and knees level.
3. Feet should be shoulder-width apart with toes pointing straight ahead.
4. Hold dumbbells in each hand, with elbows pointing toward the sky.

Movement
5. Draw abs in and activate glutes.
6. Extend elbows until arms are straight up in the air.
7. Return dumbbells slowly toward chest, by flexing elbows.
8. Regression
   a. On bench
9. Progression
   a. Alternating-arms
   b. Single-arm

Prone Ball Dumbbell Tricep Extension

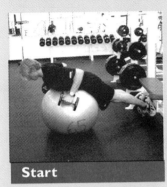

Start

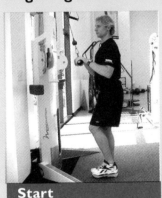

Finish

Preparation

1. Lie in a prone position, with stability ball under abdomen.
2. Keep feet pointed down and legs completely straight.
3. Hold dumbbells in each hand with elbows bent and shoulder blades retracted and depressed.

Movement

4. Draw abs in and activate glutes.
5. Maintaining a retracted position, extend elbows, so that they are parallel to the side of body.
6. Hold.
7. Slowly return dumbbells to original position, by flexing elbows.
8. Regression
   a. Standing
9. Progression
   a. Alternating-arms
   b. Single-arm

Single-leg Cable Pushdown

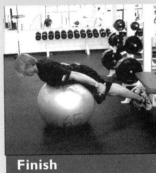

Start

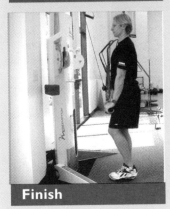

Finish

Preparation

1. Stand with feet shoulder-width apart, pointed straight ahead, and knees slightly flexed over second and third toes.
2. Grasp a cable, palm facing the ground and elbow flexed at a 90-degree angle.
3. Keep shoulder blades retracted and depressed.

Movement

4. Draw abs in and activate glutes.
5. Extend elbow, by pushing hand toward the ground until arm is fully extended.
6. Hold.
7. Slowly lower the cable back to 90 degrees of elbow flexion.
8. Regression
   a. Two-leg
9. Progression
   a. Alternating-arm
   b. Single-arm

Push-up with Rotation (Close Grip)

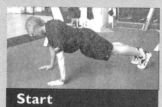

Start

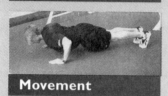

Movement

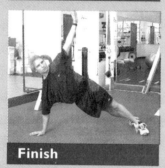

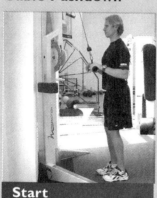

Finish

Preparation

1. Begin in a push-up position with legs fully extended and back flat.
2. Hands should be at chest level, slightly narrower than shoulder-width apart.

Movement

3. Draw abs in and activate glutes.
4. Perform a regular push-up, lowering body to ground. Do not allow back to arch.
5. Push-up to original position.
6. Rotate entire body, so that it is turned 90 degrees from the ground.
7. Both arms should be fully extended, one in the air and one stabilizing on the ground.
8. Bring the arm in the air back to its original position.
9. Repeat, alternating the direction of rotation.
10. Regression
    a. On knees
    b. Hands on bench, feet on floor
11. Progression
    a. Legs stacked on one another during the rotation

TRICEP STRENGTH EXERCISES

Cable Pushdown

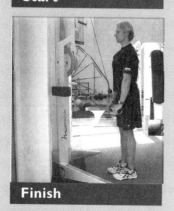

Start

Finish

Preparation

1. Stand with feet shoulder-width apart, pointed straight ahead, and knees slightly flexed over second and third toes.
2. Grasp a cable, with palms facing each other and elbows flexed at 90-degree angles.
3. Keep shoulder blades retracted and depressed.

Movement

4. Draw abs in and activate glutes.
5. Extend triceps, by pushing hands toward the ground until arms are fully extended.
6. Hold.
7. Slowly lower the cable back to 90 degrees of elbow flexion.
8. Repeat.

Supine Bench Dumbbell Tricep Extension

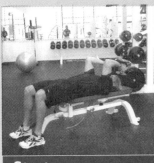
Start

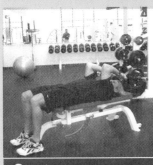
Finish

Preparation

1. Lie on flat bench, with knees bent.
2. Feet should be flat on the bench, shoulder-width apart, with toes pointing straight ahead.
3. Hold dumbbells in each hand, with elbows pointing toward the sky.

Movement

4. Draw abs in and activate glutes.
5. Extend elbows until arms are straight up in the air.
6. Hold.
7. Slowly lower dumbbells toward the side of the head, by flexing the elbows.
8. Repeat.

Supine Bench Barbell Tricep Extension

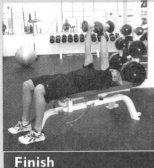
Start

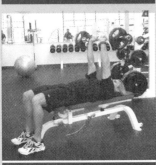
Finish

Preparation

1. Lie on flat bench, with knees bent.
2. Feet should be flat on the bench, shoulder-width apart, with toes pointing straight ahead.
3. Hold barbell, with elbows pointing up.

Movement

4. Draw abs in and activate glutes.
5. Extend elbows until arms are straight up in the air.
6. Hold.
7. Slowly lower barbell toward forehead, by flexing the elbows.
8. Repeat.

Leg Exercise Descriptions
LEG STABILIZATION EXERCISES
Ball Squat

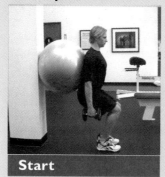
Start

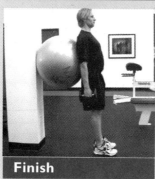
Finish

Preparation

1. Stand with feet shoulder-width apart, toes pointing forward and knees over second and third toes.
2. Rest back against a stability ball which is placed on a wall.
3. Ideally, keep feet under the knees. For individuals who lack ankle dorsiflexion (tight calves), place the feet slightly in front of the knees.

Movement

4. Draw abs in and activate glutes.
5. Slowly begin to squat down, bending knees and flexing hips, keeping feet straight (as if sitting into a chair). Do not allow any internal rotation at the hips or knees.
6. Allow the pelvis to sit back under the ball while maintaining a neutral spine.
7. Keep the chest up and put pressure through the heels. Do not rely solely on the ball for support.
8. To rise back up, contract glutes and place pressure through the heels as knees are extended.
9. Stand up straight until hips and legs are fully extended. Avoid compensation in the low back or lower extremities.
10. Regression
    a. Decrease range of motion
    b. Holding on to a stable support
11. Progression
    a. Squat without stability ball

Cable Squat

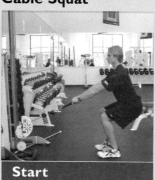
Start

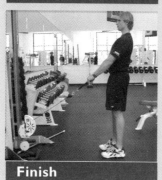
Finish

Preparation

1. Stand with feet shoulder-width apart, toes pointing forward and knees over second and third toes.
2. Hold cables to the side of the body.

Movement

3. Draw abs in and activate glutes.
4. Slowly begin to squat down, bending knees and flexing hips, keeping feet straight (as if sitting into a chair). Do not allow any internal rotation at the hips or knees.
5. Allow the pelvis to sit back while maintaining a neutral spine.
6. Keep the chest up and put pressure through the heels.
7. To rise back up, contract glutes and place pressure through the heels as knees are extended.
8. Stand up straight until hips and legs are fully extended. Avoid compensation in the low back or lower extremities.
9. Regression
    a. Decrease range of motion
    b. Ball Squat
10. Progression
    a. Squat without cables

Body Weight Squat to Calf Raise

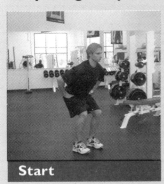

Start

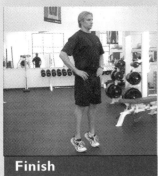

Finish

Preparation

1. Stand with feet shoulder-width apart, toes pointing forward and knees over second and third toes.
2. Keep hands on hips or behind the ears.

Movement

3. Draw abs in and activate glutes.
4. Slowly begin to squat down, bending knees and flexing hips, keeping feet straight (as if sitting into a chair). Do not allow any internal rotation at the hips or knees.
5. Allow the pelvis to sit back while maintaining a neutral spine.
6. Keep the chest up and put pressure through the heels.
7. To rise back up, contract glutes and place pressure through the heels as knees are extended.
8. Stand up straight until hips, knees and feet are fully extended (up on to toes). Avoid compensation in the low back or lower extremities.
9. Regression
   a. Omit calf raise
   b. Holding on to a stable support
10. Progression
   a. Unstable surface

Multiplanar Step-up to Balance

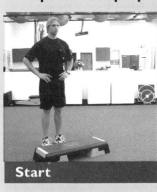

Start

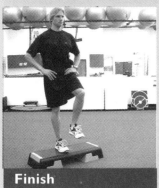

Finish

Preparation

1. Stand in front of box (six to 24 inches high), with feet shoulder-width apart and pointed straight ahead.

Movement

2. Draw abs in and activate glutes.
3. Step onto a box with one leg, keeping foot pointed straight ahead and knee lined up over midfoot.
4. Push through heel and stand up straight, balancing on one leg.
5. Flex the other leg at the hip and knee.
6. Dorsiflex the foot.
7. Return "floating" leg to the ground and step off the box, maintaining optimal alignment.
8. Repeat on other leg.
9. Regression
   a. Omit balance
   b. Decrease step height
10. Progression
   a. Frontal Plane Step-up
   b. Transverse Plane Step-up

Multiplanar Lunge to Balance

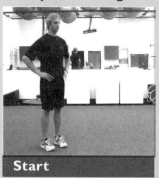

Start

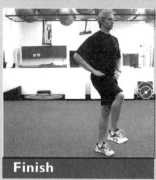

Finish

Preparation

1. Begin with both feet shoulder-width apart and pointed straight ahead.
2. Hold dumbbells in each hand.

Movement

3. Draw abs in and activate glutes.
4. Lunge forward, landing on the heel of lunge foot.
5. Then, come to a stabilized position with front foot pointing straight ahead and knee directly over second and third toes.
6. Both knees should now be bent at 90-degree angles, front foot should be flat on the ground and the back foot should have the heel lifted off the ground.
7. From this position, drive off of front foot (heel first) onto back leg.
8. Stand directly up into a balance position with balance leg straight and "floating" leg flexed 90 degrees at the hip and knee.
9. Dorsiflex foot.
10. Return "floating" leg to the ground, maintaining optimal alignment.
11. Repeat on other leg.
12. Regression
    a. Omit balance
    b. Stationary lunge
    c. Step-up
13. Progression
    a. Frontal Plane Lunge
    b. Transverse Plane Lunge

Single-leg Romanian Deadlift

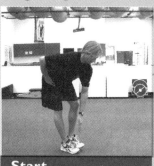

Start

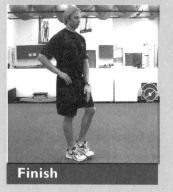

Finish

Preparation

1. Place one hand on hip.
2. Balance on same leg (where hand is on hip), with knee flexed at five degrees and aligned over second and third toes.

Movement

3. Draw abs in and activate glutes.
4. Keep "floating" leg directly beside stance leg and slowly bend over at the waist, maintaining five degrees of knee flexion.
5. Reach with the free hand toward stabilizing foot. While lowering, maintain optimal alignment of lower extremity.
6. Lower to the first point of compensation.
7. Then, activate glutes and stand back upright until hip is extended.
8. Regression
    a. Decrease range of motion
       i. Touch knee
       ii. Touch shin
9. Progression
    a. Unstable surface

Single-leg Squat

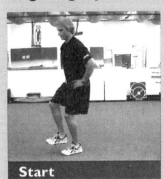

Start

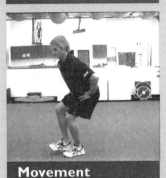

Movement

Preparation
1. Stand on one foot with foot pointing straight ahead, and knee slightly flexed and over second and third toes.
2. Clasp hands at chest.

Movement
3. Draw abs in and activate glutes.
4. Keeping foot straight ahead, perform a squat as if sitting in a chair.
5. Move "floating" leg in front of body.
6. While lowering, extend arms, moving hands away from body and to the outside of balance leg.
7. Lower to the first point of compensation.
8. Then, push through heel, activate glutes and stand back upright, bringing hands back in toward chest.
9. Regression
   a. Decrease range of motion
   b. Use outside support
10. Progression
    a. Single-leg Squat Touchdown

Single-leg Squat Touchdown

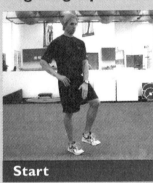

Start

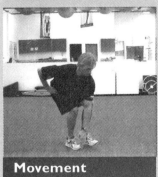

Movement

Preparation
1. Stand on one foot with foot pointing straight ahead, and knee slightly flexed and over second and third toes.

Movement
2. Draw abs in and activate glutes.
3. Keep "floating" leg directly beside body.
4. Slowly squat down.
5. Reach with free hand toward stabilizing foot.
6. Keep chest up while lowering body and maintain optimal alignment of lower extremity.
7. Lower to the first point of compensation.
8. Then, push through heel, activate glutes and stand back upright, until hip and knee are extended.
9. Regression
   a. Single-leg Squat
10. Progression
    a. Unstable surface

LEG STRENGTH EXERCISES

Hip Sled

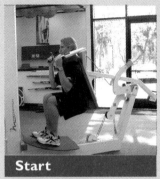

Start

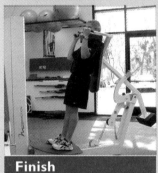

Finish

Preparation

1. Stand in machine and position back and glutes flat against support pads.
2. Make any adjustments necessary to fit body.
3. Place feet shoulder-width apart, with toes pointing forward and knees directly over second and third toes.

Movement

4. Draw abs in and activate glutes.
5. Slowly lower weight toward body, by flexing at the knees and hips. Keep optimal alignment of the lower extremity throughout the movement.
6. Before any compensation occurs, activate glutes and apply pressure through heels to push body upward and extend legs.

Multiplanar Dumbbell Step-up

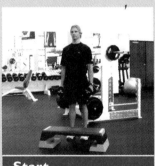

Start

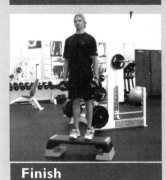

Finish

Preparation

1. Stand in front of a box (six to 24 inches high), with feet shoulder-width apart and pointed straight ahead.

Movement

2. Draw abs in and activate glutes.
3. Step onto a box with one leg, keeping foot pointed straight ahead and knee lined up over midfoot.
4. Push through heel and stand up straight
5. Step off the box, maintaining optimal alignment.
6. Repeat on other leg.

Barbell Squat

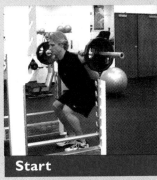

Start

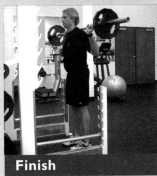

Finish

Preparation

1. Stand with feet shoulder-width apart, toes pointing straight ahead, and knees over second and third toes.
2. Rest barbell on shoulders, behind neck, with hands grasping the bar wider than shoulder-width apart.

Movement

3. Draw abs in and activate glutes.
4. Slowly begin to squat down, bending knees and flexing hips, keeping feet straight. Do not allow any internal rotation at the hips or knees.
5. Allow glutes to "stick" out behind body.
6. Keep the chest up and put pressure through the heels.
7. Squat to a three-quarter position.
8. To rise back up, contract glutes and place pressure through the heels as knees are extended.
9. Stand up straight until hips and legs are fully extended. Avoid compensation in the low back or lower extremities.

Barbell Step-up

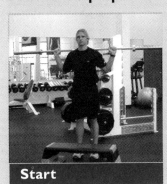

Start

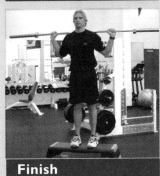

Finish

Preparation

1. Stand in front of a box (six to 24 inches high), with feet shoulder-width apart and pointed straight ahead.

Movement

2. Draw abs in and activate glutes.
3. Step onto a box with one leg, keeping foot pointed straight ahead and knee lined up over mid foot.
4. Push through heel and stand up straight
5. Step off the box, maintaining optimal alignment.
6. Repeat on other leg.

Dumbbell Lunge

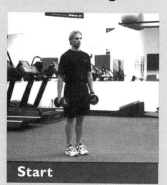

Start

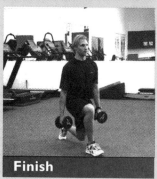

Finish

Preparation

1. Begin with both feet shoulder-width apart and pointed straight ahead.
2. Hold dumbbells in each hand.

Movement

3. Draw abs in and activate glutes.
4. Lunge forward, landing on the heel of lunge foot.
5. Then, come to a stabilized position with front foot pointing straight ahead and knee directly over second and third toes.
6. Both knees should now be bent at 90-degree angles, front foot should be flat on the ground and the back foot should have the heel lifted off the ground.
7. From this position, drive off of front foot (heel first) onto back leg.
8. Stand back up to a balanced position on both legs.
9. Repeat on other leg.

Barbell Lunge

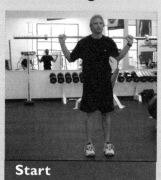

Start

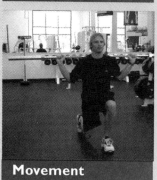

Movement

Preparation

1. Begin with both feet shoulder-width apart and pointed straight ahead.
2. Keep barbell across the shoulders while maintaining neutral cervical spine.

Movement

3. Draw abs in and activate glutes.
4. Lunge forward, landing on the heel of lunge foot.
5. Then, come to a stabilized position with front foot pointing straight ahead and knee directly over second and third toes.
6. Both knees should now be bent at 90-degree angles, front foot should be flat on the ground and the back foot should have the heel lifted off the ground.
7. From this position, drive off of front foot (heel first) onto back leg.
8. Stand back up to a balanced position on both legs.
9. Repeat on other leg.

Barbell Russian Deadlift

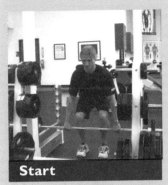

Start

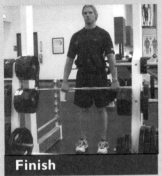

Finish

Preparation
1. Barbell should be on the ground.
2. Begin with both feet shoulder-width apart, with toes pointing forward and knees over second and third toes.

Movement
3. Draw abs in and activate glutes.
4. Squat down and grab the barbell with both hands (grip slightly wider than shoulder-width).
5. Drive through the heels, contract the glutes and lift the barbell until in a fully upright position.
6. Return to original position and repeat.

LEG POWER EXERCISES

Squat Jump

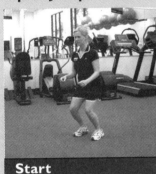

Start

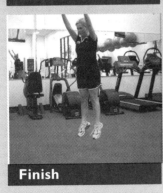

Finish

Preparation
1. Stand with feet shoulder-width apart and pointed straight ahead and knee slightly flexed over second and third toes.
2. Place arms by sides.

Movement
3. Draw abs in and activate glutes.
4. Squat down slightly.
5. Jump up into the air, using arms and extending them overhead (as if reaching for the sky).
6. Bring arms back to sides during landing.
7. Land softly on the balls of feet in a controlled manner with feet straight, knees over mid-foot. Maintain control of the entire body.

Tuck Jump

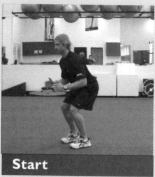

Start

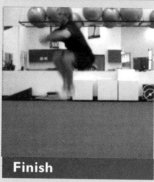

Finish

Preparation

1. Stand with feet shoulder-width apart and pointed straight ahead, and knees aligned over mid-foot with arms by sides

Movement

2. Draw abs in and activate glutes.
3. Jump up off the ground and, while in the air, bring knees up to chest.
4. Land softly on the mid-point of the feet, in a controlled manner, with feet straight and knees over mid-foot. Maintain control of your entire body.
5. Repeat immediately, as quickly as can be controlled

Butt Kick

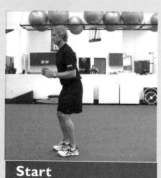

Start

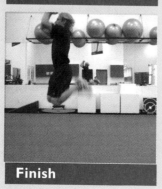

Finish

Preparation

1. Stand with feet shoulder-width apart and pointed straight ahead, and knees aligned over mid-foot with arms by sides

Movement

2. Draw abs in and activate glutes.
3. Jump up off the ground and attempt to touch your heels to your glutes. Do not allow the lower back to arch.
4. Land softly on the mid-point of the feet, in a controlled manner, with feet straight and knees over mid-foot. Maintain control of your entire body.
5. Repeat immediately, as quickly as can be controlled

Power Step-up

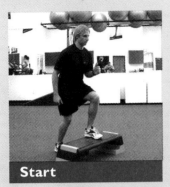

Start

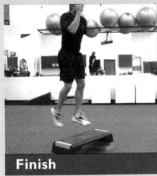

Finish

Preparation

1. Stand with one foot on a box (six to 18 inches high), and the other foot on ground, with both feet pointing straight ahead and knee aligned over second and third toes.

Movement

2. Draw abs in and activate glutes.
3. Forcefully push off step leg and put leg into full extension, stepping up on to the box. Keep body weight on step leg.
4. Switch legs for the landing. For example, if you push off right leg, land on left leg.
5. Land with feet, knees and hips in optimal alignment.
6. Repeat as quickly as can be controlled, alternating legs.

Ice Skater

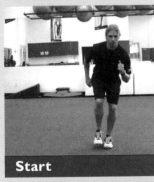

Start

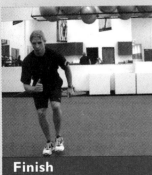

Finish

Preparation

1. Start by standing on one foot, keeping the chest up and knee aligned over mid-foot. Hands should be on hips.

Movement

2. Draw abs in and activate glutes.
3. Rapidly hop from side to side, switching legs, keeping both feet pointed straight ahead.
4. Without compensation, perform as quickly as can be controlled.
5. Repeat as instructed.

Lunge Jump

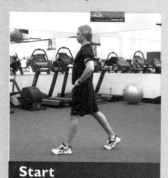

Start

Preparation

1. Stand with feet in a staggered stance.
2. Feet should be pointed straight ahead and knees over second and third toes.
3. Place arms by sides.

Movement

4. Draw abs in and activate glutes.
5. Lunge down slightly.
6. Jump up into the air, using arms and extending them overhead (as if reaching for the sky).
7. While in the air, switch legs so the back leg moves up and the front leg moves back.
8. Land softly in a controlled manner back into the lunge position with the legs now in an opposite position (back leg now in front and vice versa). Keep feet straight, knees over mid-foot. Maintain control of the entire body and repeat.

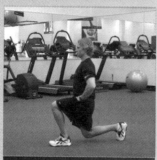

Movement

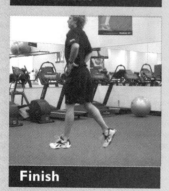

Finish

Speed Squat

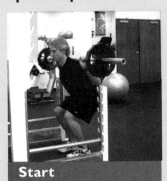

Start

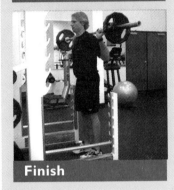

Finish

Preparation

1. Stand with feet shoulder-width apart, toes pointing straight ahead and knees over second and third toes.
2. Rest barbell on shoulders, behind neck, with hands grasping the bar wider than shoulder-width apart. Use light weight.

Movement

3. Draw abs in and activate glutes.
4. In a quick yet controlled fashion, squat down, bending knees and flexing hips, keeping feet straight. Do not allow any internal rotation at the hips or knees.
5. Sit back as if sitting into a chair.
6. Keep the chest up and put pressure through the heels.
7. Quickly rise back up by contracting the glutes and place pressure through the heels as knees are extended.
8. Stand up straight until hips and legs are fully extended. Avoid compensation in the low back or lower extremities. Quickly squat up and down for the appropriate repetitions.
9. Repeat as quickly as can be controlled.

References

1. Fleck SJ, Schutt RC. Types of strength training. *Clin Sports Med* 1985;4:159-67.

2. Pearson D, Faigenbaum A, Conley M, Kraemer WJ. The NSCA basic guidelines for the resistance training of athletes. *Strength Cond J* 2000; 22(4):14-27.

3. Stone MH, Collins D, Plisk S, Haff G, Stone ME. Training principles: evaluation of modes and methods of resistance training. *Strength Cond J* 2000; 22(3):65-76.

4. Tan B. Manipulating resistance training program variables to optimize maximum strength in men: a review. *J Strength Cond Res* 1999;13(3):289-304.

5. Brooks GA, Fahey TD, White TP. *Exercise physiology: human bioenergetics and its application.* 2nd edition. Mountain View, CA: Mayfield Publishing Company; 1996.

6. Selye H. *The stress of life.* New York: McGraw Hill; 1976.

7. Kraemer WJ, Ratamess NA. Physiology of resistance training. *Ortho Phys Ther Clin North Am* 2000;9(4):467-513.

8. Alter MJ. *Science of flexibility.* 2nd edition. Champaign, IL: Human Kinetics; 1996.

9. Gross J, Fetto J, Rosen E. *Musculoskeletal examination.* Malden, MA: Blackwell Sciences, Inc.; 1996.

10. Nordin M, Lorenz T, Campello M. Biomechanics of tendons and ligaments. Chapter 4. In: Nordin M, Franklel VH (eds.). *Basic biomechanics of the musculoskeletal system.* 3rd edition. Philadelphia: Lippincott Williams & Wilkins; 2001.

11. Kannus P. Structure of the tendon connective tissue. *Scand J Med Sci Sports* 2000; 10(6):312-20.

12. Adams K, O'Shea JP, O'Shea KL, Climstein M. The effect of six weeks of squat, plyometric and squat-plyometric training power production. *J Appl Sports Sci Res* 1992;6:36-41.

13. Bompa TO. *Theory and methodology of training.* Dubuque, IA: Kendall/Hunt; 1983.

14. Bompa TO. Variations of periodization of strength. *Strength Cond J* 1996;18:58-61.

15. Canavan PK, Garret GE, Armstrong LE. Kinematic and kinetic relationships between an olympic style lift and the vertical jump. *J Strength Cond Res* 1996;10:127-30.

16. Ebben WP, Watts PB. A review of combined weight training and plyometric training modes: complex training. *Strength Cond J* 1998;20(5):18-27.

17. Fees MA. Complex training. *Athl Ther Tod* 1997;2(1):18.

18. Fleck S, K Kontor. Complex training. *Strength Cond J* 1986;8(5):66-8.

19. Graves JE, Pollock ML, Jones AE, Colvin AB, Leggett SH. Specificity of limited range of motion variable resistance training. *Med Sci Sports Exerc* 1989;21:84-9.

20. Haff GG, Stone MH, O'Bryant HS, et al. Force-time dependent characteristics of dynamic and isometric muscle contractions. *J Strength Cond Res* 1997;11:269-72.

21. Hakkinen K, Allen M, Komi PV. Changes in isometric force and relaxation time, electromyographic and muscle fiber characteristics of human skeletal muscle during strength training and detraining. *Acta Physiol Scand* 1985;125:573-85.

22. Hennessey LC, Watson AW. The interference effects of training for strength and endurance simultaneously. *J Strength Cond Res* 1994;8:12-19.

23. Hickson RC. Interference of strength development by simultaneously training for strength and endurance. *Eur J App Physiol* 1980;45:255-63.

24. Hickson RC, Rosenkoetter MA, Brown MM. Strength training effects on aerobic power and short term endurance. *Med Sci Sports Exerc* 1980;12:336-9.

25. Hurley BF, Seals DR, Ehsani AA, Cartier LJ, Dalsky GP, Hagberg JM, Hollososzy JO. Effects of high-intensity strength training on cardiovascular function. *Med Sci Sports Exerc* 1984;16:483-8.

26. Kaneko M, Fuchimoto T, Toji H, Suei K. Training effect of different loads on the force-velocity relationship and mechanical power output in human muscle. *Scand J Sports Sci* 1983;5(2):50-5.

27. Lyttle AD, Wilson GJ, Ostrowski KJ. Enhancing performance: maximal power versus combined weights and plyometric training. *J Strength Cond Res* 1996;10:173-9.

28. Mateeva L. The speed strength correlation with the explosive strength development (Abstract). *Teniorska-missal* 1988;6:23-4.

29. McBride J, Triplett-McBride T, Davie A, Newton RU. A comparison of strength and power characteristics between power lifters, olympic lifters, and sprinters. *J Strength Cond Res* 1999;13:58-66.

30. Morrissey MC, Harman EA, Johnson MJ. Resistance training modes; specificity and effectiveness. *Med Sci Sports Exerc* 1986;18:612-24.

31. Moss BM, Refsnes PE, Abildgaard A, Nicolayysen K, Jensen J. The effects of maximal effort strength training with different loads on dynamic strength, cross-sectional area, load-power and load-velocity relationships. *Eur J Appl Physiol* 1997;75:193-9.

32. Newton RU, Kraemer WJ. Developing explosive muscular power: implications for a mixed methods training strategy. *Strength Cond J* 1994;16(5):20-31.

33. Newton, RU, Kraemer WJ, Hakkinene K, Humphries BJ, Murphy AJ. Kinematics, kinetics and muscle activation during explosive upper body movements. *J Appl Biomech* 1996;12:31-43.

34. Newton RU, Murphy AJ, Humphries BJ, Wilson GJ, Kraemer WJ, Hakkinen K. Influence of load and stretch shortening cycle on the kinematics, kinetics and muscle activation that occurs during explosive upper-body movements. *Eur J Appl Physiol* 1997;75:333-42.

35. O'Shea P. Effects of selected weight training programs on the development of strength and muscle hypertrophy. *Res Q* 1966;37:95-102.

36. Paavolainen L, Hakkinen K, Hamalainen I, et al. Explosive strength training improves 5-Km running time by improving running economy and muscle power. *J Appl Physiol* 1999;86:1527-33.

37. Polhemus R, Burkherdt E, Osina M, Patterson M. The effect of plyometric training with ankle and vest weights on conventional weight training programs for men. *Track Field Q Rev* 1980;80(4):59-61.

38. Robinson JM, Stone MH, Johnson RL, Penland CM, Warren BJ, Lewis RD. Effects of different weight training exercise/rest intervals on strength, power, and high intensity exercise endurance. *J Strength Cond Res* 1995;9:216-21.

39. Rutherford OM, Greig CA, Sargent AJ, Jones DA. Strength training and power output: transference effects in the human quadriceps muscle. *J Sport Sci* 1986;4:101-7.

40. Sale DG. Influence of exercise and training on motor unit activation. *Exer Sport Sci Rev* 1987;15:95-151.

41. Schmidtbleicher D. Training for power events. Chapter 18. In: Komi PV (ed). *Strength and power in sports*. Boston: Blackwell Scientific; 1992.

42. Schmidtbleicher D, Haralambie G. Changes in contractile properties of muscle after strength training in a man. *Eur J App Physiol* 1981;46:221-8.

43. Sforzo GA, Touey PR. Manipulating exercise order affects muscular performance during a resistance exercise training session. *J Strength Cond Res* 1996;10:20-4.

44. Verkhoshansky Y. Perspectives in the improvement of speed-strength preparation of jumpers. *Track Field* 1966;9:11-2.

45. Verkhoshansky Y. Speed-strength preparation and development of strength endurance of athletes in various specializations. *Sov Sports Rev* 1986;21:120-4.

46. Verkhoshansky Y, Tatyan V. Speed-strength preparation of future champions. *Legkaya Atletika* 1973;2:12-3.

47. Wenzel RR, Perfetto EM. The effect of speed versus non-speed training in power development. *J Appl Sport Sci Res* 1992;6:82-7.

48. Wilson GJ, Newton RU, Murphy AJ, Humphries BJ. The optimal training load for the development of dynamic athletic performance. *Med Sci Sports Exerc* 1993;25:1279-86.

49. Yessis M. Integrating plyometrics with strength training. *Fitness Sports Rev Int* 1995;28(4):113-6.

50. Young WB. Training for speed-strength: heavy versus light loads. *Strength Cond J* 1993;15(5):34-42.

51. Zatsiorsky VM. *Science and practice of strength training.* Champaign, IL: Human Kinetics; 1995.

52. Behm DG. Neuromuscular implications and applications of resistance training. *J Strength Cond Res* 1995;9:264-74.

53. Kovaleski JE, Heitman RH, Trundle TL, Gilley WF. Isotonic preload versus isokinetic knee extension resistance training. *Med Sci Sports Exerc* 1995;27:895-9.

54. Noose LJ, Hunter GR. Free weights: A review supporting their use in rehabilitation. *Athlet Train* 1985 Fall:206-9.

55. Sale DG. Neural adaptation in strength and power training. In: Jones NL, McCartney N, McComas AJ (eds). *Human muscle power.* Champaign, IL: Human Kinetics; 1986.

56. Wilson GJ, Murphy AJ, Walshe A. The specificity of strength training: the effect of posture. *Euro J Appl Physiol* 1996; 73:346-52.

57. Siff MC, Verkhoshansky Y. *Supertraining.* Escondido, CA: Sports Training; 1994.

58. Rutherford OM, Jones DA. The role of learning and coordination in strength training. *Eur J Appl Physiol* 1986;55:100-5.

59. Hakkinen K. Neuromuscular adaptation during strength training, aging, detraining and immobilization. *Crit Rev Phys Rehab Med* 1994;6:161-98.

60. Siff MC, Verkhoshansky Y. *Supertraining.* Escondido, CA: Sports Training; 1994.

61. McEvoy KP, Newton RU. Baseball throwing speed and base running speed: the effects of ballistic resistance training. *J Strength Con Res* 1998;12(4):216-21.

62. Moritani T, Muro M, Ishida K, Taguchi S. Electrophysiological analyses of the effects of muscle power training. *Res J Phys Educ Jap* 1987;1:23-32.

63. Miller J. Medicine ball training for throwers. *Strength Cond J* 1987;9(1):32-3.

64. Hamilton MT, Booth FW. Skeletal muscle adaptation to exercise: a century of progress. *J Appl Physiol* 2000;88(1):327-31.

65. Franklin BA, Roitman JL. Cardiorespiratory adaptations to exercise. Chapter 17. In American College of Sports Medicine (ed). *ACSM's resource manual for guidelines for exercise testing and prescription.* 3rd edition. Baltimore, MD: Williams & Wilkins; 1998.

66. Viru A, Viru M. Nature of training effects. Chapter 6. In: Garrett WE, Kirkendall DT (eds.). *Exercise and sport science.* Philadelphia: Lippincott Williams & Wilkins; 2000.

67. MacDougall JD, Hicks AL, MacDonald JR, McKelvie RS, Green HJ, Smith KM. Muscle performance and enzymatic adaptations to sprint interval training. *J Appl Physiol* 1998;84(6):2138-42.

68. Harmer AR, McKenna MJ, Sutton JR, Snow RJ, Ruell PA, Booth J, Thompson MW, Mackay NA, Stathis CG, Crameri RM, Carey MF, Eager DM. Skeletal muscle metabolic and ionic adaptations during intense exercise following sprint training in humans. *J Appl Physiol* 2000;89(5):1793-803.

69. Parra J, Cadefau JA, Rodas G, Amigo N, Cusso R. The distribution of rest periods affects performance and adaptations of energy metabolism induced by high-intensity training in human muscle. *Acta Physiol Scand* 2000;169(2):157-65.

70. Ogita F, Stam RP, Tazawa HO, Toussaint HM, Hollander AP. Oxygen uptake in one-legged and two-legged exercise. *Med Sci Sports Exerc* 2000;32(10):1737-42.

71. Williford HN, Olson MS, Gauger S, Duey WJ, Blesing DL. Cardiovascular and metabolic costs of forward, backward, and lateral motion. *Med Sci Sports Med* 1998;30(9):1419-23.

72. Heus R, Wertheim AH, Havenith G. Human energy expenditure when walking on a moving platform. *Eur J Sppl Physiol Occup Physiol* 1998;100(2):133-48.

73. Clark MA. *Integrated training for the new millennium.* Thousand Oaks, CA: National Academy of Sports Medicine; 2001.

74. Clark MA. *Integrated strength training.* Thousand Oaks, CA: National Academy of Sports Medicine; 2001.

75. Fleck SJ, Kraemer WJ. *Designing resistance training programs.* 2nd edition. Champaign, IL: Human Kinetics, 1997.

76. Sale DG. Neural adaptation to resistance training. *Med Sci Sports Exerc* 1988;20(5):S135-45.

77. Sale, DG, MacDougall JD, Upton AR, McComas AJ. Effect of strength training upon motorneuron excitability in man. *Med Sci Sports Exerc* 1983;15(1):57-62.

78. Enoka RM. Muscle strength and its development: new perspectives. *Sports Med* 1988;6:146-68.

79. Henneman E. Relation between size of motor neurons and their susceptibility to discharge. *Sci* 1957;126:1345-7.

80. Cosio-Lima LM, Reynolds KL, Winter C, Paolone V, Jones MT. Effects of physioball and conventional floor exercises on early adaptations in back and abdominal core stability and balance in women. *J Strength Cond Res* 2003;17(4):721-5.

81. Behm DG, Anderson K, Curnew RS. Muscle force and activation under stable and unstable conditions. *J Strength Cond Res* 2002;16(3):416-22.

82. Heitkamp HC, Horstmann T, Mayer F, Weller J, Dickhuth HH. Gain in Strength and Muscular Balance After Balance Training. *Int J Sports Med* 2001;22:285-90.

83. Bellew JW, Yates JW, Gater DR. The initial effects of low-volume strength training on balance in untrained older men and women. *J Strength Cond Res* 2003;17(1):121-8.

84. MacDougall JD, Sale DG, Always SE, Sutton JR. Muscle ultrastructural characteristics of elite powerlifters and bodybuilders. *Eur J Appl Physiol* 1982;48:117-26.

85. Always SE, Grumby WH, Stray-Gunderson J, Gonyea WJ. Efects of resistance training on elbow flexors of highly competitive bodybuilders. *J Appl Physiol* 1992;72:1512-21.

86. Thorstenson A, Hultren B., von Dobeln W, Karlsson J. Effect of strength training on enzyme activities and fibre characteristics in human skeletal muscle. *Acta Physiol Scand* 1976;96:392-8.

87. MacDougal JD, Elder GCB, Sale DG, Moroz JR, Sutton JR. Effects of strength training and immobilization on human muscle fibers. *Eur J Appl Physiol* 1980;43:25-34.

88. Abernathy PJ, Jurimae J, Logan PA, Taylor AW, Thayer RE. Acute and chronic response of skeletal muscle to resistance exercise. *Sports Med* 1994;17(1):22-38.

89. McDonagh MJM, Davies CTM. Adaptive response to mammalian muscle to exercise with high loads. *Eur J Appl Physiol* 1984;52:139-59.

90. Hakkinen K, Komi PV. Electromyographic changes during strength training and detraining. *Med Sci Sports Exerc* 1983;15(6):455-60.

91. Narici MV, Roi GS, Landoni L, Minetti AE, Cerretelli P. Changes in force, cross-sectional area and neural activation during strength training and detraining of the human quadriceps. *Euro J Appl Physiol* 1989;59:310-9.

92. Moritani T, deVries HA. Neural factors versus hypertrophy in the time course of muscle strength gain. *Amer J Phys Med* 1979;58(3):115-29.

93. Komi PV, Viitasalo JT, Rauramaa R, Vihko V. Effect of isometric strength training on mechanical, electrical, and metabolic aspects of muscle function. *Euro J Appl Physiol* 1978;40:45-55.

94. Mayhew TP, Rothstein JM, Finucane SD, Lamb RL. Muscular adaptation to concentric and eccentric exercise at equal power levels. *Med Sci Sports Exerc* 1995;27:868-73.

95. Staron RS, Karapondo DL, Kraemer WJ et al. Skeletal muscle adaptations during early phase of heavy resistance training in men and women. *J Appl Physiol* 1994;76:1247-55.

96. Chelsey A, Macdougal JD, Tarnopolsky MA, Atkinson SA, Smith K. Changes in human muscle protein synthesis after resistance exercise. *J Appl Physiol* 1992;73:1383-8.

97. Booth FW, Thomason DB. Molecular and cellular adaptation of muscle in response to exercise: perspectives of various models. *Physiol Rev* 71:541-85.

98. Fry AC, Allemeier CA, Staron CS. Correlation between percentage fiber type area and myosin heavy chain content in human skeletal muscle. *Eur J Appl Physiol* 1994;68:246-51.

99. Kraemer WJ, Fleck SJ, Evans WJ. Strength and power training: physiological mechanisms of adaptation. In: Holloszy JO (ed). *Exercise and sport science reviews*. Volume 24. Baltimore: Williams & Wilkins; 1998. pp. 363-97.

100. Staron RS, Leonardi MJ, Karapondo DL et al. Strength and skeletal muscle adaptations in heavy-resistance-trained women after detraining and retraining. *J Appl Physiol* 1991:70:631-40.

101. Enoka RM. *Neuromechanical basis of kinesiology.* 2nd edition. Champaign, IL: Human Kinetics; 1994.

102. Enoka RM. *Neuromechanics of human movement.* 3rd edition. Champaign, IL: Human Kinetics; 2002.

103. Brown HS, Stein RB, Yemm R. Changes in firing rate of human motor units during linearly changing voluntary contractions. *J Physiol* 1973;230:371-90.

104. Marx JO, Kraemer WJ, Nindl BC, Gotshalk LA, Duncan ND, Volek JS, Hakkinen K, Newton RU. The effect of periodization and volume of resistance training in women [abstract]. *Med Sci Sports Exerc* 1998;30(5):S164. Abstract 935.

105. Kraemer WJ, Ratamess N, Fry et al. Influence of resistance training volume and periodization on physiological and performance adaptations in college women tennis players. *Am J Sports Med* 2000;28(5):626-33

106. Starkey DB, Pollock ML, Ishida Y et al. Effect of resistance training volume on strength and muscle thickness. *Med Sci Sports Exerc* 1996;28:1311-20.

107. Jacobson BH. A comparison of two progressive weight training techniques on knee extensor strength. *Athl Train* 1986;21:315-9.

108. Reid CM, Yeater RA, Ullrich IH. Weight training and strength, cardiorespiratory functioning and body composition of men. *Br J Sports Med* 1987;21:40-4.

109. American College of Sports Medicine. Position stand: the recommended quantity and quality of exercise for developing and maintaining cardiorespiratory and muscular fitness in healthy adults. *Med Sci Sports Exerc* 1990;22:265-74.

110. Stone MH, Plisk SS, Stone ME, Schilling BK, O'Bryant HS, Pierce KC. Athletic performance development: volume load-1 set vs. multiple sets, training velocity and training variation. *Strength Cond J* 1998;20(6): 22-31.

111. Logan GA. *Differential applications of resistance and resultant strength measured at varying degrees of knee flexion.* Doctoral Dissertation. Los Angeles: University of Southern California; 1960.

112. Harris GR, Stone MH, O'Bryant H, Proulx CM, JohnsonR. Short-term performance effects of high speed, high force and combined weight training. *J Strength Cond Res* 2000;14:14-20.

113. Kraemer WJ. A series of studies: the physiological basis for strength training in American football: fact over philosophy. *J Strength Cond Res* 1997;11:131-42.

114. Kraemer WJ, Newton RU, Bush J, Volek J, Triplett NT, Koziris LP. Varied multiple set resistance training produces greater gains than single set program [Abstract]. *Med Sci Sports Exerc* 1995;27(5):S195.

115. O'Bryant H, Byrd R, Stone MH. Cycle ergometer and maximum leg and hip strength adaptations to two different methods of weight training. *J Appl Sports Sci Res* 1988;2(2):27-30.

116. Schoitz MK, Potteiger JA, Huntsinger PG, Denmark DC. The short-term effects of periodized and constant-intensity training on body composition, strength and performance. *J Strength Cond Res* 1998;12(3):173-8.

117. Hakkinen K, Pakarinen A, Alen M, et al. Relationships between training volume, physical performance capacity, and serum hormone concentrations during prolonged training in elite weight lifters. *Int J Sports Med* 1987;8(suppl):61-5.

118. Hakkinen K, Pakarinen A, Alen M, et al. Neuromuscular and hormonal responses in elite athletes to two successive strength training sessions in one day. *Eur J Appl Physiol* 1988;57:133-9.

119. Haltom RW, Kraemer R, Sloan R, Hebert EP, Frank K, Tryniecki JL. Circuit weight training and its effects on postexercise oxygen consumption. *Med Sci Sports Exerc* 1999;31(11):1613-8.

120. Burleson MA, O'Bryant HS, Stone MH, Collins MA, Triplett-McBride T. Effect of weight training exercise and treadmill exercise on post-exercise oxygen consumption. *Med Sci Sports Exerc* 1998;30(4):518-22.

121. Gambetta V. *The gambetta method; common sense training for athletic performance.* Sarasota, FL: Gambetta Sports Training Systems; 1998.

Program Design Concepts

MODULE 13-1: Program Design

Introduction to Program Design

Traditionally, most training programs are based on the experiences of the health and fitness professional (whether he/she is a bodybuilder, group exercise instructor, powerlifter, Olympic lifter or an athlete). This has lead to many scientifically unsupported training programs that have created confusion for the health and fitness professionals. Indeed, science has been slow to validate anecdotal evidence that still continues to be used in the fitness world.[1,2]

In order to be safe, effective and productive, all health and fitness professionals must be competent at designing resistance-training programs for a variety of clients. This entails the proper utilization of acute variables (repetitions, sets, etc.) and exercises in a structured, progressive manner. For many health and fitness professionals, this can become a daunting task, causing them to ask, "How many exercises should I use? How many sets and repetitions should I utilize? How many days per week should my client train?" When using a structured, scientifically based program design model, answers to these questions become very simple.

What is Program Design?

PROGRAM DESIGN: A purposeful system or plan put together to help an individual achieve a specific goal.

Program design simply means creating a purposeful system or plan to achieve a specific goal. The key words here are "purposeful system." The purpose of a training program is to provide a path for the client to achieve his/her goal. Providing a path requires the health and fitness professional to have a comprehensive understanding of a few key concepts:

Acute Variables

- What are they?
- How do they affect the desired adaptation?
- How do they affect the overall training program?

The OPT™ Model (Planned Fitness Training — Periodization)

- How and why must the physiological, physical and performance adaptations of stabilization, strength and power take place in a planned, progressive manner to establish the proper foundation for each subsequent adaptation?

The Seven Phases of Training in the OPT™ Model

- How do these phases promote specific adaptations?
- What are the acute variables for each of the phases?

Application

- Selecting the right exercises,
- Selecting the right acute variables, and
- Applying both in a systematic manner to different populations with different goals.

Is There an Easier Way?
Taking the Guesswork Out

If a health and fitness professional has a proven system that he/she can follow, the needed information can simply be plugged in, without the worry of using the correct formula for success. This is exactly what the OPT™ model provides (Figure 13-1).

NASM designed the OPT™ model as a planned, systematic, periodized training program. It was established to concurrently improve all functional abilities such as flexibility, core stabilization, balance, power, strength and

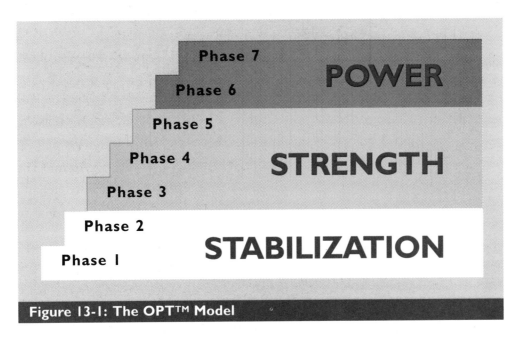

Figure 13-1: The OPT™ Model

cardiorespiratory endurance. The OPT™ program has been extremely successful in helping all populations to reduce body fat, increase lean muscle mass and/or strength, and improve performance and overall health.

The remaining modules of this chapter will detail acute variables of planned fitness training (or periodization) as it relates to the OPT™ model, the seven phases of the OPT™ model, and how to apply the OPT™ program design model to various goals.

MODULE 13-1 Summary

Health and fitness professionals must be competent at designing training programs for a variety of clients, using acute variables and exercises in a structured, progressive manner. A structured, scientifically based program design model makes this easy. The Optimum Performance Training (OPT™) model provides the health and fitness professional with a proven system where a client's information can simply be plugged in. Program design is creating a purposeful system or plan to achieve a specific goal. To do so, the health and fitness professional must understand acute variables, the OPT™ model and its phases, as well as how to apply it all.

MODULE 13-1 Quiz

1. The OPT™ model has been extremely successful in helping all populations to reduce body fat, increase lean muscle mass and/or strength, improve performance and improve overall health.

   ☐ True   ☐ False

MODULE 13-2:
Acute Variables of Training

Acute variables are the most fundamental components of designing a training program. They determine the amount of stress placed upon the body and, ultimately, what adaptation the body will incur.

The body will specifically adapt to the demands placed upon it (known also as the Principle of Specificity). The acute variables dictate these demands.

The OPT™ model takes the guesswork out of program design and allows for a planned, systematic progression by pre-assigning specific acute variables for each of the seven phases of training to elicit the desired adaptation.[3-11] Collectively, the acute variables are the foundation of program design and fall within the Program Design Continuum seen in Table 13-1.

Table 13-1: Program Design Continuum				
Adaptation	**Reps**	**Sets**	**Intensity**	**Rest Period**
Power	1-10	3-6	30% to 45% of one rep max or up to 10% of body weight	3-5 min.
Strength	1-12	2-6	70-100%	45 sec.-5 min.
Stabilization	12-25	1-3	40-70%	0 sec.-1.5 min.

As discussed in Chapter 12 (Resistance Training), the stabilization adaptation includes both endurance and stability; the strength adaptation includes hypertrophy and maximal strength; and the power adaptation includes power (rate of force production).

To ensure proper development and progression of an integrated training program, the health and fitness professional must understand the acute training variables, which are shown in Figure 13-2. Each of the acute variables will be explained in this module, as they relate to the OPT™ model.

Repetitions	**Repetition Tempo**	**Training Frequency**
Sets	**Training Volume**	**Training Duration**
Training Intensity	**Rest Interval**	**Exercise Selection**

Figure 13-2: Acute Variables of Training

Repetitions

A **repetition** is one complete movement of a particular exercise. Most repetitions will involve the three muscle actions: concentric, isometric and eccentric (not necessarily in that order).

These muscle actions can be seen in the example of a biceps curl. Starting with a weight at one side, a single repetition includes raising the dumbbell up against the direction of resistance (a concentric contraction), pausing for any specified amount of time (an isometric contraction) and then lowering the dumbbell with the direction of resistance back to its starting position (an eccentric contraction).

Another example of this can be seen when performing a squat. Starting from a standing position, one repetition includes lowering the body (with the direction of resistance) toward the ground (eccentric), pausing for any specified amount of time (isometric) and then rising back up (against the direction of resistance) to the starting position (concentric).

Repetitions are simply a means to count the number of movements performed in a given amount of time. They can therefore be a means to count the time the muscles are under tension (*time under tension*).

Each phase of training in the OPT™ model has specific goals and therefore requires a specific number of repetitions to achieve these goals. The number of repetitions performed in a given set is dependent upon the client's work capacity, intensity of the exercise and the specific phase of training.

The health and fitness professional must keep in mind that all acute variables are interdependent. This means that the specific use of one will affect the others. For example, the more intense the exercise or heavier the load, the fewer the number of repetitions that the individual can perform.[11-17]

Research demonstrates that training in a specific repetition range yields specific adaptations.[11-15,17,19] Therefore, depending on the goal of the individual and the phase of training, it is possible to define a specific repetition range (Table 13-2).

> **REPETITION (OR REP):**
> One complete movement of a single exercise.

Table 13-2: Repetition Continuum	
Training Adaptation	**Repetition Range**
Power	1-10
Strength	1-12
Stabilization	12-25

- Power adaptations require one to 10 repetitions at 30-45 percent of the one-repetition maximum (1RM) or up to 10 percent of body weight.

- If maximal strength adaptations are desired, the repetition range is one to five at 85-100 percent of the 1RM.

- Hypertrophy is best achieved utilizing eight to 12 repetitions at 70-85 percent of the 1RM.

■ Endurance is best achieved by performing 12-25 repetitions at 50-70 percent of the IRM.[11-17]

The OPT™ model utilizes the specified repetition continuum to provide the desired adaptations in a systematic manner. The beginning phases consist of higher repetition schemes necessary to build proper connective tissue strength, stability and endurance. This is especially important for the beginning client. However, a common mistake of many advanced clients is to not utilize a planned training program that provides periods of low repetition training alternated with periods of high repetition training. Higher intensities of training (lower repetitions) can only be sustained for a short period of time without running the risk of over-training.[20,21] Utilizing the OPT™ model enables the health and fitness professional to employ a systematic training approach to prevent over-training and yield specific results by using planned intervals of training.[22]

Sets

A **set** is a group of consecutive repetitions.[14,16,17,23] The quantities of the other acute variables (i.e. repetitions, training intensity, number of exercises, training level and recoverability) determine the number of sets an individual performs.[14,16,17,23]

There is an inverse relationship between sets, repetitions and intensity. The individual usually performs fewer sets when performing higher repetitions at a lower intensity (endurance and hypertrophy adaptations) and more sets when performing lower repetitions at a higher intensity (strength and power adaptations), as seen in Table 13-3.[11,13,23]

> **SET:**
> **A group of consecutive repetitions.**

Table 13-3: Set Continuum	
Training Adaptation	**Set Range**
Power	3-6
Strength	2-6
Stabilization	1-3

■ For power adaptations, three to six sets of between one and 10 repetitions at an intensity of 30-45 percent of IRM or up to 10 percent of body weight are recommended.

■ For maximal strength adaptation, four to six sets of between one and five repetitions at an intensity of 85-100 percent IRM are recommended.

■ Hypertrophy adaptations require three to four sets of eight to 12 repetitions at 70-85 percent IRM intensity level.

■ Endurance is best developed with one to three sets of 12-25 repetitions at 40-70 percent IRM intensity.[11,13,16,17,23]

It has been suggested that in order to prevent over-training, 24-36 total sets should be performed in a given workout (24 total sets for low volume or up to 36 total sets for high volume).[15] For the beginning client, this number may be as low as five to 12 total sets (one set of five to 12 exercises).

As a training program advances, and the desired adaptations change from stabilization and endurance to hypertrophy and/or maximal strength, the number of sets capable of being performed will also change.

When training for strength adaptations, the number of sets performed needs to increase to place enough stress on the tissues to provoke the desired changes.[11,12,15] As shown in Table 13-4, a beginning client may perform one to two exercises per body part for two to three sets per exercise, while an advanced client may perform three to four exercises per body part for three to five sets per exercise. This manipulation will have a large impact on the total training volume and must be planned (periodized) with phases that include a higher and lower number of sets over the course of the training program. Also, using the numbers in Table 13-4 in conjunction with the total number of sets per workout discussed above (24-36 sets), it is clear that the intermediate and advanced client may only train two to three body parts per workout, due to the total volume of training in a given workout and time constraints.

Table 13-4: Set Manipulations per Body Part

Client Level	Exercises per Body Part	Sets Each Exercise	Total Sets per Body Part
Beginning	1-2	2-3	2-6
Intermediate	2-3	3-4	6-12
Advanced	3-4	3-5	9-20

Training Intensity

Training intensity is one of the most important acute variables to consider when designing an integrated training program.[11,13,16,17,23] **Training intensity** is defined as an individual's level of effort compared to their maximum effort.[11,13]

The specific training phase and an individual's training goal will determine the number of sets and repetitions for an exercise. Intensity is then determined by the number of sets and repetitions to be performed, which is based on the individual's specific training goals (Table 13-5).

- Power (high velocity) adaptations are best attained with 30-45 percent of 1RM when using conventional weight training or up to 10 percent of body weight, when using medicine balls.

- Maximum strength adaptations require training with 85-100 percent of 1RM.

> **TRAINING INTENSITY:**
> An individual's level of effort, compared to their maximal effort, which is usually expressed as a percentage.

- Hypertrophy is best achieved by training with 70-85 percent of IRM.
- Endurance is best developed with a training intensity of 40-70 percent of IRM.[8,14,24-34]

Training intensity can also be derived from the percent of maximal oxygen consumption, as in the case of cardiorespiratory training programs.[35,36]

Training in an unstable environment, as seen in the stabilization phases of the OPT™ model, can also increase the training intensity because it requires more motor unit recruitment. This leads to more energy expenditure per exercise.[37-40] This allows for optimum development of neuromuscular efficiency. Changing other acute training variables such as rest periods and tempo also changes the training intensity. In short, intensity is a function of more than just external resistance. An integrated training program must focus on a holistic approach to force continued adaptations.[33,41]

Table 13-5: Intensity Continuum	
Training Adaptation	**Repetition Range**
Power	30% to 45% of IRM or up to 10% of body weight
Strength	70-100% of IRM
Stabilization	40-70% of IRM

Repetition Tempo

REPETITION TEMPO:
The speed with which each repetition is performed.

Repetition tempo refers to the speed with which each repetition is performed. This is an important variable that can be manipulated to achieve specific training objectives such as power, hypertrophy, stability and endurance.[11,13,16,17,42-48]

Movements also occur at different velocities. Therefore, to get the appropriate results from training, the health and fitness professional must select the appropriate speed of movement for the exercise, based on the Repetition Tempo Spectrum (Table 13-6).[48]

Table 13-6: Repetition Tempo Spectrum	
Training Adaptation	**Repetition Tempo (Eccentric/Isometric/Concentric)**
Power	Explosive (x/x/x)
Strength	Moderate (3/2/1-1/1/1)
Stabilization	Slow (4/2/2-4/2/1)

The amount of time that a muscle is under tension yields a specific result *(time under tension)*. For example, the optimum tempo for hypertrophy is approximately 20-70 seconds per set (eight to 10 repetitions in a range between 4/2/1 and 2/0/2 tempos).[49] The optimum tempo for power is as fast as the individual can move.[42-45,48] Therefore, based on the client's specific goals, the health and fitness professional must utilize the entire repetition tempo spectrum to achieve the desired results.[11,15-17,43,44]

The OPT™ model places a major emphasis on the Repetition Tempo Spectrum as it has a significant impact on the functional outcome of the stressed tissues. By emphasizing eccentric and isometric muscle actions at slower velocities during the initial stabilization phases of training, more demand is placed upon the connective tissue (as well as the stabilizing muscles) and better prepares the nervous system for functional movements. This is important for building the appropriate structural and functional foundation for more specific forms of strength and power training that will follow.

Rest Interval

The **rest interval** is the time taken to recuperate between sets and/or exercises and has a dramatic effect on the outcome of the training program.[11,16,17,23,34,48] Each exercise that is performed requires energy. The primary type of energy used during training depends on the training phase, intensity and goal (Table 13-7).[13,14]

REST INTERVAL:
The time taken to recuperate between sets.

Table 13-7: Rest Interval Continuum		
Training Adaptation	**Rest Interval**	**Energy Source**
Power	3-5 minutes	ATP-CP
Strength	45 sec.-5 minutes	ATP-CP/Glycolosis
Stabilization	0 sec.-1.5 minutes	Oxidative/Glycolosis

Power and maximal strength adaptations may require up to five minutes of rest between sets and exercises, depending on the client's level of fitness. Hypertrophy adaptations are maximized by decreasing the rest interval to 45-90 seconds between sets and exercises, but are dependent on the load being used. Stability and endurance adaptations should involve 30-90 seconds of rest.

Dynamic resistance training, as well as isometric training, can significantly reduce ATP and creatine phosphate (CP) supplies.[50,51] The ability to replenish these supplies is crucial for optimal performance and/or the desired adaptation. By adjusting the rest interval, energy supplies can be regained according to the goal of the training program. Rest intervals of:[52]

- 20-30 seconds will allow approximately 50 percent recovery of ATP/CP

- 40 seconds will allow approximately 75 percent recovery of ATP/CP

- 60 seconds will allow approximately 85-90 percent recovery of ATP/CP

- Three minutes will allow approximately 100 percent recovery of ATP/CP

The rest interval between sets determines to what extent the energy resources are replenished prior to the next set.[13,14,48] The shorter the rest interval, the less ATP-CP will be replenished and consequently less energy will be available for the next set.[11] In the beginner client, this can result in fatigue, which can lead to decreased neuromuscular control, force production and stabilization by decreasing motor unit recruitment.[53,54] Therefore, inadequate rest intervals can decrease performance and could lead to excessive compensation and even injury. As the client advances, this can be used as a means to increase the intensity of the workout and promote better adaptations especially for stability, endurance and hypertrophy.

Conversely, if rest periods are too long between sets or exercises, the potential effects include decreased neuromuscular activity and decreased body temperature. If the beginner client is then asked to perform an intense bout of exercise, this could entail a potential increased risk of injury. For the advanced client, this may be necessary if heavy weight is being used repetitively. The goal of the training program should establish the appropriate rest periods.[11,14,15] There are several factors to consider when prescribing appropriate rest intervals (Figure 13-3).[11,13,15]

- **Training experience**
- **Training intensity**
- **Tolerance of short rest periods**
- **Muscle mass**
- **General fitness level**
- **Training goals**
- **Nutritional status**
- **Recoverability**

Figure 13-3: Factors for Appropriate Rest Intervals

Individuals who are beginning an integrated training program may respond better to longer rest periods (60-90 seconds) until they adjust to the demands of their program. This also helps to ensure proper neuromuscular efficiency. By decreasing the amount of fatigue experienced by the client, that individual will be able to recruit the appropriate motor units and perform each exercise with greater precision. Individuals who are at advanced levels of training, have larger muscle mass and/or higher fitness levels, may respond better to shorter rest periods, but it is still dependent on the phase of training and the goal.

Training Volume

Training volume is the total amount of work performed within a specified time period.[13,16-17,23,34] It is extremely important to plan and control training volume to prevent over-training, as all training is cumulative.[20-22] Training volume varies among individuals and is based on:

- Training phase
- Goals
- Age
- Work capacity
- Recoverability
- Nutritional status
- Injury history

For an individual to achieve optimum results from an integrated training program, the program must provide them with the appropriate planned training volume over extended periods of time (Table 13-8).[22]

Table 13-8: Volume Continuum	
Training Adaptation	**Total Volume of Reps per Exercise (Sets x Repetitions)**
Power	6-30
Strength	8-36
Stabilization	36-75

One of the most important training concepts to remember is that volume is always inversely related to intensity. In other words, you cannot safely perform high volumes of high intensity exercises for any extended length of time.[13,14,24,25] For example, when working with loads exceeding 90 percent of an individual's maximum, one rarely exceeds a workout volume of 20 repetitions (four sets of three to five repetitions) per exercise. However, when working with loads of 60 percent of maximum, the trainee can easily perform a workout volume of 36-60 repetitions per exercise (three sets of 12-20 repetitions). The exception here is the beginning client who may only perform 12-25 total repetitions per exercise (one set of each exercise).

The training phase and the training goal dictate the repetitions, sets, intensity, rest, tempo and these, combined, dictate the volume.[11,13-17,22,23] Research demonstrates that higher volume training (three to four sets of nine to 20 repetitions) produces cellular adaptations (Table 13-9).[55-60] Conversely, high intensity training with low training volumes (four to six sets of one to five repetitions) produces greater neurological adaptations (Table 13-9).[11,13,15-17,33]

Table 13-9: Training Volume Adaptations	
High Volume (Low Intensity)	**Low Volume (High Intensity)**
Increased muscle cross-sectional area	Increased neuromuscular efficiency
Improved blood lipid serum profile	Increased rate of force production
Improved lean body mass	Increased motor unit recruitment
Decreased body fat	Increased rate coding
Increased metabolic rate	Increased motor unit synchronization

Training Frequency

TRAINING FREQUENCY: The number of training sessions performed over a specified time period (usually one week).

Training frequency refers to the number of training sessions that are performed over a given time period (usually one week). There is considerable debate concerning the adequate number of training sessions per body part, per week necessary for optimum results.[13,14,17,23] The number of training sessions per week, per body part is determined by many factors including training goals, age, general health, work capacity, nutritional status, recoverability, lifestyle and other stressors.[16,17]

For example, a first time client may begin by training his/her entire body two times a week.[11,13,14,61] However, an experienced bodybuilder with the specific goal of hypertrophy may have a training cycle where he/she trains with a split routine of six sessions per week, training each body part two times per week with a larger volume per session.

The specific training goal dictates the program design. Research on training frequency indicates that the optimum training frequency for improvements in strength is three to five times per week. There is no significant difference noted between three days and five days.[11,13,16,17,61,62] Other research indicates that training at least one to two times per week is sufficient to maintain the physical, physiological and performance improvements that were achieved during other phases of training.[11,13,16,17,61]

Training Duration

TRAINING DURATION: The timeframe of a workout (including warm-up and cool-down) or the length of time spent in one phase of training.

Training duration has two prominent meanings:
1. The timeframe from the start of the workout to the end of the workout, including the warm-up or cool-down
2. The length of time (number of weeks) spent in one phase (or period) of training.

The training duration for a workout is a function of the number of repetitions, number of sets, number of exercises and the length of the rest intervals (Table 13-10).

Table 13-10: Durations for a General Fitness Program	
Sets	3
Reps	12
Tempo	4/2/1
Rest Interval	30 sec. between sets
Number of Exercises	7
TOTAL DURATION	**25-40 min. of workout (excluding warm-up and cool-down)**

Training programs that exceed 60-90 minutes (excluding warm-up/cool-down) are associated with rapidly declining energy levels.[11,19,23,63,64] This causes alterations in hormonal and immune system responses that can have a negative effect on a training program.[19,48,63,64]

The training duration for a phase of training is dictated by the client's level of physical ability, goal and compliance to the program. Typically, a phase of training will last between four and eight weeks as this is the amount of time it generally takes for the body to adapt to a given stimulus.[65-75]

Exercise Selection

Exercise selection is the process of choosing exercises for program design that allow for the optimal achievement of the desired adaptation. It has a tremendous impact on the outcome of the training program.[13,16,17,23,34,48]

The kinetic chain is a highly adaptable organism and readily adjusts to the imposed demands of training (Principle of Specificity). Therefore, exercises should be specific to the training goals and based on the principles of the Exercise Selection Continuum (Table 13-11).[13,16,17,23,34,48]

In the OPT™ model, exercises from all components (core, balance, reactive and resistance training) are categorized by the adaptation for which they are primarily used. For example, exercises that are used in Phases 1 and 2 (stabilization) of the OPT™ model are termed *stabilization level* exercises because they are used and progressed for the stabilization adaptation. Similarly, the

EXERCISE SELECTION:
The process of choosing appropriate exercises for a client's program.

Table 13-11: The Exercise Selection Continuum		
Training Adaptation	**Training Level**	**Exercise Selection**
Power	Power Level	Total-body; Multi-joint (explosive)
Strength	Strength Level	Total-body; Multi-/single-joint
Stabilization	Stabilization Level	Total-body; Multi-/single-joint; Controlled Unstable

exercises used in Phases 3-5 are termed *strength level* exercises and exercises used in Phases 6 and 7 are termed *power level* exercises (Table 13-11).

Exercises can be broken down simplistically into three different types based upon the number of joints used, movements performed and adaptation desired (Table 13-12)[48]

Table 13-12: Exercise Selection Examples			
Level	**Total Body**	**Multi-joint**	**Single-joint**
Power	Squat Jump	Two-arm Medicine Ball Chest Pass Medicine Ball Pullover Medicine Ball Oblique Throw Leg Circuit	N/A
Strength	Squat to Two-arm Dumbbell Press	Bench Press Seated Row Machine Standing Two-arm Dumbbell Press Squat	Standing Two-arm Dumbbell Curl
Stabilization	Step-up, Balance to Overhead Press	Ball Dumbbell Chest Press Ball Dumbbell Row Standing Scaption Step-up	Single-leg Dumbbell Curl

1. Total-body: These exercises include multiple joint movements such as a squat, bicep curl to a shoulder press (squat, curl and press).

2. Multi-joint: These exercises utilize the involvement of two or three joints.

3. Single-joint: These exercises focus on isolating one major muscle group or joint.

The OPT™ model enables the health and fitness professional to effectively select the appropriate exercise for each client. Completing a fitness assessment and reviewing the specific training goals will allow the health and fitness professional to implement these exercises into a properly planned integrated training program.

For example, to develop optimum stability, traditional exercises can be *progressed* to a more unstable environment, such as standing up (two-leg, staggered-stance, single-leg) or from a stable bench to an unstable surface (stability ball). Research has shown that exercises performed in unstable environments produce superior results for the goal of stabilization and training the core stabilizing muscles.[65,66,67] Stabilization exercise examples include:

- Ball Crunch
- Ball Cobra

- Chest Press (stability ball or standing using a cable)
- Row (stability ball or standing using a cable)
- Shoulder Press or Lateral Raise (stability ball or standing)
- Step-up to Balance

To develop optimum strength, the use of total-body and multi-joint exercises has been shown most beneficial.[10,17] Strength exercise examples include:

- Russian Deadlift
- Bench Press (barbell or dumbbell)
- Row (machine or free weight; seated or bent over)
- Shoulder Press (barbell or dumbbell, seated or standing)
- Squat

To develop optimum power, explosive medicine ball and body weight exercises can be performed during functional movement patterns.[13,16,17,23,34,48] Power exercise examples include:

- Overhead Medicine Ball Throw
- Medicine Ball Chest Pass
- Medicine Ball Soccer Throw
- Squat Jump
- Tuck Jump
- Box Jump

All exercises, once selected, can be progressed or regressed in a systematic fashion, by following the Progression Continuum (Table 13-13).

Table 13-13: The Progression Continuum		
Stabilization Continuum	**Lower Body**	**Upper Body**
Floor	Two-leg	Two-arm
	Staggered-stance	Alternating-arm
Sport beam	Single-leg	Single-arm
Reebok Core Board **Half Foam Roll** **Airex Pad** **BOSU** **Dyna Disc**	Single/Two-leg Unstable	Single-arm with Trunk Rotation

MODULE 13-2 Summary

Designing the appropriate program for a client is the primary function of the health and fitness professional. Programs should be individualized to meet the needs and goals of each client. Therefore, it is important that a scientifically based, systematic and progressive model is used. The OPT™ model provides the health and fitness professional with all the necessary tools to properly utilize acute variables (repetitions, sets, etc.), scientific concepts and exercises to design programs.

Acute variables determine the amount of stress placed upon the body and, ultimately, what adaptation the body will incur. The acute variables to consider when designing a program are as follows:

- **Repetitions:** The more intense the exercise, the fewer the number of repetitions that the individual should perform.
- **Sets:** The individual usually performs fewer sets when performing higher repetitions at a lower intensity (endurance and hypertrophy adaptations) and more sets when performing lower repetitions at a higher intensity (strength and power adaptations). 24-36 total sets should be performed in a given workout.
- **Training intensity:** Should be determined after sets and reps. Altering other variables (such as environment stability, rest periods and tempo) changes the training intensity.
- **Repetition tempo:** Different times under tension yield specific results. By emphasizing eccentric and isometric muscle actions at slower velocities, more demand is placed upon the connective tissue.
- **Rest interval:** Has a dramatic effect on the outcome of the training program. By adjusting the rest interval, energy supplies can be regained according to the goal of the training program. The shorter the rest interval, the less ATP-CP will be replenished and consequently less energy will be available for the next set. In order to avoid making rests too long or short, consider the following factors: training experience, training intensity, tolerance to short rest periods, muscle mass, general fitness level, training goals, nutritional status and recoverability.
- **Training volume:** Plan and control training volume to prevent over-training. Volume is always inversely related to intensity.
- **Training frequency:** Optimum training frequency for improvements in strength is three to five times per week. Training at least one to two times per week is sufficient to maintain improvements achieved during other phases of training.

■ **Training duration:** Programs should not exceed 90 minutes. Typically, a phase of training will last between four and eight weeks.

■ **Exercise selection:** Exercises should be specific to the training goals and based on the principles of the Exercise Selection Continuum.

MODULE 13-2 Quiz

1. Beginning clients should perform lower repetition schemes.

   ☐ True   ☐ False

2. In order to prevent over-training, what is the range of total sets that should be performed in a given workout?

   _____

3. How long does it take for the body to replenish 100 percent of its ATP and creatine phosphate (CP) supplies?

   _____

4. Training volume is always inversely related to intensity.

   ☐ True   ☐ False

5. Determine whether the following exercises are primarily stabilization, strength or power exercises.

   Russian Deadlift:_____

   Squat Jump:_____

   Chest Press on a Stability Ball:_____

   Bench Press:_____

   Step-up:_____

   Squat:_____

MODULE 13-3:
Periodization and the OPT™ Model (Planned Fitness Training)

Understanding the need for program design and the purpose of acute variable manipulation is important fundamental information for all health and fitness professionals. Applying this knowledge will determine the success of a health and fitness professional. A system is required to properly organize this base level of information.

The science behind the OPT™ model of program design lies in the concept of periodization. As discussed in Chapter 11 (Resistance Training), periodization is a systematic approach to program design that uses the General Adaptation Syndrome and Principle of Specificity to vary the amount and type of stress placed on the body to produce adaptation and prevent injury. Periodization (or planned fitness training) varies the focus of a training program at regularly planned periods of time (weeks, months, etc.) to produce optimal adaptation. It involves two primary objectives:

1. Dividing the training program into distinct periods (or phases) of training

2. Training different forms of strength in each period (or phase) to control the volume of training and to prevent injury.[11-14,76,77]

Training Plans

To accomplish these objectives, a client's training program should be organized into a training plan that involves long-term and short-term planning. A **training plan** is a specific plan that a health and fitness professional uses to meet the client's goal. It will determine the forms of training to be used, how long it will take, how often it will change and what specific exercises will be performed. The long-term plan of a training plan in the OPT™ model is known as an *annual* plan while the short-term plans are termed *monthly* and *weekly* plans. By providing a training plan, the client will be able to see the future achievement of his/her goal, in a timely, organized fashion.

An **annual plan** organizes the training program over a one-year period (Figure 13-4). The annual plan allows the health and fitness professional to provide the client with a blueprint (or map) that specifically shows how the OPT™ training program will progress over the long term, from month-to-month, to meet the desired goal. This gives the client a clear representation of how the health and fitness professional plans to get the client to his/her goal and how long it will take to get there.

TRAINING PLAN:
The specific outline, created by a Fitness Professional to meet a client's goals, that details the form of training, length of time, future changes and specific exercises to be performed.

ANNUAL PLAN:
Generalized training plan that spans one year to show when the client will progress between phases.

		JAN	FEB	MAR	APR	MAY	JUN	JUL	AUG	SEP	OCT	NOV	DEC
Stabiliz-ation	CET												
	IST												
Strength	SET												
	MDT												
	MST												
Power	EET												
	MPT												
Cardio													

Figure 13-4: Annual Plan

In Figure 13-4, the column on the far left represents the period or main strength adaptation. The second column shows the specific phases of the OPT™ model that make up each specific adaptation of training.

Each month within the annual plan is further broken down into periods of training called monthly plans (Figure 13-5). The **monthly plan** details the specific days of each workout, showing the client exactly what phase of the OPT™ model (type of training) will be required each day of the week as well as when the reassessment will occur. The monthly plan also shows the client the necessary cardiorespiratory and flexibility requirements.

MONTHLY PLAN: Generalized training plan that spans one month and shows which phases will be required each day of each week.

Week		1							2							3							4						
Day	M	T	W	T	F	S	S	M	T	W	T	F	S	S	M	T	W	T	F	S	S	M	T	W	T	F	S	S
CET																												
IST																												
SET																												
MDT																												
MST																												
EET																												
MPT																												
Cardio																												
Flexibility																												
KCA																												

Figure 13-5: Monthly Plan

Each monthly plan is then simplified into **weekly plans** which are the specific workouts that the client will do for that week. The weekly plan gives the client a picture of exactly what exercises will be used in his/her workout for that period of time. The weekly plan is the OPT™ workout that the client will follow for that day or week. It is divided into the components of cardiorespiratory, flexibility, core, balance, reactive, speed-agility-quickness and resistance training with areas for the specific acute variables. This allows the health and fitness professional to properly track each client's workout routine, noting progress and any pertinent comments.

WEEKLY PLAN: Training plan of specific workouts that spans one week, to show which exercises are required each day of the week.

Much of the literature regarding periodization refers to dividing the training program into specific cycles termed macro-, meso- and microcycles (Figure 13-6). For ease of understanding, a *macrocycle* is the largest cycle and typically, covers a year-long period of training (or annual plan). The macrocycle is divided into *mesocycles*, which are typically one to three months in length (or monthly plans). Each mesocycle in turn is divided into *microcycles*, which are usually a week in length (or weekly plans).[49,78]

Annual Plan   =   Macrocycle
Monthly Plan   =   Mesocycle
Weekly Plan   =   Microcycle

Figure 13-6: Periodization Cycles

Periodization has been shown to be an effective form of program design for many fitness-related goals and yet, to date, it is not a common practice among fitness professionals.[49,79,80,81] It provides for the repeated use of different forms of training at specific times in an annual training program to elicit different adaptations in the body (stabilization, strength and power). By intentionally cycling through different periods (or phases) of training, the acute variables are manipulated to adjust the volume of training. By controlling the volume of training over time in any given program, periodization allows for maximal levels of adaptation, while minimizing over-training. This is a primary benefit of periodization, because over-training will lead to fatigue and eventual injury.[49,76,79,80]

MODULE 13-3 Summary

Planned fitness training (or periodization) shifts the focus of a training program at regularly planned intervals of time to vary stress placed on the body in order to produce adaptation and prevent injury.

A training plan clarifies what forms of training will be used, how long it will take, how often it will change and what specific exercises will be performed. An annual plan organizes the training program over a one year period to show when the client is in which phase. The annual plan is further broken down into periods of training called monthly plans, which detail the specific days of each workout, showing the client exactly what type of training will be required each day of the month. Weekly plans are the specific workouts and exercises that the client will do for that week.

MODULE 13-3 Quiz

1. Which type of plan shows cardio and flexibility requirements as well as when re-assessments will occur?

    ☐ Weekly plan

    ☐ Monthly plan

    ☐ Annual plan

2. The two primary objectives of periodization is dividing the training program into distinct periods (or phases) of training, and training different forms of strength in each period (or phase) to control the volume of training and to prevent injury.

    ☐ True   ☐ False

3. In periodization, cycling through different phases of training, the acute variables are manipulated to adjust the _____ of training?

MODULE 13-4: The OPT™ Model

The different periods (or phases) of training seen in a traditional periodization model include a preparatory period (termed *anatomical adaptation*), a hypertrophy period, a maximum strength period and a power period.

In the OPT™ model, these are simplified into stabilization (anatomical adaptation), strength (hypertrophy and maximum strength) and power. The OPT™ model seen in a phase-specific model of training includes seven different phases of training. These phases systematically progress all clients through the three main adaptations of stabilization, strength and power (Figure 13-1).

Think of the OPT™ model as a staircase, guiding a client to different adaptations. This journey will involve going up and down the stairs, stopping at different steps and moving to various heights, depending on the client's goals, needs and abilities. This module will detail the various phases of training in the OPT™ model.

Stabilization

The first level of training in the OPT™ model focuses on the main adaptation of stabilization (or anatomical adaptation) and is designed to prepare the body for the demands of higher levels of training that may follow. This period is crucial for all beginners. It is also necessary to cycle back through after periods of strength and power training in order to maintain a high degree of core and joint stability. In addition, it allows the body to rest from more intense bouts of training. The focus of stabilization training includes:[76,78]

- Correcting muscle imbalances
- Improving stabilization of the core musculature
- Preventing tissue overload by preparing muscles, tendons, ligament and joints for the upcoming imposed demands of training
- Improving overall cardiorespiratory and neuromuscular condition
- Establishing proper movement patterns or exercise technique

The above goals are accomplished through low intensity, high repetition training programs, emphasizing core and joint stabilization (as opposed to increasing the strength of the arms and legs). This will incorporate exercises that progressively challenge the body's stability requirements (or proprioception), as opposed to how much weight is being used.[76,78]

Therefore, the primary means of progressing (or increasing the intensity of training) in this period is by increasing the proprioceptive demands of the exercises. This form of training has been shown to be extremely effective for increasing neuromuscular efficiency in the healthy,[82] elderly[83] and unhealthy populations.[84-87] Another important component of stabilization training is that it may help to ensure activity-specific strength adaptations (such as standing on one leg to kick a ball, climbing up stairs or simply walking).[88]

The stabilization period of training in the OPT™ model consists of two phases: Phase 1: Corrective Exercise Training and Phase 2: Integrated Stabilization Training (Figure 13-1).

Corrective Exercise Training (Phase 1)

Corrective Exercise Training is the first step of the OPT™ model and should be utilized for first-time clients (with none or little training background), clients who display prominent muscle imbalances, elderly clients, clients with joint discomfort or those coming from the care of a medical professional. It is also beneficial to cycle back through this phase of training after prolonged periods of high-intensity training, or following extended periods of no training. This phase of training focuses on increasing core stability and endurance strength of all major muscles.

Table 13-14: Phase 1: Corrective Exercise Training Acute Variables Corrective Exercise Training								
	Reps	Sets	Tempo	% Intensity	Rest Interval	Frequency	Duration	Exercise Selection
Flexibility	1	1-2	30 sec. hold	n/a	n/a	3-7x/week	1-6 weeks	SMR and static
Core	10-15	1-3	3-10 sec.	n/a	0-90 sec.	1-5x/week	1-6 weeks	1-3 5-10 sec. hold
Balance	10-15	1-3	3-10 sec.	n/a	0-90 sec.	1-5x/week	1-6 weeks	1-2 stabilization
Reactive	3-5	0-2	3-5 sec. hold	n/a	0-90 sec.	1-5x/week	1-6 weeks	0-1 stabilization
Resistance	15-25	1-3	4-2-2	40-60%	0-90 sec.	1-5x/week	1-6 weeks	0-2 stabilization progression
Comments:	Total of 7-10 exercises in each workout							

The low-intensity, high-repetition scheme used in this phase of training is designed to optimize the amount of continuous blood flow in the muscles during exercise. When intensities become too high during resistance training, muscle contractions are extreme enough to restrict blood flow.[89] This decreases the amount of oxygen that can be transported to the muscle and tissues by the blood during concentric contraction. Clients who have evident muscle imbalances already have decreased blood flow to those tissues. Thus, the use of heavier intensities may not be the most beneficial application. By using intensities of 50 percent or less of a maximal effort as well as emphasizing eccentric and isometric muscle actions, muscle contractions will not be extreme enough to restrict blood flow during the workout. This will increase oxygen delivery to tissues and promote better recovery.[90]

Acute variables can be slowly progressed, if the client is deconditioned and has minimal training background (Table 13-15). The health and fitness professional should slowly increase the number of repetitions with these clients in order to establish the necessary levels of endurance in stabilizing muscles. However, the intensity will remain low in order to promote better blood flow to the muscles.

A client in this category will generally stay in this phase of training for four to six weeks. This will prepare the client for the demands of Phase 2. This progression can be beneficial for any client, but especially for the elderly and those with the goal of body fat reduction and/or general fitness.

Table 13-15: Phase 1: Corrective Exercise Training Progressions for Beginning or Deconditioned Clients

Weekly Progression		Week 1	Week 2	Week 3	Week 4
Core	Sets	1	2	2	3
	Reps	10	10	12	15
Balance	Sets	1	2	2	3
	Reps	10	10	12	15
Reactive	Sets	0	0	0	0
	Reps	0	0	0	0
Strength	Sets	1	2	2	3
	Reps	15	15	20	25
	Intensity	40-50%	40-50%	40-50%	40-50%

If a client is fairly conditioned and has good level of training background, acute variables can be progressed differently. The health and fitness professional should slowly increase the intensity level and decrease the repetitions in order to establish the necessary levels of endurance and strength in stabilizing muscles.

This progression is beneficial for clients with the goal of increasing lean body mass and general performance. A client in this category will generally stay in this phase of training for a four-week duration.

Table 13-16:	Phase 1: Corrective Exercise Training Progressions for Clients that are Fairly Conditioned with Good Training Background				

Weekly Progression		Week 1	Week 2	Week 3	Week 4
Core	Sets	1	2	3	3
	Reps	15	12	10	10
Balance	Sets	1	2	3	3
	Reps	15	12	10	10
Reactive	Sets	1	1	2	2
	Reps	5	5	5	5
Strength	Sets	1	2	3	3
	Reps	25	20	20	15
	Intensity	40%	50%	50%	60%

Integrated Stabilization Training (Phase 2)

Integrated Stabilization Training should be used for the beginning client who has some prior training history and exhibits good postural control with minimal muscle imbalances (Table 13-17). It will also be important to cycle back through this phase of training between periods of higher intensity training seen in Phases 3 through 7. This will allow for proper recovery and maintenance of high levels of stability that will ensure optimal strength and/or power adaptations. This phase of training focuses on:

- Increasing stability
- Endurance strength
- Increasing neuromuscular efficiency of the core musculature
- Improving inter- and intramuscular coordination.

The higher intensity and volume of this phase (in comparison to Phase 1) also allows for the promotion of strength and hypertrophy at a lower level. However, the primary focus is on increasing the proprioception of the exercises, rather than just the load.

Acute variables can be progressed if the client is starting in the Integrated Stabilization Training phase, with minimal to no training background and is also fairly conditioned, with no major muscle imbalances (Table 13-18). The health and fitness professional will want to increase repetitions and challenge proprioception to establish the necessary levels of endurance in core muscles. The intensity of the weight will remain low, to allow the client to focus on proprioception.

Table 13-17: Phase 2: Integrated Stabilization Training (IST) Acute Variables

Integrated Stabilization Training								
	Reps	Sets	Tempo	% Intensity	Rest Interval	Frequency	Duration	Exercise Selection
Flexibility	1	1-2	30 sec. hold	n/a	n/a	2-4x/week		SMR and static
Core	12-20	1-3	5-10 sec. hold	n/a	0-90 sec.	2-4x/week	4-6 weeks	1-4 stabilization level
Balance	12-20	1-3	5-10 sec. hold	n/a	0-90 sec.	2-4x/week	4-6 weeks	1-4 stabilization level
Reactive	5-8	1-30	3-5 sec. hold	n/a	0-90 sec.	2-4x/week	4-6 weeks	0-2 stabilization level
Resistance	12-20	1-3	4-2-1	60-70%	0-90 sec.	2-4x/week	4-6 weeks	1-2 stabilization progression
Comments:	Total of 7-10 exercises in each workout							

A client in this category will generally stay in this phase of training for a four-week duration. This will prepare the client for the demands of the Stabilization Equivalent Training phase. This progression is beneficial for any client, but especially for those with the goal of body fat reduction and/or general fitness.

Table 13-18: Phase 2: Integrated Stabilization Training Progressions for Beginning Clients with No Major Muscle Imbalances

Weekly Progression		Week 1	Week 2	Week 3	Week 4
Core	Sets	1	2	2	3
	Reps	12	15	20	20
Balance	Sets	1	2	2	3
	Reps	12	15	20	20
Reactive	Sets	1	2	2	2
	Reps	5	5	6	8
Strength	Sets	1	2	2	3
	Reps	12	15	20	20
	Intensity	60%	60%	60%	60%

Acute variables can also be progressed if the client is fairly conditioned and has good level of training background (Table 13-19). The health and fitness professional should slowly progress by increasing intensity and decreasing the repetitions, to establish the necessary levels of endurance and strength in stabilizing muscles.

Table 13-19: Phase 2: Integrated Stabilization Training Progressions for Clients that are Fairly Conditioned with Good Training Background

Weekly Progression		Week 1	Week 2	Week 3	Week 4
Core	Sets	1	2	3	3
	Reps	20	20	15	15
Balance	Sets	1	2	3	3
	Reps	20	20	15	15
Reactive	Sets	1	2	3	3
	Reps	6	6	6	8
Strength	Sets	1-2	2	3	3
	Reps	20	15	15	12
	Intensity	60%	65%	65%	70%

This progression is beneficial for the client who has the goal of increasing lean body mass and general performance. A client in this category will generally stay in this phase of training for a four-week duration.

Strength

The second level of training in the OPT™ model focuses on the main adaptation of strength, which includes hypertrophy and maximal strength. It is designed to increase the amount of stress placed upon the body for increased muscle size and strength. This period of training is a necessary progression from stabilization for anyone who desires to increase caloric expenditure, muscle size, muscle strength and bone mineral density. The focus of the strength period of training is to:

■ Increase the ability of the core musculature to stabilize the pelvis and spine under heavier loads, through more complete ranges of motion

■ Increase the load bearing capabilities of muscles, tendons, ligaments and joints

■ Increase the volume of training with more reps, sets and intensity

■ Increase metabolic demand by taxing the ATP/CP and glycolosis energy systems to induce cellular changes in muscle (weight loss and/or hypertrophy)

■ Increase motor unit recruitment, frequency of motor unit recruitment and motor unit synchronization (maximal strength)

The strength period of training in the OPT™ model consists of three phases: Phase 3: Stabilization Equivalent Training, Phase 4: Muscular Development Training and Phase 5: Maximal Strength Training (Figure 13-1).

Stabilization Equivalent Training (Phase 3)

Stabilization Equivalent Training is a hybrid form of training that promotes increased stabilization endurance, hypertrophy and strength. This form of training entails the use of superset techniques where a more stable exercise (such as a bench press) is immediately followed with a stabilization exercise with similar biomechanical motions (such as a ball push-up). Thus, for every set of an exercise/body part performed according to the acute variables, there are actually two exercises or two sets being performed. High amounts of volume can be generated in this phase of training.

Table 13-20: Phase 3: Stabilization Equivalent Training Acute Variables

Stabilization Equivalent Training

	Reps	Sets	Tempo	% Intensity	Rest Interval	Frequency	Duration	Exercise Selection
Flexibility	5-10	1-2	2-4 sec. hold	n/a	n/a	3-7x/week	4-6 weeks	SMR and active
Core	8-12	2-4	3-2-1	n/a	0-60	2-4x/week	4-6 weeks	1-3 strength
Balance	8-12	2-4	3-2-1	n/a	0-60	2-4x/week	4-6 weeks	1-3 strength
Reactive	8-12	2-4	Repeating	n/a	0-60	2-4x/week	4-6 weeks	1-3 strength
Resistance	8-12	2-4	(Str) 2-0-2 (Stab) 3-2-1	70-80%	0-60	2-4x/week	4-6 weeks	1 strength superset 1 stabilization
Comments:	Each resistance training exercise is a superset of a strength level exercise immediately followed by a stabilization level exercise							

Acute variables can be progressed if a client with the goal of general fitness and/or body fat reduction has properly progressed through Phases 1 and 2 of the OPT™ model (Table 13-21). Because the goal does not require maximal hypertrophy, sets, repetition and intensity ranges will remain moderate.

Acute variables can also be progressed if a client with the goal of increasing lean body mass and general performance has properly progressed through Phases 1 and 2 of the OPT™ model (Table 13-22). Because the goal for this client is strength and hypertrophy, the health and fitness professional will want to increase intensity and decrease the repetitions to establish the necessary levels of strength. A client in this category will generally stay in this phase of training for a four-week duration.

**Table 13-21: Phase 3: Stabilization Equivalent Training
Progressions for Clients with Goals of Body Fat Reduction or General Fitness**

Weekly Progression		Week 1	Week 2	Week 3	Week 4
Core	Sets	2	2	2	2
	Reps	12	12	12	12
Balance	Sets	2	2	2	2
	Reps	12	12	12	12
Reactive	Sets	2	2	2	2
	Reps	8	8	8	8
Strength	Sets	2	2	2	2
	Reps	12 strength	12 strength	10 strength	10 strength
		12 stabilization	12 stabilization	10 stabilization	10 stabilization
	Intensity	70%	70%	75%	75%

**Table 13-22: Phase 3: Stabilization Equivalent Training
Progressions for Clients with Goals of Increased Lean Body Mass
and/or General Performance**

Weekly Progression		Week 1	Week 2	Week 3	Week 4
Core	Sets	2	2	3	3
	Reps	12	12	10	8
Balance	Sets	2	2	3	3
	Reps	12	12	10	8
Reactive	Sets	2	3	3	3
	Reps	8	8	10	10
Strength	Sets	2	3	3	4
	Reps	12 strength	10 strength	8 strength	8 strength
		12 stabilization	10 stabilization	8 stabilization	8 stabilization
	Intensity	70%	75%	80%	80%

Muscular Development Training (Phase 4)

Muscular Development Training is specific for the adaptation of maximal hypertrophy, focusing on high levels of volume with minimal rest periods to force cellular changes that result in an overall increase in muscle size (Table 13-23).

Table 13-23: Phase 4: Muscular Development Training Acute Variables

Muscular Development Training

	Reps	Sets	Tempo	% Intensity	Rest Interval	Frequency	Duration	Exercise Selection
Flexibility	5-10	1-2	2-4 sec hold	n/a	n/a	3-7x/week	4 weeks	SMR and active
Core	8-12	2-4	2-0-2	n/a	0-60 s.	3-6x/week	4 weeks	0-4 strength
Balance	8-12	2-4	2-0-2	n/a	0-60 s.	3-6x/week	4 weeks	0-4 strength
Reactive	8-12	2-4	Repeating	n/a	0-60 s.	3-6x/week	4 weeks	0-4 strength
Resistance	6-12	3-5	2-0-2	75-85%	0-60 s.	3-6x/week	4 weeks	2-4 strength level exercises/body part
Comments:	Total of 24-36 sets per workout Light day = 20-24 total sets Moderate day = 24-30 total sets Heavy day = 30-36 total sets							

Acute variables can be progressed if a client with the goal of increasing lean body mass and/or general performance has properly progressed through Phases 1, 2 and 3 of the OPT™ model (Table 13-24). Because the goal of this phase of training is primarily hypertrophy, the health and fitness professional will want to increase intensity and volume.

Table 13-24: Phase 4: Muscular Development Training Progressions for Clients with Goals of Increased Lean Body Mass and/or General Performance

Weekly Progression		Week 1	Week 2	Week 3	Week 4
Core	Sets	2	2	3	3
	Reps	12	12	10	8
Balance	Sets	2	2	3	3
	Reps	12	12	10	8
Reactive	Sets	2	3	3	3
	Reps	8	8	10	10
Strength	Sets	3	3	4	5
	Reps	12	10	8	6
	Intensity	75%	80%	80%	85%

A client in this category will generally stay in this phase of training for a four-week duration, before cycling back through Phases 2 or 3, or progressing on to Phases 5 or 6.

Maximal Strength Training (Phase 5)

The Maximal Strength Training Phase focuses on increasing the load placed upon the tissues of the body. Maximal intensity improves:

- Recruitment of more motor units
- Rate of force production
- Motor unit synchronization

Maximal Strength Training has also been shown to help increase the benefits of forms of power training used in Phase 6.[61]

Acute variables can be progressed if the client with the goal of increasing lean body mass and/or general performance has properly progressed through Phases 1, 2, 3 (and possibly Phase 4) (Table 13-26). Because the goal of this phase of training is primarily maximal strength, the health and fitness professional will want to increase load.

Table 13-25: Phase 5: Maximal Strength Training Acute Variables

Maximal Strength Training

	Reps	Sets	Tempo	% Intensity	Rest Interval	Frequency	Duration	Exercise Selection
Flexibility	5-10	1-2	2-4 sec hold	n/a	n/a	3-7x/week	4 weeks	SMR and active
Core	8-12	2-4	1-1-1	n/a	0-60 s.	2-4x/week	4 weeks	0-3 strength
Balance	8-12	2-4	1-1-1	n/a	0-60 s.	2-4x/week	4 weeks	0-3 strength
Reactive	8-10	2-4	Repeating	n/a	0-60 s.	2-4x/week	4 weeks	0-3 strength
Resistance	1-5	4-6	X-X-X	85-100%	3-5 min.	2-4x/week	4 weeks	1-3 strength
Comments								

A client in this category will generally stay in this phase of training for a four-week duration before cycling back through Phases 2 or 3 or progressing on to Phase 6.

Table 13-26: Phase 5: Maximal Strength Training Progressions for Clients with Goals of Increased Lean Body Mass and/or General Performance

Weekly Progression		Week 1	Week 2	Week 3	Week 4
Core	Sets	2	2	3	3
	Reps	12	12	10	8
Balance	Sets	2	2	3	3
	Reps	12	12	10	8
Reactive	Sets	2	3	3	3
	Reps	8	8	10	10
Strength	Sets	4	5	5	6
	Reps	5	5	4	3
	Intensity	85%	85%	89%	93%

Power

The third level of training is power and is designed to increase the rate of force production (or speed of muscle contraction). This form of training uses the adaptations of stabilization and strength acquired in the previous phases of training and applies them with more realistic speeds and forces that the body will encounter in everyday life and/or sport.

Power training is usually not common practice in the fitness environment, but has a very viable and purposeful place in a properly planned training program. Power is simply defined as force multiplied by velocity $(P = F \times V)$.[61] Therefore, any increase in either force and/or velocity will produce an increase in power. This is accomplished by either increasing the load (or force) as in progressive strength training or increasing the speed with which you move a load (or velocity). The combined effect is a better rate of force production in daily activities and sporting events.[61]

To develop optimum levels of power, it has been shown that individuals must train both with heavy loads (85-100 percent) and light loads (30-45 percent) at high speeds.[8,26,27,30,32,65] The focus of power training is to increase the rate of force production by increasing the number of motor units activated, the synchrony between them and the speed at which they are excited.[62,91,92]

The power level of training in the OPT™ model consists of two phases of training: Phase 6: Elastic Equivalent Training and Phase 7: Maximal Power Training (Figure 13-1).

Table 13-27: Phase 6: Elastic Equivalent Training Acute Variables

Elastic Equivalent Training

	Reps	Sets	Tempo	% Intensity	Rest Interval	Frequency	Duration	Exercise Selection
Flexibility	10-15	1-2	Controlled	n/a	n/a	2-4x/week		SMR and static
Core	8-12	2-4	1-0-1	n/a	0-90 sec.	2-4x/week	4-6 weeks	1-4 stabilization
Balance	8-12	2-4	Controlled	n/a	0-90 sec.	2-4x/week	4-6 weeks	1-4 stabilization
Reactive	8-12	2-4	x-x-x	n/a	0-90 sec.	2-4x/week	4-6 weeks	0-2 stabilization
Resistance	1-5(S) 8-10 (P)	3-5	x-x-x (S) x-x-x (P)	85-100% (S) up to 10% BW or 30-45% 1RM (P)	1-2 min. b/w pairs 3-5 min. b/w circuits	2-4x/week	4 weeks	1 strength superset 1 power
Comments:	BW = body weight 1 RM = 1 repetition maximum							

Elastic Equivalent Training (Phase 6)

The Elastic Equivalent Training Phase focuses on both high force and velocity to increase power (Table 13-27). This is accomplished by super-setting a strength exercise with a power exercise for each body part (such as performing a barbell bench press superset with a medicine ball chest pass.)

Don't let the intensities confuse you. The 85-100 percent refers to the intensity for traditional strength training exercises. It increases power by increasing the *force* side of the power equation (force multiplied by velocity).

The 30-45 percent intensity, on the other hand, is used for "speed" exercises such as speed squats where the squats are performed as fast as possible with a low load.[93] The approximately 10 percent intensity is used for medicine ball training that will require the throwing or release of a medicine ball. These last two forms of training affect the *velocity* side of the power equation (force multiplied by velocity).

By using heavy weight with explosive movement and low resistance with a high velocity, you can produce high power outputs.[12,93-96]

Acute variables can be progressed if the client with the goal of increasing general performance has properly progressed through the rest of the OPT™ model (Table 13-28). Because the goal of this phase of training is primarily power, the health and fitness professional will want to progress by increasing load and velocity.

A client in this category will generally stay in this phase of training for a four-week duration, before cycling back through Phases 2 or 3, or progressing on to Phase 7.

Table 13-28: Phase 6: Elastic Equivalent Training Progressions for Clients with Goals of Increased Lean Body Mass and/or General Performance

Weekly Progression		Week 1	Week 2	Week 3	Week 4
Core	Sets	2	2	3	3
	Reps	12	12	10	8
Balance	Sets	2	2	3	3
	Reps	12	12	10	8
Reactive	Sets	2	3	3	3
	Reps	8	8	10	10
Strength	Sets	3	4	4	5
	Reps	5 strength 10 power	4 strength 10 power	4 strength 8 power	3 strength 8 power
	Intensity	Strength 85% Power 2% BW	Strength 89% Power 3% BW	Strength 89% Power 4% BW	Strength 93% Power 4% BW
Comments	BW = body weight 1RM = 1 repetition maximum				

Maximal Power Training (Phase 7)

The Maximal Power Training phase focuses on velocity of movement through a complete range of motion (Table 13-29). Maximal power is developed by training with 30-45 percent of an individual's one repetition maximum (1RM) and/or up to 10 percent of a person's body weight (BW) and accelerating through the entire range of motion.[12,26,65,66]

Traditional training techniques (such as Olympic-style lifting, bench pressing and squatting) are unable to allow maximal acceleration throughout the entire range of motion. It has been demonstrated that approximately half of a traditional lift is deceleration.[48,65] Therefore, the individual performing the exercise is unable to express high velocity throughout the entire range of motion, which prevents optimum power improvements.

Maximal Power Training is a very specialized form of training and should be implemented only for those that require maximum power and who have developed optimum levels of stabilization and eccentric strength, prior to this phase of training.

Acute variables can be progressed if the client with the goal of increasing general performance has properly progressed through rest of the OPT™ model (Table 13-30). Because the goal of this phase of training is power, the health and fitness professional will want to progress by increasing intensity and velocity.

Table 13-29: Phase 7: Maximal Power Training Acute Variables

Maximal Power Training

	Reps	Sets	Tempo	% Intensity	Rest Interval	Frequency	Duration	Exercise Selection
Flexibility	10-15	1-2	Controlled	n/a	n/a	3-7x/week	4-6 weeks	SMR and dynamic 3-5 exercises
Core	8-12	2-4	X-X-X	75-85%	0-90 sec.	1-2x/week	2 weeks	0-2 power
Balance	8-12	2-4	Controlled	75-85%	0-90 sec.	1-2x/week	2 weeks	0-3 power
Reactive	8-12	2-4	X-X-X		0-90 sec.	1-2x/week	2 weeks	0-2 power
Resistance	1-5	4-6	X-X-X	30-45% Max 10% BW	3-5 min.	1-2x/week	2 weeks	Power level
Comments:	4-6 total exercises Include 1 EET and 1 SET workout during each week							

A client in this category will generally stay in this phase of training for a four-week duration, before cycling back through Phases 2 or 3.

Table 13-30: Phase 7: Maximal Power Training Progressions for Clients with Goals of Increased Lean Body Mass and/or General Performance

Weekly Progression

		Week 1	Week 2	Week 3	Week 4
Core	Sets	2	2	3	3
	Reps	12	12	10	8
Balance	Sets	2	2	3	3
	Reps	12	12	10	8
Reactive	Sets	2	3	3	3
	Reps	8	8	10	10
Strength	Sets	3	4	4	5
	Reps	5	5	4	4
	Intensity	30% or 5% of BW	33% or 6% of BW	35% or 7% of BW	38% or 8% of BW
Comments	BW = body weight 1RM = 1 repetition maximum				

MODULE 13-4 Summary

Period of Training (Main Adaptation)	Specific Adaptation	Phases Used	Method of Progression
Stabilization	Endurance Stability	1 and 2	Proprioception
Strength	Strength Endurance Hypertrophy Maximal Strength	3, 4 and 5	Volume/Load
Power	Power	6 and 7	Speed

Figure 13-7: Summary of the OPT™ System

The different levels of training seen in a traditional periodization model include anatomical adaptation, hypertrophy, maximum strength and power. In the OPT™ model, these are simplified into stabilization, strength and power. These are further broken down into seven different phases of training.

The first level, stabilization, is crucial for all beginners as it is designed to prepare the body for the demands of higher levels of training. For advanced clients, this level allows for rest from more intense bouts of training. It involves low intensity, high repetition training, emphasizing core and joint stabilization (as opposed to increasing the strength of the arms and legs). Exercises progressively challenge proprioception.

The stabilization level of consists of two Phases: Phase 1: Corrective Exercise Training and Phase 2: Integrated Stabilization Training. Corrective Exercise Training focuses on increasing core stability and endurance strength of all major muscles. It also optimizes the amount of continuous blood flow in the muscles during exercise to reduce tissue adhesions. The phase usually lasts for four weeks. Integrated Stabilization Training should be used for the beginning client who has some prior training history and exhibits good postural control with minimal muscle imbalances. It focuses on increasing stability, endurance strength and integrating the core into all of the exercises. The phase usually lasts for four weeks.

The second level, strength, is designed to increase muscle size and strength. The strength period of training in the OPT™ model consists of three phases: Phase 3: Stabilization Equivalent Training, Phase 4: Muscular Development Training and Phase 5: Maximal Strength Training. Stabilization Equivalent Training uses superset techniques with high volume, for about four weeks. Muscular Development Training stresses maximal hypertrophy, focusing on high levels of volume with minimal rest periods, for about four weeks. Maximal Strength Training focuses on increasing the load placed upon the tissues of the body, for about four weeks.

The third period of training, power, is designed to increase the rate of force production. To develop optimum levels of power, it has been shown that individuals must train both with heavy and light loads at high speeds. The power period consists of two phases of training: Phase 6: Elastic Equivalent Training and Phase 7: Maximal Power Training. Elastic Equivalent Training focuses on both high force and velocity to increase power and lasts about four weeks. Maximal Power Training should be implemented only for those that require maximum power and who have developed optimum levels of stabilization and eccentric strength, prior to this phase of training. It focuses on velocity of movement through a complete range of motion and lasts about four weeks.

MODULE 13-4 Quiz

1. How many different periods and phases are there in the OPT™ model?
   _____ levels and _____ phases?

2. Phase 1: Corrective Exercise Training uses ☐ **low**   ☐ **high** intensity and ☐ **low**   ☐ **high** repetitions to optimize the amount of continuous blood flow in the muscles during exercise.

3. Which phase(s) of training use(s) superset techniques?

   _____

   _____

4. Power is defined as force multiplied by _____.

MODULE 13-5:
Applying the OPT™ Model

The concepts of program design, periodization and the OPT™ model have all been described. Program design was defined as creating a purposeful system or plan to achieve a goal. Periodization is the scientific basis that allows health and fitness professionals to strategically plan, design programs and achieve goals, without the risk of placing improper stresses on the body.

The OPT™ model is a proven, easy-to-use system of periodization that can be used to create programs for clients with various goals. While the understanding of these concepts is paramount, what matters the most is the ability to apply the information in multiple situations, to a variety of clients. This module will demonstrate how to specifically apply the OPT™ model to goals. These include body fat reduction, increase in lean body mass and general performance.

Applying the Model for the Goal of Body Fat Reduction

The goal of reducing body fat requires clients to follow the simple principle of burning more calories than they consume (see Chapter 15 — Nutrition). The best way to increase the calories burned is to move more. Weight training provides an extremely potent means to burn calories, when it is combined with cardiorespiratory training. It also provides the added benefit of increased muscle strength.[97-100]

The following program is a general representation of how the OPT™ model is used for clients with the goal of body fat reduction. Figure 13-8 shows the annual plan. Because the goal is not for hypertrophy or to gain maximal strength and power, the client only needs to be cycled through the first three

		JAN	FEB	MAR	APR	MAY	JUN	JUL	AUG	SEP	OCT	NOV	DEC
Stabiliz- ation	CET	X											
	IST		X		X		X		X		X		X
Strength	SET			X		X		X		X		X	
	MDT												
	MST												
Power	EET												
	MPT												
Cardio		X	X	X	X	X	X	X	X	X	X	X	X

Figure 13-8: Annual Plan for the Goal of Body Fat Reduction

phases of the OPT™ model. The client will start in January in Phase 1, to ensure proper muscle balance and endurance of the stabilization muscles. He/she will remain there for approximately four weeks before moving onto Phases 2 and 3. It will not necessary for the client to return to Phase 1 unless an extended amount of time is taken off (30-60 days), such as a long vacation during the summer or holiday seasons.

The remainder of the annual plan shows the client cycling back and forth between phases 2 and 3 (Figure 13-8). Phase 3 will promote times of greater metabolic demand and more volume for increased caloric expenditure. Phase 2 will allow the client proper recovery time before entering back into Phase 3. Cardiorespiratory training can be performed each month. During Phases 1 and 2, the client may be inclined to do more cardiorespiratory work (in conjunction with weight training) to sustain good caloric expenditure, without the higher intensity of weight training seen in Phase 3. This will also provide proper periodization of the client's cardiorespiratory training.

Figure 13-9 illustrates the monthly plan for January. This plan demonstrates a three-day-per-week workout plan, with scheduled workouts on Mondays, Wednesdays and Fridays. This monthly plan can easily be performed twice a week. The client can perform flexibility exercises every day of the week, if desired. Cardio can be done on the workout days (or any other day during the week, depending on the client's schedule).

Week	1							2							3							4						
Day	M	T	W	T	F	S	S	M	T	W	T	F	S	S	M	T	W	T	F	S	S	M	T	W	T	F	S	S
CET	X		X		X			X		X		X			X		X		X			X		X		X		
IST																												
SET																												
MDT																												
MST																												
EET																												
MPT																												
Cardio	X		X		X			X		X		X			X		X		X			X		X		X		
Flexibility	X	X	X	X	X	X	X	X	X	X	X	X	X	X	X	X	X	X	X	X	X	X	X	X	X	X	X	X
KCA																												

Figure 13-9:   **Monthly Plan for the Goal of Body Fat Reduction
January - Phase 1: Corrective Exercise Training**

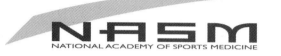

Optimum Performance Training™

NATIONAL ACADEMY OF SPORTS MEDICINE

NAME:	JOHN SMITH	DATE:	February 10, 2004
TRAINER:	CHERE	PHASE:	1: Corrective Exercise Training
DAYS/WEEK:		GOAL:	Fat Loss

CARDIO TRAINING: Stage 1	TIME: 20 min	EQUIPMENT: Elliptical Trainer

WARMUP/FLEXIBILITY	Sets	Reps	Duration	Rest	Notes
1. SMR: Calves, IT band, adductors	1				Hold tender spots 20-30 secs
2. Cardio: Elliptical trainer			5 min.		
3. Static Stretching: Calves, hip flexors, lats	1		30 sec.		

CORE & BALANCE	Sets	Reps	Tempo	Rest	Notes
1. Marching	2	12	3-10 sec hold	0	Circuit training
2. Two-leg Floor bridge	2	12	3-10 sec hold	0	
3. Single-leg Balance	1-3	6-10/leg	5-10 sec hold	90 sec.	

REACTIVE	Sets	Reps	Tempo	Rest	Notes
1. N/A					
2.					

SPEED, AGILITY, QUICKNESS	Sets	Reps	Time	Rest	Notes
1. N/A					
2.					

STRENGTH	Exercise	Sets	Reps	Intensity	Tempo	Rest	Notes
TOTAL BODY	Optional						
CHEST	Standing Cable Chest Press	2	20	50%	4-2-2	0	
BACK	Standing Cable Row	2	20	50%	4-2-2	0	
SHOULDERS	Standing Dumbbell Shoulder Press	2	20	50%	4-2-2	0	
BICEPS	Seated Dumbbell Curls	2	20	50%	4-2-2	0	
TRICEPS	Supine Dumbbell Extensions	2	20	50%	4-2-2	0	
LEGS	Step-up to Balance	2	20	50%	4-2-2	90 sec	

COOL-DOWN	
POST-WORKOUT FLEXIBILITY	Static Stretching: Calves, adductors, hip flexors, pectorals

Week	1							2							3							4						
Day	M	T	W	T	F	S	S	M	T	W	T	F	S	S	M	T	W	T	F	S	S	M	T	W	T	F	S	S
CET																												
IST	X		X		X			X		X		X			X		X		X			X		X		X		
SET																												
MDT																												
MST																												
EET																												
MPT																												
Cardio	X		X		X			X		X		X			X		X		X		X	X	X	X	X	X	X	X
Flexibility	X	X	X	X	X	X	X	X	X	X	X	X	X	X	X	X	X	X	X	X	X	X	X	X	X	X	X	X
KCA																												

**Figure 13-10: Monthly Plan for the Goal of Body Fat Reduction
February - Phase 2: Integrated Stabilization Training**

Figure 13-10 illustrates the monthly plan for February. As with the previous month, this plan demonstrates a three-day-per-week workout plan with scheduled workouts on Mondays, Wednesdays and Fridays. Again, this monthly plan could easily be performed twice a week. The client can perform flexibility exercises every day of the week, if desired. Cardio can be done on the workout days (or any other day during the week depending on the client's schedule).

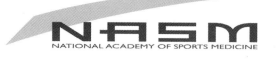

Optimum Performance Training™

NAME: _____

TRAINER: _____

DAYS/WEEK: _____

DATE: _____

PHASE: <u>2: Integrated Stabilization Training</u>

GOAL: <u>Fat Loss</u>

CARDIO TRAINING: Stage 1	TIME: 20 min	EQUIPMENT: Elliptical Trainer

WARMUP/FLEXIBILITY	Sets	Reps	Duration	Rest	Notes
1. SMR: Calves, IT band, adductors, piriformis	1				Hold tender spots 20-30 sec.
2. Cardio: Elliptical trainer			5 min.		
3. Static Stretching: Calves, adductors, hip flexors, lats	1		30 sec.		

CORE & BALANCE	Sets	Reps	Tempo	Rest	Notes
1. Ball Bridge	2	20	5-10 sec.hold	0 sec.	Circuit training
2. Quadruped Opposite Arm/Leg Reach	2	20	5-10 sec.hold	0 sec.	
3. Single-leg Balance Reach (Sagittal Plane)	2	20	5-10 sec.hold	90 sec.	

REACTIVE	Sets	Reps	Tempo	Rest	Notes
1. Squat Jump with Stabilization	2	5-8	3 sec hold	60 sec.	
2.					

SPEED, AGILITY, QUICKNESS	Sets	Reps	Time	Rest	Notes
1. Optional					
2.					

STRENGTH	Exercise	Sets	Reps	Intensity	Tempo	Rest	Notes
TOTAL BODY	Optional						
CHEST	Ball Dumbbell Chest Press	2	20	60%	4-2-1	0 sec.	Circuit
BACK	Ball Dumbbell Row	2	20	60%	4-2-1	0 sec.	
SHOULDERS	Single-leg Scaption	2	20	60%	4-2-1	0 sec.	
BICEPS	Single-leg Dumbbell Curl	2	20	60%	4-2-1	0 sec.	
TRICEPS	Ball Dumbbell Tricep Extension	2	20	60%	4-2-1	0 sec.	
LEGS	Single-leg Squat	2	20	60%	4-2-1	90 sec.	

COOL-DOWN	
POST-WORKOUT FLEXIBILITY	Static Stretching: Calves, adductors, hip flexors, pectorals

Figure 13-11 illustrates the monthly plan for March. As with the previous month, this plan demonstrates a three-day-per-week workout plan, with scheduled workouts on Mondays, Wednesdays and Fridays. This monthly plan could easily be performed either two or four times per week. The client can perform flexibility exercises every day of the week, if desired. In this phase of training, the workouts require more time and energy, so cardio can be done on the days opposite the workout days. This does not mean, however, that the client should not also do cardio on their workout days.

Week	1							2							3							4						
Day	M	T	W	T	F	S	S	M	T	W	T	F	S	S	M	T	W	T	F	S	S	M	T	W	T	F	S	S
CET																												
IST																												
SET	X		X		X			X		X		X			X		X		X			X		X		X		
MDT																												
MST																												
EET																												
MPT																												
Cardio		X		X		X			X		X		X			X		X		X			X		X		X	
Flexibility	X	X	X	X	X	X	X	X	X	X	X	X	X	X	X	X	X	X	X	X	X	X	X	X	X	X	X	X
KCA																												

Figure 13-11: Monthly Plan for the Goal of Body Fat Reduction March - Phase 3: Stabilization Equivalent Training

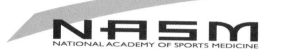

Optimum Performance Training™

NAME: _____

TRAINER: _____

DAYS/WEEK: _____

DATE: _____

PHASE: 3: Stabilization Equivalent Training

GOAL: Fat Loss

CARDIO TRAINING: Stage II and III	TIME: 30-60 min	EQUIPMENT: Elliptical Trainer

WARMUP/FLEXIBILITY	Sets	Reps	Duration	Rest	Notes
1. SMR: Calves, IT band, adductors, piriformis	1				Hold tender spots 20-30 sec.
2. Cardio: Elliptical trainer			10 min.		
3. Active Stretching: Calves, adductors, hip flexors, lats	1		2-4 sec.		

CORE & BALANCE	Sets	Reps	Tempo	Rest	Notes
1. Ball Long-lever Crunch	2	12	3-2-1	0 sec.	Circuit training
2. Back Extension	2	12	3-2-1	0 sec.	
3. Single-leg Squat Touchdown	2	12	3-2-1	0 sec.	

REACTIVE	Sets	Reps	Tempo	Rest	Notes
1. Power Step-up	2	8	Repeating	60 sec.	
2.					

SPEED, AGILITY, QUICKNESS	Sets	Reps	Time	Rest	Notes
1. Optional					
2.					

STRENGTH	Exercise	Sets	Reps	Intensity	Tempo	Rest	Notes
TOTAL BODY	Optional						
CHEST	1. Seated Machine Chest Press 2. Ball Push-up	2	12	70%	2-0-2 3-2-1	0 sec.	Circuit
BACK	1. Seated Machine Row 2. Prone Ball Cobra	2	12	70%	4-2-1	0 sec.	
SHOULDERS	1. Seated Dumbbell Shoulder Press 2. Prone Ball Scaption	2	12	70%	2-0-2 3-2-1	0 sec.	
BICEPS	Optional						
TRICEPS	Optional						
LEGS	1. Dumbbell Squat 2. Step-up to Balance	2	12	70%	2-0-2 3-2-1	0 sec. 60 sec.	

COOL-DOWN	
POST-WORKOUT FLEXIBILITY	Static Stretching: Calves, adductors, hip flexors, pectorals

Applying the Model for the Goal of Increasing Lean Body Mass

The goal of increasing lean body mass (or hypertrophy) requires the client to increase caloric intake to exceed the amount that is burned, in order to put weight on. The training will need to be progressed to higher volumes (more sets, reps and intensity) to force muscles to increase their cellular makeup and produce increased size.

The following program is a general representation of how the OPT™ model is used for clients with the goal of increased lean body mass. With the goal of hypertrophy the client can be cycled through the first five phases of the OPT™ model, depending on the needs and wants of the client.

Figure 13-12 shows the annual plan. The client will start January in Phase 1 to ensure proper muscle balance and endurance of the stabilization muscles. He/she will remain there for approximately four weeks before moving into Phase 2. Once the client has completed Phase 1 and moves on to Phase 2, it will not necessary to return to Phase 1, unless an extended amount of time is taken off (30-60 days), such as a long vacation during the summer or holiday seasons. Phases 1 and 2 are vital for this client, since each will prepare the connective tissues and muscles for the high demands of training required for this goal. Without proper preparation, injury will be eminent.

		JAN	FEB	MAR	APR	MAY	JUN	JUL	AUG	SEP	OCT	NOV	DEC
Stabilization	CET	X											
	IST		X						X				
Strength	SET			X		X				X		X	
	MDT				X		X				X		X
	MST							X					
Power	EET												
	MPT												
Cardio													

Figure 13-12: Annual Plan for the Goal of Increasing Lean Body Mass

The remainder of the annual plan shows the client cycling through Phases 2 through 5. Phase 3 will promote greater strength endurance and more volume to prepare the client for the greater demands of Phases 4 and 5.

Phase 4 is specific for maximal hypertrophy and will place larger volumes of stress through the body to force cellular changes that result in muscle hypertrophy. Phase 5 is used to increase the strength capacity to allow the client to train with heavier weights in the future. This will equate to higher volumes of training and greater hypertrophy.

Returning to Phase 2 will allow the client proper recovery time before entering back into Phases 3 through 5. Cardiorespiratory training can be performed each month to ensure the cardiorespiratory system is efficient and promoting optimal tissue recovery.

Figure 13-13 illustrates the monthly plan for January. This plan demonstrates a three-day-per-week workout plan, with scheduled workouts on Mondays, Wednesdays and Fridays. The client can perform flexibility exercises every day of the week, if desired. Cardio can be done on the workout days (or any other day during the week, depending on the client's schedule).

Week	1							2							3							4						
Day	M	T	W	T	F	S	S	M	T	W	T	F	S	S	M	T	W	T	F	S	S	M	T	W	T	F	S	S
CET	X		X		X			X		X		X			X		X		X			X		X		X		
IST																												
SET																												
MDT																												
MST																												
EET																												
MPT																												
Cardio																												
Flexibility	X	X	X	X	X	X	X	X	X	X	X	X	X	X	X	X	X	X	X	X	X	X	X	X	X	X	X	X
KCA																												

**Figure 13-13: Monthly Plan for the Goal of Increasing Lean Body Mass
January — Phase 2: Integrated Stabilization Training**

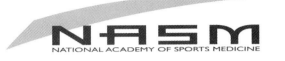

Optimum Performance Training™

NAME: _____   DATE: _____

TRAINER: _____   PHASE: 1: Corrective Exercise Training

DAYS/WEEK: _____   GOAL: Lean Body Mass Gain

CARDIO TRAINING: Optional	TIME:	EQUIPMENT:

WARMUP/FLEXIBILITY	Sets	Reps	Duration	Rest	Notes
1. SMR: Calves, IT band, adductors, thoracic Spine	1				Hold tender spots 20-30 sec.
2. Cardio: Elliptical trainer			5 min.		
3. Static Stretching: Calves, adductors, hip flexors, lats, pecs	1		30 sec.		

CORE & BALANCE	Sets	Reps	Tempo	Rest	Notes
1. Floor Cobra	2	12	3-10 sec. hold	0 sec.	Circuit training
2. Floor Bridge	2	12	3-10 sec. hold	0 sec.	
3. Single-leg Balance	2	12	3-10 sec. hold	0 sec.	

REACTIVE	Sets	Reps	Tempo	Rest	Notes
1. N/A					
2.					

SPEED, AGILITY, QUICKNESS	Sets	Reps	Time	Rest	Notes
1. N/A					
2.					

STRENGTH	Exercise	Sets	Reps	Intensity	Tempo	Rest	Notes
TOTAL BODY	Optional						
CHEST	Seated Machine Chest Press	2	20	50%	4-2-1	30 sec.	
BACK	Seated Machine Row	2	20	50%	4-2-1	30 sec.	
SHOULDERS	Seated Dumbbell Shoulder Press	2	20	50%	4-2-1	30 sec.	
BICEPS	Seated Machine Bicep Curl	2	20	50%	4-2-1	30 sec.	
TRICEPS	Supine Machine Tricep Extension	2	20	50%	4-2-1	30 sec.	
LEGS	Ball Squat	2	20	50%	4-2-1	30 sec.	

COOL-DOWN	
POST-WORKOUT FLEXIBILITY	Static Stretching: Calves, adductors, hip flexors, pectorals

Figure 13-14 illustrates the monthly plan for February. As with the previous month, this plan demonstrates a three-day-per-week workout plan with scheduled workouts on Mondays, Wednesdays and Fridays. The client can perform flexibility exercises every day of the week, if desired. Cardio can be done on the workout days (or any other day during the week depending on the client's schedule).

Week	1							2							3							4						
Day	M	T	W	T	F	S	S	M	T	W	T	F	S	S	M	T	W	T	F	S	S	M	T	W	T	F	S	S
CET																												
IST	X		X		X			X		X		X			X		X		X			X		X		X		
SET																												
MDT																												
MST																												
EET																												
MPT																												
Cardio																												
Flexibility	X	X	X	X	X	X	X	X	X	X	X	X	X	X	X	X	X	X	X	X	X	X	X	X	X	X	X	X
KCA																												

Figure 13-14: Monthly Plan for the Goal of Increasing Lean Body Mass February — Phase 2: Integrated Stabilization Training

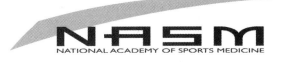

Optimum Performance Training™

NAME: _____   DATE: _____

TRAINER: _____   PHASE: 2: Integrated Stabilization Training

DAYS/WEEK: _____   GOAL: Lean Body Mass Gain

CARDIO TRAINING: Optional	TIME:	EQUIPMENT:

WARMUP/FLEXIBILITY	Sets	Reps	Duration	Rest	Notes
1. SMR: Calves, IT band, adductors, thoracic spine	1				Hold tender spots 20-30 sec.
2. Cardio: Elliptical trainer			5 min.		
3. Static Stretching: Calves, adductors, hip flexors, lats, pecs	1		30 sec.		

CORE & BALANCE	Sets	Reps	Tempo	Rest	Notes
1. Quadruped Opposite Arm/Leg Raise	2	20	5-10 sec. hold	0 sec.	Circuit training
2. Ball Bridge	2	20	5-10 sec. hold	0 sec.	
3. Single-leg Balance Reach	2	20	5-10 sec. hold	60 sec.	

REACTIVE	Sets	Reps	Tempo	Rest	Notes
1. Squat Jump with Stabilization	2	5	3 sec. hold	60 sec.	
2.					

SPEED, AGILITY, QUICKNESS	Sets	Reps	Time	Rest	Notes
1. Optional					
2.					

STRENGTH	Exercise	Sets	Reps	Intensity	Tempo	Rest	Notes
TOTAL BODY	Optional						
CHEST	Standing Cable Chest Press	2	15	65%	4-2-1	60 sec.	
BACK	Seated Cable Row	2	20	65%	4-2-1	60 sec.	
SHOULDERS	Seated Dumbbell Shoulder Press	2	20	65%	4-2-1	60 sec.	
BICEPS	Seated Dumbbell Bicep Curl	2	20	65%	4-2-1	60 sec.	
TRICEPS	Supine Ball Dumbbell Tricep Extension	2	20	65%	4-2-1	60 sec.	
LEGS	Dumbbell Squat	2	20	65%	4-2-1	60 sec.	

COOL-DOWN	
POST-WORKOUT FLEXIBILITY	Static Stretching: Calves, adductors, hip flexors, lats, pectorals

Figure 13-15 illustrates the monthly plan for March. As with the previous month, this plan demonstrates a three-day-per-week workout plan, with scheduled workouts on Mondays, Wednesdays and Fridays. This monthly plan could easily be performed four times per week, with a split routine for the body parts. The client can perform flexibility exercises every day of the week, if desired. In this phase of training, the workouts require more time and energy, so cardio can be done on the days opposite the workout days. This does not mean, however, that the client should not also do cardio on workout days.

Week	1							2							3							4						
Day	M	T	W	T	F	S	S	M	T	W	T	F	S	S	M	T	W	T	F	S	S	M	T	W	T	F	S	S
CET																												
IST																												
SET	X		X		X			X		X		X			X		X		X			X		X		X		
MDT																												
MST																												
EET																												
MPT																												
Cardio																												
Flexibility	X	X	X	X	X	X	X	X	X	X	X	X	X	X	X	X	X	X	X	X	X	X	X	X	X	X	X	X
KCA																												

**Figure 13-15: Monthly Plan for the Goal of Increasing Lean Body Mass
March — Phase 3: Stabilization Equivalent Training**

Figure 13-16 illustrates the monthly plan for April. As with the previous month, this plan demonstrates a four-day-per-week workout plan with scheduled workouts on Mondays, Wednesdays and Fridays. This monthly plan could easily be performed four times per week, with a split routine for the body parts. The client can perform flexibility exercises every day of the week, if desired. In this phase of training, the workouts require more time and energy, so cardio can be done on the days opposite the workout days. This does not mean, however, that the client should not also do cardio on workout days.

Week	1							2							3							4						
Day	M	T	W	T	F	S	S	M	T	W	T	F	S	S	M	T	W	T	F	S	S	M	T	W	T	F	S	S
CET																												
IST																												
SET																												
MDT	X	X		X	X			X	X		X	X			X	X		X	X			X	X		X	X		
MST																												
EET																												
MPT																												
Cardio																												
Flexibility	X	X	X	X	X	X	X	X	X	X	X	X	X	X	X	X	X	X	X	X	X	X	X	X	X	X	X	X
KCA																												

**Figure 13-16: Monthly Plan for the Goal of Increasing Lean Body Mass
April — Phase 4: Muscular Development Training**

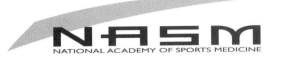

Optimum Performance Training™

NAME: _____

TRAINER: _____

DAYS/WEEK: _____

DATE: _____

PHASE: 3: Stabilization Equivalent Training

GOAL: Lean Body Mass Gain

CARDIO TRAINING: Optional	TIME:	EQUIPMENT:

WARMUP/FLEXIBILITY	Sets	Reps	Duration	Rest	Notes
1. SMR: Calves, IT band, adductors	1				Hold tender spots 20-30 sec.
2. Cardio: Elliptical trainer			5 min.		
3. Active Stretching: Calves, adductors, hip flexors, lats, pecs	1	5-10	2-4 sec.		

CORE & BALANCE	Sets	Reps	Tempo	Rest	Notes
1. Supine Ball Crunch	2	10	3-2-1	0 sec.	Circuit training
2. Back Extension	2	10	3-2-1	0 sec.	
3. Single-leg Squat	2	10	3-2-1	60 sec.	

REACTIVE	Sets	Reps	Tempo	Rest	Notes
1. Squat Jump	2	10	Repeating	60 sec.	
2.					

SPEED, AGILITY, QUICKNESS	Sets	Reps	Time	Rest	Notes
1. Optional					

STRENGTH	Exercise	Sets	Reps	Intensity	Tempo	Rest	Notes
TOTAL BODY	Optional						
CHEST	1. Bench Dumbbell Chest Press 2. Ball Push-up	3	8	80%	2-0-2 3-2-1	0 sec. 60 sec.	
BACK	1. Lat Pulldown 2. Single-leg Cable Row	3	8	80%	2-0-2 3-2-1	0 sec. 60 sec.	
SHOULDERS	1. Seated Dumbbell Shoulder Press 2. Single-leg Scaption	3	8	80%	2-0-2 3-2-1	0 sec. 60 sec	
BICEPS	1. Barbell Curl 2. Single-leg Dumbbell Curl	3	8	80%	2-0-2 3-2-1	0 sec. 60 sec	
TRICEPS	1. Cable Pressdown 2. Ball Dumbbell Extension	3	8	80%	2-0-2 3-2-1	0 sec. 60 sec	
LEGS	1. Barbell Squat 2. Single-leg Romanian Deadlift	3	8	80%	2-0-2 3-2-1	0 sec. 60 sec	

This workout can be split into a 2-, 3-, or 4-day workout routine.
Sample 3-day routine: Day 1 (chest and back), Day 2 (shoulders and legs), day 3 (biceps and triceps).

COOL-DOWN	
POST-WORKOUT FLEXIBILITY	Static Stretching: Calves, adductors, hip flexors, lats, pectorals

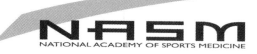

NATIONAL ACADEMY OF SPORTS MEDICINE

Optimum Performance Training™

NAME: _____

TRAINER: _____

DAYS/WEEK: <u>Days 1 and 3</u>

DATE: _____

PHASE: <u>4: Muscular Development Training</u>

GOAL: <u>Lean Body Mass Gain</u>

CARDIO TRAINING:	TIME:	EQUIPMENT:

WARMUP/FLEXIBILITY	Sets	Reps	Duration	Rest	Notes
1. SMR: Calves, IT band, adductors	1				Hold tender spots 20-30 sec.
2. Cardio: Elliptical trainer			5 min.		
3. Active Stretching: Calves, hip flexors, lats	1	5-10	2-4 sec.		

CORE & BALANCE	Sets	Reps	Tempo	Rest	Notes
1. Reverse Crunch	3	10	3-2-1	60 sec.	
2. Ball Crunch with Rotation	3	10	3-2-1	60 sec.	
3.					

REACTIVE	Sets	Reps	Tempo	Rest	Notes
1. Optional					
2.					

SPEED, AGILITY, QUICKNESS	Sets	Reps	Time	Rest	Notes
1. Optional					

STRENGTH	Exercise	Sets	Reps	Intensity	Tempo	Rest	Notes
TOTAL BODY							
CHEST	1. Barbell Bench Press 2. Incline Dumbbell Chest Press	3	8	85%	2-0-2	60 sec.	
BACK							
SHOULDERS	1. Dumbbell Shoulder Press 2. Shoulder Press Machine	3	8	85%	2-0-2	60 sec.	
BICEPS							
TRICEPS	1. Cable Pushdown 2. Supine Bench Dumbbell Tricep Extension	3	8	80%	2-0-2	0 sec. 60 sec	
LEGS							

COOL-DOWN	
POST-WORKOUT FLEXIBILITY	Static Stretching: Calves, adductors, hip flexors, pectorals

NASM
NATIONAL ACADEMY OF SPORTS MEDICINE

Optimum Performance Training™

NAME: _____ DATE: _____

TRAINER: _____ PHASE: <u>4: Muscular Development Training</u>

DAYS/WEEK: <u>Days 2 and 4</u> GOAL: <u>Lean Body Mass Gain</u>

CARDIO TRAINING:	TIME:	EQUIPMENT:

WARMUP/FLEXIBILITY	Sets	Reps	Duration	Rest	Notes
1. SMR: Calves, IT band, adductors	1				Hold tender spots 20-30 sec.
2. Cardio: Elliptical trainer			5 min.		
3. Active Stretching: Calves, hip flexors, lats	1	5-10	2-4 sec.		

CORE & BALANCE	Sets	Reps	Tempo	Rest	Notes
1. Ball Bridge	2	12	2-0-2	60 sec.	
2. Back Extension	2	12	2-0-2	60 sec.	
3.					

REACTIVE	Sets	Reps	Tempo	Rest	Notes
1. Optional					
2.					

SPEED, AGILITY, QUICKNESS	Sets	Reps	Time	Rest	Notes
1. Optional					

STRENGTH	Exercise	Sets	Reps	Intensity	Tempo	Rest	Notes
TOTAL BODY							
CHEST							
BACK	1. Lat Pulldown 2. Seated Cable Row	3	8	85%	2-0-2	60 sec.	
SHOULDERS							
BICEPS	1. Standing Barbell Curl 2. Bicep Curl Machine	3	8	85%	2-0-2	60 sec.	
TRICEPS							
LEGS	1. Barbell Squat 2. Dumbbell Lunge	3	8	85%	2-0-2	60 sec.	

COOL-DOWN	
POST-WORKOUT FLEXIBILITY	Static Stretching: Calves, adductors, hip flexors, pectorals

Applying the Model for the Goal of General Performance

The goal of improving general performance requires the client to increase overall proprioception, strength and power output (or rate of force production). The training will need to be progressed from stabilization through power phases of training and utilize the entire OPT™ model.

The following program is a general representation of how the OPT™ model is used for clients with the goal of improving general performance. The client can be cycled through the entire OPT™ model, depending on the needs and wants of the client. However, for the typical client, Phases 1, 2, 3, 5 and 6 will be the most important.

Because Phase 4 is dedicated to maximal hypertrophy, it will not be necessary for the goal of general performance (as is also the case with Phase 7). Typical fitness clients will not need to train at the extreme intensity seen in Phase 7 to make necessary gains in their overall performance. Phase 5 can be used in moderation to help increase the initial strength levels required to optimize the adaptation in Phase 6, if necessary.

Figure 13-17 shows the annual plan. The client will start January in Phase 1 to ensure proper muscle balance and endurance of the stabilization muscles. He/she will remain there for approximately four weeks before moving onto Phase 2. Once the client has completed Phase 1 and moves on to Phase 2 it will not necessary to return to Phase 1, unless an extended amount of time is taken off (30-60 days), such as a long vacation during the summer, holiday seasons or injury. Phases 1 and 2 are vital for this client, as each will prepare the connective tissues and muscles for the high demands of training required for this goal. Without proper preparation, injury will be eminent for the athletic client.

		JAN	FEB	MAR	APR	MAY	JUN	JUL	AUG	SEP	OCT	NOV	DEC
Stabiliz-ation	CET	X											
	IST		X		X		X		X		X		X
Strength	SET			X	X	X	X	X	X	X	X	X	X
	MDT												
	MST												
Power	EET				X	X	X	X	X	X	X	X	X
	MPT												
Cardio		X	X	X	X	X	X	X	X	X	X	X	X

Figure 13-17: Annual Plan for the Goal of General Performance

The remainder of the annual plan shows the client cycling through Phases 2, 3 and 6. Phase 3 will promote greater overall strength and more volume to prepare the client for the greater demands of Phase 6. As previously mentioned, Phase 5 can be used to increase the strength capacity of the client, but is not vitally necessary for general performance.

From April on, Phases 2 and/or 3 and 6 are used in the same month/week. This is a hybrid form of periodization known as *undulating periodization*. Undulating periodization allows the client to train at various intensities over the course of a week, eliciting multiple adaptations once a certain level of fitness is achieved.[77,81] In this program, stabilization (Phase 2), strength (Phase 3) and power (Phase 6) are all being trained together. Cardiorespiratory training can be performed each month to ensure the cardiorespiratory system is efficient and promoting optimal tissue recoverability.

Figure 13-18 illustrates the monthly plan for January. This plan demonstrates a three-day-per-week workout plan with scheduled workouts on Mondays, Wednesdays and Fridays. The client can perform flexibility exercises every day of the week, if desired. Cardio can be done on the workout days (or any other day during the week, depending on the client's schedule).

Week	1							2							3							4						
Day	M	T	W	T	F	S	S	M	T	W	T	F	S	S	M	T	W	T	F	S	S	M	T	W	T	F	S	S
CET	X		X		X			X		X		X			X		X		X			X		X		X		
IST																												
SET																												
MDT																												
MST																												
EET																												
MPT																												
Cardio	X		X		X			X		X		X			X		X		X			X		X		X		
Flexibility	X	X	X	X	X	X	X	X	X	X	X	X	X	X	X	X	X	X	X	X	X	X	X	X	X	X	X	X
KCA																												

**Figure 13-18: Monthly Plan for the Goal of General Performance
January - Phase 1: Corrective Exercise Training**

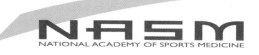
NATIONAL ACADEMY OF SPORTS MEDICINE

Optimum Performance Training™

NAME: _____

TRAINER: _____

DAYS/WEEK: _____

DATE: _____

PHASE: 1: Corrective Exercise Training

GOAL: General Performance

CARDIO TRAINING:	TIME:	EQUIPMENT:

WARMUP/FLEXIBILITY	Sets	Reps	Duration	Rest	Notes
1. SMR: Calves, IT band, adductors	1				Hold tender spots 20-30 sec.
2. Cardio: Elliptical trainer			5 min.		
3. Static Stretching: Calves, hip flexors, lats	1		30 sec.		

CORE & BALANCE	Sets	Reps	Tempo	Rest	Notes
1. Floor Cobra	2	12	3-10 sec. hold	0 sec.	Circuit
2. Floor Bridge	2	12	3-10 sec. hold	0 sec.	
3. Single-leg Balance	2		3-10 sec.hold	30 sec.	

REACTIVE	Sets	Reps	Tempo	Rest	Notes
1. N/A					
2.					

SPEED, AGILITY, QUICKNESS	Sets	Reps	Time	Rest	Notes
1. N/A					

STRENGTH	Exercise	Sets	Reps	Intensity	Tempo	Rest	Notes
TOTAL BODY	Optional						
CHEST	Seated Machine Chest Press	2	20	50%	4-2-2	0 sec.	
BACK	Seated Machine Row	2	20	50%	4-2-2	0 sec.	
SHOULDERS	Seated Machine Shoulder Press	2	20	50%	4-2-2	0 sec.	
BICEPS	Seated Machine Bicep Curl	2	20	50%	4-2-2	0 sec.	
TRICEPS	Seated Machine Tricep Extension	2	20	50%	4-2-2	0 sec.	
LEGS	Ball Squat	2	20	50%	4-2-2	0 sec.	

COOL-DOWN	
POST-WORKOUT FLEXIBILITY	Static Stretching: Calves, adductors, hip flexors, lats, pectorals

**Program Design
Concepts**

Week	1							2							3							4						
Day	M	T	W	T	F	S	S	M	T	W	T	F	S	S	M	T	W	T	F	S	S	M	T	W	T	F	S	S
CET																												
IST	X		X		X			X		X		X			X		X		X			X		X		X		
SET																												
MDT																												
MST																												
EET																												
MPT																												
Cardio	X		X		X			X		X		X			X		X		X			X		X		X		
Flexibility	X	X	X	X	X	X	X	X	X	X	X	X	X	X	X	X	X	X	X	X	X	X	X	X	X	X	X	X
KCA																												

**Figure 13-19: Monthly Plan for the Goal of General Performance
February — Phase 2: Integrated Stabilization Training**

Figure 13-19 illustrates the monthly plan for February. As with the previous month, this plan demonstrates a three-day-per-week workout plan with scheduled workouts on Mondays, Wednesdays and Fridays. The client can perform flexibility exercises every day of the week, if desired. Cardio can be done on the workout days (or any other day during the week depending on the client's schedule).

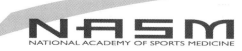

Optimum Performance Training™

NAME: _____   DATE: _____

TRAINER: _____   PHASE: 2: Integrated Stabilization Training

DAYS/WEEK: _____   GOAL: General Performance

CARDIO TRAINING: Stage I and II	TIME: 30 minutes	EQUIPMENT: Elliptical trainer

WARMUP/FLEXIBILITY	Sets	Reps	Duration	Rest	Notes
1. SMR: Calves, IT band, adductors, thoracic spine	1				Hold tender spots 20-30 sec.
2. Cardio: Elliptical trainer			10 min.		
3. Static Stretching: Calves, adductors, hip flexors, lats, pecs	1		30 sec.		

CORE & BALANCE	Sets	Reps	Tempo	Rest	Notes
1. Quadruped Opposite Arm/Leg Reach	2	20	5-10 sec. hold	0 sec.	Circuit
2. Ball Bridge	2	20	5-10 sec. hold	0 sec.	
3. Single-leg Balance Reach (Multiplanar)	2	20	5-10 sec.hold	60 sec.	

REACTIVE	Sets	Reps	Tempo	Rest	Notes
1. Box Jump with Stabilization	2	5	3 sec. hold	30 sec.	
2.					

SPEED, AGILITY, QUICKNESS	Sets	Reps	Tempo	Rest	Notes
1. Speed Ladder	1-2		Controlled	60 sec.	4 exercises
2. Box Drill	1-2		Controlled	60 sec.	1-2 drills

STRENGTH	Exercise	Sets	Reps	Intensity	Tempo	Rest	Notes
TOTAL BODY	Optional						
CHEST	Standing Cable Chest Press	2	20	60%	4-2-1	0 sec.	Circuit
BACK	Standing Cable Row	2	20	60%	4-2-1	0 sec.	
SHOULDERS	Staggered-stance Dumbbell Shoulder Press	2	20	60%	4-2-1	0 sec.	
BICEPS	Standing Dumbbell Bicep Curl	2	20	60%	4-2-1	0 sec.	
TRICEPS	Supine Ball Dumbbell Tricep Extension	2	20	60%	4-2-1	0 sec.	
LEGS	Step-up to Balance	2	20	60%	4-2-1	90 sec.	

COOL-DOWN	
POST-WORKOUT FLEXIBILITY	Static Stretching: Calves, adductors, hip flexors, lats, pectorals

Week	1							2							3							4						
Day	M	T	W	T	F	S	S	M	T	W	T	F	S	S	M	T	W	T	F	S	S	M	T	W	T	F	S	S
CET																												
IST																												
SET	X		X		X			X		X		X			X		X		X			X		X		X		
MDT																												
MST																												
EET																												
MPT																												
Cardio		X		X		X			X		X		X			X		X		X			X		X		X	
Flexibility	X	X	X	X	X	X	X	X	X	X	X	X	X	X	X	X	X	X	X	X	X	X	X	X	X	X	X	X
KCA																												

Figure 13-20: Monthly Plan for the Goal of General Performance
March — Phase 3: Stabilization Equivalent Training

Figure 13-20 illustrates the monthly plan for March. As with the previous month, this plan demonstrates a three-day-per-week workout plan with scheduled workouts on Mondays, Wednesdays and Fridays. This monthly plan could easily be four times a week, with a split routine for the body parts. The client can perform flexibility exercises every day of the week, if desired. In this phase of training, the workouts require more time and energy so cardio can be done on the days opposite the workout days. This does not mean, however, that the client should not also do cardio on workout days.

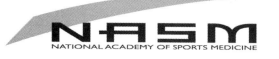

Optimum Performance Training™

NAME: _____   DATE: _____

TRAINER: _____   PHASE: <u>3: Stabilization Equivalent Training</u>

DAYS/WEEK: _____   GOAL: <u>General Performance</u>

CARDIO TRAINING: Stage II and III	TIME: 30 minutes	EQUIPMENT: Elliptical trainer

WARMUP/FLEXIBILITY	Sets	Reps	Duration	Rest	Notes
1. SMR: Calves, IT band, adductors, thoracic spine	1				Hold tender spots 20-30 sec.
2. Cardio: Elliptical trainer			5 min.		
3. Static Stretching: Calves, adductors, hip flexors, lats, pecs	1	5-10	2-4 sec.		

CORE & BALANCE	Sets	Reps	Tempo	Rest	Notes
1. Ball Crunch with Rotation	2	10	3-2-1	0 sec.	Circuit
2. Back Extension	2	10	3-2-1	0 sec.	
3. Step-up to Balance	2	10	3-2-1	60 sec.	

REACTIVE	Sets	Reps	Tempo	Rest	Notes
1. Squat Jump	2	10	Repeating	30 sec.	

SPEED, AGILITY, QUICKNESS	Sets	Reps	Tempo	Rest	Notes
1. Speed Ladder	3		Controlled	60 sec.	6 exercises
2. Box Drill	2		Controlled	60 sec.	2 drills

STRENGTH	Exercise	Sets	Reps	Intensity	Tempo	Rest	Notes
TOTAL BODY	Optional						
CHEST	1. Bench Dumbbell Chest Press 2. Ball Push-up	3	8	80%	2-0-2 3-2-1	0 sec.	Circuit
BACK	1. Lat Pulldown 2. Ball Dumbbell Row	3	8	80%	2-0-2 3-2-1	0 sec.	
SHOULDERS	1. Seated Dumbbell Shoulder Press 2. Single-leg Scaption	3	8	80%	2-0-2 3-2-1	0 sec.	
BICEPS	1. Machine Bicep Curl 2. Single-leg Single-arm Dumbbell Curl	3	8	80%	2-0-2 3-2-1	0 sec.	
TRICEPS	1. Standing Tricep Extension 2. Ball Alternating-arm Tricep Extension	3	8	80%	2-0-2 3-2-1	0 sec.	
LEGS	1. Lunge 2. Single-leg Romanian Deadlift	3	8	80%	2-0-2 3-2-1	60 sec.	

COOL-DOWN	
POST-WORKOUT FLEXIBILITY	Static Stretching: Calves, adductors, hip flexors, lats, pectorals

Week	1							2							3							4						
Day	M	T	W	T	F	S	S	M	T	W	T	F	S	S	M	T	W	T	F	S	S	M	T	W	T	F	S	S
CET																												
IST			X							X							X							X				
SET	X							X							X							X						
MDT																												
MST																												
EET					X							X							X							X		
MPT																												
Cardio		X		X					X		X					X		X					X		X			
Flexibility	X	X	X	X	X	X	X	X	X	X	X	X	X	X	X	X	X	X	X	X	X	X	X	X	X	X	X	X
KCA																												

**Figure 13-21: Monthly Plan for the Goal of General Performance
April — Phase 4: Elastic Equivalent Training**

Figure 13-21 illustrates the monthly plan for April. As with the previous month, this plan demonstrates a three-day-per-week workout plan with scheduled workouts on Mondays, Wednesdays and Fridays. In this month, however, Phases 2, 3 and 6 are all used in the same week. This helps to introduce power training at a slower, more moderate pace, with low weekly volumes, while ensuring optimal levels of stabilization and strength necessary to increase power. The client can perform flexibility exercises every day of the week, if desired.

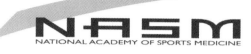

Optimum Performance Training™

NAME: _____

TRAINER: _____

DAYS/WEEK: _____

DATE: _____

PHASE: 6: Elastic Equivalent Training

GOAL: General Performance

CARDIO TRAINING: Stage II and III	TIME: 30-60 minutes	EQUIPMENT: Elliptical trainer

WARMUP/FLEXIBILITY	Sets	Reps	Duration	Rest	Notes
1. SMR: Calves, IT band, adductors, thoracic spine	1				Hold tender spots 20-30 sec.
2. Cardio: Elliptical trainer			5 min.		
3. Static Stretching: Calves, adductors, hip flexors, lats, pecs	1	10	2-4 sec.		Prisoner Squat, Lateral Tube Walking, Walking Lunge with Twist

CORE & BALANCE	Sets	Reps	Tempo	Rest	Notes
1. Ball Medicine Throw	2	12	Explosive	0 sec.	
2. Rotation Chest Pass	2	12	Explosive	0 sec.	
3. Hop to Balance (Multiplanar)	2	12	Controlled	60 sec.	

REACTIVE	Sets	Reps	Tempo	Rest	Notes
1. Optional					

SPEED, AGILITY, QUICKNESS	Sets	Reps	Tempo	Rest	Notes
1. Speed Ladder	3			60 sec.	6 exercises
2. Box Drill	3			60 sec.	2 drills

STRENGTH	Exercise	Sets	Reps	Intensity	Tempo	Rest	Notes
TOTAL BODY	Optional						
CHEST	1. Incline Dumbbell Chest Press	3	5	85%	x-x-x	0 sec.	Circuit
	2. Plyometric Push-up		10	BW		60 sec.	
BACK	1. Seated Row	3	5	85%	x-x-x	0 sec.	
	2. Soccer Throw		10			60 sec.	
SHOULDERS	1. Standing Dumbbell Shoulder Press	3	5	85%	x-x-x		
	2. Medicine Ball Scoop Toss		10			60 sec.	
BICEPS	Optional						
TRICEPS	Optional						
LEGS	1. Barbell Squat	3	5	85%	x-x-x	0 sec.	
	2. Squat Jump		10			60 sec.	

COOL-DOWN	
POST-WORKOUT FLEXIBILITY	Static Stretching: Calves, adductors, hip flexors, lats, pectorals

Filling in the Template

Now that all the necessary components of the OPT™ template have been discussed, Section 5 (strength) can be completed. The beauty of the OPT™ system is that is eliminates the guesswork. When filling in the resistance training portion of the OPT™ template, simply choose which phase of training the client will work in. In this manner, all of the major acute variables are already predetermined. Therefore, *sets*, *reps*, *intensity*, *tempo* and *rest interval* are already given.

In the *exercises* box, simply choose an exercise that fits the desired body part as well as the guidelines of the specific Phase of training. For example, Phase 3: Stabilization Equivalent Training consists of a strength exercise, followed by a stabilization exercise. Thus, in the *chest* section, a bench press followed by a single-leg alternating-arm cable chest press would be appropriate exercise selections.

Using information from the Chapter 12 (Resistance Training), the health and fitness professional can choose a particular system of training (such as using a circuit training or vertical loading method) to increase the intensity of the workout. If the client works out two to six days a week, a split routine may be utilized with varying body parts. Essentially, the possibilities are endless and only limited by creativity. The most important thing, however, is to follow the physiological guidelines of the OPT™ model. After becoming more familiar with the system and the information, begin to experiment and try new approaches.

Fill in the template according to the example in Figure 13-22.

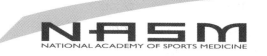

Optimum Performance Training™

NAME: _____   DATE: _____

TRAINER: _____   PHASE: <u>2: Integrated Stabilization Training</u>

DAYS/WEEK: _____   GOAL: <u>General Performance</u>

CARDIO TRAINING: Stage I	TIME: 20 minutes	EQUIPMENT: Elliptical trainer

WARMUP/FLEXIBILITY	Sets	Reps	Duration	Rest	Notes
1. SMR: Calves, IT band, adductors	1				Hold tender spots 20-30 sec.
2. Cardio: Elliptical trainer			5 min.		
3. Static Stretching: Calves, hip flexors, lats	1	10	2-4 sec.		

CORE & BALANCE	Sets	Reps	Tempo	Rest	Notes
1. Quadruped Arm Opposite Leg Raise	1-3	12-20	3-10 sec. hold	0 sec.	Circuit training
2. Floor Bridge	1-3	12-20	3-10 sec. hold	0 sec.	
3. Single-leg Flexion/Extension	1-3	12-20	3-10 sec. hold	60 sec.	

REACTIVE	Sets	Reps	Tempo	Rest	Notes
1. Jump with Stabilization	1-3	5-8	3 sec. hold	60 sec.	

SPEED, AGILITY, QUICKNESS	Sets	Reps	Tempo	Rest	Notes
1. Speed Ladder	1-2			60 sec.	4 exercises
2. Box Drill	1-2			60 sec.	1-2 drills

STRENGTH	Exercise	Sets	Reps	Intensity	Tempo	Rest	Notes
TOTAL BODY							
CHEST	Standing Cable Chest Press	1-3	12-20	60-70%	4-2-1	0	Circuit training
BACK	Standing Cable Row	1-3	12-20	60-70%	4-2-1	0	
SHOULDERS	Standing Dumbbell Shoulder Press	1-3	12-20	60-70%	4-2-1	0	
BICEPS							
TRICEPS							
LEGS	Step-up to Balance	1-3	12-20	60-70%	4-2-1	90 sec.	

COOL-DOWN	
POST-WORKOUT FLEXIBILITY	Static Stretching: Calves, adductors, hip flexors, lats, pectorals

Figure 13-22: OPT™ Template

MODULE 13-5 Summary

The OPT™ model is a planned fitness training system that can be used to create programs for clients with various goals. Health and fitness professionals must be able to apply the information in multiple situations, to a variety of clients. The OPT™ model can be used to reduce body fat, increase in lean body mass and increase general performance.

In order to reduce body fat, clients must burn more calories than they consume by moving more with resistance and cardiorespiratory training. The client will work in Phase 1 for four weeks, to ensure proper muscle balance and endurance of the stabilization muscles. The remainder of the annual plan shows the client cycling back and forth between Phases 2 and 3 (metabolic demand and more volume for increased caloric expenditure).

In order to increase lean body mass, clients must consume more calories than are burned by working with higher volumes to increase muscle size. The client will work in Phase 1 for four weeks, to ensure proper muscle balance and endurance of the stabilization muscles. The remainder of the annual plan shows the client cycling through Phase 2 (recovery time), Phase 3 (greater strength endurance and more volume), Phase 4 (larger volumes of stress for hypertrophy) and Phase 5 (increase strength capacity with even higher volumes of training and more hypertrophy). Cardiorespiratory training can be performed each month to ensure the cardiorespiratory system is efficient and promoting optimal tissue recoverability.

In order to improve general performance, clients must increase overall proprioception, strength and rate of force production. The training will utilize the entire OPT™ model, although for the typical client, Phases 1, 2, 3, 5 and 6 will be the most important. The client will work in Phase 1 for four weeks, to ensure proper muscle balance and endurance of the stabilization muscles. The remainder of the annual plan shows the client cycling through Phases 2, 3 (greater overall strength and more volume) and 6. After the first four months, undulating periodization is utilized and stabilization (Phase 2), strength (Phase 3) and power (Phase 6) are used in the same month/week. Cardiorespiratory training can be performed each month as well.

MODULE 13-5 Quiz

1. A client with the goal of body fat reduction will only need to be cycled through the first _____ phases of the OPT™ model.

2. A typical client with the goal of improving general performance should specifically be cycled through which phases?

   _____

3. A client with the goal of increasing lean body mass must eventually return to Phase 1.

   ☐ True   ☐ False

4. Undulating periodization allows the client to train at various intensities over what period of time?

   _____

References

1. Rose DL, Radzyminski SF, Beaty RR. Effect of brief maximal exercise on the strength of the quadriceps femoris. *Arch Phys Med Rehabil* Mar 1957:157-64.

2. Rutherford OM, Jones DA. The role of learning and coordination in strength training. *Eur J Appl Physiol* 1986;55:100-5.

3. Hickson RC. Interference of strength development by simultaneously training for strength and endurance. *Eur J Appl Physiol* 1980;45:255-63.

4. Hickson RC, Rosenkoetter MA, Brown MM. Strength training effects on aerobic power and short term endurance. *Med Sci Sports Exerc* 1980;12:336-9.

5. Issurin VB, Liebermann DG, Tenenbaum G. Effect of vibratory stimulation training on maximal force and flexibility. *J Sports Sci* 1994;12:561-6.

6. O'Shea P. Throwing speed. *Sports Fitn* Aug 1985;66-7, 89-90.

7. Ostrowski KJ, Wilson GJ, Weatherby R, Murphy PW, Lyttle AD. The effect of weight training volume on hormonal output and muscular size and function. *J Strength Cond Res* 1997;11:148-54.

8. Ploutz LL, Tesch PA, Biro RL, Dudley GA. Effect of resistance training on muscle use during exercise. *J Appl Physiol* 1994;76:1675-81.

9. Stone MH, O'Bryant HS, Schilling BK, Johnson RL, Pierce KC, Haff GG, Koch AJ, Stone M. Periodization: effects of manipulating volume and intensity. Part 2. *NSCA J* 1999;21(3):54-60.

10. Stone MH, Plisk SS, Stone ME, Schilling BK, O'Bryant HS, Pierce KC. Athletic performance development: Volume load-1 set vs. multiple sets, training velocity and training variation. *NSCA J* 1998;20(6):22-31.

11. Tan B. Manipulating resistance training program variables to optimize maximum strength in men: a review. *Strength Cond Res* 1999;13(3):289-304.

12. Baker D, Wilson G, Carlyon R. Periodization: the effect on strength of manipulating volume and intensity. *J Strength Cond Res* 1994;8(4):235-42.

13. Bompa TO. *Theory and methodology of training.* Dubuque, IA: Kendall/Hunt; 1983.

14. Bompa TO. Variations of periodization of strength. *Strength Cond* 1996;18:58-61.

15. Poliquin C. Five steps to increasing the effectiveness of you strength training program. *Natl Stren Cond Assoc J* 1998;10:34-9.

16. Siff MC, Verkhoshansky Y. *Supertraining.* Escondido, CA: Sports Training; 1994.

17. Fleck SJ, Kraemer WJ. *Designing resistance training programs.* 2nd edition. Champaign, IL: Human Kinetics; 1997.

19. Kraemer WJ, Patton JF, Gordon SE, Harman EA, Deschenes KR, Reynolds K, Newton RU, Triplett NT, Dziados JE. Compatibility of high-intensity strength and endurance training on hormonal and skeletal muscle adaptations. *J Appl Physiol* 1995; 78:976-89.

20. Hakkinen K, Pakarinen A, Alen M, et al. Relationships between training volume, physical performance capacity, and serum hormone concentrations during prolonged training in elite weight lifters. *Int J Sports Med* 1987;8(suppl):61-5.

21. Hakkinen K, Pakarinen A, Alen M, et al. Neuromuscular and hormonal responses in elite athletes to two successive strength training sessions in one day. *Eur J Appl Physiol* 1988;57:133-9.

22. Stone MH, Fry AC. Responses to increased resistance training volume. In: Kreider R, Fry AL, O'Toole M (eds). *Overtraining and overreaching in sport.* Champaign, IL: Human Kinetics; 1997.

23. Zatsiorsky VM. *Science and practice of strength training.* Champaign, IL: Human Kinetics; 1995.

24. Berger RA. Effect of varied weight training programs on strength. *Res Q* 1962;33:169-81.

25. Hakkinen K. Neuromuscular adaptation during strength training, aging, detraining and immobilization. *Crit Rev Phys Rehab Med* 1994;6:161-98.

26. Kaneko M, Fuchimoto T, Toji H, Suei K. Training effect of different loads on the force-velocity relationship and mechanical power output in human muscle. *Scand J Sport Sci* 1983;5(2):50-5.

27. Sale DG. Neural adaptation in strength and power training. In: Jones NL, McCartney N, McComas AJ (eds). *Human muscle power.* Champaign, IL: Human Kinetics; 1986. pp. 289-307.

28. Sale DG. Influence of exercise and training on motor unit activation. *Exer Sport Sci Rev* 1987;15:95-151.

29. Sale DG. Neural adaptation to strength training. In: Komi PV (ed). *Strength and power in sport.* London: Blackwell Scientific; 1992. pp 249-65.

30. Schmidtbleicher D. Training for power events. In: Chem PV (ed). *Strength and power in sports.* Boston: Blackwell Scientific; 1992. pp 381-96.

31. Schmidtbleicher D, Haralambie G. Changes in contractile properties of muscle after strength training in a man. *Eur J Appl Physiol* 1981;46:221-8.

32. Stone MH. Considerations in gaining a strength power training effect. *NSCA J* 1982;4(1):22-4, 54.

33. Stone MH., Borden RA. Modes and methods of resistance training. *Strength Cond* 1997;19(4):18-24.

34. Stone MH O'Bryant HS. *Weight training: a scientific approach.* Minneapolis: Burgess; 1987.

35. Holly RG, Shaffrath JD. Cardiorespiratory endurance. Chapter 52. In: American College of Sports Medicine (ed.). *ACSM's resource manual for guidelines for exercise testing and prescription.* 3rd edition. Baltimore, MD: Williams & Wilkins; 1998.

36. American College of Sports Medicine. *ACSM's guidelines for exercise testing and prescription.* 5th edition. Philadelphia: Williams & Wilkins; 1995.

37. Heus R, Wertheim AH, Havenith G. Human energy expenditure when walking on a moving platform. *Eur J Appl Physiol Occup Physiol* 1998;100(2):133-48.

38. Williford HN, Olson MS, Gauger S, Duey WJ, Blessing DL. Cardiovascular and metabolic costs of forward, backward, and lateral motion. *Med Sci Sports Exerc* 1998;30(9)1419-23.

39. Ogita F, Stam RP, Tazawa HO, Toussaint HM, Hollander AP. Oxygen uptake in one-legged and two-legged exercise. *Med Sci Sports Exerc* 2000;32(10):1737-42.

40. Willoughby DS. Training volume equated: a comparison of periodized and progressive resistance weight training programs. *J Hum Move Studies* 1991;21233-48.

41. Gambetta V. *The gambetta method; common sense training for athletic performance.* Sarasota, FL: Gambetta Sports Training Systems; 1998.

42. Hakkinen K, Komi PV, Allen M. Effect of explosive type strength training on isometric force- and relaxation-time, electromyographic and muscle fiber characteristics of leg extensor muscles. *Acta Physiol Scand* 1985;125:587-600.

43. Bauer T, Thayer TE, Boras G. Comparison of training modalities for power development in the lower extremity. *J Appl Sports Sci Res* 1990;4:115-21.

44. Burkhardt E, Barton B, Garhammer J. Maximal impact and propulsion forces during jumping and explosive lifting exercise. *J Appl Sport Sci Res* 1990;4(3):107.

45. Chu DA. Plyometrics: the link between strength and speed. *NSCA J* 1983;5(2):20-1.

46. Housh DJ, Housh TJ, Johnson GO, et al. Hypertrophic response to unilateral concentric isokinetic resistance training. *J Appl Physiol* 1992;73:65-70.

47. Ballor DL, Becque MD, Katch VL, et al. Metabolic responses during hydraulic resistance exercise. *Med Sci Sports Exerc* 1987;19:363-7.

48. Kraemer WJ, Ratamess NA. Physiology of Resistance training. *Ortho Phys Ther Clin North Am* 2000;9(4):467-513.

49. Stone MH, O'Bryant H, Garhammer H. A hypothetical model for strength training. *J Sport Med Phys Fitn* 1981;21:341-52.

50. Tesch PA, Colliander EB, Kaiser P. Muscle metabolism during intense, heavy resistance exercise. *Eur J Appl Physiol* 1986;55:362-6.

51. Tesch PA, Karlsson J. Lactate and fast and slow twitch skeletal muscle fibers of man during isometric contraction. *Acta Physiol Scand* 1977;99:230-6.

52. Fleck SJ. Bridging the gap: interval training physiological basis. *NSCA J* 1983;5:57-62.

53. Brooks GA, Fahey TD, White TP. *Exercise physiology: human bioenergetics and its application.* 2nd edition. Mountain View, CA: Mayfield Publishing Company; 1996.

54. Fitts RH. Cellular mechanisms of muscle fatigue. *Physiol Rev* 1994;74:49.

55. Thorstenson A, Hultren B., von Dobeln W, Karlsson J. Effect of strength training on enzyme activities and fibre characteristics in human skeletal muscle. *Acta Physiol Scand* 1976;96:392-8.

56. MacDougal JD, Elder GCB, Sale DG, Moroz JR, Sutton JR. Effects of strength training and immobilization on human muscle fibers. *Eur J Appl Physiol* 1980;43:25-34.

57. Abernathy PJ, Jurimae J, Logan PA, Taylor AW, Thayer RE. Acute and chronic response of skeletal muscle to resistance exercise. *Sports Med* 1994;17(1):22-38.

58. Kim JR, Oberman A, Fletcher GF, Lee JY. Effect of exercise intensity and frequency on lipid levels in men with coronary heart disease: training Level Comparison Trial. *Am J Cardiol* 2001;87(8):942-6.

59. Tsukui S, Kanda T, Nara M, Nishino M, Kondo T, Kobayashi I. Moderate-intensity regular exercise decreases serum tumor necrosis factor-alpha and HbA1c levels in healthy women. *Int J Obes Relat Metab Disord* 2000;24(9):1207-11.

60. Van Etten LMLA, Westerterp KR, Verstappen FTJ, et al. Effect of an 18-week training program on energy expenditure and physical activity. *J Appl Physiol* 1997;82:298-304.

61. Gillam GM. Effects of frequency of weight training on muscle strength enhancement. *J Sport Med Phys Fitn* 1981;21:432-6.

62. Hunter GR. *Changes in body composition, body build and performance associated with weight training frequencies in males and females.*

63. Kraemer WJ, Marchitelli L, Gordon SE, Harman E, Dziados JE, Mello M, Frykman P, McCrury D, Fleck SJ. Hormonal growth factor responses to heavy resistance protocols. *J Appl Physiol* 1990;69:1442-50.

64. Kraemer WJ, Fleck SJ, Callister R, Shealy M, Dudley GA, Maresh CM, Marchitelli L, Cruthirds C, Murray T, Falkel JE. Training responses of plasma beat-endorphin, adrenocorticotrophin, and cortisol. *Med Sci Sport Exerc* 1989;21:146-53.

65. Cosio-Lima LM, Reynolds KL, Winter C, Paolone V, Jones MT. Effects of physioball and conventional floor exercises on early adaptations in back and abdominal core stability and balance in women. *J Strength Cond Res* 2003;17(4):721-5.

66. Behm DG, Anderson K, Curnew RS. Muscle force and activation under stable and unstable conditions. *J Strength Cond Res* 2002;16(3):416-22.

67. Heitkamp HC, Horstmann T, Mayer F, Weller J, Dickhuth HH. Gain in strength and muscular balance after balance training. *Int J Sports Med* 2001;22:285-90.

68. Haff GG, Stone MH, O'Bryant HS, et al. Force-time dependent characteristics of dynamic and isometric muscle contractions. *J Strength Cond Res* 1997;11:269-72.

69. Schmidt RA. *Motor learning performance*. Champaign, IL: Human Kinetics; 1991.

70. Sale DG. Neural adaptation to resistance training. *Med Sci Sport Exerc* 1988;20(5): S135-45.

71. Enoka RM. Muscle strength and its development: new perspectives. *Sport Med* 1988;6:146-68.

72. Henneman E. Relation between size of motor neurons and their susceptibility to discharge. *Sci* 1957;126:1345-7.

73. Sale DG. Neural adaptation to resistance training. *Med Sci Sports Exerc* 1988;20(5):S135-45.

74. Enoka RM. Muscle strength and its development. New perspectives. *Sport Med* 1988;6:146-68.

75. Westerterp KR, Meijer GAL, Janssen GME, Saris WHM, Hoor F. Long-term effect of physical activity on energy balance and body composition. *Br J Nutr* 1992;68(1):21-30.

76. Bompa TO. *Periodization of strength: The new wave in strength training*. Toronto, ON: Verita Publishing Inc.; 1993.

77. Plisk SS, Stone MH. Periodization strategies. *Strength Cond J* 2003;25(6):19-37.

78. Graham J. Periodization research and an example application. *Strength Cond J* 2002;24(6):62-70.

79. Herrick AB, Stone WJ. The effects of periodization versus progressive resistance exercise on upper and lower body strength in women. *J Strength Cond Res* 1996;10:72-6

80. Dolezal BA, Potteiger JA. Concurrent resistance and endurance traininginfluence basal metabolic rate (BMR) in non-dieting individuals. *J Appl Physiol* 1998;85:695-700

81. Rhea MR, Ball SD, Phillips WT, Burkett LN. A comparison of linear and daily undulating periodized programs with equated volume and intensity for strength. *J Strength Cond Res* 2002; 16(2): 250-5.

82. Heitkamp HC, Horstmann T, Mayer F, Weller J, Dickhuth HH. Gain in strength and muscular balance after balance training. *Int J Sports Med* 2001;285-90.

83. Wolf B, Feys H, Weerdt D, Van der Meer J, Noom M, Aufdemkampe G, Noom M. Effect of a physical therapeutic intervention for balance problems in the elderly: a single-blind, randomized, controlled multicentre trial. *Clin Rehab* 2001:15(6):624-36.

84. Fitzgerald GK, Childs JD, Ridge TM, Irrgang JJ. Agility and perturbation training for a physically active individual with knee osteoarthritis. *Phys Ther* 2002;82(4):372-82

85. Luoto S, Aalto H, Taimela S, Hurri H, Pyykko I, Alaranta H. One footed and externally disturbed two footed postural control in patients with chronic low back pain and health control subjects. A controlled study with follow-up. *Spine* 1998 Oct 1;23(19)2081-9.

86. Borsa PA, Lephart SM, Kocher MS, Lephart SP. Functional assessment and rehabilitation of shoulder proprioception for glenohumeral instability. *J Sport Rehab* 1994;3:84-104

87. Hirsch M, Toole T, Maitland CG, Rider RA. The effects of balance training and high-intensity resistance training on persons with idiopathic Parkinson's disease. *Arch Phys Med Rehab* 2003;84:1109-17.

88. Behm DG, Anderson K, Curnew RS. Muscle force and activation under stable and unstable conditions. *J Strength Cond Res* 2002;16(3):416-22.

89. Meyer K, Steiner R, Lastayo P, Lippuner K, Allemann Y, Eberli F, Schmid J, Saner H, Hoppeler H. Eccentric exercise incoronary patients: central hemodynamic and metabolic responses. *Med Sci Sports Exerc* 2003;35(7):1076-82.

90. Duthie GR, Young WB, Aitken DA. The acute effects of heavy loads on jump squat performance: an evaluation of the complex and contrast methods of power development. *J Strength Cond Res* 2002;16(4):530-8

91. DeRenne C, Hetzler RK, Buxton BP, Ho KW. Effects of training frequency on strength maintenance in pubescent baseball players. *J Strength Cond Res* 1996;10:8-14.

92. Hoffman JR, Fry AC, Howard R, Maresh CM, Armstrong LE, Kraemer WJ. Effects of off-season and in-season resistance training programs on a collegiate male basketball team. *J Hum Muscle Perform* 1991;1:48-55.

93. Baker D. Selecting the appropriate exercises and loads for speed-strength development. *Strength Cond Coach* 1995;3(2):8-16

94. Ebben WP, Watts PB. A review of combined weight training and plyometric training modes: complex training. *Strength Cond* 1998;20(5):18-27.

95. Fleck S, Kontor K. Complex training. *NSCA J* 1986;8(5):66-8.

96. Ebben WP, Blackard DO. Complex training with combined explosive weight and plyometric exercises. *Olymp Coach* 1997;7(4):11-2.

97. Kaikkonen H, Yrlama M, Siljander E, Byman P, Laukkanen R. The effect of heart rate controlled low resistance circuit weight training and endurance training on maximal aerobic power in sedentary adults. *Scand J Med Sci Sports* 2000;10(4):211-5.

98. Jurimae T, Jurimae J, Pihl E. Circulatory response to single circuit weight and walking training sessions of similar energy cost in middle-aged overweight females. *Clin Physiol* 2000;20(2):143-9.

99. Burleson MA, O'Bryant HS, Stone MH, Collins MA, Triplett-McBride T. Effect of weight training exercise and treadmill exercise on post-exercise oxygen consumption. *Med Sci Sports Exerc* 1998;30(4):518-22.

100. Gillette CA, Bullough RC, Melby CL. Postexercise energy expenditure in response to acute aerobic or resistive exercise. *Int J Sport Nutr* 1994;4(4):347-60.

CHAPTER FOURTEEN

Special Populations

Objectives

After studying this chapter, you will be able to:

- Define and describe conditions, dysfunctions or pathologies common in the special populations of clients.
- Understand how these conditions affect the acute training variables within the OPT™ model.
- Alter program design for clients with various conditions.

Key Terms

- Obesity
- Diabetes
- Hypertension
- Osteopenia
- Osteoporosis
- Arthritis

- Osteoarthritis
- Rheumatoid arthritis
- Cancer
- Pregnancy
- Restrictive lung disease
- Obstructive lung disease

Introduction to Special Populations

Up to this point, information studied has been based on the assumption that the clients being worked with are apparently healthy adults. These individuals do not seem to have conditions, dysfunctions or pathologies that would necessitate an alteration in their assessment or program design.

However, in some cases, application of exercise principles for the apparently healthy adult could be potentially dangerous. This could easily be the case for an individual with underlying coronary heart disease, or osteoporosis. In other instances, such as obesity, application of these principles might not harm the participant, but may not be the optimal course of exercise treatment. Thus, the consideration of individuals with special needs is twofold: to provide a margin of safety and to optimize training.

In this chapter, a variety of common conditions and pathologies encountered in exercise training programs will be reviewed. The list is by no means inclusive. There are considerably more pathologies that may require different assessment techniques or altered program design (those with neuromuscular disease, for example). Additional excellent resources are available for other special populations.[1-3]

MODULE 14-1: Age Considerations

Youth Training

Health and fitness professionals are confronted with an increasing variance in clientele seeking assistance in fitness venues. One such growing population is youth clients. Realistically, this population can range between the ages of six and 20 years of age. However, due to biomechanical and physiological variations in growth, it is difficult to precisely determine maturity and the exact age of "youth" training. A 1994 consensus paper by Sallis and colleagues defines adolescence as ages 11-21 years. As such, the guidelines for youth training are largely based on that age range, although physical development and maturation can vary.[4]

Most established guidelines for exercise in the youth population have previously been focused on sport training. Given the alarming increase in childhood obesity and diabetes, increased attention has recently been directed to the development of guidelines to promote a healthy threshold for physical activity (including federal guidelines for school and community programs).[5] Consistent with the recommendations made for adults, adolescents should engage in moderate to vigorous physical activity for a minimum of 20 minutes, three or more days of the week, in order to promote health and chronic disease prevention as adults.[2] Emphasizing the need to initiate high levels of physical activity in even younger children, the National Association for Sport and Physical Education promotes physical activity of at least 30-60 minutes on most, or all, days of the week for elementary school children, focusing on developmentally appropriate activities.[6] The American College of Sports Medicine has published a summary of appropriate field fitness tests for children, as well as specific exercise testing protocols.[7]

Physiological Differences between Children and Adults

It is important to appreciate that there are fundamental physiological differences between children and adults. Children are not miniature adults. While they may experience similar effects to training, they do not demonstrate the same capabilities or progressions. Therefore, the youth population will still use the OPT™ model for training purposes, but will progress in a fashion more specific to their physiological capabilities.

The fitness professional should be aware of some simple physiological differences between children and adults that impact physical performance and include (Table 14-1):[8]

- **Peak oxygen uptake** — The term "maximum oxygen uptake" should not be used to describe peak assessed values in children, since they do not exhibit a plateau in oxygen uptake at maximum exercise. Thus, "peak" is a more appropriate term. When adjusted for body weight, peak oxygen consumption is similar for young and mature males, and slightly higher for young females (compared to mature females). A similar interpretation can be made for force production, or strength.

- **Sub-maximal oxygen demand** — Economy of movement

- **Glycolytic enzymes** — Enzymes used in the glycolysis energy pathway

- **Sweating rate**

The similarity in peak oxygen uptake values between children and adults allows for children to perform endurance related tasks fairly well. This enables youths to train in the stabilization level of training (Phase 1 and 2 of the OPT™ model).

A higher sub-maximal oxygen demand, combined with a lower absolute sweating rate (and other factors beyond the scope of this text) contribute to children having less of a tolerance for temperature extremes. Vigorous exercise in the presence of high temperature and humidity should be restricted to less than 30 minutes. As in adults, adequate hydration is important.

The lower glycolytic enzymes seen in children decrease their ability (or efficiency) to perform higher intensity (or anaerobic) tasks for prolonged periods of time (10-90 seconds). This requires that children have adequate rest intervals when training at high intensities.

Resistance Training in the Youth Population

Overcoming the perception that resistance training is inappropriate for children has resulted in research, which has demonstrated that resistance training is both safe and effective in children.[9,10,11] It has been shown that resistance training for health and fitness conditioning in the youth population results in a lower risk of injury, when compared to many popular sports (including soccer, football and basketball).[12] Furthermore, resistance training in the five-to-14-year-old age group has been associated with a decrease in the number of common injuries.[13] The most common injuries related to resistance training in the youth population have been sprains and strains.[14] These injuries have been attributed to lack of qualified supervision, poor technique and improper progression.[15]

Table 14-1: Physiological and Training Considerations for Youth

Physiological Considerations	Implication of Exercise Compared to Adult	Considerations for Health and Fitness	Considerations in Sport and Athletic Training
"VO$_2$ peak" is similar to adult when adjusted for body weight.	Able to perform endurance tasks relatively well	Physical activity of 30-60+ minutes on most or all days of the week for elementary school children, emphasizing developmentally appropriate activities.[5]	Progression of aerobic training volume should not exceed 10% per period of adaptation. (If weekly training volume was 200 minutes per week, increase to 220 minutes, prior to further increases in intensity.)
Sub-maximal oxygen demand is higher compared to adults for walking and running.	Greater chance of fatigue and heat production in sustained higher intensity tasks	Moderate to vigorous physical activity for adolescents, for a minimum of 20 minutes three or more days of the week[3]	Intensive anaerobic exercise exceeding 10 seconds is not well tolerated. (If using Stage II or III training, provide sufficient rest/recovery intervals between intense bouts of training.)
Glycolytic enzymes are lower than adult	Decreased ability to perform longer duration (10-90 sec.), high-intensity tasks	Resistance exercise for muscular fitness: 1-2 sets of 8-10 exercises 8-12 reps per exercise[7]	Resistance exercise should emphasize proprioception, skill and controlled movements. Repetitions should not exceed: 6-8 per set for strength development, 20 for enhanced muscular endurance
Sweating rate	Decreased tolerance to environmental extremes, particularly heat and humidity	2-3 days per week Duration = 30 minutes, with added time for warm-up and cool-down	2-3 days per week, with increases in overload occurring through increases in reps first, then resistance

This information reiterates the importance of following a systematic approach to exercise training. To promote a safe and effective training environment, health and fitness professionals must first use a simple movement assessment to observe a youth's movement ability.

This movement assessment can easily be done by having the youth perform 10 body-weight squats and 10 push-ups. Follow the kinetic chain checkpoints from Chapter 5 (Fitness Assessment) to gather information regarding movement imbalances. This information will allow for the selection of exercises that are appropriate for each individual youth client. Adherence to these kinetic chain checkpoints during regular exercise will also ensure safe and effective training technique and proper progression.

Results in youth physiological adaptation are similar to those in adults.[16] A review of literature by Faigenbaum and colleagues suggests that, on average, untrained children have increased strength by 30 to 40 percent. It has also been suggested that resistance training has positive effects on motor skills (sprinting and jumping), body composition and bone mineral density.[9,16,17] The source of strength gains and improvements in performance for this population appear to be attributed to neural adaptations in contrast to hypertrophy.[11,18] Relating to flexibility in youth populations, it has been shown that there is a decline as they get older.[19,20]

Collectively, this information is extremely important for a health and fitness professional to understand, in regard to program design. It suggests the importance of assessing each youth for movement deficiencies, incorporating the flexibility continuum and training in the stabilization level (Phase 1 and 2) of the OPT™ model. Progression into Phases 3 through 7 should be predicated on maturity level, dynamic postural control (flexibility and stability) and advice from a licensed physician. Perhaps the most important aspect of training, especially for the youth population, is to make it fun.

Recommendations for youth training parameters are outlined in Tables 14-1 and 14-2. An example youth training program can be found in the appendix of the textbook.

Table 14-2: Basic Exercise Guidelines for Youth Training	
Mode	Walking, jogging, running, games, activities, sports, water activity, resistance training
Frequency	2-5 days per week
Intensity	50-90% of maximum heart rate for cardiorespiratory training
Duration	30-120 minutes per day (for sports)
Movement Assessment	10 body-weight squats. 10 push-ups (if 10 cannot be performed, do as many can be tolerated. Single-leg stance (if can tolerate perform 3-5 single-leg squats per leg)
Flexibility	Follow the Flexibility Continuum specific for each phase of training
Resistance Training	1-5 sets of 6-20 repetitions at 40-70% on 2-3 days per week. Phases 1 and 2 of OPT™ model should be mastered prior to moving on Phases 3-7 should be reserved for mature adolescents based on dynamic postural control and a licensed physician's recommendation.
Special Considerations	Progression for the youth population should be based upon postural control and not on the amount of weight that can be used. Make exercising fun!

Older Adults

By the middle of this century, it is estimated that the number of Americans over the age of 65 will reach approximately 70 million (nearly one in five residents will be considered elderly). As America's population ages, it is increasingly faced with the issue of mortality, longevity and quality of life.[21] This upward drift in average age has significant implications for health and fitness professionals. As the importance of exercise for functional independence becomes more widely known and accepted, opportunities to evaluate and provide meaningful physical training for older adults will increase.

Unfortunately, aging has come to be associated with degeneration and the limited functional ability of the older adult.[22] Typical forms of degeneration in the older adult include osteoporosis, arthritis (osteoarthritis),[23,24] low back pain (LBP)[25,26] and obesity.[27] While special considerations for those specific diseases will be addressed in subsequent modules, considerations for apparently healthy older adults help provide the fitness professional with the fundamental knowledge to effectively evaluate and design programs for this population.

With this being said, it is important to draw a distinction between what is observed in older adults and what is abnormal. For example, it is not unusual to find increased blood pressure at rest and during exercise, due to a combination of physiological aging and behavioral factors. However, blood pressure reaching pre-hypertensive (135 mm HG systolic, 85 mm HG diastolic) or higher levels should be referred to a physician, for further evaluation and treatment, regardless of the client's age.

Likewise, an important observation about older adults lies in the adaptive capability for physiological improvement in fitness. It is known that as adults age all of the following functions decrease:[28,29]

- Maximum attainable heart rate
- Cardiac output
- Muscle mass
- Balance
- Coordination (neuromuscular efficiency)
- Connective tissue elasticity
- Bone mineral density

This obviously affects the central component to fitness. These degenerative processes can lead to a decrease in the functional capacity of the older adult, as defined by overall strength (cardiorespiratory and muscular) and proprioceptive responses.[30,31] Perhaps the most important functional capacity affected is walking. The decreased ability to move freely in one's own

Table 14-3: Physiological and Training Considerations for Older Adults	
Physiological Considerations	**Implications of Health and Fitness Training**
Maximum oxygen uptake, maximum exercise heart rate and measures of pulmonary function will all decrease with increasing age.	Initial exercise workloads should be low and progressed more gradually. 3-5 days per week Duration = 20-45 minutes Intensity = 45-80% of VO_2 max.
Percentage of body fat will increase, and both bone mass and lean body mass will decrease with increasing age.	Resistance exercise is recommended, with lower initial weights and slower progression. (For example: 1-3 set of 8-10 exercises, 8-20 reps Session length = 20-30 minutes)
Balance, gait and neuromuscular coordination may be impaired.	Exercise modalities should be chosen and progressed to safeguard against falls and foot problems. Cardio options include stationary or recumbent cycling, aquatic exercise, or treadmill with handrail support. Resistance options include seated machines progressing to standing exercises
There is a higher rate of both diagnosed and undetected heart disease in the elderly.	Knowledge of pulse assessment during exercise is critical, as is monitoring for chronic disease signs and symptoms.
Pulse irregularity is more frequent.	Careful analysis of medication use and possible exercise effects

environment not only reduces the physical and emotional independence of an individual, it also can lead to an increase in the degenerative cycle.[16]

Many people who exhibit one or more of these degenerative conditions may tend to shy away from known remedies (such as resistance training) out of fear of injury, or feelings of inadequacy.[32] However, research shows that musculoskeletal degeneration may not be entirely age-related and that certain measures can be taken to prevent functional immobility.[33-36] It has also been demonstrated that many of the structural deficits responsible for decreased functional capacity in the older adult (loss of muscle strength and proprioception) can be slowed and even reversed.

By adhering to the OPT™ model, health and fitness professionals can make a dramatic impact on the overall health and well being of the older adult. Training must begin with a PAR-Q and movement assessment such as a squat, sitting and standing from a seated position, or a single-leg stance. This assessment will provide information about quality of movement as well as a person's functional capacity for activities of daily living. Flexibility will be paramount, as older adults lose the elasticity of their connective tissue. Self-myofascial release and static stretching are advised for this population, provided there is sufficient ability to perform the necessary movements. Otherwise, simple forms of active or dynamic stretching may be required to simply get the client to move their joints and "warm-up."

Stages I and II will be appropriate levels of cardiorespiratory training for this population and should progress slowly, however, medications and other co-morbidities must be taken into consideration. Phases 1, 2 and 3 of the OPT™ model will be applicable for this population and should be progressed slowly, with an emphasis on stabilization training (core, balance and progression to standing resistance exercises). As always, consult with a licensed physician for specific information regarding the older adult client.

The physiological considerations and their implications for training apparently healthy older adults are listed in Table 13-2. Resources that further detail the physiological changes that occur in the older adult are available.[37] Refer to the appendix of the textbook for an example program for an older adult.

Table 14-4: Basic Exercise Guidelines for Older Adults	
Mode	Stationary or recumbent cycling, aquatic exercise, or treadmill with handrail support
Frequency	2-5 days per week
Intensity	40-85% of VO$_2$ max.
Duration	30-60 minutes per day or 8-10 min bouts.
Movement Assessment	Push, pull or 5-10 body-weight squats or sitting and standing into a chair. Single-leg balance
Flexibility	Self-myofascial release and static stretching (see Special Considerations)
Resistance Training	1-3 sets of 8-20 repetitions at 40-80% on 2-3 days per week. Phases 1, 2 and 3 of OPT™ model should be mastered prior to moving on. Phases 4-6 should be based on dynamic postural control and a licensed physician's recommendation.
Special Considerations	Progression should be slow, well monitored and based upon postural control. Exercises should be progressed if possible toward free sitting (no support) or standing. Make sure client is breathing in normal manner and avoid holding breath as in a Valsalva maneuver. If client cannot tolerate self-myofascial release or static stretches due to other conditions, perform slow rhythmical active or dynamic stretches.

MODULE 14-1 Summary

The guidelines for youth training are largely based on an 11-21 age range, although physical development and maturation can vary. Adolescents should engage in moderate to vigorous physical activity for a minimum of 20 minutes, three or more days of the week. Elementary school children should engage in 30-60 minutes of physical activity on most days of the week.

Children have lower body weight and peak oxygen uptake than adults. Special considerations must be given to musculoskeletal growth issues as well as children's lower tolerance for temperature extremes. High volume aerobic training is not advisable in children. Instead, physiological adaptations should be developed through resistance training that emphasizes skill and controlled movements.

In older adults, it is important to draw a distinction between what is observed and what is abnormal. These individuals may have increased blood pressure, due to a combination of physiological aging and behavioral factors. In addition, maximum attainable heart rate decreases and cardiac output declines, although peripheral adaptation remains in tact. Resistance training is recommended three to five days per week, using lighter weights and slower progressions.

MODULE 14-1 Quiz

1. Why shouldn't the term the term "maximum oxygen uptake" be used to describe peak assessed values for children?

   _____

   _____

2. In youth populations, the progression of aerobic training volume should not exceed what percentage per period of adaptation.

   ☐ 10   ☐ 20   ☐ 50

3. In older adults, which of the following items will decrease with age:

   ☐ Maximum oxygen uptake   ☐ Bone mass

   ☐ Percentage of body fat   ☐ Measures of pulmonary function

   ☐ Maximum exercise heart rate   ☐ Lean body mass

MODULE 14-2: Obesity

OBESITY:
The condition of subcutaneous fat exceeding the amount of lean body mass.

Obesity is the fastest growing health problem in America and most other industrialized cultures. The trends in the United States are especially alarming. Currently, it is estimated that approximately 33 percent of the adult population and 15 percent of children over the age of six are obese.[38,39] However, it has been demonstrated that perhaps two-thirds of the adult population may be considered overweight.[40] Not only is obesity associated with many chronic diseases discussed in this chapter, it is emotionally difficult as well.

Body Mass Index

The most reliable measure of overweight and obesity in adults is body mass index (BMI). BMI is defined as total body weight in kilograms divided by the height in meters squared. For example, a client with a body weight of 200 pounds (91 kg) and is 70 inches tall (178 cm, or 3.16 m^2) would have a BMI of 29.8 (91/3.16). This is not to suggest that body composition measurements (such as skin fold calipers and/or circumference measurements) cannot be used to assist in developing goals and providing realistic feedback to clients. However, in the obese population, the actual computation of body fat is less clinically accurate or relevant. While BMI is not a perfect measure, it does provide reliable values for comparison and for reasonable goal setting. For example, once the BMI is established, setting a goal of a weight associated with a BMI that is two units less, is easy to derive and monitor.

When BMI is considered, a value of 18.5-24.9 is considered within normal limits, 25-29.9 overweight, and greater than 30 obese. It is estimated that over two-thirds of adults in the United States have a BMI greater than 25. Risk of chronic disease increases in proportion to BMI in the obese population. Yet, radical treatment for obesity (such as medically-supervised fasting, pharmacological or surgical intervention) is generally reserved for individuals with a BMI above 40.

Causes of Obesity

The causes of obesity are the subject of considerable debate, but virtually all experts agree that the fundamental problem (with respect to both prevention and treatment) is energy balance. As such, it is critically important for health and fitness professionals to refer clients to a registered dietitian and/or nutritionist who can provide reasonable and achievable dietary recommendations to coincide with their exercise regimen. Evans and Rosenburg suggest that adults who are not involved in exercising regimens will lose approximately five pounds of muscle per decade, while simultaneously adding 15 pounds of fat per decade.[41] This is exacerbated by the fact that the average person will have an approximate 15 percent decrease in fat-free mass (FFM) between the ages of 30 and 80. When the concept of age-related fat gain was investigated, it was determined that body fat was not an age-related issue, but rather was attributed to the number of hours individuals spent exercising per week.[42] It has also been shown in sedentary individuals that the daily-activity level accounts for more than 75 percent of the variability of body-fat storage in men.[43]

Obesity and Training

With respect to functional movement, research has also shown a correlation between the weight of an individual and the functional capacity of their gait. In a study involving more than two hundred 75-year-old women, the relationship between balance, muscular strength and gait was investigated. It was shown that the heavier individuals exhibited poorer balance, slower gait velocity and shorter steps, regardless of their higher level of muscular strength.[44] It can be inferred that, due to the higher level of strength in the heavier individuals, strength training alone is not the prime issue. Rather, emphasis on balance or proprioceptive training may better facilitate the obese individual, as demonstrated by lack of balance and stepping parameters.

For effective weight loss, caloric expenditure should approximate 200-300 kcal per day, with a minimum weekly output greater than 1,250 kcal associated with exercise.[2] This should be progressively increased to 2,000 calories per week of exercise expenditure. Resistance training should be part of any exercise regimen to promote weight loss. In Chapter 7 (Cardiorespiratory Training), it was shown that circuit style resistance training (when compared to walking at a fast pace) produced near identical caloric expenditure for the same given time span.[45] Other researchers have noted much higher values in similar studies.[46,47] Furthermore, resistance training helps to produce lean body mass. Lean body mass helps to maintain basic metabolic rate, which improves the effectiveness of an energy-balance weight loss program. The same guidelines that are used for adults with normal weight should be employed for resistance training in the obese population, with emphasis on correct form and breathing.

This points to the importance of following the OPT™ model for the obese client. When working with this population, it may be advisable to use exercises in a standing or seated position. Health and movement assessments should always be performed to establish pertinent program design parameters. However, assessing the obese client can be challenging. Following the fitness assessment seen in Chapter 5, using a pushing, pulling and squatting exercise is suggested. These may be best performed with cables, exercise tubing and/or body weight from a standing or seated position. Also, using a single-leg balance assessment is suggested. Flexibility exercises should also be performed from a standing or seated position. For example, using the standing hip flexor (rather than the kneeling hip flexor stretch), standing hamstring, calf stretch and seated adductor stretch would be advised. Self-myofascial release should be used with caution and may need to be done from a standing position or at home (see Psychosocial Aspects of Working with Obese Clients). This population can progress through the Flexibility Continuum as needed.

Core and balance training will be very important for this population, based on their lack of balance and walking speed. Health and fitness professionals must be cautious when placing a client in a prone or supine position to perform many of these exercises, due to the high probability that these clients will also exhibit hypertension. These positions may be contraindicative. Performing many of these exercises in the standing position may be more appropriate. For example, performing prone iso-abs on an incline or cobras in a standing position would be suggested. Other examples include performing crunches or back extensions from a standing position, using a cable resistance. Resistance training should be performed in a seated or standing position as well.

Phases 1, 2 and 3 of the OPT™ model will be appropriate for the obese population. The health and fitness professional should always ensure that the client is breathing normally and not straining to exercise or over-gripping (squeezing too tightly) the exercise equipment, as this can increase blood pressure.

Psychosocial Aspects of Working with Obese Clients

Obesity is a unique chronic disease because it brings with it many issues that affect a person's sense of emotional well-being.[48] It can alter the emotional and social aspects of a person's life just as much as the physical. Health and fitness professionals must be very aware of this when training an obese client in order to ensure that the client feels socially and emotionally safe. This will help to create trust between the client and professional and assist the client in adhering to a program.

Proper exercise selections and positions will be very important to the client's sense of well-being. For example, machines are often not the best choice for exercises because they may require a fair amount of mobility to get in and out of. Using dumbbell, cable or exercise tubing exercises work quite well. The use of self-myofascial release should be done with caution, as many clients will not feel comfortable rolling or lying on the floor. This may be done in the privacy of their own home if they agree. In addition, it is commonly recommended that obese clients engage in weight-supported exercise (such as cycling or swimming) to decrease orthopedic stress. However, walking is often both a preferred activity for many clients and one that is more easily engaged in. Thus, if the benefits of walking, particularly adherence, exceed the perceived risk of an orthopedic injury, walking might well be a primary exercise recommendation. When working with this population, the health and fitness professional must make sure to be aware of the situations, positions and locations in the training facility they are placing the client. Exercise considerations are given in Table 14-5. For an example program for the obese client, please refer to the appendix of the textbook.

Table 14-5:	Basic Exercise Guidelines for Individuals who are Overweight or Obese
Mode	Low-impact or step aerobics (such as treadmill walking, rowing, stationary cycling and water activity)
Frequency	At least 5 days per week
Intensity	60-80% of maximum heart rate. Use the Talk Test* to determine exertion. Stage I cardiorespiratory training progressing to Stage II (intensities may be altered to 40-70% of maximum heart rate if needed).
Duration	40-60 minutes per day, or 20-30 minute sessions twice each day
Movement Assessment	Push, pull, squat Single-leg balance (if tolerated)
Flexibility	Self-myofascial release (only if comfortable to client) Flexibility Continuum
Resistance Training	1-3 sets of 10-15 repetitions on 2-3 days per week. Phases 1-3 will be appropriate performed in a circuit training manner. Higher repetitions such as 20 may be used.
Special Considerations	Make sure client is comfortable — Be aware of positions and locations in the facility your client is in. Exercises should be performed in a standing or seated position. May have other chronic diseases.

*The "**Talk Test**" is a method of measuring intensity, if the health and fitness professional is unable to assess intensity via heart rate. If the client can comfortably carry on a conversation while exercising, he/she is probably at the lower ranges of training heart rate. If he/she is having difficulty finishing a sentence, the client is probably at the high range. Depending on the individual's response and exercise status, adjust intensity accordingly.

Table 14-6: Physiological and Training Considerations for Individuals who are Overweight or Obese	
Physiological Considerations	**Considerations for Health and Fitness**
May have other co-morbidities (diagnosed or undiagnosed), including hypertension, cardiovascular disease or diabetes	Initial screening should clarify the presence of potential undiagnosed co-morbidities.
Maximum oxygen uptake and ventilatory (anaerobic) threshold is typically reduced.	Consider testing and training modalities that are weight-supported (such as cycle ergometer, swimming). If a client does not have these limitations, consider a walking program to improve compliance.
Co-existing diets may hamper exercise ability and result in significant loss of lean body mass.	Initial programming should emphasize low intensity, with a progression in exercise duration (up 60 minutes as tolerable) and frequency (5-7 days per week), before increases are made in intensity of exercise. Exercise intensity should be no greater than 60-80% of work capacity (RPE 11-13), with weekly caloric volume a minimum of 1,250 kcal per week and a progression to 2,000, as tolerable.
Measures of body composition (hydrostatic weighing, skin fold calipers) may not accurately reflect degree of overweight or obesity.	Body mass index (BMI) is recommended as the measure of weight loss. Also use skin fold caliper measurements as a method of monitoring progress and absolute regional loss of body fat.

MODULE 14-2 Summary

Obesity is the fastest growing health problem in the United States. Health and fitness professionals must be prepared to work with obese clients. First, body mass must be measured in order to chart progress. The most reliable measure of overweight and obesity in adults is body mass index (BMI). Once BMI is established, setting a goal weight associated with it is easy to derive and monitor.

When designing programs for overweight and obese clients, their adherence to the type of exercise should be considered. Walking is often a good recommendation if there is little risk of orthopedic injury. For effective weight loss, aerobic exercise should approximate 200-300 kcal per day, with a minimum weekly output of greater than 1,250 kcal associated with exercise. In addition, resistance training should be part of any exercise regimen to promote weight loss. Although it burns fewer calories than aerobic exercise, it preserves lean body mass, which is important for maintaining metabolism. The same resistance training guidelines used for adults with normal weight should be employed in the obese population, focusing on correct form and breathing.

MODULE 14-2 Quiz

1. BMI is defined as total body weight (in kilograms) divided by_____.

2. It is estimated that more than _____ of adults in the United States are overweight, with a BMI above 25?

   ☐ One-fourth   ☐ Half   ☐ Two-thirds

3. In overweight or obese adults, exercise capacity should be no greater than:

   ☐ 10-30% of work capacity   ☐ 40-70% of work capacity

   ☐ 25-55% of work capacity   ☐ 60-90% of work capacity

MODULE 14-3: Diabetes

DIABETES:
Chronic metabolic disorder, caused by insulin deficiency, which impairs glucose usage.

Diabetes is a metabolic disorder in which the body's ability to produce *insulin* (a hormone secreted by the pancreas to help deliver glucose to cells) or to utilize *glucose* (blood sugar) is altered. It is estimated that nearly six percent of the U.S. population has diabetes, with about one million new cases per year. This number is expected to double in the next 15-20 years. Diabetes is also the seventh leading cause of death in the United States.[49] It has been shown that people who develop diabetes prior to the age of 30 are twenty times more likely to die by age 40 than those who do not have diabetes.[50]

There are two primary forms of diabetes: Type I (Insulin Dependent Diabetes) and Type II (Adult-onset Diabetes). Type II is also referred to as "Non-Insulin Dependent Diabetes," although that is technically incorrect. Some Type II diabetics cannot manage their blood glucose levels and do require additional insulin. Coupled with an increase in obesity is the risk of Type II diabetes.

Type I diabetes is typically found in normal (or even underweight) younger individuals and is rooted in a primary disease that impairs normal glucose management. Due to this lack of insulin, blood sugar is not optimally delivered into the cells (particularly muscle and fat cells), resulting in *hyperglycemia* (high levels of blood sugar). To control this high level of blood sugar, the Type I diabetic must inject insulin to compensate for what their pancreas cannot produce. This is important to note because exercise increases the rate in which cells utilize glucose. If the Type I diabetic does not control his/her blood-glucose levels (via insulin injections and dietary carbohydrates) before, during and after exercise, blood-sugar levels can drop rapidly and cause a condition called *hypoglycemia* (low blood sugar), leading to weakness, dizziness and fainting. Although insulin, proper diet and exercise are the primary components prescribed for Type I diabetics, these individuals must still be monitored throughout exercise, to ensure safety.

Type II is associated with obesity, particularly abdominal obesity. The incidence and prevalence of adult Type II diabetes in the United States has increased sharply in recent years. There is significant public health concern about the rising incidence of Type II diabetes in children, associated with both the increase in abdominal obesity and decrease in voluntary physical activity.

Type II diabetics usually produce adequate amounts of insulin; however, their cells are resistant to the insulin (that is, they don't allow insulin to bring adequate amounts of blood sugar into the cell). This condition can lead to *hyperglycemia* (high blood sugar). Chronic hyperglycemia is associated with a number of diseases associated with damage to the kidneys, heart, nerves, eyes, and circulatory system. Although Type II diabetics do not experience the same fluctuations in blood sugar as Type I diabetics, it is still important to be aware of the symptoms, particularly with Type II diabetics using insulin medications.

Exercise and Diabetes

The overriding issue in diabetes is glucose control. Exercise training is effective in that regard, since it acts much like insulin by enhancing the uptake of circulating glucose by skeletal muscle. Studies show that exercise improves a variety of glucose measures including tissue sensitivity, improved glucose tolerance and even a decrease in insulin requirements.[51,52] Thus, exercise has been shown to have a substantial positive effect on the prevention of Type II diabetes.

There are fairly specific recommendations to follow in this population to prevent hypo- and hyperglycemic events during or after exercise, as well as when to defer exercise, based on blood glucose levels or symptoms. In most cases, the exercise management and goals should be the same as would be

Table 14-7: Basic Exercise Guidelines for Individuals with Diabetes	
Mode	Low impact activities (such as cycling, treadmill walking, low impact or step aerobics)
Frequency	4-7 days per week
Intensity	50-90% of maximum heart rate Stage I cardiorespiratory training progressing to stage II and III (may be adjusted to 40-70% of maximum heart rate if needed)
Duration	20-60 minutes
Movement Assessment	Push, pull, overhead squat Single-leg balance
Flexibility	Flexibility Continuum
Resistance Training	1-3 sets of 10-15 repetitions 2-3 days a week Phases 1-3 of the OPT™ model Higher repetitions such as 20 may be used.
Special Considerations	Make sure client has appropriate footwear and have client or physician check feet for blisters or abnormal wear patterns. Advise client or class participant to keep a snack (quick source of carbohydrate) available during exercise, to avoid sudden hypoglycemia. Use self-myofascial release with special care and licensed physician's advise. Avoid excessive reactive training and higher intensity training is not recommended for typical client.

Table 14-8: Physiological and Training Considerations for Individuals with Diabetes

Physiological Considerations	Considerations for Health and Fitness	Considerations in Sport and Athletic Training
Frequently associated with co-morbidities (including cardiovascular disease, obesity and hypertension)	Program should target weekly caloric goal of 1,000-2,000 kcal, progressing as tolerable, to maximize weight loss and cardio protection.	Screening for co-morbidities is important.
Exercise exerts an effect similar to that of insulin.	Increased risk of exercise-induced hypoglycemia	Be cognizant of signs and symptoms of hypoglycemia.
Hypoglycemia may occur several hours after exercise, as well as during exercise.	For those recently diagnosed, glucose should be measured before, during and after exercise.	Restoration of glucose post-event may be necessary to prevent nocturnal hypoglycemia.
Clients taking beta-blocking medications may be unable to recognize signs and symptoms of hypoglycemia.	Some reduction in insulin and increase in carbohydrate intake may be necessary and proportionate to exercise intensity and duration.	Substantial insulin dose reduction may be necessary prior to exercise. Carbohydrate intake, before and during exercise, may be necessary.
Exercise in excessive heat may mask signs of hypoglycemia.	Post-exercise carbohydrate consumption is advisable.	Initial exercise prescription should emphasize low intensity, with a progression in exercise duration (up 60 minutes as tolerable) and frequency (5-7 days per week), for consistent glucose control. Intensity should be no greater than 50-90% of work capacity to start with.
Increased risk for retinopathy	Be cognizant of signs and symptoms of hypoglycemia.	Resistance training guidelines may follow those for normal weight healthy adults (e.g. 1-3 sets of 8-10 exercises, 10-15 reps per set, 2-3 days per week).
Peripheral neuropathy may increase risk for gait abnormalities and infection from foot blisters that may go unnoticed.	Utilize weight-bearing exercise cautiously and wear appropriate footwear.	Check daily for blisters or skin injury and appropriate footwear.

developed to treat the underlying causes of inactivity and excess body weight. However, in contrast to the obesity recommendation to emphasize walking as the primary mode, care must be taken to prevent blisters and foot micro-trauma that could result in foot infection. Special note should be taken with respect to advice about carbohydrate intake or insulin use, not only before exercise, but afterwards, to reduce the risk of a hypoglycemic event post exercise.

The parameters for exercise generally follow those advised for obese adults, since many Type II diabetic patients are obese, and since daily exercise is recommended for more stable glucose management. Lower impact exercise modalities reduce the risk of injury and resistance exercise is advised as part of an overall exercise plan for health and fitness. Assessment procedures should follow those outlined in Chapter 5 (Fitness Assessments). Flexibility exercises can be used as suggested; however, special care should be given to self-myofascial release and may be contraindicated for anyone with peripheral neuropathy (loss of protective sensation in feet and legs). Obtain the advice of a licensed physician concerning self-myofascial release (foam rolling) and specific clients. Phases 1, 2 and 3 of the OPT™ model are appropriate for this population; however, the use of reactive training may be inappropriate. For an example program for the diabetic client, please refer to the appendix of this textbook.

MODULE 14-3 Summary

Diabetes impairs the body's ability to produce insulin. Type I Diabetes (Insulin Dependent Diabetes) is typically found in younger individuals. If the Type I diabetic does not control blood-glucose levels (via insulin injections and dietary carbohydrates) before, during and after exercise, blood-sugar levels can drop rapidly and cause hypoglycemia leading to weakness, dizziness and fainting. Type II Diabetes (Adult-onset Diabetes), is associated with obesity, particularly abdominal obesity. Type II diabetics usually produce adequate amounts of insulin; however, their cells are resistant to the insulin, which can lead to hyperglycemia.

Exercise is effective for glucose control. Exercise recommendations generally follow those advised for obese adults, since many Type II diabetic patients are obese and daily exercise is recommended for more stable glucose management. However, weight-bearing activities may need to be avoided to prevent blisters and foot micro-trauma that could result in foot infection. Carbohydrate intake or insulin use should be stressed before exercise as well as afterwards, to reduce the risk of a post-exercise hypoglycemic event.

Follow exercise guidelines for obese adults, using lower impact exercise modalities. Special care should be given to self-myofascial release and may be contraindicated for anyone with a loss of protective sensation in feet and legs. Phases 1, 2 and 3 of the OPT™ model are appropriate for this population, but reactive training may be inappropriate.

MODULE 14-3 Quiz

1. Due to a lack of insulin in Type I diabetes, blood sugar is not optimally delivered to the cells, which results in:

   ☐ Hyperglycemia   ☐ Hypoglycemia

2. Because peripheral neuropathy may increase the risk of gait abnormalities and infection, what is it important to check for?

   _____

3. Clients taking beta-blocking medications may be unable to recognize signs and symptoms of hypoglycemia.

   ☐ True   ☐ False

MODULE 14-4: Hypertension

The definition of **hypertension** is blood pressure with the systolic (top number) reading greater than or equal to 140 mmHg and the diastolic (bottom number) reading greater than or equal to 90 mmHg. (Of course, if a client is taking medication to control blood pressure, that individual is considered hypertensive, regardless of a normal tension reading at rest.) More recent guidelines emphasize that a measurement of 135/85 mmHG should be considered 'pre-hypertensive' and should be lowered through appropriate lifestyle modifications. Average, healthy blood pressure is 120/80. Some of the most common contributors to hypertension include smoking, a diet high in fat (particularly saturated fat) and excess weight. The health risks of hypertension are well known and include increased risk for stroke, cardiovascular disease, chronic heart failure and kidney failure.

> **HYPERTENSION:** Raised systemic arterial blood pressure, which, if sustained at a high enough level, is likely to induce cardiovascular or end-organ damage.

One traditional method of controlling hypertension is through anti-hypertensive medications. Although medications have been proven effective, proper cardiorespiratory exercise and diet have also been shown to reduce blood pressure, potentially allowing for the elimination of medications. Fortunately, there is ample evidence to suggest that exercise can have a significant impact on the lowering of elevated blood pressure.[53,54,55] It may also cause the body to produce a more appropriate response to exercise or other physiological stressors. The changes appear mild, on the order of 3-4 mmHG (or more with higher resting blood pressure) but any lowering of pressure conveys a lowered overall health risk, and is important. Interestingly, low to moderate cardiorespiratory exercise has been shown to be just as effective as high-intensity activity in reducing blood pressure. This is important for elderly or obese individuals with high blood pressure and who are not physically capable of performing high-intensity cardiorespiratory exercise.

It is important to emphasize the importance of an overall plan to reduce blood pressure that includes exercise, diet, weight loss (if appropriate) and, importantly, compliance with the medical regimen prescribed by a physician. Often, compliance with medicating is a serious problem with hypertensive individuals, since they do not "feel sick." The health and fitness professional must monitor and stress medication compliance.

It is also important for the health and fitness professional to evaluate the client's heart rate response to exercise, as measured during a sub-maximal exercise test or even a simple assessment of heart rate, during a comfortable exercise load. Hypertensive clients frequently take medications (most commonly beta-blockers, but others may have similar effects) that blunt the

Table 14-9: Basic Exercise Guidelines for Individuals with Hypertension	
Mode	Stationary cycling, treadmill walking, rowers
Frequency	3-7 days per week
Intensity	50-85% of maximum heart rate Stage I cardiorespiratory training
Duration	30-60 minutes
Movement Assessment	Push, pull, overhead squat Single-leg balance (squat if tolerated)
Flexibility	Static and active in a standing or seated position
Resistance Training	1-3 sets of 10-20 repetitions 2-3 days a week Phases 1-2 of the OPT™ model Tempo should not exceed 1 sec for isometric and concentric portions (e.g. 4/1/1 instead of 4/2/2 or 4/2/1 or 3/2/1). Utilize circuit and/or PHA weight training as an option, with appropriate rest intervals.
Special Considerations	Avoid heavy lifting and Valsalva maneuvers — make sure client breathes normally. Do not let client over-grip weights or clinch fists when training. Modify tempo to avoid extended isometric and concentric muscle action. Perform exercises in a standing or seated position. Allow client to stand up slowly to avoid possible dizziness. Progress client slowly.

heart rate response to exercise, thus invalidating prediction equations or estimates of exercise heart rate.

When training the hypertensive client, it is imperative that the health and fitness professional also monitor the body position. Similar to the obese and diabetic client, body position can dramatically increase the effects of hypertension. Often, supine or prone positions (especially when the head is lower in elevation than the heart) can increase tension. These positions may be contraindicated.

For assessment of a hypertensive client, the health and fitness professional should follow the guidelines in Chapter 5 (Fitness Assessment). Use of a single-leg balance (or squat) exercise can also be beneficial, if tolerated by the client. If possible, all other exercises should be performed in a seated or standing position. Clients may use the full flexibility continuum; however, static and active stretching may be the easiest and safest. Self-myofascial release may be contraindicated, since it requires lying down. Consult with specific clients' physicians for specific recommendations. Cardiorespiratory training should focus on Stage I and progress only upon physician's approval.

Table 14-10: Physiological and Training Considerations for Individuals with Hypertension	
Physiological Considerations	**Considerations for Health and Fitness, Sport and Athletic Training**
Blood pressure response to exercise may be variable and exaggerated, depending on the mode and level of intensity.	A program of continuous, lower-intensity (50-85% of work capacity) aerobic exercise is initially recommended. Frequency and duration parameters should be at minimum 3-5 days per week, 20-45 minutes per day, with additional increases on overall volume of exercise if weight loss is also desired.
Despite medication, clients may arrive with pre-exercise hypertension.	Resistance exercise should consist of a peripheral-heart-action and/or circuit training style. Avoid Valsalva maneuvers, emphasize rhythmic breathing and a program design for muscular fitness (e.g. 1-3 sets of 8-10 exercises, 10-20 reps, 2-3 days per week).
Hypertension frequently is associated with other co-morbidities, including obesity, cardiovascular disease and diabetes.	Screening for co-morbidities is important. Exercise should target a weekly caloric goal of 1,500-2,000 kcal, progressing as tolerable, to maximize weight loss and cardio protection.
Some medications, such as beta-blockers, for hypertension will attenuate the heart rate at rest and its response to exercise.	For clients taking medications that will influence heart rate, do not use predicted maximum heart rate or estimates for the exercise. Instead, use actual heart rate response.
	Accepted blood pressure contraindications for exercise include a SBP of 200 mm HG and a DBP of 115 mm HG. Always check with any other lower guidelines the fitness facility may have in place.

Core exercises in the standing position would include performing prone iso-abs on an incline, or cobras in a standing position (two-leg or single-leg). Other examples include performing crunches or back extensions from a standing position using a cable resistance. Reactive training would not be recommended for this population.

Resistance training should be performed in a seated or standing position as well. Phases 1, 2 and 3 of the OPT™ model will be appropriate for this population. The programs should be performed in a circuit style and/or using the Peripheral Heart Action (PHA) training system (see Chapter 12 Resistance Training). The health and fitness professional should always ensure that the client is breathing normally and not straining to exercise or over-gripping (squeezing too tightly) the exercise equipment as this can increase blood pressure. In addition, the health and fitness professional should monitor the client when rising from a seated or lying position as he/she may experience dizziness. For an example program for the hypertensive client, please refer to the appendix of this textbook.

MODULE 14-4 Summary

Normal blood pressure is 120/80 mmHG. Hypertension is defined as a blood pressure greater than 140/90, although 135/85 is considered pre-hypertensive. Hypertension can be controlled through cardiorespiratory exercise and diet. However, clients must also be sure to follow any prescribed medication or physician's recommendations.

Individuals with hypertension should engage in low intensity aerobic exercise, but may want to avoid resistance training. Health and fitness professionals should measure hypertensive clients' heart rate response to exercise, instead of relying on estimates or equations.

Monitoring body position is very important. Supine or prone positions (especially when the head is lower in elevation than the heart) may be contraindicated. Most exercises should be performed in a seated or standing position. The full flexibility continuum can be used, but static and active stretching may be easiest and safest. Self-myofascial release may be contraindicated. Cardiorespiratory training should focus on Stage 1 and progress only upon physician's approval. Reactive training would not be recommended for this population. Resistance training should be performed in a seated or standing position as well. Phases 1 and 2 of the OPT™ model are appropriate. Programs should be performed in a circuit style and/or using the Peripheral Heart Action (PHA) training system.

MODULE 14-4 Quiz

1. What are some of the most common contributors to hypertension?

   _____

2. Exercise may only lower blood pressure by _____ to _____ mmHG, but any lowering of pressure conveys a lowered overall health risk, and is important.

3. Clients who take beta-blockers may display a skewed heart rate response to exercise.

   ☐ True   ☐ False

MODULE 14-5:
Coronary Heart Disease

Since reaching epidemic proportions in the mid-20th century, deaths from heart disease have steadily declined in the United States, but still account for approximately 40 percent of all deaths annually. Importantly, most recent statistics suggest nearly 18 million individuals in the United States have coronary artery disease or chronic heart failure, with another 50 million diagnosed with high blood pressure.[56]

For individuals with coronary artery disease, the underlying pathology of concern has traditionally been the plaque accumulation in the coronary arteries, and the eventual obstruction of the artery, resulting in a myocardial infarction (or heart attack). The procedures that have evolved over the years have all been designed with this in mind.

In recent years, there has been increased emphasis on improving the health of the internal lining of the coronary artery, resulting in plaque "stabilization." More recent research has suggested that it is unstable coronary lesions that rupture and precipitate most coronary events. Not surprisingly, factors such as stress and smoking are known to destabilize arterial endothelium. Exercise is a major factor that appears to improve the stability of the endothelium.

It is logical that in increasing numbers, individuals with diagnosed heart disease (as well as a small percentage of individuals with undiagnosed heart disease) engage in regular exercise in health and fitness facilities and/or seek the advice of the health and fitness professional. The cardiovascular complication rate is low in exercise programs, probably owing to the fact that the clients are well managed by their physicians and that healthier clients are more likely to engage in exercise. Nonetheless, health and fitness professionals must be aware of the presence of clients with heart disease and help design effective exercise programs with the knowledge that exercise can pose a risk for clients with heart disease.

In some cases, clients will begin a fitness program after completing a cardiac rehabilitation program. However, research shows that less than 30 percent of heart patients (and a far lower percentage of women) are referred to and participate in cardiac rehabilitation programs.[57] In any case, the health and fitness professional must have a clear understanding about the client's disease, medication use and most importantly, the upper safe limit of exercise — and any other restrictions — imposed by the client's physician. The health and fitness professional must not compromise on obtaining this information, and client participation must not proceed until the information is received. In many cases, the client can facilitate obtaining this information.

Clients must be able to find and monitor their own pulse rate and/or use an accurate monitor in order to stay below their safe upper limit of exercise. (Heart rate should never be estimated from existing prediction formulas for clients with heart disease.) It is important to note that the heart rate response to exercise will almost always vary considerably from age-predicted formulas, and will often be lower. While symptoms should always supersede anything else as a sign to decrease or stop exercising, some clients may not have this warning system, so monitoring of heart rate becomes increasingly important.

Clients with stable coronary artery disease (and especially those that have participated in a cardiac rehabilitation program) understand the essential benefits of exercise, which include an increase in mortality, increased exercise tolerance, muscle strength, reduction in angina and heart failure symptoms, and

Table 14-11:	Basic Exercise Guidelines for Individuals with Coronary Heart Disease
Mode	Large muscle group activities, such as stationary cycling, treadmill walking or rowing
Frequency	At least 3 days/week
Intensity	40-85% of maximum heart rate reserve Stage 1 cardiorespiratory training
Duration	5-10 minute warm up, followed by 20-40 minutes of exercise, followed by a 5-10 minute cool-down
Movement Assessment	Push, pull, overhead squat Single-leg balance (squat if tolerated)
Flexibility	Static and active in a standing or seated position
Resistance Training	1-3 sets of 10-20 repetitions 2-3 days a week Phases 1-2 of the OPT™ model Tempo should not exceed 1 sec for isometric and concentric portions (e.g. 4/1/1 instead of 4/2/2 or 3/2/1). Utilize circuit and/or PHA weight training as an option, with appropriate rest intervals.
Special Considerations	Be aware that clients may have other diseases to consider as well, such as diabetes, hypertension, peripheral vascular disease or obesity. Modify tempo to avoid extended isometric and concentric muscle action. Avoid heavy lifting and Valsalva maneuvers — make sure client breathes normally. Do not let client over-grip weights or clinch fists when training. Perform exercises in a standing or seated position. Progress exercise slowly.

Table 14-12: Physiological and Training Considerations for Individuals with Coronary Heart Disease	
Physiological Considerations	**Considerations for Health and Fitness, Sport and Athletic Training**
The nature of heart disease may result in a specific level of exercise, above which it is dangerous to perform.	The upper safe limit of exercise, preferably by heart rate, must be obtained. Heart rate should never be estimated from existing prediction formulas for clients with heart disease. Consult their physician.
Clients with heart disease may not have angina (chest pain equivalent) or other warning signs.	Clients must be able to monitor pulse rate and/or use an accurate monitor, to stay below the upper safe limit of exercise.
Between the underlying disease and medication use, the heart rate response to exercise will nearly always vary considerably from age-predicted formulas, and will almost always be lower.	While symptoms should always supercede anything else as a sign to decrease or stop exercising, some clients may not have this warning system, so monitoring of heart rate becomes increasingly important.
Clients may have other co-morbidities (such as diabetes, hypertension, peripheral vascular disease or obesity).	Screening for co-morbidities is important and modifications to exercise made based on these diagnoses.
Peak oxygen uptake (as well as ventilatory threshold) are often reduced due to the compromised cardiac pump and peripheral muscle deconditioning.	The exercise prescription should be low intensity, to start, and based on recommendations provided by a certified exercise specialist or physical therapist with specialty training. Aerobic training guidelines should follow, at minimum, 20-30 minutes 3-5 days per week at 40-85% of maximum capacity, but below the upper safe limits prescribed by the physician.
	A weekly caloric goal of 1,500-2,000 kcal is usually recommended, progressing as tolerable, to maximize cardio protection.
	Resistance training may be started after the patient has been exercising asymptomatically and comfortably for >3 months in the aerobic exercise program. A circuit training format is recommended, 8-10 exercises, 1-3 set of 10-20 reps per exercise, emphasizing breathing control and rest as needed between sets.

improved psychological status and social adjustment.[58] There is also evidence that heart disease may be slowed (or even reversed) when a multifactor intervention program of intensive education, exercise, counseling and lipid lowering medications are used, as appropriate.[59-61]

Health and fitness professionals must be careful to not overstate the benefits of exercise as a singular intervention and must emphasize to clients the importance of a multidisciplinary approach to heart disease. That said, exercise is critically important and can be safely conducted in most health and fitness settings.

The health and fitness professional should follow the guidelines in Chapter 5 (Fitness Assessment) for assessment of these clients. Use of a single-leg balance (or squat) exercise can also be beneficial, if tolerated by the client. If possible, all other exercises should be performed in a seated or standing position. Clients should stay with static and active stretching in a standing or seated position, since they may be the easiest and safest to perform. Consult with a licensed physician for specific recommendations concerning self-myofascial release. Cardiorespiratory training should focus on Stage I and only progress upon physician's advice.

Core exercises in the standing position would include performing prone iso-abs on an incline or cobras in a standing position (two-leg or single-leg). Other examples include performing crunches or back extensions from a standing position, using a cable resistance. Reactive training would not be recommended for this population in the initial months of training.

Resistance training should be performed in a seated or standing position, as well. Phases 1 and 2 of the OPT™ model will be appropriate for this population. The programs should be performed in a circuit style and/or using the Peripheral Heart Action (PHA) training system (see Chapter 12, Resistance Training). The health and fitness professional should always ensure that the client is breathing normally and not straining to exercise or over-gripping (squeezing too tightly) the exercise equipment, as this can increase blood pressure. For an example program for the client with coronary heart disease, please refer to the appendix of this textbook.

MODULE 14-5 Summary

Nearly 18 million individuals in the United States have coronary artery disease or chronic heart failure, with another 50 million diagnosed with high blood pressure The cardiovascular complication rate is low in exercise programs, however health and fitness professionals must be aware of the presence of clients with heart disease and help design effective exercise programs with the knowledge that exercise can pose a risk for clients with heart disease

A health and fitness professional must have a clear understanding about a client's disease, medication use and upper safe limit of exercise imposed by the client's physician. Participation must not proceed until the information is received.

Clients must be able to find and monitor their own pulse rate to stay below the safe upper limit of exercise. Heart rate should *never* be estimated from existing prediction formulas since it will almost often be lower than age-predicted formulas.

Aerobic low-intensity exercise is recommended, with a weekly caloric expenditure goal of 1,500-2,000 kcal. Resistance training should not be started until the client has been exercises without any problems for at least three months.

Most exercises should be performed in a seated or standing position. Flexibility exercises should be limited to static and active stretching in a seated position. Self-myofascial release should be pre-approved by a physician. Cardiorespiratory training should focus on Stage 1 and progress only upon physician's approval. Reactive training would not be recommended for this population in the initial months of training. Resistance training should be performed in a seated or standing position as well. Phases 1 and 2 of the OPT™ model are appropriate. Programs should be performed in a circuit style and/or using the Peripheral Heart Action (PHA) training system.

MODULE 14-5 Quiz

1. Annual deaths from heart disease account for _____% of all deaths in the United States?

   ☐ 40   ☐ 10   ☐ 75

2. Symptoms should always supersede anything else as a sign to decrease or stop exercising.

   ☐ True   ☐ False

3. Peak oxygen uptake is often _____ in clients with heart disease.

   ☐ Increased   ☐ Decreased

MODULE 14-6: Osteoporosis

OSTEOPENIA:
A decrease in the calcification or density of bone as well as reduced bone mass.

OSTEOPOROSIS:
Condition in which these is a decrease in bone mass and density as well as an increase in the space between bones, resulting in porosity and fragility.

Osteopenia is the precursor to osteoporosis and is indicated upon screening by a lowered bone mass. **Osteoporosis** is divided into two types (I and II) and in the vast majority of cases, fitness professionals are much more likely to see clients with Type I, as the onset of Type II is typically 70 years and older. Health and fitness professionals will encounter an increasing number of clients with osteopenia and osteoporosis. While the vast majority of clients will be female, males can, in fact, have either of these diseases.[62]

Type I osteoporosis is most commonly associated with, and is most prevalent in, postmenopausal women. A principal observation in Type I osteoporosis is a deficit in estrogen (usually secondary to menopause). The disease is characterized by an increase in bone re-absorption (removal of old bone) with a decrease in bone remodeling (formation of new bone). This leads to a decrease in bone mineral density.

Osteoporosis commonly affects the neck of the femur and the lumbar vertebrae. These structures are considered part of the core and are located in the region of the body where all forces come together. Thus, decreased bone mineral density places the core in a weakened state and thus, more susceptible to injury, such as a fracture.[62] Research has shown that the risk of hip fractures doubles every five years in postmenopausal women over the age of 50.[62] Furthermore, osteoporosis affects more than 25 million people each year, resulting in approximately 1.5 million hip fractures. Of these 1.5 million hip fractures, only 20 percent of the patients return to a normal functional status.[63]

There are a variety of risk factors that influence osteoporosis. One of the most important is the amount of peak bone mass (or density). Peak bone mass is the highest amount of bone mass a person is able to achieve during his/her lifetime.[64] New bone formation (remodeling) occurs as the result of stress placed upon the musculoskeletal system. In order to maintain consistent bone remodeling, people must remain active enough to ensure adequate stress is being placed on their bodies. This is imperative for adolescents and young adults in order to reach a high peak bone mass.

Other risk factors include a lack of physical inactivity, smoking, excess alcohol consumption and low dietary calcium intake. The key for the health and fitness professional is to recognize that these factors can be influenced through a comprehensive health and fitness program. In addition to exercise programs, clients should be encouraged to modify increased dietary intake of calcium, decrease alcohol intake and to cease smoking.

With respect to physical activity, it is important to know whether the diagnosis is osteopenia or osteoporosis, and if the latter, to what degree the client may engage in weight bearing activities or resistive exercise training. That is, there is a balance between the benefit of providing exercises that are designed to increase bone through the provision of bone stress (weight bearing exercise or heavier resistive exercises) and the risk of fracture that might be precipitated by advanced osteoporosis.

It has been demonstrated that individuals who partake in resistance training have a higher bone mineral density than those who do not.[65-67] Resistance training, however, has been shown to improve bone mineral density by no more than five percent and some researchers believe that this does not represent a high enough increase to prevent fractures from occurring.[68] In fact, it has been estimated that a 20-percent increase in bone mineral density is necessary to offset fractures.[68] Thus, it has been suggested that training which focused on the prevention of falls, rather than strength alone, is more advantageous for the elderly.[30,68] Therefore, exercise regimens that combine resistance training to increase bone mineral density with flexibility, core and balance training to enhance proprioception (as seen in the OPT™ model) might better facilitate the needs of this population.[65-67,69]

When using the OPT™ model with this population, the health and fitness professional must follow some precautionary measures. If the client

Table 14-13: Basic Exercise Guidelines for Individuals with Osteoporosis	
Mode	Stationary or recumbent cycling, aquatic exercise, or treadmill with handrail support
Frequency	2-5 days per week
Intensity	40-85% of VO$_2$ peak. Stage I cardiorespiratory training progressing to Stage II
Duration	30-60 minutes per day or 8-10 min bouts
Movement Assessment	Push or pull 5-10 body weight squats or sitting and standing into a chair
Flexibility	Static and active stretching
Resistance Training	1-3 sets of 8-20 repetitions at up to 85% on 2-3 days per week. Phases 1, 2 and 3 of OPT™ model should be mastered prior to moving on.
Special Considerations	Progression should be slow, well monitored and based upon postural control. Exercises should be progressed if possible toward free sitting (no support) or standing. Focus exercises on hips, thighs, back and arms. Avoid excessive spinal loading on squat/leg press exercises. Make sure client is breathing in normal manner and avoid holding breath as in a Valsalva maneuver.

Table 14-14: Physiological and Training Considerations for Individuals with Osteoporosis

Physiological Considerations	Considerations for Health and Fitness, Sport and Athletic Training
Maximum oxygen uptake and ventilatory threshold is frequently lower, due to chronic deconditioning.	Typical exercise loads prescribed are consistent with fitness standards: 40-70% of maximum work capacity, 3-5 days per week, approximately 20-30 minutes per session.
Gait and balance may be negatively affected.	Physiological and physical limitations point to low-intensity, weight-supported exercise programs that emphasize balance training.
Chronic vertebral fractures may result in significant lower back pain.	For clients with osteopenia (and no contraindications to exercise), resistance training is recommended to build bone mass. For clients who can engage in resistance exercise, recommended loads are relatively high intensity (>75% of 1RM). A circuit training format is recommended, 8-10 exercises, 1 set of 8-12 reps per exercise, with rest as needed between sets.
Age, disease, physical stature and deconditioning may place the client at risk for falls.	For clients with severe osteoporosis, exercise modality should be shifted to water exercise to reduce risk of loading fracture. If aquatic exercise is not feasible, use other weigh supported exercise, such as cycling, and monitor signs and symptoms. Reinforce other lifestyle behaviors that will optimize bone health, including smoking cessation, reduced alcohol intake and increased dietary calcium intake.

demonstrates the ability to move fairly well without assistance, the fitness assessment reviewed in Chapter 5 may be followed. If the client is not able to get around very well, use more stable, machine-based equipment. Follow the kinetic chain checkpoints as closely as possible with this population, but realize that there may be degenerative deformations in their posture that cannot be corrected. Get clients to their own ideal position, not a general ideal position. Exercises should be performed in a seated or standing position.

Flexibility should be limited to static and active stretching. The use of self-myofascial release may be contraindicated for this population. Cardiorespiratory training should begin in Stage 1 (with a walking program, if tolerated). Weight bearing activities may be more beneficial to increasing bone mineral density. Progression to Stage II cardiorespiratory training should be based upon physician's advice and client's ability.

Example core exercises in the standing position would include performing prone iso-abs on an incline, or cobras in a standing position (two-leg or single-leg). Other examples include performing back extensions from a standing position, using a cable resistance (being cautious of excessive extension). Care should be taken with crunches or movements with a lot of spinal flexion. Monitor range of motion and check with a licensed physician. Reactive training would not be recommended for this population.

Resistance training should be performed in a seated or standing position, as well. Phases 1, 2 and 3 of the OPT™ model will be appropriate for this population. Research has indicated that higher intensities (75-85 percent) are needed to stimulate bone formation. Furthermore, it appears that the load (rather than the amount of repetitions) is the determining factor in bone formation.[70] However, to ensure proper kinetic chain preparation for these higher intensities, the health and fitness professional should progress clients through the OPT™ model. Stabilization training (especially balance exercises) will be just as important to counter a lack of balance that can lead to falls and hip fractures. For training to have an effect on bone mass it will require approximately six months of consistent exercise at high enough intensities. This means that the client will be making a long-term commitment to the exercise program. If the client is not progressed appropriately (following the OPT™ model), he/she may acquire injuries that will be a setback. The programs may be performed in a circuit style and/or using the Peripheral Heart Action (PHA) training system (see Chapter 12 Resistance Training), focusing on hips, thighs, back and arms. Progressing exercises to the standing position will help increase stress to the hips, thighs and back as well as increase the demand for balance. Both components are necessary to overcome the effects of osteoporosis. For an example program for the osteoporotic client, please refer to the appendix in the textbook.

MODULE 14-6 Summary

Clients with osteopenia show a lowered bone mass. This is the precursor to osteoporosis. Osteoporosis is divided into two types. Fitness professionals are much more likely to see clients with Type I, the vast majority of these being female.

Physical inactivity, smoking, excess alcohol consumption and low dietary calcium intake are factors that contribute to the risk of osteoporosis. In addition to exercise, clients should be encouraged to modify increased dietary intake of calcium, alcohol intake and to quit smoking.

If the diagnosis is osteoporosis, a physical must dictate to what degree the client may engage in weight bearing activities or resistance training. The benefit of exercises designed to increase bone density may be outweighed by the risk of fracture. Exercise regimens that combine resistance training to increase bone mineral density with flexibility, core and balance training to enhance proprioception might better facilitate the needs of this population.

Clients who can move fairly well, without assistance, can use the fitness assessment reviewed in Chapter 5. Those not able to get around very well, should use more stable, machine-based equipment. Kinetic chain checkpoints should be followed, taking into consideration that degenerative deformations in posture may not be ale to be corrected. Exercises should be performed in a seated or standing position.

Flexibility exercises should be limited to static and active stretching in a seated position. Self-myofascial release may be contraindicated for this population. Cardiorespiratory training should focus on Stage I (with a walking program, if tolerated). Progression to Stage II cardiorespiratory training should be based upon physician's advice and client's ability. Care should be taken with crunches or movements with a lot of spinal flexion. Reactive training would not be recommended for this population. Resistance training should be performed in a seated or standing position. Phases 1 and 2 of the OPT™ model are appropriate. Six months of consistent exercise at high intensities, progressed appropriately, will be required for training to have an effect on bone mass. This means that the client will be making a long-term commitment to the exercise program. Programs should be performed in a circuit style and/or using the Peripheral Heart Action (PHA) training system, focusing on hips, thighs, back and arms and progressing exercises to the standing position.

MODULE 14-6 Quiz

1. The onset of Type II osteoporosis is generally seen in individuals over the age of _____.

2. A principal observation in Type I osteoporosis is a deficit in testosterone.
    ☐ True   ☐ False

3. For clients with osteoporosis who can engage in resistance exercise, the recommended loads are relatively _____ in intensity.
    ☐ Low   ☐ Moderate   ☐ High

MODULE 14-7: Arthritis

Arthritis is an inflammatory condition that mainly affects the joints of the body. It is estimated that arthritis is the most common chronic condition, affecting 50 percent of persons over the age of 65 and more than 15 percent of the American population.[71] By the year 2020, arthritis is predicted to reach approximately 18 percent of the American population.[72] Two of the most common types of arthritis are *osteoarthritis* and *rheumatoid arthritis*.

Osteoarthritis is caused by degeneration of cartilage in joints. This lack of cartilage creates a wearing on the surfaces of articulating bones, causing inflammation and pain at the joint. Some of the most commonly affected joints are in the hands, knees, hips and spine.

Rheumatoid arthritis is a degenerative joint disease in which the body's immune system mistakenly attacks its own tissue (in this case, tissue in the joint or organs). This can cause an inflammatory response in multiple joints leading to pain and stiffness. The condition is systemic and may affect both a variety of joints and organ systems. Joints most commonly affected by this condition include the hands, feet, wrists and knees. It is usually characterized by morning stiffness, lasting over a half hour, which can be both acute and chronic, with eventual loss of joint integrity.

It is important for the health and fitness professional to understand the difference between rheumatoid arthritis and osteoarthritis, and be aware of the signs and symptoms of an acute rheumatoid arthritis exacerbation. In the presence of an arthritic flare-up, even flexibility exercises may be curtailed.

In addition, health and fitness professionals should monitor the progress of clients with arthritis to assess the effects of the exercise program on joint pain. Pain persisting for more than one hour after exercise is an indication that the exercise should be modified or eliminated from the routine. Moreover, exercises of higher intensity and/or involving high repetitions are to be avoided, to decrease joint aggravation. In that regard, a circuit program or multiple session format are suitable for clients with arthritis.

Health and fitness professionals need to be aware of the medications being taken by clients with arthritis. Clients taking oral corticosteroids, particularly over time, may have osteoporosis, increased body mass and (if there is a history of gastrointestinal bleeding) anemia. Steroids also increase fracture risk.

Research indicates that people exhibiting osteoarthritis have a decrease in strength and proprioception.[73,74] Wegner and colleagues have demonstrated that individuals with arthritis have a decreased ability to balance while standing.[57] In addition, Slemenda and colleagues noted that loss in knee-

ARTHRITIS: Chronic inflammation of the joints.

OSTEOARTHRITIS: Arthritis in which cartilage becomes soft, frayed, or thins out, due to trauma or other conditions.

RHEUMATOID ARTHRITIS: Arthritis primarily affecting connective tissues, in which there is a thickening of articular soft tissue, and extension of synovial tissue over articular cartilages that have become eroded.

extensor strength was a strong predictor of osteoarthritis.[73,74] Furthermore, researchers have shown that patients with osteoarthritis exhibit increased muscle inhibition of knee extensors and were not able to effectively activate their knee-extensor musculature to optimal levels.[75,76]

Balance (or proprioception) and muscle strength are vital components of walking and, therefore, any deficit in these areas could potentially have a negative affect one's ability to exercise and perform activities of daily living. This claim was supported by a study that showed a significant decrease in dynamic balance for elderly people who had a history of falling.[77]

It used to be common practice for arthritic patients to avoid strenuous exercise. However, research on the effects of training on the symptoms of arthritis have begun a paradigm shift.[78,79] Tufts University shows that a 12-week strength-training program provided relief from arthritic symptoms.[79] Hurley and colleagues demonstrated that a four-week training regimen (including proprioceptive training) decreased muscle inhibition and increased muscle strength in patients with moderate muscle inhibition.

Therefore, individuals with arthritis are advised to participate in a regular exercise program that follows the OPT™ methodology for increasing

Table 14-15: Basic Exercise Guidelines for Individuals with Arthritis	
Mode	Treadmill walking, stationary cycling, rowers, low impact or step aerobics
Frequency	3-5 days per week
Intensity	60-80% of maximum heart rate Stage I cardiorespiratory training progressing to Stage II (May be reduced to 40-70% of maximum heart rate if needed)
Duration	30 minutes
Movement Assessment	Push, pull, overhead squat Single-leg balance
Flexibility	*Self-myofascial release, static and active stretching
Resistance Training	1-3 sets of 10-12 repetitions 2-3 days per week. Phases 1 and 2 of OPT™ model with reduced repetitions (10-12). May use a circuit or PHA training system.
Special Considerations	Avoid heavy lifting and high repetitions. Stay in pain free ranges of motion. *Only use self-myofascial release if tolerated by the client. There may be a need to start out with only 5 minutes of exercise and progressively increase, depending on the severity of conditions.

Table 14-16: Physiological and Training Considerations for Individuals with Arthritis

Physiological Considerations	Considerations for Health and Fitness, Sport and Athletic Training
Maximum oxygen uptake and ventilatory threshold is frequently lower, due to decreased exercise associated with pain and joint inflammation.	Multiple sessions or a circuit format, using treadmill, elliptical trainer, arm and leg cycles are a better alternative than higher intensity, single modality exercise formats. The usual principles for aerobic exercise training apply (60-80% peak work capacity, 3-5 days per week). Duration of exercise should be an accumulated 30 minutes, following an intermittent or circuit format, 3-5 days per week.
Medications may significantly influence bone and muscle health.	Incorporate functional activities in the exercise program wherever possible.
Tolerance to exercise may be influenced by acute arthritic flare-ups.	Awareness of the signs and symptoms that may be associated with acute arthritic flare-ups should dictate a cessation or alteration of training, and joint pain persisting for more than one hour should result in an altered exercise format.
Rheumatoid arthritis results, in particular, in early morning stiffness.	Avoid early morning exercise for clients with rheumatoid arthritis.
Evaluate for presence of co-morbidities, particularly osteoporosis.	Resistive exercise training is recommended, as tolerable, using pain as a guide. Start with very low number of repetitions and gradually increase to the number usually associated with improved muscular fitness (e.g. 10-12 reps, before increasing weight, 1 set of 8-10 exercises, 2-3 days per week).

stabilization and strength, while also increasing activities of daily living. In spite of the risks associated with exercise in the arthritic client, it is very important in restoring functional mobility and endurance in a deconditioned client who has joint limitations secondary to arthritis. Symptoms of arthritis (such as joint pain and stiffness) are heightened through inactivity due to muscle atrophy and lack of tissue flexibility. Progressing exercises so that they are performed in the seated position (without support) and standing position will increase functional capacity and balance of clients.

A methodical approach is important in the assessment and activity recommendations to reduce symptoms of flare-ups. Follow the guidelines for assessment in Chapter 5 (Fitness Assessment) and note the pain-free range of motion that clients exhibit during these exercises. Improving muscle strength and enhancing flexibility through exercise can assist in decreasing symptoms associated with arthritis. Static and active forms of stretching can be used and may be better tolerated from a seated or standing position. The use of self-myofascial release can be used if tolerated. Cardiorespiratory training should begin in Stage I and may progress to Stage II and/or Stage III, depending on client's capabilities and a physician's advice. Core and balance exercises will be very important for this population to increase levels of stability. Reactive training is not recommended for arthritic clients. Phases 1 and 2 of the OPT™ model will be used for this population with modified repetitions (10-12) to avoid heavy, repetitive joint loading that increases stress to the affected joints. For an example program for the arthritic client, please refer to the appendix of this textbook.

MODULE 14-7 Summary

Arthritis is an inflammatory condition that mainly affects the joints of the body. Two of the most common types of arthritis are *osteoarthritis* and *rheumatoid arthritis*. Osteoarthritis is caused by degeneration of cartilage in joints. Rheumatoid arthritis is a systemic, degenerative joint disease in which the body's immune system mistakenly attacks it own as tissues in the joint or organs, causing an inflammatory response, leading to pain and stiffness.

Improving muscle strength and enhancing flexibility through exercise can decrease arthritis symptoms. However, health and fitness professionals must be aware of the signs and symptoms of an acute rheumatoid arthritis exacerbation. In the case of an arthritic flare-up, even flexibility exercises may not be able to be performed. In addition, exercises that cause pain to persist for more than one hour after exercise should be modified or eliminated from the routine. Health and fitness professionals need to be aware of the medications being taken by clients, especially oral corticosteroids and steroids.

Clients with osteoarthritis have a decrease in strength and proprioception. A loss of knee-extensor strength is a strong predictor of osteoarthritis. Symptoms of arthritis (such as joint pain and stiffness) are heightened through inactivity due to muscle atrophy and lack of tissue flexibility. Functional capacity and balance can be increased by progressing exercises so that they are performed in the seated position (without support) and standing.

Flexibility exercises should improve muscle strength and enhance joint motion. Static and active forms of stretching can be used and may be better tolerated from a seated or standing position. The use of self-myofascial release can be used, if tolerated. Cardiorespiratory training should begin in Stage I and may progress to Stage II and/or Stage III, depending on client's capabilities and a physician's advice. Core and balance exercises will be very important. Reactive training is not recommended. Phases 1 and 2 will be used for this population with modified repetitions (10-12) to avoid heavy, repetitive joint loading that increases stress to the affected joints.

MODULE 14-7 Quiz

1. Clients with rheumatoid arthritis should exercise first thing in the morning.

   ☐ True   ☐ False

2. Clients taking oral corticosteroids may have which of the following?

   ☐ Muscle atrophy   ☐ Increased body mass

   ☐ Anemia   ☐ Osteoporosis

   ☐ Fracture risk

3. Arthritic clients may need to start out with only _____ minutes of exercise and progressively increase, depending on the severity of conditions.

MODULE 14-8: Cancer

CANCER:
Any of various types of malignant neoplasms, most of which invade surrounding tissues, may metastasize to several sites and are likely to recur after attempted removal and to cause death of the patient unless adequately treated.

Cancer is the second leading cause of death in the United States with more than one-half million deaths annually, behind cardiovascular disease. It has been estimated that American males have about a 44 percent probability and women have a 38 percent probability of developing cancer over their lifetime.[80]

Because of better detection and treatment strategies, those living with cancer have increased substantially. Moreover, in recent years there have been a variety of studies that have documented the positive benefits of exercise in the treatment of cancer, including: improved aerobic and muscular fitness, retention of lean body mass, less fatigue, improved quality of life and positive effects on mood and self-concept.[81] Because cancer is not a single disease, but a collection of diseases that share the same description (with respect to cell division, accumulation and death), its signs and symptoms vary widely. This chapter cannot do justice to the complexity of cancer. There are several excellent and descriptive resources that can be reviewed for more information.[1,3]

Medications used by clients with cancer can result in substantial adverse effects, including peripheral nerve damage, cardiac and pulmonary problems, skeletal muscle myopathy and anemia. Clients may also experience frequent nausea. In addition, the combination of the disease and its treatments frequently result in a diminished quality of life. Health and fitness professionals must have a knowledge and appreciation for the varied adverse effects of the treatments for cancer, since they can be substantially greater than the treatments prescribed for most other chronic diseases.

Exercise is an important intervention for clients recovering from cancer. It can improve exercise tolerance, reduce the cellular risks associated with cancer and also improve quality of life. Specifically, exercise at low to moderate intensities for moderate durations appears to have a more positive effect on the immune system (when compared to higher intensities for longer durations).[82] Research indicates that moderate to high levels of physical activity seem to be associated with decreased incidence and/or mortality rates for certain forms of cancer.[83]

That said, exercise programs for this population should follow the OPT™ model. Assessment procedures for the individual with cancer can follow the guidelines in Chapter 5 (Fitness Assessment). The specific push, pull and overhead squat exercise should be representative of the client's ability level. A single-leg balance assessment would also be advised, if the client is capable. Flexibility should include static and active stretching. Self-myofascial release can be used if no complications exist that would prevent its use. Check with a physician if there is any question. Cardiorespiratory training for this population is very important, but may have to start with five minutes of Stage I training progressing up to 30 minutes, three to five days per week. Stage II and/or Stage III training may be used upon agreement of the client's physician.

Core and balance exercises will be essential for this population. These exercises will help in regaining stabilization necessary for activities of daily living that may have been lost (due to the lack of activity caused by treatments). Clients should be progressed slowly using the stabilization, strength and power continuum. Reactive training is not recommended until the client has sufficiently progressed to performing three complete Phase 2 workouts per week. Resistance training for this population will include Phase 1 and 2 of the OPT™ model. Other phases may be used as client progresses and is approved by his/her physician. For an example program for the client with cancer, please refer to the appendix of this textbook.

Table 14-17: Basic Exercise Guidelines for Individuals with Cancer	
Mode	Treadmill walking, stationary cycling, rowers, low impact or step aerobics
Frequency	3-5 days per week
Intensity	60-80% of maximum heart rate Stage I cardiorespiratory training progressing to Stage II (May be reduced to 40-70% of maximum heart rate if needed)
Duration	15-30 minutes per session (may only start with 5 min)
Movement Assessment	Push, pull, overhead squat Single-leg balance (if tolerated)
Flexibility	*Self-myofascial release, static and active stretching
Resistance Training	1-3 sets of 10-15 repetitions 2-3 days per week. Phases 1 and 2 of OPT™ model. May use a circuit or PHA training system
Special Considerations	Avoid heavy lifting in initial stages of training. Allow for adequate rest intervals and progress client slowly. *Only use self-myofascial release if tolerated by the client. There may be a need to start out with only 5 minutes of exercise and progressively increase, depending on the severity of conditions and fatigue.

Table 14-18: Physiological and Training Considerations for Individuals with Cancer

Physiological Considerations	Considerations for Health and Fitness, Sport and Athletic Training
Fatigue and weakness is common.	Aerobic exercise should be done at low-moderate intensity (40-50% of peak capacity), 3-5 days per week, using typical aerobic modes (treadmill, elliptical trainer, cycle, depending on patient preference). In particular, avoid higher intensity training during periods of cancer treatment.
Excessive fatigue may result in overall diminished activity.	Use intermittent bouts of exercise bouts to accumulate 20-30 minutes of total aerobic exercise
Diminished immune function.	Resistance training can be performed (1 set of 8-10 exercises, 10-15 repetitions to fatigue, 2-3 days per week).
Decreased lean muscle mass.	Assess and provide intervention for decreased range of motion and balance

Module 14-8 Summary

Cancer is the second leading cause of death in the United States, although the number of individuals living with cancer has increased substantially. There are several the positive benefits of exercise in the treatment of cancer. Exercise is an important intervention in terms of improving exercise tolerance, reducing cellular risks associated with cancer and improving quality of life.

Medications used by clients with cancer can result in substantial adverse effects. In addition, the combination of the disease and its treatments frequently result in a diminished quality of life. The adverse effects of the treatments for cancer can be substantially greater than the treatments prescribed for most other chronic diseases.

For clients recovering from cancer, exercise that follows the OPT™ model at low to moderate intensities for moderate durations has a positive effect on the immune system. Research indicates that moderate to high levels of physical activity seems to be associated with decreased incidence and/or mortality rates for certain forms of cancer.

Assessment procedures for the individual with cancer can follow fitness assessment guidelines. The specific push, pull and overhead squat exercise should be representative of the client's ability level. A single-leg balance assessment would also be advised, if the client is capable. Flexibility should include static and active stretching. Self-myofascial release can be used if no complications exist that would prevent its use. Cardiorespiratory training for this population is very important, but may have to start with five minutes of Stage I training progressing up to 30 minutes, three to five days per week. Stage II and/or Stage III training may be used upon agreement of the client's physician. Core and balance exercises are essential for this population. Reactive training is not recommended until the client has progressed to three Phase 2 workouts per week. Resistance training for this population will include Phase 1 and 2 of the OPT™ model. Other phases may be used as client progresses and is approved by his/her physician.

MODULE 14-8 Quiz

1. In clients with excessive fatigue, health and fitness professionals can design programs that do what?

   _____

   _____

2. What is the probability that an American male will develop cancer in his lifetime?

   ☐ 44%   ☐ 38%   ☐ 15%

3. Medications used by clients with cancer can result in frequent nausea.

   ☐ True   ☐ False

MODULE 14-9: Women and Pregnancy

The physiological differences between men and women have been well studied. The majority of observed disparities in athletic performance between males and females are explained by differences in body structure, muscle mass and lean-body-mass-to-fat and to a lesser extent, blood chemistry. When measures are adjusted for body composition, both physiological and performance parameters narrow considerably or completely vanish. Nonetheless, women have lower absolute measures for aerobic capacity and measures of muscular fitness.

PREGNANCY: The condition of a female who contains an unborn child within the body.

With regard to **pregnancy**, there has been substantial research evaluating the effects of exercise on the physiology and health of both mother and developing fetus. Fears that the fetus may be harmed by increased blood circulation, thermoregulatory changes or decreased oxygen supply can be minimized with appropriate precautions. The general consensus is that most recreational pursuits are appropriate for all pregnant women. Those already engaged in an exercise program prior to pregnancy may continue with moderate levels of exercise until the third trimester, when a logical reduction in activity is recommended.[84]

The gradual growth of the fetus can alter the posture of pregnant women, making flexibility and core-stabilization training important. As the mother-to-be progresses to the more advanced stages of pregnancy (second and third trimesters, or after 12 weeks), performing exercises in a prone (on stomach) or supine (on back) position is not advised. Changes also occur in the cardiovascular system, decreasing work capacity and leading to necessary alterations in the cardiorespiratory program.

In the postpartum period, there may be a tendency to rush an exercise program in an effort to return to pre-pregnancy physiological and morphological status. Fitness professionals must be careful to advise clients that the changes that occurred during pregnancy may persist for a month to a month and a half. A return to a more vigorous program should be deferred and entered into gradually.

Health and fitness professionals should follow the assessment guidelines in Chapter 5 (Fitness Assessment), using seated and/or standing exercises. A single-leg balance assessment may be performed as well, if a woman is capable. Flexibility exercises should be performed in a seated and standing position, especially in the second and third trimesters. Static and active stretching should be used and self-myofascial release may also be used as tolerated. However, the health and fitness professional is strongly cautioned to avoid using the foam roll on the inside of the lower leg (calves) as this may be linked to a premature uterine contraction. Also, self-myofascial release should not be performed on varicose veins that are sore, or where there is swelling (such as the calves). Cardiorespiratory training should consist primarily of Stage I and only enter Stage II upon a physician's advice. Reactive training is not advised for this population, especially after the first trimester. Phases 1, 2 and 3 of the OPT™ model may be used in the first trimester, however, in the second and third trimesters the use of only Phases 1 and 2 is advised. For an example program for the pregnant client, please refer to the appendix of this textbook.

Table 14-19: Basic Exercise Guidelines for Women and Pregnancy	
Mode	Low-impact or step aerobics that avoid jarring motions, treadmill walking, stationary cycling and water activity
Frequency	3-5 days per week
Intensity	140 beats per minute, for beginning clients. 160 beats per minute for intermediate to advanced clients. Stage I
Duration	15-30 minutes per day. There may be a need to start out with only 5 minutes of exercise and progressively increase to 30 minutes, depending on the severity of conditions
Movement Assessment	Push, pull, overhead squat Single-leg balance
Flexibility	Static, active stretching and self-myofascial release*
Resistance Training	2-3 days per week, using light loads at 12-15 repetitions. Phases 1, 2 and 3 of the OPT™ model are advised (use only Phases 1 and 2 after first trimester)
Special Considerations	Avoid exercises in a prone (on stomach) or supine (on back) position, after 12 weeks of pregnancy. *Self-myofascial release after first trimester may not be tolerated in all clients and should NOT foam roll the inside of the lower leg — stay on the lateral gastrocnemius and peroneals region and avoid sore varicose veins and areas with swelling

Table 14-20: Physiological and Training Considerations for Women and Pregnancy

Physiological Considerations	Considerations for Health and Fitness, Sport and Athletic Training
Contraindications include; persistent bleeding 2nd to 3rd trimester, medical documentation of incompetent cervix or intrauterine growth retardation, pregnancy-induced hypertension, pre-term rupture of membrane or pre-term labor during current or prior pregnancy.	Screen carefully for potential contraindications to exercise.
Decreased oxygen available for aerobic exercise.	Low-moderate intensity aerobic exercise (40-50% of peak work capacity) should be performed 3-5 days per week, emphasizing non-weight bearing exercise (e.g. swimming, cycling), although certainly treadmill or elliptical training modes may be preferred and are appropriate.
Posture can affect blood flow to uterus during vigorous exercise.	Avoid supine exercise, particularly after the first trimester.
Even in the absence of exercise, pregnancy may increase metabolic demand by 300 kcal per day to maintain energy balance.	Advise adequate caloric intake to offset exercise effect.
High risk pregnancy considerations include individuals over the age of 35, history of miscarriage, diabetes, thyroid disorder, anemia, obesity and/or a sedentary lifestyle.	There are no published guidelines for resistance, flexibility or balance training specific to pregnancy exercise. Provided exercise intensity is below the aerobic prescription of 40-50% of peak work capacity, with careful attention to special considerations and contraindications described, adding these components may be helpful. For resistance training, if cleared by the physician, a circuit training format is recommended, 1-3 sets of 12-15 reps per exercise, emphasizing breathing control and rest, as needed, between sets.
	Advise clothing that will dissipate heat easily during exercise.
	Post-partum exercise should be similar to pregnancy guidelines, as physiological changes that occur during pregnancy may persist for up to 6 weeks.

MODULE 14-9 Summary

Most disparities in athletic performance between males and females are explained by differences in body structure, muscle mass and lean-body-mass-to-fat and blood chemistry. These differences are mostly eliminated when adjustments are made for body composition.

In pregnant women, appropriate precautions can minimize the risks of increased blood circulation, thermoregulatory changes or decreased oxygen supply. Most recreational pursuits are appropriate for all pregnant women and moderate levels of exercise are encouraged until the third trimester. In the postpartum period, a return to a more vigorous program should be entered into gradually.

Fitness professionals should follow the assessment guidelines in Chapter 5 (Fitness Assessment), using seated and/or standing exercises. A single-leg balance assessment may be performed. Flexibility exercises should be performed in a seated and standing position, especially in the second and third trimesters. Static and active stretching should be used. Self-myofascial release can be used as long as the client avoids using the foam roll on the inside of the lower leg, on varicose veins, and/or anywhere there is swelling. Cardiorespiratory training should consist primarily of Stage I. Reactive training is not advised for this population. Phases 1, 2 and 3 of the OPT™ model may be used in the first trimester. In the second and third trimesters only Phases 1 and 2 are advised.

MODULE 14-9 Quiz

1. Women have lower absolute measures for aerobic capacity and measures of muscular fitness.

   ☐ True   ☐ False

2. The gradual growth of the fetus can alter the posture of pregnant women, making flexibility and _____ training important.

3. Avoid exercises in a _____ or _____ position after 12 weeks of pregnancy.

MODULE 14-10: Lung Disease

Smoking has progressively declined over the last few decades. However, it is still vitally important to reinforce a continued decrease in the number of current smokers and prevent initiation of the habit. There remains an epidemiology of lung disease and its concurrent effects on so many other diagnosed chronic diseases (heart disease, cancer and peripheral vascular disease).

Lung disease is largely broken into two major categories, obstructive and restrictive. In **restrictive lung disease** or disorders, lung tissue may be fibrotic and thus, dysfunctional (as in the cases of pulmonary fibrosis or asbestosis). More simply, the ability to expand the lungs may be decreased due to any number of causes (such as fractured ribs, a neuromuscular disease, or even obesity). In **obstructive lung disease**, the lung tissue may be normal, but flows are restricted. The major obstructive lung diseases include asthma, chronic bronchitis and emphysema. These diseases are characterized by chronic inflammation (due primarily to smoking, although in the case of asthma may be due to environmental irritants) and airway obstruction via mucous production. Cystic fibrosis is another disease that is characterized by excessive mucous production, but is instead a genetic disorder.

Regardless, both restrictive and obstructive lung diseases result in similar impairments during exercise. Problems include decreased ventilation and decreased gas exchange ability (resulting in decreased aerobic capacity, endurance, oxygen desaturation). Clients with lung disease experience fatigue at low levels of exercise and often have shortness of breath (or *dyspnea*). Those with emphysema are frequently underweight and may exhibit overall muscle wasting with hypertrophied neck muscles (which are excessively used to assist in labored breathing). Those with chronic bronchitis may be the opposite: overweight and barrel-chested.

In general, exercise for these clients is similar to what would be appropriate for the general population. Exercise can improve functional capacity and decrease the symptoms of dyspnea in this population, among many other physiological and psychological benefits.[85] The use of lower body cardiorespiratory and resistance training exercises seem to be best tolerated. Upper extremity exercises place an increased stress on the secondary respiratory muscles that are involved in stabilizing the upper extremities during exercise.[86] Therefore, caution should be used when designing programs for this population to ensure adequate rest intervals. The use of the Peripheral Heart Action (PHA) training system would be advised.

RESTRICTIVE LUNG DISEASE: The condition of a fibrous lung tissue, which results in a decreased ability to expand the lungs.

OBSTRUCTIVE LUNG DISEASE: The condition of altered air flow through the lungs, generally caused by airway obstruction, due to mucous production.

In some clients, inspiratory muscle training can specifically improve the work associated with breathing. Health and fitness professionals working with clients who have lung disease should inquire about this intervention to see if it might augment the general exercise program. For more information, read the comprehensive guidelines regarding the exercise assessment and training of individuals with lung disease published by the American Association of Cardiovascular and Pulmonary Rehabilitation.[87] For an example program for the client with lung disease, please refer to the appendix of this textbook.

Table 14-21: Basic Exercise Guidelines for Individuals with Lung Disease	
Mode	Treadmill walking, stationary cycling, steppers and elliptical trainers
Frequency	3-5 days per week
Intensity	40-60% of peak work capacity Stage 1
Duration	Work up to 20-45 minutes
Movement Assessment	Push, pull, squat Single-leg balance
Flexibility	Static, active stretching and self-myofascial release
Resistance Training	1 set of 8-15 repetitions 2-3 days per week. Phases 1 and 2 of the OPT™ model are advised. PHA training system is recommended.
Special Considerations	Upper body exercises cause increased dyspnea and must be monitored. Allow for sufficient rest between exercises.

Table 14-22: Physiological and Training Considerations for Individuals with Lung Disease

Physiological Considerations	Considerations for Health and Fitness, Sport and Athletic Training
Lung disease frequently is associated with other co-morbidities, including cardiovascular disease.	Screen for presence of other co-morbidities.
A decreased in the ability to exchange gas in the lungs may result in oxygen de-saturation and marked dyspnea, at low workloads.	Whenever possible, try to ascertain the level of oxygen saturation using a pulse oximeter. Pulse oximetry values should be above 90% and certainly above 85%. Values below this level are a contraindication to continued exercise, regardless of symptoms.
Chronic de-conditioning results in low aerobic fitness and decreased muscular performance.	The aerobic exercise prescription should be guided by the client's shortness of breath. Workloads of 40-60% of peak work capacity, 3-5 days per week, 20-45 minutes as tolerable, may be achievable. Intermittent exercise with frequent rest breaks (at a ratio of two parts exercise to one part recovery) may be necessary to achieve sufficient overall exercise duration.
Upper extremity exercise may result in earlier onset of dyspnea and fatigue than expected, when compared to lower extremity exercise.	Upper extremity exercise should be programmed carefully and modified, based on fatigue. Resistance training can be helpful; use conservative guidelines. A circuit training format is recommended (8-10 exercises, 1 set of 8-15 reps per exercise), emphasizing breathing control and rest as needed between sets.
Clients may have significant muscle wasting and be of low body weight (with a BMI <18).	If the client is very thin, be certain to recommend adequate caloric intake to offset exercise effects.
Clients may be using supplemental oxygen	Fitness professionals may not adjust oxygen flow during exercise; it is considered a medication. If a client experiences unusual dyspnea or has evidence of oxygen de-saturation during exercise, stop exercise and consult with the client's physician.

MODULE 14-10 Summary

Lung disease is largely broken into two major categories, *obstructive* and *restrictive*. In restrictive disease or disorders, lung tissue may be fibrotic and the ability to expand the lungs may be decreased due to any number of causes. In obstructive lung disease, the lung tissue may be normal, but flows are restricted. Both types cause decreased ventilation and decreased gas exchange ability.

Clients with lung disease are often short of breath (*dyspnea*) and fatigue at low levels of exercise. Exercise can improve functional capacity and decrease the symptoms of dyspnea. In some clients, inspiratory muscle training can specifically improve the work associated with breathing.

In general, exercise for this population is similar to what would be appropriate for the general population. Lower body cardiorespiratory and resistance training exercises seem to be best tolerated. Adequate rest intervals need to be maintained. The Peripheral Heart Action training system is advised.

MODULE 14-10 Quiz

1. Asthma, chronic bronchitis and emphysema are examples of which category of lung disease?

   _____

2. What is dyspnea?

   _____

3. Pulse oximetry values should be above 90 percent but at least 85 percent.

   ☐ True   ☐ False

MODULE 14-11:
Intermittent Claudication/ Peripheral Arterial Disease

INTERMITTENT CLAUDICATION: The manifestation of the symptoms caused by peripheral arterial disease.

PERIPHERAL ARTERIAL DISEASE: A condition characterized by narrowing of the major arteries that are responsible for supplying blood to the lower extremities.

Intermittent claudication is the name for the manifestation of the symptoms caused by peripheral arterial disease (PAD). (The term *peripheral vascular disease* is also commonly used to describe the activity-induced symptoms that characterize this disease.) Essentially, intermittent claudication is characterized by limping, lameness and/or pain in the lower leg during mild exercise, resulting from a decrease in blood supply (oxygen) to the lower extremities. **Peripheral arterial disease** is characterized by narrowing of the major arteries that are responsible for supplying blood to the lower extremities.

The primary limiting factor for exercise in the PAD client is, of course, leg pain. One of the problems facing the fitness professional is the ability to differentiate between those who are limited by true symptoms of true intermittent claudication, versus similar leg complaints (such as tightness, cramping and pain) that might simply be associated with deconditioning. If the client has a PAD diagnosis, the symptoms are likely to be accurate for intermittent claudication, although they still could be associated with deconditioning.[88] Consult with client's physician concerning the condition. If pain continues during exercise, the health and fitness professional must refer client to a licensed physician immediately.

While experience will improve the ability of the health and fitness professional to differentiate between disease and deconditioning, in many respects it doesn't really matter. That is, the health and fitness professional should still develop a training regimen that attempts to improve physical function in the face of limiting factors.[89] In the case of peripheral vascular disease or deconditioning, the use of an intermittent format of exercise, with rest as necessary between exercise bouts, is similar.

Since PAD is associated with coronary heart disease and diabetes, health and fitness professionals should be aware of other existing co-morbidities and be suspicious that these co-morbidities may still exist, undiagnosed. Thus, physician clearance for exercise is necessary for the PAD patient.

Exercise programming should follow the OPT™ methodology, using the suggested assessment process in Chapter 5 (Fitness Assessment). The number of repetitions for the assessment may have to be decreased to five to 10, depending on the client's abilities. It will be important to make clients feel comfortable and competent with this process in order to ensure compliance. Static and active stretching should be used for this population. Guidelines for self-myofascial release are not known at this time and it is suggested that it not be used in this population, unless approved by a licensed physician. Phases 1 and 2 of the OPT™ model are suggested. Repetitions may need to start at eight to 12 (lower than indicated by these phases) and slowly progress to 12-20. Exercise bouts may initially start with five to 10 minutes of activity and progress slowly to 20-30 minutes. For an example program for the client with PAD, please refer to the appendix of this textbook.

Table 14-23:	Basic Exercise Guidelines for Individuals with Intermittent Claudication / PAD
Mode	Treadmill walking is preferred, also stationary cycling, steppers and elliptical trainers
Frequency	3-5 days per week working up to every day
Intensity	Established heart rate upper limit or comfortable pace
Duration	Work up to 20-30 minutes
Movement Assessment	Push, pull, overhead squat Single-leg balance
Flexibility	Static, active stretching
Resistance Training	1-3 sets of 8-12 repetitions 2-3 days per week. Phases 1 and 2 of the OPT™ model are advised. PHA training system is recommended.
Special Considerations	Allow for sufficient rest between exercises. Workout may start with 5-10 minutes of activity. Slowly progress client.

Table 14-24: Physiological and Training Considerations for Individuals with Intermittent Claudication / PAD

Physiological Considerations	Considerations for Health and Fitness, Sport and Athletic Training
PAD patients frequently have co-existing coronary artery disease and/or diabetes.	For clients with co-existing coronary artery disease, do not exceed established heart rate upper limit. (Usually, this limit is established from a walking test, where leg pain is the limiting factor.) Switching modalities where leg pain will not limit exercise may result in a higher — and possibly inappropriate — cardiac workload. If possible, a continuous format of exercise utilizing walking is preferred. Exercise duration should be 20-30 total minutes, with continuous bouts of 10 minutes or greater, 5-7 days per week.
Smoking significantly worsens PAD and exercise tolerance.	Strongly recommend smoking cessation. If a client continues to smoke, do not allow smoking for at least 1 hour prior to exercise.
PAD frequently results in decreased aerobic capacity and endurance.	Focus on aerobic exercise activities, with an emphasis on walking.
Resistance training may improve overall physical function, but may not address limitations of PAD.	Resistance exercise should be complementary, but not substituted for aerobic exercise. A circuit training format is recommended, (e.g. 8-10 exercises, 1-3 sets of 8-12 reps per exercise).
	An intermittent format of exercise may be necessary, with intensity guided by pain tolerance. Typical guidelines suggest exercise into moderate to severe discomfort, rest until subsided, repeat until total exercise time is achieved (20-30 minutes).
	Always screen for co-morbidities.

MODULE 14-11 Summary

Intermittent claudication is the name for the manifestation of the symptoms caused by peripheral arterial disease (PAD). When there is increased activity of the leg muscles, PAD results in symptoms where oxygen supply does not meet demand.

Exercise for PAD should *induce* symptoms, causing a stimulus that increases local circulation. The primary limiting factor is leg pain. The health and fitness professional must differentiate between true intermittent claudication versus similar leg complaints associated with deconditioning. If the client has a PAD diagnosis, the symptoms are likely to be accurate for intermittent claudication, although they still could be associated with deconditioning.

Exercise in an intermittent format, with rest as necessary between exercise bouts, is recommended. Physician clearance for exercise is necessary for the PAD client.

Exercise programming should follow the OPT™ methodology, using the fitness assessment. The number of repetitions for the assessment may have to be decreased to five to 10, depending on the client's abilities. Static and active stretching should be used for this population. However, self-myofascial release is not recommended. Phases 1 and 2 of the OPT™ model should be used, with adherence to repetition tempos. Repetitions may need to start at eight to 12 and slowly progress to 12-20. Exercise bouts may initially start with five to 10 minutes of activity and progress slowly to 20-30 minutes

MODULE 14-11 Quiz

1. What is the primary limiting factor for exercise in clients with PAD?

   _____

2. For clients with PAD, a continuous format of exercise utilizing running is preferred.

   ☐ True   ☐ False

References

1. *ACSM's Exercise management for persons with chronic diseases and disabilities.* 2nd edition. Champaign, IL: Human Kinetics; 2003.

2. *ACSM's Resource manual for guidelines for graded exercise and prescription.* 4th edition. Philadelphia: Lippincott William & Wilkins; 2001.

3. *ACSM's Resources for clinical exercise physiology.* Philadelphia: Lippincott William & Wilkins; 2002.

4. Sallis JF, Patrick K, Long BJ. Overview of the international consensus conference on physical activity guidelines for adolescents. *Pediatr Exerc Sci* 1994;6:299-301.

5. US Department of Health and Human Services. Guidelines for school and community programs to promote lifelong physical activity among young people. *Morb Mort Week Rep* 1997;46:1-36.

6. Pate RR. *Physical activity for young children.* President's Council on Physical Fitness and Sport Research Digest, Series 3, 1998;3:1-8.

7. *ACSM's guidelines for graded exercise and prescription.* 6th edition. Philadelphia: Lippincott William & Wilkins; 2000.

8. Saltarelli W. Children. In: Ehrman JK, Gordon PM, Visich PS, Keteyian SJ (eds). *Clinical exercise physiology.* Champaign, IL: Human Kinetics; 2003. pp. 544-70.

9. Faigenbaum A, Kraemer B, Cahill B, Chandler J, Dziados J, Elfrink E, Forman M, Gaudiose M, Micheli L, Nitka M, Roberts S. Youth resistance training: position statement paper and literature review. *Strength Cond J* 1996;18:62-75.

10. Weltman A, Janney CA, Rians CB, Stand K, Berg B, Tippett S, Wise J, Cahill BR, Katch FI. The effects of hydraulic resistance strength training on pre-pubertal males. *Med Sci Sports Exerc* 1986;18:629-38.

11. Ozmun JC, Mikesky AE, Sarburg PR. Neuromuscular adaptations following prepubescent strength training. *Med Sci Sports Exerc* 1994;26(4):510-4.

12. Hamill BP. Relative safety of weightlifting and weight training. *J Strength Cond Res* 1994;8(1):53-7.

13. Jones CS, Christensen C, Young M. Weight training injury trends. *Phys Sports Med* 2000;7:61-72.

14. US Consumer Product Safety Commission. *National electronic injury surveillance system.* Washington: Director of Epidemiology, National Injury Information Clearinghouse; 1987.

15. Haff GG. Roundtable discussion: youth resistance training. *Strength Cond J* 2003;25(1):49-64.

16. Falk B, Tenenbaum G. The effectiveness of resistance training in children, a meta-analysis. *Sports Med* 1996;22:176-86.

17. Payne V, Morrow J, Johnson L. Resistance training in children and youth: a meta-analysis. *Res Q Exerc Sport* 1997;68:80-9.

18. Ramsay JA, Blimkie CJ, Smith K, Garner S, MacDougall JD, Sale DG. Strength training effects in prepubescent boys. *Med Sci Sports Exerc* 1990;22(5):605-14.

19. Milne C, Seefedlt V, Reuschlein P. Relationship between grade, sex, race, and motor development in young children. *Res Q* 1976;47:726.

20. Clark HH. Joint and body range of movement. *Phys Fit Res Digest* 1975;5:16-8.

21. Brock D, Guralnick J, Brody J. Demography and epidemiology of aging in the US. In: Schneider E, Rowe J (eds). *Handbook of the biology of aging.* San Diego: Academic Press; 1990. pp. 3-23.

22. [Anonymous] Administration on Aging 1999. http://www.aoa.dhhs.gov/aoa/stats/profile/#health

23. American Heart Association. Heart Disease and Stroke Statistics - 2003 Update. Dallas, Tex: American Heart Association; 2002.

24. [Anonymous] Arthritis Foundation. *Arthritis fact sheet.* Atlanta; 1997.

25. Bell R, Hoshizaki T. Relationships of age and sex with joint range of motion of seventeen joint actions in humans. *Can J Appl Sports Sci* 1981;6:202-6.

26. Fielding JW. Presentation. Orthopedic and physical therapy seminar. September 1979. University of Cincinnati Medical Center.

27. Evans WJ. Exercise training guidelines for the elderly. *Med Sci Sports Exerc* 1999;31(1):12-7.

28. Larsson L, Grimby G, Karlsson J. Muscle strength and speed of movement in relation to age and muscle morphology. *J Appl Physiol* 1979;46;451-6.

29. Ringsberg K, Gerghem P, Johansson J, Obrant KJ. Is there a relationship between balance, gait performance and muscular strength in 75-year-old women? *Age and Aging* [serial online] 1999;28(3):289-93. [Abstract]

30. Luoto S, Aalto H, Taimela S, Hurri H, Pyykko I, Alaranta H. One footed and externally disturbed two footed postural control in patients with chronic low back pain and health control subjects. A controlled study with follow-up. *Spine* 1998 Oct 1;23(19):2081-9.

31. Myers A, Young Y, Langlois J. Prevention of falls in the elderly. *Bone* 1996; 18:87S-101S.

32. Wescott WL, Baechle TR. *Strength training for seniors.* Champaign, IL: Human Kinetics; 1999. pp. 1-2.

33. Hides JA. Multifidus muscle recovery in acute low back patients. Ph.D. thesis. University of Queensland Department of Physiotherapy; 1996.

34. Hides JA, Richardson CA, Jull GA. Multifidus muscle rehabilitation decreases recurrence of symptoms following first episode low back pain. In: Proceedings of the National Congress of the Australian Physiotherapy Association. Brisbane; 1996.

35. Marks R. The effect of isometric quadriceps strength training in mid-range for osteoarthritis of the knee. *Arthritis Care Res* 1993; 6:52-6.

36. Quirk A, Newman R, Newman K. An evaluation of interferential therapy, shortwave diathermy and exercise in the treatment of osteo-arthritis of the knee. *Physiother* 1985;71:55-7.

37. American College of Sports Medicine. Position stand on exercise and physical activity for older adults. *Med Sci Sports Exer* 1998;30;992-1008

38. Kuczmanski RJ, Flegal JM, Campbell SM, Johnson CL. Increasing prevalence of overweight among US adults. The national health and examination survey, 1960 to 1991. *JAMA* 1994;272:205-11.

39. Schwimmer JB, Burwinkle TM, Varni JW. Health-related quality of life of severely obese children and adolescents. *JAMA* 2003;289(14):1813-9.

575

40. Must A, Spadano J, Coakley EH, Field AE, Colditz G, Dietz WH. The disease burden associated with overweight and obesity. *JAMA* 1999 Oct 27;282(16):1523-9

41. Evans W, Rosenberg I. *Biomarkers.* New York: Simon and Schuster; 1992.

42. Meredith CN, Zackin MJ, Frontera WR, Evans WJ. Body composition and aerobic capacity in young and middle-aged endurance-trained men. *Med Sci Sports Exerc* 1987;19:557-63.

43. Roberts SB, Young VR, Fuss P. What are the dietary energy needs of adults? *Int J Obesity* 1992;16:969-76.

44. Slemenda C, Heilman DK, Brandt KD, Katz BP, Mazzuca SA, Braunstein EM, Byrd D. Reduced quadriceps strength relative to body weight. A risk factor for knee osteoarthritis in women? *Arthrit Rheumatol* 1998;41:1951-9.

45. Jurimae T, Jurimae J, Pihl E. Circulatory response to single circuit weight and walking training sessions of similar energy cost in middle-aged overweight females. *Clin Physiol* 2000;20(2):143-9.

46. Kraemer WJ, Noble BJ, Clark MJ, et al. Physiological responses to heavy-resistance exercises with very short rest periods. *Int J Sports Med* 1987;8:247-51.

47. Hurley BF, Seals DR, Ehsani AA, Cartier LJ, Dalsky GP, Hagberg JM, Hollososzy JO. Effects of high-intensity strength training on cardiovascular function. *Med Sci Sports Exerc* 1984;16:483-8.

48. Murray D. Morbid obesity--psychosocial aspects and surgical interventions. *AORN J* 2003;78(6):990-5.

49. Centers for Disease Control and Prevention. *National diabetes fact sheet: national estimates and general information on diabetes in the United States.* Revised edition. Atlanta: U.S. Department of Health and Human Services, Centers for Disease Control and Prevention; 1998.

50. Portuese E, Orchard T. Mortality in insulin dependent diabetes. In: Harris MI, Cowie CC, Stern MP et al (eds). *Diabetes in America.* National Institute of Health, National Institute of Diabetes and Digestive and Kidney Diseases. Bethesda, MD: 1995.

51. Pan XP, Li GW, Hu YH, Wang J, Yang W, Hu ZX, Lin J, Xiao JZ, Cao HB, Liu P, Jiang XG, Jiang YY, Wang JP, Zheng H, Zhang H, Bennet PH, Howard BV. Effects of diet and exercise in preventing NIDDM in people with impaired glucose tolerance. *Diabet Care* 1997;20:537-44.

52. American College of Sports Medicine. Position stand on exercise and physical activity for older adults. *Med Sci Sports Exer* 1998;30;992-1008.

53. Hagberg JM, Ferrell RE, Dengel DR, Wilund KR. Exercise training-induced blood pressure and plasma lipid improvements in hypertensives may be genotype dependent. *Hyperten* 1999;34:18-23.

54. Joint National Committee of Prevention, Detection, Evaluation, and Treatment of High Blood Pressure. The sixth report of the Joint National Committee of Prevention, Detection, Evaluation, and Treatment of High Blood Pressure. *Arch Int Med* 1997;157:2413-46.

55. American College of Sports Medicine position stand. Physical activity, physical fitness, and hypertension. *Med Sci Sports Exerc* 1993;25(10):i-x.

56. American Heart Association. *Heart disease and stroke statistics — 2003 update.* Dallas: American Heart Association; 2002.

57. Centers for Disease Control and Prevention. Receipt of cardiac rehabilitation services among heart attack survivors — 19 states and the District of Columbia, 2001. *Morb Mort Week Rep* 2003;52(44):1072-5.

58. Wenger NK, Froelicher ES, Smith LK, et al. *Cardiac Rehabilitation*. Clinical Practice Guideline No. 17. Rockville, MD: US Department of Health and Human Services, Public Health Service, Agency for Health Care Policy and Research, and the National Heart, Lung, and Blood Institute. AHCPR Publication No. 96-0672. October 1995.

59. Haskell WL, Alderman EL, Fair JM, Maron DJ, Mackey SF, Superko HR, Williams PT, Johnstone IM, Champagne ME, Krauss RM, et al. Effects of intensive multiple risk factor reduction on coronary atherosclerosis and clinical cardiac events in men and women with coronary artery disease: The Stanford Coronary Risk Intervention Project (SCRIP). *Circulat* 1994;89:975-90.

60. Ornish D, Brown SE, Scherwitz LW, Billings Armstrong WT, Ports TA, McLanahan SM, Kirkeeide RL, Braud RJ, Gould KL. Can lifestyle changes reverse coronary heart disease? The Lifestyle Heart Trial. *Lancet* 1990;336:129-33.

61. Hambrecht R, Niebauer J, Marburger C, Grunze M, Kalberer B, Hauer K, Schlierf G, Kubler W, Schuler G. Various intensities of leisure time physical activity in patients with coronary artery disease: effects on cardiorespiratory fitness and progression of coronary atherosclerotic lesions. *J Am Coll Cardiol* 1993;22:468-77.

62. Cummings S, Kelsey J, Nevitt M. Epidemiology of osteoporosis and osteoporotic fractures. *Epidemol Rev* 1985;7;178-205.

63. Lindsay R. *Osteoporosis*. Chicago: National Osteoporosis Foundation; 1992.

64. Riggs BL, Melton LJ. Involutional osteoporosis. *N Eng J Med* 1986;311:1676-86.

65. Haapasalo H, Kannus P, Sievanen H, Heinonen A, Oja P, Vuori I. Long-term unilateral loading and bone mineral density and content in female squash players. *Calc Tiss Int* 1994;54:249-55.

66. Kannus P, Haapasalo H, Sievanen H, Oja P, Vuori I. Site-specific effects on long-term unilateral activity on bone mineral density and content. *Bone* 1994;15:279-84.

67. Karlsson M, Vergnaud P, Delmas P, Obrant K. Indicators of bone formation in weight lifters. *Calc Tiss Inter* 1995;56:177-80.

68. Courtney A, Watchel E, Myers E, Hayes W. Effects of loading rate on strength of the proximal femur. *Calc Tis Int* 1994;55:53-8.

69. MacRae P, Feltner M, Reinsch S. A 1-year exercise program for women: effect on falls, injury and physical performance. *J Aging Phys Activ* 1994;2:127-42.

70. Kerr N, Morton A, Dick I, Prince R. Exercise effects on bane mass in postmenopausal women are site specific and load dependent. *J Bone Miner Res* 1996;11(2):218-25.

71. Lawrence RC, Hemlick CG, Arnett FC, Deyo RA, Felson DT, Giannini EH, Heyse SP, Hirsch R, Hochberg MC, Hunder CG, Liang MH, Pillemer SR, Steen VD, Wolfe F. Estimates of the prevalence of arthritis and selected musculoskeletal disorders in the United States. *Arthritis Rheum* 1998;41(5):778-99.

72. Hemlick CG, Lawrence RC, Pollard RA, Lloyd E, Heyse SP. Arthritis and other rheumatic conditions: who is affected now, who will be affected later? National Arthritis Data Workgroup. *Arthritis Care Res* 19958(4):203-11.

73. Slemenda C, Brandt KD, Heilman DK, Mazzuca SA, Braunstein EM, Katz BP, Wolinsky FD. Quadriceps weakness and osteoarthritis of the knee. *Ann Int Med* 1997;17;97-104.

577

74. Slemenda C, Heilman DK, Brandt KD, Katz BP, Mazzuca SA, Braunstein EM, Byrd D. Reduced quadriceps strength relative to body weight. A risk factor for knee osteoarthritis in women? *Arthrit Rheumatol* 1998;41:1951-9.

75. Hurley MV, Scott DL, Rees J, Newham DJ. Sensorimotor changes and functional performance in patients with knee osteoarthritis. *Ann Rheum Disord* 1997;56:641-8.

76. O'Reilly SC, Jones A, Muir KR, Doherty M. Quadriceps weakness in knee osteoarthritis: the effect on pain and disability. *Ann Rheum Disord* 1998;57:588-94.

77. Pai YC, Rogers MW, Patton J, Cain TD, Hanke TA. Static versus dynamic predictions of protective stepping following waist-pull perturbations in young and older adults. *J Biomech* 1998;31(12);1111-8.

78. Hurley MV, Jones DW, Newham DJ. Arthrogenic quadriceps inhibition and rehabilitation of patients with extensive traumatic knee injuries. *Clin Sci* 1994; 86:305-10.

79. [Anonymous] Never too late to build up your muscle. *Tufts university diet and nutrition letter.* Tufts University 1994;12 (September):6-7.

80. American Cancer Society. *Cancer facts and figures 2003.* Atlanta: American Cancer Society; 2003.

81. Courneya KS. Exercise interventions during cancer treatment: Biopsychosocial outcomes. *Exerc Sports Sci Rev* 2001:29;60-4.

82. Woods JA, Davis JM, Smith JA, Nieman DC. Exercise and cellular innate immune function. *Med Sci Sports Exerc* 1999;31:57-66.

83. Segal R, Johnson D, Smith J, Colletta S, Guyton J, Woodard S, Wells G, Reid R. Structured exercise improves physical functioning in women with stages I and II breast cancer: results of a randomized controlled trial. *J Clin Oncol* 2001;19(3):657-65.

84. American College of Obstetricians and Gynecologists. Exercise during pregnancy and the postpartum period, ACOG Committee Opinion No. 267. *Obstet Gynecol* 2002;99:171-3.

85. Ries AL, Carlin BW, Carrieri-Kohlman V, et al. Pulmonary rehabilitation: joint ACCP/AACVPR evidence-based guidelines. *Chest* 1997;112:1363-96.

86. Celli BR, Rassulo J, Make BJ. Dyssynchronous breathing during arm but not leg exercise in patients with chronic airflow obstruction. *N Engl J Med* 1986;314:1485-90.

87. American Association of Cardiovascular and Pulmonary Rehabilitation. *Guidelines for pulmonary rehabilitation programs.* 2nd edition. Champaign: Human Kinetics; 1998.

88. Greenland PG. Clinical significance, detection, and medical treatment for peripheral arterial disease. *J Cardiopul Rehabil* 2002;22(2):73-9.

89. Falcone RA, Hirsch AT, Regensteiner JG, et al. Peripheral arterial disease rehabilitation. *J Cardiopul Rehabil* 2003;23:170-5.

CHAPTER FIFTEEN

Nutrition

Objectives

After studying this chapter, you will be able to:

- Describe the macronutrients and their functions.
- Describe how macronutrient composition of an individual's food intake can affect satiety, compliance and daily energy expenditure and weight control.
- Provide basic nutritional recommendations for optimizing health.
- Answer questions, handle issues and dispel myths regarding the relationship of macronutrients to the successful alteration of body composition.

Key Terms

- Nutrition
- Protein
- Carbohydrate
- Lipids

Introduction to Nutrition

Understanding how the kinetic chain operates and being able to design individualized integrated programs for a client is only a portion of the puzzle. NASM recognizes that a proper nutritional background is an essential component to being a well-rounded health and fitness professional. In a time when fad diets are escalating and appearance is more important than ever, it is vital that health and fitness professionals arm themselves with the hard facts about nutrition and the human body.

This text specifically explores nutritional concepts and how they relate to the kinetic chain for a variety of scenarios. This will further enable the health and fitness professional to provide a scientific rationalization for proper nutritional protocols.

MODULE 15-1:
Nutrition and Body Composition

Definition

Nutrition is defined as the sum of the processes by which an animal or plant takes in and utilizes food substances.[1] This very basic definition does not begin to illuminate the role that diet plays in the health, appearance, performance and well-being of an individual. An understanding of nutrition will be vital to the success of the health and fitness professional's clients. The proper nutrition strategy has the ability to hasten the results from the stimulus of exercise, improve health and athletic performance, reduce the risk of disease and illness, increase energy levels and favorably alter body composition. While the following section is designed to give the health and fitness professional an understanding of the basics of nutrition and its use in facilitating clients' goals, it is not designed to instruct on the use of diet to treat ill or high-risk individuals. It is recommended that the health and fitness professional have a network of qualified health-care professionals (doctors, dietitians and eating-disorder specialists) in their area, to whom they can refer when dealing with clients who have special needs. This can be mutually beneficial, as these same health-care professionals will need qualified trainers to work with their patients when recommending exercise.

Nutrition and Body Composition

There are an increasing number of overweight and obese people in the United States. A desire for a quick solution for weight loss has led to the mystification of exercise and diet and an environment ripe for promoters of quick weight-loss methods and fad diets.[2-4] Sorting through this pile of myths and inaccuracies makes the health and fitness professional's job a daunting one. Clients are coming to the health club with preconceived ideas about how they should be eating. These ideas may hinder their progress and have negative health consequences.

The facts about weight loss and gain are quite simple. Eat fewer calories than are expended and there will be a reduction in weight. Conversely, consume more calories than are expended and there will be an increase in weight.[5,6] Today's environment provides a constantly available, palatable food supply (increasing energy intake) and promotes a sedentary lifestyle (reducing energy expenditure). The facts are that we eat too much and move too little. The combination is causing America's waistline to expand.[7]

The following modules address the macronutrients (protein, carbohydrate and fat), their uses and recommendations, and will explore many common myths. These topics will be addressed as they relate to the common goals of altering body composition and increasing performance.

MODULE 15-1 Summary

Diet plays an important role in a person's health, appearance, energy and performance as well as affecting results from exercise and overall well-being. The health and fitness professional should not instruct clients on the use of diet to treat illness or high-risk cases, but rather refer clients to qualified health-care professionals.

Clients come to health and fitness professionals with misconceptions about how they should be eating. However, the fact is that eating fewer calories than are burned will result in weight loss.

MODULE 15-2: Protein

The Function of Protein

The primary function of **protein** is to build and repair body tissues and structures. It is also involved in the synthesis of hormones, enzymes and other regulatory peptides. Additionally, protein can be used for energy if calories or carbohydrate are insufficient in the diet.[12]

> **PROTEIN:** Amino acids linked by peptide bonds, which consist of carbon, hydrogen, nitrogen, oxygen and usually sulfur that have several essential biological compounds.

The Structure of Protein

Proteins are made up of amino acids linked together by peptide bonds. The body uses approximately 20 amino acids to build its many different proteins.[8] These amino acids can be compared to the letters of the alphabet. Just as specific words are formed by certain sequences of letters, arranging the amino acids in different sequences yield the body's myriad of proteins (from a muscle protein like actin to proteins that make up the lens of the eye).

There are two general classes of amino acids: *essential* and *non-essential* (Table 15-1). Essential amino acids cannot be manufactured in the body (or are manufactured in insufficient amounts); therefore, they must be obtained from the food supply or some other exogenous source. There are eight essential amino acids. The second group of amino acids is termed non-essential because the body is able to manufacture them from dietary nitrogen and fragments of carbohydrate and fat.[12]

Table 15-1: Amino Acids

Essential	Non-essential	Semi-essential
Isoleucine	Alanine	Arginine
Leucine	Asparagine	Histidine
Lysine	Aspartic acid	
Methionine	Cysteine	
Phenylalanine	Glutamic acid	
Threonine	Glutamine	
Tryptophan	Glycine	
Valine	Proline	
	Serine	
	Tyrosine	

Due to their rate of synthesis within the body, arginine and histidine are considered semi-essential amino acids. It appears that these amino acids cannot be manufactured by the body at a rate that will support growth (especially in children).

Digestion, Absorption and Utilization

Proteins must be broken down into the constituent amino acids before the body can utilize these building blocks for its own purposes. The fate of the amino acids following digestion and absorption through the intestines depends on the body's homeostatic needs, which can range from tissue replacement or tissue addition to a need for energy. Figure 15-1 depicts the digestion, absorption and synthesis sequence.

As ingested proteins enter the stomach, they encounter hydrochloric acid (HCL), which uncoils (or *denatures*) the protein so that digestive enzymes can begin dismantling the peptide bonds. In addition, the enzyme pepsin begins to cleave the protein strand into smaller polypeptides (strands of several amino acids) and singular amino acids. As these protein fragments leave the stomach and enter the small intestine, pancreatic and intestinal proteases (or *protein enzymes*) continue to dismantle the protein fragments.

The resulting di- and tri-peptides and singular amino acids are then absorbed through the intestinal wall into the enterocytes and released into the blood supply to the liver (Figure 15-2).

Once in the blood stream, the freeform amino acids have several possible fates: they can be used for protein synthesis (building and repairing tissues or structures), immediate energy or potential energy (fat storage).

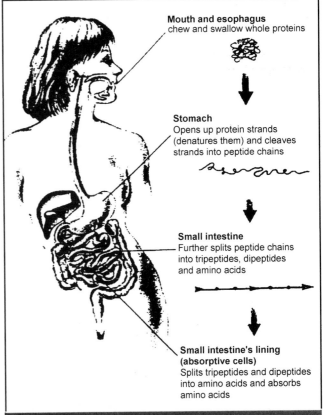

Mouth and esophagus
chew and swallow whole proteins

Stomach
Opens up protein strands (denatures them) and cleaves strands into peptide chains

Small intestine
Further splits peptide chains into tripeptides, dipeptides and amino acids

Small intestine's lining (absorptive cells)
Splits tripeptides and dipeptides into amino acids and absorbs amino acids

Figure 15-1: Protein Digestion, Absorption and Endogenous Synthesis

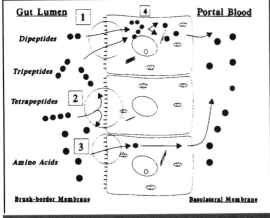

Figure 15-2: Amino-acid Absorption

Amino Acids for Immediate Energy

The body has a constant need for energy and the brain and nervous system, in particular, have a constant need for glucose. If carbohydrate or total energy intake is too low, the body has the ability to use amino acids (from dietary or body proteins) to provide energy.[9,10] The amino

583

acids are first *deaminated* (or stripped of the amine group), allowing the remaining carbon skeleton to be used for the production of glucose or ketones to be used for energy. The removed amine group produces ammonia, a toxic compound, which is converted to urea in the liver and excreted as urine by the kidneys.

Amino Acids for Potential Energy (Fat)

If protein intake exceeds the need for synthesis and energy needs are met, then amino acids from dietary protein are deaminated and their carbon fragments may be stored as fat. Among Americans, protein and caloric intakes are typically well above requirements, allowing protein to contribute significantly to individuals' fat stores.[4]

Protein in Foods

Dietary protein is the delivery vehicle for amino acids. Meats, fruits, vegetables, grains, dairy products and even supplements supply us with the valuable building blocks of protein we need. If a food supplies all of the essential amino acids in appropriate ratios, it is called a *complete protein*. If a food source is low or lacking in one or more essential amino acid, it is called an *incomplete protein*. The essential amino acid that is missing or present in the smallest amount is called the *limiting factor* of that protein. Because the process of protein synthesis works on an all-or-none principle, all amino acids must be present at the site of protein manufacture, or synthesis will be reduced to the point where the cell runs out of the limiting amino acid.[11]

The ability of a protein to satisfy these essential amino-acid requirements can be quantified in several ways. Terms used to rate dietary protein include protein efficiency ratio (PER), net protein utilization (NPU) and biological value (BV).[12]

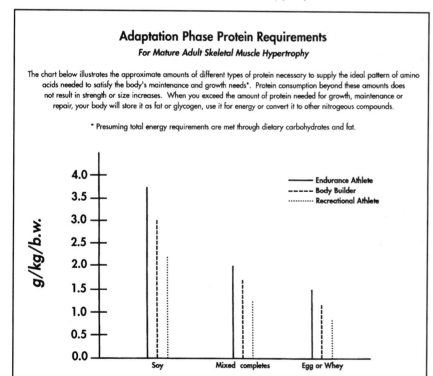

Adaptation Phase Protein Requirements
For Mature Adult Skeletal Muscle Hypertrophy

The chart below illustrates the approximate amounts of different types of protein necessary to supply the ideal pattern of amino acids needed to satisfy the body's maintenance and growth needs*. Protein consumption beyond these amounts does not result in strength or size increases. When you exceed the amount of protein needed for growth, maintenance or repair, your body will store it as fat or glycogen, use it for energy or convert it to other nitrogeous compounds.

* Presuming total energy requirements are met through dietary carbohydrates and fat.

—— Endurance Athlete
- - - Body Builder
········· Recreational Athlete

g/kg/b.w.

Soy   Mixed completes   Egg or Whey

Figure 15-3: Adaptation-phase Protein Requirements

Biological value (BV) is a measure frequently used when discussing protein sources in popular media and by supplement manufacturers. Essentially, BV is a measure of protein quality, or how well it satisfies the body's essential amino-acid needs. A protein source with a higher score provides an amino-acid profile that is more closely related to the needs of the human body. BV is a concept that is often misused, especially by marketers of protein supplements. One is led to believe that consuming specially-prepared, high-BV proteins will allow an individual who is already consuming adequate protein to build muscle to a greater degree, or more quickly. However, consuming protein above requirements will not force the body to unleash a previously untapped muscle-building capacity.[13,14] If, instead, one exclusively consumes very high BV proteins, his/her amino-acid requirements would be met with less protein. Conversely, if one chooses a diet composed of mostly lower BV protein sources, their total protein requirements will increase (Figure 15-3).

Factors Affecting Protein Requirements
Exercise

Both anaerobic and aerobic exercise affect protein requirements in different ways. Exercise increases the oxidation of amino acids as well as the rate of protein turnover in lean body mass during recovery. Because different types of exercise have specific effects, an individual participating in both types of exercise may have a need for protein greater than someone involved in only one.[15,16]

Caloric Intake

Because protein can be used for tissue repair and synthesis as well as for energy, protein requirements will increase as total energy intake decreases.[17,30] As total caloric intake is reduced, energy needs may no longer be satisfied by carbohydrate and fat intake alone, necessitating that protein be used to provide energy. The goal is to satisfy the majority of energy needs with carbohydrate and fat, saving protein for tissue repair and growth. This is why carbohydrates are often referred to as protein sparing. If one does not eat adequate amounts of carbohydrate and/or fat (as is often seen in low-calorie or low-carbohydrate diets or during physique-competition preparation), more protein will be used for energy by default. Individuals interested in general fat loss or muscle hypertrophy have erroneously mimicked the acceptable use of a high-protein diet by a physique competitor. However, under the proper circumstances, these diets, when used temporarily, can be effective.

Negative Energy Balance

For clients pursuing body-fat reduction, body-fat-loss goals require that a caloric deficit be maintained, until the goal is reached. These individuals seek to modify their body composition. During a negative energy balance, amino acids are used to assist in energy production. This is called *gluconeogenesis.* Anaerobic or aerobic exercise depletes glycogen, increasing gluconeogenesis. The increase in gluconeogenesis is supported by the release of branched-chain and other amino acids from structural proteins in order to maintain glucose homeostasis during exercise.[18-21] The hypocaloric diet establishes less-than-optimal glycogen stores. When this is combined with increased glycogen demand during exercise, protein's energy utilization is increased.[22,23] The amount of lean body mass lost in persons on a negative energy balance can be reduced by increasing the amount of protein in the diet, leading to a more rapid return to nitrogen balance. A number of studies show that an increase in protein utilization during a hypocaloric diet will produce effects that can be exacerbated by exercise.[24-30]

Protein and the Bodybuilder

Bodybuilders during positive energy balance (off-season) should follow the same protein recommendations as strength athletes. However, during negative energy balance (used to create competition-level body-fat percentages), protein requirements may dramatically increase. To reach competitive body-fat levels, calorie intake is continually lowered while exercise (such as cardiorespiratory, weight training and posing) is increased.

Competitive levels of body fat are generally unhealthy and impossible to maintain for prolonged periods. Each component of this regime may have additive effects on protein requirements. The body's survival mechanisms, related to increases in energy expenditure and decreases in food supply, are probably highly active during this period, forcing a continued reduction in food intake to achieve the goal.[31,32] However, because of its anabolic requirements, protein intake cannot be lowered. In fact, protein intake may have to be increased in the final weeks before competition. During this period, the body must have the option to use available food either for energy or muscle support. The body does not have a choice with dietary carbohydrate or fat, making them the only dispensable calories. Therefore, protein intake could be dramatically increased to theoretically lessen the obligatory loss of lean tissue during these drastic measures.[18-30]

It is quite common to see clients consuming the majority of their calories from protein in the final weeks before competition. However, during the off-season, athletes return to normal food intake (or protein at anabolic requirements and energy needs met primarily with carbohydrate and fats) and normal energy balance. This return to normal eating habits enables greater muscular gains than would be achieved by maintaining a high-protein intake year-round.[33-35] In fact, it appears that carbohydrate (1g/kg), not protein, consumed within an hour after heavy resistance training inhibits muscle-protein breakdown, resulting in a positive protein balance.[36]

Protein's Effect on Satiety

In addition to the above factors, protein intake may be adjusted to aid in *satiety* (or feeling of fullness). Protein's role in satiety is an important consideration. As with all macronutrients, protein activates specific satiety mechanisms and may be more satiating than fat and carbohydrate. Protein-induced suppression of food intake in animals and humans is greater than its energy content alone. This suggests that protein has a direct effect on satiety.[37] In studies of rats and humans, a pre-load of protein suppressed their food intake for several hours and to a greater extent than a similar energy load of fat and carbohydrate.[38-42] Individuals seeking fat loss may benefit from the satiating properties of protein in order to feel full and energized throughout the day. This can assist clients in program adherence.[43,44]

Protein-intake Recommendations

The above factors can now be added to the Recommended Dietary Allowance (RDA) for protein (0.8g/kg/d or 15-30 percent of total caloric intake), providing a range of protein recommendations for exercisers. Table 15-2 lists the appropriate recommendations for most athletes and exercisers.

The protein recommendations listed for adaptation periods are for anabolic, not necessarily total-metabolic, purposes (e.g., satiety, performance). These protein recommendations may range from 10 to 25 percent of total caloric intake. This not only allows for differences in goals and activity, but also

Table 15-2: Protein Recommendations (gm/kg/day)			
	Bodybuilder	**Active Recreational Athlete**	**Endurance Athlete**
Minimum Acceptable Intake	1.0	1.0	1.4
Adaptation Period	1.6 - 2.0	1.2 - 1.8	1.6 - 2.0

for bio-individuality in terms of satiety and performance. Some people respond better to slightly higher or lower protein intakes, which may help with adherence to the amount of calories required to reach and maintain goals. Individuals eating lower amounts of protein may need supplementation. Whatever the percentage of protein ends up being, in relation to total caloric intake, the protein intake should still fall approximately within the above ranges of g/kg. In other words, a small person losing fat (or hypocaloric) and exercising using strength and aerobic training, may have a high percentage of protein (around 25 percent) but still fall in the appropriate range of absolute protein (1.2 - 2.0 gm/kg/day).

Negative Side Effects Associated with Chronic Use of High-protein Diets

For our purposes, a high-protein diet is defined as one that consists of more than 30 percent of total caloric intake from protein, or three times the protein RDA for athletes. Chronic consumption of a high-protein diet is generally associated with a higher intake of saturated fat and low fiber intake, both of which are risk factors for heart disease and some types of cancer.[45,46] Also, the kidneys are required to work harder to eliminate the increased urea produced.

Of genuine concern is the effect of high-protein diets on calcium status. For every gram of protein consumed above tissue maintenance, between 1 and 1.5 mg of calcium is excreted.[47-50] America's intake of calcium is notoriously poor. A high-protein diet, consumed by many sedentary Americans, certainly does not help in achieving calcium-intake goals.

In addition, the need for fluids is increased by high-protein intake. Protein requires approximately seven times the water for metabolism than carbohydrate or fat.[51] Typically accompanying high-protein diets is low-carbohydrate consumption (especially for weight loss). This can lead to decreased glycogen stores, which inhibit performance and contribute to dehydration. Both of these situations will negatively affect athletic performance and overall functioning of the individual.

Protein Supplementation

Because of protein's structure and function, protein supplementation may be the easiest to rationalize. However, in a healthy population, protein supplementation is difficult to defend, at least in its general use among athletes. The concept that "more is better" is the conventional thinking of many users of protein supplements, especially in the bodybuilding community.[52] Athletes tend to base their diet decisions on nutritional advice from their peers, nonscientific mentors, heroes or idols, rather than the peer-reviewed, scientific literature.[53-56] No evidence has shown a constant, linear increase in muscle mass or performance related to protein intake. Thus, there is a physiological threshold for incorporating dietary protein into fat-free mass (FFM), or for using protein as an immediate energy substrate.

Enhanced Recovery After Exercise

One defensible reason to ingest supplemental protein is to quickly get amino acids into the blood following exercise. Research has shown that the use of protein and carbohydrate supplements before and after weight training can enhance anabolic hormones compared to a non-supplemented state.[57-59] Theoretically, this would enhance recovery, allowing the body to spend more time on building muscle rather than repair.[60-63]

Weight-Reduction Programs

Protein supplements replace whole-food proteins, eliminating unwanted calories in order to maintain equal or positive nitrogen balance during body-fat reduction for competitive cosmetic athletes.

Convenience

Protein supplements are used in situations when whole food is not available or is not an option (e.g. early-morning workouts).

Cost

Marketers often promote protein supplements as a lower-cost-per-gram nitrogen source when compared to whole foods. In recent years, marketers have focused on building "the perfect protein." Their objective has been to enhance protein synthesis, as opposed to food protein or standard protein supplements.

Whey protein hydrolysates are the current protein-product "rage." Special processing of whey protein, which has the highest BV of any protein, yields small peptides that are absorbed faster into the enterocyte than free-form amino acids.[64] In addition, these special blends have been found to provide greater nitrogen retention and protein synthesis in starved animals, burn patients and during enteral feeding of hospitalized patients, when compared to other proteins.[65-68] The amino-acid profile of whey protein (very high in branched-chain amino acids), combined with a manufacturing process that yields the ideal peptide lengths for rapid absorption, probably gives this special blend its benefits to injured, diseased or starved recipients. The relevance of this to well-fed, healthy athletes is probably non-existent. However, for bodybuilders, wrestlers or other weight-conscious athletes preparing for competition (these athletes are generally underfed and over-trained at this point), these formulas offer a viable way to meet protein requirements with fewer calories.

The timing of available amino acids (pre- and post-training), reduction of calories (while sparing nitrogen losses), convenience and cost are all defensible benefits of protein supplements. On the other hand, if individuals meet their protein requirements (Table 15-2) and maintain desired body-fat levels, no substantial evidence exists that either using protein supplements to replace food or increasing protein intake above requirements will enhance performance or adult skeletal muscle hypertrophy.

Review of Properties of Protein

One gram of protein yields four calories. Protein must be broken down completely (into constituent amino acids) before it can be utilized.

Amino acids from protein are used by the body for the following:
- Synthesizing body-tissue protein,
- Providing glucose for energy (many can be converted to glucose),
- Providing nitrogen in the form of amine groups to build non-essential amino acids and
- Contributing to fat stores.

Amino acids are not utilized to build protein under the following conditions:
- Not enough available energy from carbohydrate and fat;
- Consistently low or lacking essential dietary amino acids, due to the exclusive consumption of incomplete proteins; and
- An excess of necessary protein.

The following conditions are necessary for the body to synthesize endogenous protein:
- Availability of all essential and non-essential amino acids in proper amounts,
- An adequate supply of exogenous protein (supplying amine groups, which synthesize the non-essential amino acids) and
- Adequate energy-yielding carbohydrate and fat (sparing the protein).

Recommended protein intake for athletes and exercisers:
- 1 to 2.0 gm per kg/wt depending on goal, activity, protein source and total caloric intake

- Typically falls in a range of 15 to 30 percent of total caloric intake

Chronic high-protein intake (greater than 2.5 times the RDA) diets can lead to:
- Calcium depletion,
- Fluid imbalance,
- Eventual hunger,
- Slower metabolism,
- Weight rebound and
- Energy loss.

MODULE 15-2 Summary

Protein primarily builds and repairs body tissues and structures. It also helps to synthesize hormones, enzymes and other peptides, and can also be used for energy in diets lacking calories or carbohydrates.

Proteins are made up of about 20 essential and non-essential amino acids linked together by peptide bonds. Proteins must be broken down into the amino acids before the body can use them for its own purposes. The eight essential amino acids cannot be manufactured in the body. The remaining non-essentials are manufactured by the body from dietary nitrogen and fragments of carbohydrate and fat. Protein can be used by the body to create immediate energy or potential energy.

Dietary protein is the delivery vehicle for amino acids. One gram of protein yields four calories. Complete proteins supply all of the essential amino acids in appropriate ratios, while incomplete proteins are low or lacking in one or more essential amino acid. Biological value (BV) is a measure of how well a protein satisfies the body's essential amino-acid needs. One with a higher score is more closely related to the needs of the human body.

Protein requirements can be affected by anaerobic and aerobic exercise, total energy intake, caloric intake and carbohydrate intake. During a negative energy balance (or caloric deficit), amino acids are used to assist in energy production (or gluconeogenesis), wherein protein requirements may dramatically increase. Protein intake may also be adjusted to aid in satiety in individuals seeking fat loss, who may benefit from protein by feeling full and energized throughout the day. The Recommended Dietary Allowance for protein is 0.8 g/kg/day, or 15-30 percent of total caloric intake. However, this may be vary among athletes from 1.0 - 2.0 g/kg/day.

A high-protein diet consisting of more than 30 percent of total caloric intake from protein is associated with heart disease and some types of cancer (due to a higher intake of saturated fat and low fiber intake), overworked kidneys (due to elimination of the increased urea), inadequate calcium intake and possible dehydration.

Protein supplementation is not typically recommended in general use among athletes. No substantial evidence exists that either using protein supplements to replace food or increasing protein intake above requirements will enhance performance or adult skeletal muscle hypertrophy. However, supplemental protein may be useful:

- To quickly get amino acids into the blood before and after weight training,
- To replace whole-food proteins for weight loss,
- In situations when whole food is not available and
- For bodybuilders, wrestlers or other weight-conscious athletes preparing for competition.

MODULE 15-2 Quiz

1. Why are arginine and histidine considered semi-essential amino acids?

_____

_____

_____

2. The essential amino acid that is missing (or present in the smallest amount) is called the _____ _____ of that protein.

3. A person who consumes very high BV proteins will have amino-acid requirements that are met with ☐ **more** ☐ **less** protein.

4. Recommended protein intake for athletes and exercisers is:

   ☐ 5-20 percent of total caloric intake

   ☐ 15-30 percent of total caloric intake

   ☐ 30-45 percent of total caloric intake

MODULE 15-3: Carbohydrates

The Structure and Function of Carbohydrates

Carbohydrates are compounds containing carbon, hydrogen and oxygen and are generally classified as sugars (simple), starches (complex) and fiber. The definition of sugar, as it would appear on a food label, is any mono- or disaccharide.[69]

A *monosaccharide* is a single sugar unit, many of which are connected to make starches (the storage form of carbohydrates in plants) and glycogen (the storage form of carbohydrates in humans). Monosaccharides include glucose (commonly referred to as blood sugar), fructose (or fruit sugar) and galactose. *Disaccharides* (two sugar units) include sucrose (or common sugar), lactose (or milk sugar) and maltose.

Carbohydrates are a chief source of energy for all body functions and muscular exertion. This leads to a rapid depletion of available and stored carbohydrate and creates a continual craving for this macronutrient. Carbohydrates also help to regulate the digestion and utilization of protein and fat.[82,83]

> **CARBOHYDRATES:** Neutral compounds of carbon, hydrogen and oxygen (such as sugars, starches and celluloses), which make up a large portion of animal foods.

Digestion, Absorption and Utilization

The principal carbohydrates present in food occur in the form of simple sugars, starches and cellulose. Simple sugars, such as those in honey and fruits, are very easily digested. Double sugars, such as table sugar, require some digestive action but are not nearly as complex as starches, such as those found in whole grain. Starches require prolonged enzymatic action in order to be broken down into simple sugars (i.e., glucose) for utilization. Cellulose, commonly found in the skins of fruits and vegetables, is largely indigestible by humans and contributes little energy value to the diet. It does, however, provide the bulk necessary for intestinal motility and aids in elimination.[70,71]

The rate at which ingested carbohydrate raises blood sugar and its accompanying effect on insulin release is referred to as the *glycemic index* (GI). The GI for a food is determined when the particular food is consumed by itself and on an empty stomach. Mixed meals of protein, other carbohydrate and fat can alter the glycemic effect of single foods.[72] Some fad diets place too much emphasis on the GI, stating that foods with a higher GI lead to fat storage, regardless of caloric intake. This leads to categorizing foods as "good" or "bad" based solely on their GI value. As stated earlier, weight gain or loss is related to total energy intake, not the source of the food eaten. However, as one can see in Table 15-3, foods lower on the glycemic index are good sources of complex carbohydrates, as well as being high in fiber and overall nutritional value.

Table 15-3: Glycemic Index of Select Foods	
Foods	**GI %**
Soy beans (fresh/canned), peanuts	10-19
Kidney beans, lentils, fructose	20-29
Milk (skim or whole), yogurt, tomato soup, ice cream, chick peas, apples (Golden Delicious)	30-39
Spaghetti, sweet potato, navy beans (canned), dried peas, oranges, orange juice, porridge, oats	40-49
Sweet corn, All-Bran cereal, peas (frozen), sucrose, potato chips	50-59
Bread (white), rice (brown), muesli, bananas, raisins	60-69
Bread (whole wheat), millet, rice (white), potato	70-79
Corn Flakes, carrots, honey, potatoes (instant, mashed)	80-90
Glucose	100

Through the processes of digestion and absorption, all disaccharides and polysaccharides are ultimately converted into simple sugars such as glucose or fructose (Figure 15-4). However, fructose must be converted to glucose in the liver before it can be used for energy. Some of the glucose (or blood sugar) is used as fuel by tissues of the brain, nervous system and muscles. Because humans are periodic eaters, a small portion of the glucose is converted to glycogen after a meal and stored within the liver and muscles. Any excess is converted to fat and stored throughout the body as a reserve source of energy. When total caloric intake exceeds output, any excess carbohydrate, dietary fat or protein may be stored as body fat until energy expenditure once again exceeds energy input.

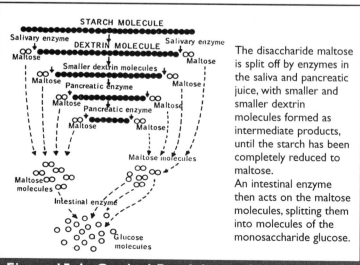

The disaccharide maltose is split off by enzymes in the saliva and pancreatic juice, with smaller and smaller dextrin molecules formed as intermediate products, until the starch has been completely reduced to maltose.

An intestinal enzyme then acts on the maltose molecules, splitting them into molecules of the monosaccharide glucose.

Figure 15-4: Gradual Breakdown of Large Starch Molecules by Enzymes in Digestion

Fiber and its Role in Health

One of the greatest contributions made by dietary complex carbohydrate is fiber. Higher intakes of dietary fiber are associated with lower incidence of heart disease and certain types of cancer.[73,74] Additional benefits of fiber include:[74-78]

- Provides bulk in the diet, thus increasing the satiety value of foods.
    - Some fibers also delay the emptying of the stomach, further increasing satiety.[79]

- Prevents constipation and establishes regular bowel movements.

- Maintains good intestinal motility.
    - Helps to retain the health and tone of the digestive-tract muscles, therefore preventing diverticulosis, which causes the weakening of intestinal walls, then causing them to swell and distend.

- Aids in the prevention of bacterial infections of the appendix (or appendicitis).

- Helps to lower the risk of colon cancer.

- May reduce the risks of heart and artery disease by lowering blood cholesterol.
    - Certain soluble fibers bind with cholesterol compounds and are excreted from the body in the feces, lowering the body's cholesterol content.
    - Additionally, the substances produced by the bacteria's digestion of soluble fiber may help inhibit the production of cholesterol and eliminate cholesterol from the blood.

- Regulates the body's absorption of glucose (diabetics included) perhaps because fiber is believed to be capable of controlling the rate of digestion and assimilation of carbohydrates.
    - High-fiber meals have been shown to exert regulatory effects on blood-glucose levels for up to five hours after eating.

Carbohydrate and Performance

Carbohydrate availability is vital for maximal sports performance. When performing high-intensity, short-duration activity (anaerobic), muscular demand for energy is provided for and dependent upon muscle glycogen. During endurance exercise (aerobic) performed at a moderate intensity (60 percent of VO_2 max), muscle glycogen provides approximately 50 percent of energy needs. During high-intensity aerobic exercise (over 79 percent of VO_2 max), it yields nearly all of the energy needs.[80]

Duration of exercise also affects the amount of glycogen used for energy. As duration of activity increases, available glucose and glycogen diminish, increasing the reliance on fat as a fuel source. In addition, one could presume that if there is an appreciable increase in duration, there must also be a decrease in intensity, decreasing the use of glycogen.

However, this does not mean that the best way to lose body fat is to perform low-intensity activities for a long duration. If the workout contributes to a caloric deficit, the body will draw on its fat stores at some point to make up for the deficit.[81]

However, the limiting factor for exercise performance is carbohydrate availability: "Fat burns in a carbohydrate flame." That is to say, maximal fat utilization cannot occur without sufficient carbohydrate to continue Kreb's Cycle activity.[82,83] When an endurance athlete "hits the wall," it is due to fatigue caused by severely lowered liver and muscle glycogen. This occurs even though there is sufficient oxygen being delivered to the muscles and an abundance of potential energy from fat stores.[84]

Recommendations

Endurance Exercise

The amount of carbohydrate in the diet can affect performance. High-carbohydrate diets increase the use of glycogen as fuel; whereas a high-fat diet increases the use of fat as fuel.[81] However, a high-fat diet results in lower glycogen synthesis.[85,86] This is of particular concern if the individual is consuming a reduced-energy diet.[87] For the endurance athlete, a carbohydrate-rich diet will build glycogen stores and aid in performance and recovery.[88,89] Although some studies show an increase in performance associated with the consumption of a high-fat diet, these improvements are seen in exercise performed at a relatively low intensity (less than 70 percent of VO_2 max).[86,90] As the intensity of exercise increases, performance of high-intensity exercise will ultimately be impaired.[91-93]

A diet containing between six and 10 g/kg/day of carbohydrate, or approximately 60 percent of caloric intake, is recommended for individuals participating in endurance exercise. Complex carbohydrates (such as whole grains and fresh fruits and vegetables) should comprise the majority of calories, due to their nutrient-dense (providing B vitamins, iron and fiber) nature.

Pre-exercise

It is recommended that the individual consume a high-carbohydrate meal two to three hours prior to exercising for more than an hour. This will allow time for appropriate gastric emptying before exercise. This is especially helpful for morning workouts when glycogen stores are lowered by as much as 80 percent.[81] If this is not feasible due to time constraints, a liquid meal such as a meal-replacement formula may be used. One advantage to such formulas is their quick gastric emptying time.

Some research recommends a carbohydrate intake of 1 - 4.5 g/kg, between one and four hours prior to exercise, respectively.[94] In this study, the group ingesting 4.5 g/kg of carbohydrate four hours prior to exercise saw performance improved by 15 percent.[95] To avoid gastrointestinal distress, smaller meals should be consumed closer to the exercise session.

Carbohydrate Loading

In endurance exercise of greater than a 90-minute duration (e.g. marathon running), muscle-glycogen stores become depleted. This depletion limits the performance of endurance exercise. Carbohydrate loading, also called glycogen supercompensation, is a technique used to increase muscle glycogen prior to an endurance event. This practice can nearly double muscle-glycogen stores, increasing endurance potential.[96]

Historically, the week-long program includes four days of glycogen depletion (through a low-carbohydrate diet and exhaustive exercise), followed by three days of rest and a high-carbohydrate diet. This method had many drawbacks, including periods of hypoglycemia, irritability, increased susceptibility to injury and difficulty in compliance. In 1981, one study proposed a revised method (Table 15-4) that accomplishes the same goal with greater ease of compliance and fewer side effects.[97]

Table 15-4: Glycogen-Loading Schedule		
Days Before the Event	**Exercise Intensity and Duration**	**Carbohydrate Intake**
6 days out	**70-75% of VO$_2$ max, for 90 min.**	4 g/kg of body weight
4-5 days out	**70-75% of VO$_2$ max, for 40 min.**	4 g/kg of body weight
2-3 days out	**70-75% of VO$_2$ max, for 20 min.**	10 g/kg of body weight
1 day out	**Rest**	10 g/kg of body weight

Athletes with diabetes or high triglycerides should consult a physician before using this plan.

During Exercise

For exercise lasting more than one hour, carbohydrate feedings during exercise can help supply glucose to working muscles whose glycogen stores are dwindling. This technique also maintains blood-glucose levels, increasing time to exhaustion by 20-60 minutes.[98-101] It is recommended that endurance athletes consume between 30 and 60 grams of carbohydrate every hour to accomplish this. Popular sports beverages are perfect for this goal and have the added benefit of replacing fluid losses, also benefiting performance. The replacement of carbohydrate and water has individual benefits that together are additive.

One study showed that performance during one hour of intense cycling was improved by 12 percent with the consumption of 1,330 ml (53 oz.) of water containing 79 g of carbohydrate.[102] NASM concurs that consuming 600-1,200 ml (20-40 oz.) per hour of fluid that contains between four and eight percent carbohydrate will contribute to better performance for the endurance athlete.[101]

After Exercise

Repeated days of strenuous exercise take a toll on an individual's glycogen stores. A high-carbohydrate intake helps to replenish glycogen stores; however, the timing of carbohydrate ingestion can also be important to maximizing recovery. Consuming 1.5 g/kg/wt of carbohydrate within 30 minutes of completing exercise is recommended to maximize glycogen replenishment.[103] Delaying carbohydrate intake by even two hours can decrease total muscle glycogen synthesis by 66 percent.[104] The post-workout environment may hasten glycogen repletion due to increased blood flow to the muscles and an increased sensitivity of the cells to the effects of insulin.[81] Additional meals of 1.5 g/kg of carbohydrate every two hours are recommended to completely restore muscle glycogen.[103]

For Altering Body Composition

Carbohydrate should generally make up the highest percentage of macronutrient calories when one is attempting fat loss or muscle gain. Carbohydrates provide variety, valuable nutrients and volume to the diet. The satiating value of complex carbohydrate is especially important when one is in a caloric deficit for the goal of fat loss.[105-107] For most moderately active adults, a carbohydrate intake of between 50 and 70 percent is recommended. This will provide sufficient food volume and the fuel necessary for energy and productive workouts.

Despite the popularity of low-carbohydrate diets and the perpetuation of erroneous claims regarding type or time of carbohydrate intake, there is no need for one to reduce carbohydrate percentage to lose fat (see Carbohydrate and Weight Gain below). Weight loss or gain is related to total caloric intake, not the macronutrient profile of the diet. The weight lost on a low-carbohydrate diet can be attributed to two factors: low caloric intake and loss of fat-free mass (FFM).[108] When one begins dropping carbohydrate-rich foods from their diet, it is inevitable that caloric intake is reduced. Added to the caloric reduction are dwindling glycogen stores. For every gram of glucose taken out of glycogen, it brings with it 2.7 g of water.[109] This loss of muscle glycogen (including water) can be quite significant in the first week of a low-carbohydrate diet, and adds to the pounds lost on the scale. This is how low-carbohydrate fad diets can promise dramatic weight loss in such a short period of time. Long-term success in weight loss is associated with a realistic eating style, not one that severely limits or omits one of the macronutrients.[110]

Carbohydrate and Weight Gain: The Facts

A significant amount of time, energy and resources are spent investigating the link between carbohydrate intake and the increased prevalence of obesity in Americans. The accusations are familiar: "carbohydrates make you fat;" "Americans are getting fatter, despite lower fat intakes."

Data available from the Third National Health and Nutrition Examination Survey (NHANES III), which catalogs Americans' nutrition patterns for the years 1988-1991, shows that percentage of calories consumed from fat has indeed dropped, from 36 percent (NHANES II 1976-1980) to 34 percent of total energy intake.[111] However, when total fat intake (grams per person per day) is measured, and not simply the percentage contributed, the data shows that fat intake has remained quite constant over the past several years.[112] Additionally this data may not accurately reflect fat consumption in America, as many people underreport fat consumption due to its negative health connotations.[69] The data from NHANES III also shows an increase in total energy intake. This would support the relationship between excessive energy intake, leading to increased fat stores.

When reviewing the data on Americans' food intake, it is interesting to note that in the early 1900s, the percentage of carbohydrates consumed as energy intake was higher and consumption of fat lower than it is today, without the prevalence of obesity we now experience.[113] Only over the last two decades has there been a significant increase in obesity. Data supports two primary variables responsible for this dramatic rise in obesity: an increased energy intake and a reduction in energy expenditure.[111,114] Data published in 1996 by the U.S. Department of Health and Human Services found that 60 percent of American adults are not regularly active and that 25 percent participate in no physical activity at all.[114]

In summary, at the turn of the century, carbohydrate intake as a percentage of total energy was higher, fat as a percentage was lower and obesity was not the problem it is today. Currently, total fat intake is higher, carbohydrate is lower and obesity has reached epidemic proportions.[115] In addition, energy intake has increased and energy expenditure has decreased. The facts are very clear: America's increasing problem of obesity is not a direct result of carbohydrate intake, but rather of energy imbalance.

Review of the Properties of Carbohydrates

One gram of carbohydrate yields four calories.

Carbohydrates provide the body with:

- Nutrition that fat and protein cannot (from complex carbohydrates);
- Satiety by keeping glycogen stores full and adding bulk to the diet;
- Proper cellular-fluid balance, maximizing cellular efficiency;
- Proper blood-sugar levels, if there is a consistent intake of low-glycemic carbohydrates; and
- Spare protein for building muscle.

The body needs carbohydrates because:

- They are the perfect and preferred form of energy,
- They constantly need to be replaced, causing a craving that must be satisfied,
- Parts of the central nervous system rely exclusively on carbohydrate,
- They efficiently burn and utilize fat and protein.

Recommended carbohydrate intake:

- Daily diet should include 25 grams of fiber.
- Carbohydrate intake typically should be between 50 and 70 percent of total caloric intake according to preference, performance and satiety.
- Carbohydrate recommendations should be estimated after protein and fat requirements are met.
- Fruits, whole grains and vegetables are all excellent sources of fiber.

MODULE 15-3 Summary

Carbohydrates are a chief source of energy for all body functions and muscular exertion. They are compounds containing carbon, hydrogen and oxygen and are generally classified as sugars (simple), starches (complex) and fiber. A monosaccharide is a single sugar unit (such as glucose, fructose or galactose), many of which are connected to make starches and glycogen. Disaccharides (two sugar units) include sucrose, lactose and maltose. Carbohydrates help to regulate the digestion and utilization of protein and fat.

Glycemic index (GI) is the rate at which ingested carbohydrate raises blood sugar and affects insulin release. Foods lower on the glycemic index are good sources of complex carbohydrates, as well as being high in fiber and overall nutritional value. When total caloric intake exceeds output, any excess carbohydrate, dietary fat or protein may be stored as body fat, until needed.

Fiber is one of the greatest contributions made by dietary complex carbohydrate. Higher intakes of dietary fiber are associated with lower incidence of heart disease and certain types of cancer. In addition, fiber provides many other benefits including: satiety, intestinal health and regulation of the body's absorption of glucose.

The availability of carbohydrate is vital for maximal sports performance because the demand for energy is provided for and dependent upon muscle glycogen. Duration and intensity of exercise affects the amount of glycogen used for energy. Maximal fat utilization cannot occur without sufficient carbohydrate. For the endurance athlete, a daily carbohydrate-rich diet (containing between six and 10 g/kg/day of carbohydrate, or approximately 60 percent of caloric intake) will build glycogen stores and aid in performance and recovery. It is recommended that the individual consume a high-carbohydrate meal two to three hours prior to exercising for more than an hour. In endurance exercise of greater than a 90-minute duration, carbohydrate loading can be used to increase muscle glycogen, prior to an endurance event. For exercise lasting more than one hour, endurance athletes should consume between 30 and 60 grams of carbohydrate every hour (which may consist of sports beverages). After exercise, consuming 1.5 g/kg/wt of carbohydrate within 30 minutes is recommended. Additional meals of 1.5 g/kg of carbohydrate every two hours are recommended to completely restore muscle glycogen.

For fat loss or muscle gain, carbohydrates should generally make up the highest percentage of macronutrient calories. An intake between 50 and 70 percent is recommended. There is no need for one to reduce carbohydrate percentage to lose fat. America's increasing problem of obesity is not a direct result of carbohydrate intake, but rather one of energy imbalance.

MODULE 15-3 Quiz

1. Match the following words to their meanings:

   a. Carbohydrate _____ Starches

   b. Simple carbohydrates _____ Storage form of carbohydrates in humans

   c. Complex carbohydrates _____ Fruit sugar

   d. Starches _____ Milk sugar

   e. Glycogen _____ Sugars

   f. Monosaccharide _____ Common sugar

   g. Disaccharide _____ Storage form of carbohydrates in plants

   h. Glucose _____ Two sugar units

   i. Fructose _____ Blood sugar

   j. Sucrose _____ Compounds containing carbon, hydrogen and oxygen

   k. Lactose _____ Single sugar unit

2. The limiting factor for exercise performance is _____ availability.

3. Foods with a higher GI lead to fat storage, regardless of caloric intake.

   ☐ True   ☐ False

4. Recommended carbohydrate intake for adults is _____ percent of total caloric intake, according to preference, performance and satiety.

   ☐ 10-30   ☐ 30-50   ☐ 50-70

MODULE 15-4: Lipids

The Structure of Lipids

Lipids are a group of compounds that include *triglycerides* (fats and oils), *phospholipids* and *sterols*. Of the lipids contained in food, 95 percent are fats and oils. In the body, 99 percent of the stored lipids are also triglycerides.[116] Structurally, triglycerides are three fatty acids attached to a glycerol backbone (Figure 15-5).

> **LIPIDS:**
> **Various substances that make up the principal structural components of living cells.**

Mixed triglycerides are typical of those found in foods. The fat in a food is a mixture of many different mixed triglycerides. (The shape of the fatty acids is shown for ease of viewing.)

Figure 15-5: The Triglyceride

Fatty Acids

These fatty acids may be *saturated* or *unsaturated* (Figure 15-6). Unsaturated fatty acids may be further classified according to their degree of unsaturation. If the fatty acid has one double bond in its carbon chain, it is called a *mono-unsaturated* fatty acid. If there is more than one point of unsaturation, it is classified as a *polyunsaturated* fatty acid.

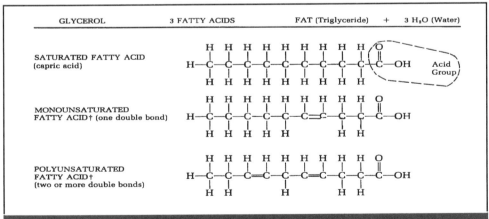

Figure 15-6: Fatty Acids

Polyunsaturated fatty acids provide important essential fatty acids (or fats that cannot be manufactured by the body but are essential for proper health and functioning).[117]

Saturated fatty acids are implicated as a risk factor for heart disease because they raise bad cholesterol levels (LDL), while unsaturated fats are associated with increases in good cholesterol (HDL) and decreased risk of heart disease.[118,119]

Mono-unsaturated fatty acids (found in olive and canola oils) and polyunsaturated fatty acids such as Omega-3 fatty acids (found in cold-water fish, like salmon) are considered to have favorable effects on blood-lipid profiles and may play a role in the treatment and prevention of heart disease, hypertension, arthritis and cancer.[118,119]

Another prevalent fatty acid in today's food supply is trans-fatty acids, the result of *hydrogenation* (or the process of adding hydrogen to unsaturated fatty acids to make them harder at room temperature and increase food shelf life). Trans-fatty acids have been shown to increase LDL cholesterol and decrease HDL cholesterol, much like saturated fats.[120-122]

The Function of Lipids

Lipids (or fats) are the most concentrated source of energy in the diet. One gram of fat yields approximately nine calories when oxidized, furnishing more than twice the calories per gram of carbohydrates or proteins. In addition to providing energy, fats act as carriers for the fat-soluble vitamins A, D, E and K. Vitamin D aids in the absorption of calcium, making it available to body tissues, particularly to the bones and teeth. Fats are also important for the conversion of carotene to vitamin A.[123] Fats are involved in the following:[123]

- Cellular-membrane structure and function;
- Precursors to hormones;
- Cellular signals;
- Regulation and excretion of nutrients in the cells;
- Surrounding, protecting and holding in place organs, such as the kidneys, heart and liver;
- Insulating the body from environmental temperature changes and preserving body heat;
- Prolonging the digestive process by slowing the stomach's secretions of hydrochloric acid, creating a longer lasting sensation of fullness after a meal; and
- Initiating the release of the hormone cholecystokinin (CCK), which contributes to satiety.

Digestion, Absorption and Utilization

Digestion of dietary fat starts in the mouth, moves to the stomach and is completed in the small intestine. In the intestine, the fat interacts with bile to become emulsified, where pancreatic enzymes can break the triglycerides down into two fatty acids and a monoglyceride.

Absorption of these constituents occurs through the intestinal wall into the blood. In the intestinal wall, they are reassembled into triglycerides that are then released into the lymph in the form of a lipoprotein, called the *chylomicron*. Chylomicrons from the lymph move to the blood. The triglyceride content of the chylomicron is removed by the action of the enzyme lipoprotein lipase (LPL) and the released fatty acids are taken up by the tissues (Figure 14-6).

Throughout the day, triglycerides are constantly cycled in and out of tissues, including muscles, organs and adipose.

Recommendations

Clients must be satiated by the amount of calories necessary to allow fat loss or energy balance or they will eventually overeat. Our goal is to keep the client's diet within the guidelines for health. If the goal is fat loss or to enhance overall health, a diet containing 10-30 percent of calories from fat is recommended. Higher fat diets are not conducive to successful weight loss or maintenance and appear to increase the ease with which the body converts ingested calories to body fat.[124-126]

Fat has a lower *thermic effect* than other macronutrients.[127] The thermic effect of a food (TEF) is the rise in metabolic rate that occurs after the food is ingested. Typically, TEF amounts to 10 percent of ingested calories.[117] As fat percentage in the diet increases, the amount of heat given off (TEF) decreases. Conversely, as carbohydrate percentage in the diet increases, so does the TEF. It is metabolically inexpensive to convert dietary fat to body-fat stores. Only three percent of the calories in fat are required to store it as fat. In contrast, it takes 23 percent of the calories in carbohydrate to convert it to body fat.[127]

Fat and Satiety

Dietary fats stimulate the release of CCK, a hormone that signals satiety. Additionally, fats slow the digestion of foods (and thus the nutrient content in the bloodstream), assisting in blood-sugar stabilization. Reducing blood-sugar fluctuations can contribute to satiety.

However, diets containing more than 30 percent of calories from fat lose the volume of food provided by higher carbohydrate diets. In other words, both a tablespoon of oil and a large salad with nonfat dressing may contain the same amount of calories.

Because satiety is achieved by more than just total caloric intake, this low-volume/high-calorie contribution of fat may not satisfy other peripheral satiation mechanisms (chewing, swallowing, stomach distention) leading to *hyperphagia* (or overeating).[128]

Fat Supplementation During Exercise

In general, fat is digested and absorbed quite slowly. Long-chain triglycerides (LCT), which make up the majority of dietary fatty acids (16-18 carbons), must go through the process of digestion and absorption described earlier. Medium-chain triglycerides (MCT), however, are more rapidly absorbed. Additionally, they do not require incorporation into chylomicrons for transport, but can enter systemic circulation directly through the portal vein, providing a readily-available, concentrated source of energy.[129] It has been suggested that MCT could benefit endurance performance by supplying an exogenous energy source in addition to carbohydrate during exercise and increase plasma free fatty acids (FFA), sparing muscle glycogen.[130,131] Currently, there is insufficient evidence to recommend MCT supplementation for the goal of improving endurance exercise.

Insulin Resistance and Obesity

Proponents of high-protein/low-carbohydrate diets have profited from the erroneous assertion that carbohydrates are to blame for the increasing prevalence of metabolic syndrome (MS) (or Syndrome X) and therefore lead to weight gain. Metabolic syndrome is a cluster of symptoms characterized by obesity, insulin resistance, hypertension and dyslipidemia, leading to an increased risk of cardiovascular disease. Syndrome X is usually associated with obesity (especially abdominal), a high-fat diet and a sedentary lifestyle.[132-135]

A common denominator associated with these factors is high levels of circulating free fatty acids (FFA). In the presence of high FFA concentrations, the body will favor their use as energy, decreasing glucose oxidation, glycogen synthesis, and inhibiting glucose transport.[132] The result of this is hyperglycemia. When blood-sugar levels are chronically high, insulin will also be elevated, leading to the conversion of the excess blood sugar to other products such as sugar proteins and fatty acids.

These facts alone seem to bolster the idea that carbohydrates lead to health problems. The truth is that a healthy person would need to eat an extremely high percentage of simple carbohydrates (such as sucrose) and fat, maintain a constant energy excess or be overweight in order to have chronically-elevated blood sugar. Although there is some evidence that there may be a genetic component that contributes to insulin resistance (IR), the condition itself will not allow for weight gain without an energy intake in excess of expenditure.[5,136,137] In fact, obesity itself is a risk factor for development of IR, not the other way around.[138]

So, what is the common cause of IR? If one constantly overeats, excess calories are stored as fat. Fat cells then increase in size. The growing fat cell itself becomes insulin resistant and the resulting prevalence of FFA will cause the body to favor the use of fat for energy at the expense of glucose.[139] This becomes a vicious cycle.

The overweight condition leads to IR, which in turn leads to impaired glucose use. Blood-sugar levels rise; insulin levels rise; cholesterol, TG and blood pressure rise as well. To make matters worse, the impaired ability of glucose to enter muscle cells keeps glycogen stores lower, which can increase appetite, motivating the individual to eat more, increasing fat stores, exacerbating IR, and so on.

As numerous studies point out, high-fat diets are strongly associated with obesity, thus insulin resistance and diabetes.[139-141] Of course, eating fat does not make one fat (the same applies to carbohydrate), unless it is consumed in excess of energy requirements. However, it is easier to consume excess energy (or hyperphagia) on a high-fat diet, due to fat's high caloric density. When this high intake of dietary fat is combined with excess calories and a sedentary lifestyle, it is easy to envision an abundance of fatty acids floating around in the blood stream.

It is much more likely that a high-fat diet leads to excess consumption of calories, obesity, IR and eventually non-insulin dependent diabetes mellitus, than it is that carbohydrates cause insulin resistance and, as a result, obesity. The only solution is a diet containing the appropriate amount of energy, high in fibrous or starchy carbohydrates, and exercise. In fact, a study of Type II diabetics, those with insulin resistance, and people of normal weight found that three weeks of a high-carbohydrate, low-fat diet and exercise program significantly lowered insulin levels.[142]

Perhaps it is convenient to place blame on carbohydrates. With obesity continuing to rise, a simple solution to the problem of America's weight gain would be welcomed. Our current environment has created a Petri dish that encourages the growth of the human organism. Highly palatable and caloric-rich food is available to most and today's work and recreational demands do not call for much physical movement.

On the surface, the cure for obesity is simple: move more and eat less. However, the influence of societal, psychological and physiological factors can make putting this simple plan into action very difficult. Be that as it may, any solution will ultimately provide a way to increase energy expenditure, decrease energy consumption or a combination of both.

Review of the Properties of Lipids

One gram of fat yields nine calories. It is generally insoluble in water. Fat is present in all cells: high in adipose and nerve tissue, low in epithelial and muscle tissue. Fatty acids can be saturated, polyunsaturated and monounsaturated.

The body needs fats for:

- Energy,
- Structure and membrane function,
- Precursors to hormones,
- Cellular signals and
- Regulation of uptake and excretion of nutrients in the cells.

Recommended fat intake:

- Fat intake can range from 10 to 30 percent, according to performance, satiety and palatability.
- A high polyunsaturated-to-saturated-fat ratio is desirable.
- The average American's fat consumption is between 32 and 42 percent of total caloric intake.
- More than 30 percent leads to overeating (lack of food volume) and often slows metabolism.

MODULE 15-4 Summary

Lipids are a group of compounds that include triglycerides (fats and oils), phospholipids and sterols. Most lipids in food and in the body are triglycerides, which are three fatty acids (saturated or unsaturated) attached to a glycerol backbone. Polyunsaturated fatty acids provide important essential fatty acids. Saturated fatty acids and trans-fatty acids are implicated as a risk factor for heart disease because they raise bad cholesterol levels (LDL), while unsaturated fats are associated with increases in good cholesterol (HDL) and decreased risk of heart disease.

Lipids are the most concentrated source of energy in the diet. One gram of fat yields approximately nine calories. Lipids also regulate and excrete nutrients and act as carriers for vitamins A, D (which aids in the absorption of calcium), E and K. Fats have many other benefits including cellular-membrane structure and function, body insulation, aid in the digestive process and satiety.

Digestion of dietary fat starts in the mouth, moves to the stomach and is completed in the small intestine. Throughout the day, triglycerides are constantly cycled in and out of tissues.

A diet containing 10-30 percent of calories from fat is recommended for fat loss or to enhance overall health. Fat has a lower thermic effect than other macronutrients, only taking three percent of its calories to store it in the body as fat. Fat is digested and absorbed quite slowly. Thus, medium-chain triglycerides are not recommended as supplements for the goal of improving endurance exercise.

Metabolic syndrome is a cluster of symptoms characterized by obesity and insulin resistance. However, insulin resistance alone will not allow for weight gain without an energy intake in excess of expenditure. Obesity itself is a risk factor for development of insulin resistance, not the other way around.

MODULE 15-4 Quiz

1. Which kind(s) of fatty acids is/are considered to have favorable effects on blood-lipid profiles and may play a role in the treatment and prevention of heart disease, hypertension, arthritis and cancer?

   ☐ Monounsaturated ☐ Polyunsaturated ☐ Trans-fatty

2. The _____ _____ of a food is the rise in metabolic rate that occurs after the food is ingested.

3. A study of Type II diabetics (with insulin resistance) and people of normal weight found that three weeks of a high-carbohydrate, low-fat diet and exercise program significantly lowered insulin levels.

   ☐ True ☐ False

MODULE 15-5: Water

The Importance of Water

Water is the soup of life. It constitutes approximately 60 percent of the adult human body, by weight. Whereas deficiencies of nutrients such as the macronutrients, vitamins and minerals may take weeks or even years to develop, one can only survive for a few days without water. Consuming an adequate amount of water will benefit the body in the following ways:[143]

- Endocrine-gland function improves.
- Fluid retention is alleviated.
- Liver functions improve, increasing percentage of fat used for energy.
- Natural thirst returns.
- Appetite decreases significantly.
- Metabolic functions improve.
- Nutrients are distributed throughout the body.
- Body-temperature regulation improves.
- Blood volume is maintained.

On average, an individual should drink approximately 96 ounces (three quarts) of water per day. Those participating in a fat-loss program should drink an additional eight ounces of water for every 25 pounds they carry above their ideal weight. Water intake should also be increased if an individual is exercising briskly or residing in a hot climate.

Water and Performance

The importance of proper hydration cannot be stressed enough. The body cannot adapt to dehydration, which impairs every physiological function. Table 15-5 shows the effects of dehydration.

Studies have shown that a fluid loss of even two percent of body weight will adversely affect circulatory functions and decrease performance levels.[144]

Table 15-5: Effects of Dehydration	
Decreased blood volume	Increased heart rate
Decreased performance	Sodium retention
Decreased blood pressure	Decreased cardiac output
Decreased sweat rate	Decreased blood flow to the skin
Increased core temperature	Increased perceived exertion
Water retention	Increased use of muscle glycogen

However, if a fairly regular daily pattern of exercise and water and food consumption is followed, average body weight will provide a very good index of the body's state of hydration. Realizing this, the organizers of certain ultra-distance running events make it mandatory for competitors to weigh themselves at stations along the course and require each runner to consume enough fluid to regain a predetermined body weight before being allowed to continue.

Thirst alone is a poor indicator of how much water is needed. Athletes consistently consume inadequate fluid, managing to replace approximately 50 percent of sweat losses.[145] A good way to keep track of how much one needs to drink is to first determine his or her average daily weight (e.g., weight upon waking). Use this number as the standard for the person's *euhydrated* (or normal) state. Don't begin a practice session or endurance competition until the body is at, or slightly above, its standard weight. Drink enough water, juice or sports drinks during exercise in order to maintain the starting weight.

Guidelines for fluid replacement in the athlete are as follows:[146,147]

- Consume 16 oz. of fluid two hours prior to exercise. An additional eight to 16 oz. may be needed if exercising in warmer weather.
- Drink 20-40 oz. of fluid for every hour of exercise.
- Fluids should be cold, due to more rapid gastric emptying.
- If exercise exceeds 60 minutes, use of a sports drink (containing up to eight percent carbohydrate) can replace both fluid and dwindling muscle-glycogen stores.
- When exercising for less than 60 minutes, water is the experts' choice for fluid replacement.
- The goal is to replace sweat and urine losses.
- Ingest 20 oz. of fluid for every pound of body weight lost after an exercise bout, especially if rapid rehydration is necessary, as in twice-a-day training.

MODULE 15-5 Summary

On average, an individual should drink approximately 96 ounces (three quarts) of water per day. Those on fat-loss programs should drink an additional eight ounces of water for every 25 pounds carried above ideal weight. Water intake should also be increased if an individual is exercising briskly or residing in a hot climate. The body cannot adapt to dehydration, which impairs every physiological function. A fluid loss of even two percent of body weight will adversely affect circulatory functions and decrease performance levels.

Consuming an adequate amount of water will improve body temperature regulation, metabolic function, endocrine gland and liver function. In addition, nutrients are distributed throughout the body, blood volume is maintained, fluid retention is alleviated and appetite decreases significantly.

Thirst alone is a poor indicator of how much water is needed. Instead, determine average daily weight and use this number as the standard for a euhydrated state. Consume 16 oz. of fluid two hours prior to exercise and drink 20-40 oz. of fluid for every hour of exercise. Finally, ingest 20 oz. of fluid for every pound of body weight lost after an exercise bout.

MODULE 15-5 Quiz

1. Water constitutes approximately _____ percent of the adult human body, by weight.

2. When exercising for more than 60 minutes, water is the experts' choice for fluid replacement.

   ☐ True ☐ False

MODULE 15-6:
Altering Body Composition

Basic Nutrition Guidelines for Altering Body Composition

For Fat Loss

- Distribute protein, carbohydrate and fat throughout the day and at each meal.

- Choose whole grains and fresh vegetables over refined grains and simple sugars (as the fiber and complexity of the starch will aid in hunger control).

- Schedule no fewer than four and as many as six meals a day. This helps to control hunger, minimize blood-sugar fluctuations and increase energy levels throughout the day.

- Avoid empty calories and highly processed foods, which contain many calories and do little to provide satiety.

- Drink a lot of water (eight to 12 cups per day).

- Have clients weigh and measure food for at least one week. This will make them more aware of caloric values and serving sizes, as well as decrease the likelihood of underreporting calories.

For Lean Body Mass Gain

- Eat four to six meals a day. Insulin response to a meal stimulates protein synthesis.

- Spread protein intake throughout the day to take advantage of the previous tip.

- Keep in mind the post-workout window of opportunity. Ingestion of protein and carbohydrate within 90 minutes of a workout will increase recovery and protein synthesis, maximizing gains. This may be most easily accomplished with a liquid meal-replacement formula that can be absorbed quickly due to being predigested. Food may take several hours to digest and absorb, missing the window.

- Do not neglect the importance of carbohydrate and fat. It takes more than protein to increase lean body mass.

References

1. *Webster's ninth new collegiate dictionary.* Springfield, MA: Merriam-Webster Inc.;1991. 1564 p.

2. [Anonymous] Clinical guidelines on the identification, evaluation, and treatment of overweight and obesity in adults — the evidence report. National Institutes of Health. *Obesity Res* Sep 1998;6(suppl 2):51S-209S.

3. Walsh MF, Flynn TJ. A 54-month evaluation of a popular very low calorie diet program. *J Fam Pract* Sep 1995;41(3):231-6.

4. Position of the American Dietetic Association: weight management. *J Am Diet Assoc* Jan 1997;97(1):71-4.

5. Faires VM. *Thermodynamics.* New York: Macmillan Company; 1967.

6. Jensen, MD. Diet effects on fatty acid metabolism in lean and obese humans. *Am J Clin Nutr* 1998(67 suppl):531-4.

7. Agricultural Research Service. Fat intake continues to drop; veggies, fruits still low in the US diet. *Res News* 1996.

8. Rose WC, Haines WJ, Warner DT. The amino acid requirements of man. V. The role of lysine, arginine, and tryptophan. *J Biol Chem* 1954;206:421-30.

9. Martineau A, Lecavalier L, Falardeau P, Chiasson JL. Simultaneous determination of glucose turnover, and gluconeogenesis in human using a double stable-isotope-labeled tracer infusion and gas chromatography-mass spectrometry analysis. *Anal Biochem* Dec 1985;151(2):495-503.

10. Berdanier CD. *Advanced nutrition: macronutrients.* Boca Raton, FL: CRC Press; 1995. pp. 277.

11. Block RJ, Mitchell HH. *Nut Ab Rev* 1946;16:249-78.

12. Shils ME, Young VR. *Modern nutrition in health and disease.* 7th edition. Philadelphia, PA: Lea & Febiger; 1988. pp. 1694.

13. Tarnopolsky MA, Atkinson SA, MacDougall JD, Chesley A, Phillip S, Schwarcz HP. Evaluation of protein requirements for trained strength athletes. *J Appl Phys* 1992;73(5):1986-95.

14. Lemon PW, Tarnolpolsky MA, MacDougall JD, Atkinson SA. Protein requirements and muscle mass/strength changes during intensive training in novice bodybuilders. *J Appl Phys* 1992;73(2):767-75.

15. Keul J. The relationship between circulation and metabolism during exercise. *Med Sci Sports* 1973;5:209.

16. Keul J, Doll E, Keppler D. *Energy metabolism of human muscle.* Baltimore, MD: University Park; 1972.

17. Wahlberg JL, Leidy MK, Sturgill DJ, Hinkle DE, Ritchey SJ, Sebolt DR. Macronutrient content of a hypoenergy diet affects nitrogen retention and muscle function in weight lifters. *Int J Sports Med* Aug 1988; 9(4):261-6.

18. Ruderman NB. Muscle amino acid metabolism and gluconeogenesis. *Ann Rev Med* 1975;26:245-58.

19. Harper AE, Miller RH, Block KP. Branched-chain amino acid metabolism. *Ann Rev Nutr* 1984;4:409-54.

20. Hood DA, Terjung RL. Amino acid metabolism during exercise and following endurance training. *Sports Med* Jan 1990;9(1):23-35.

21. Ahlborg G, Felig P, Hagenfeldt L, Hendler R, Wahren J. Substrate turnover during prolonged exercise in man. Splanchnic and leg metabolism of glucose, free fatty acids, and amino acids. *J Clin Invest* Apr 1974; 53(4):1080-90.

22. Lemon PW, Mullin JP. Effect of initial muscle glycogen levels on protein catabolism during exercise. *J Appl Physiol* Apr 1980;48(4):624-9.

23. White TP, Brooks GA. [U-14C] glucose, -alanine, and -leucine oxidation in rats at rest and two intensities of running. *Am J Physiol* Feb 1981;240(2):E155-65.

24. Knapik J, Meredith C, Jones B, Fielding R, Young V, Evans W. Leucine metabolism during fasting and exercise. *J Appl Physiol* Jan 1991;70(1):43-7.

25. Youn VR. Metabolic and nutritional aspects of physical exercise. *Fed Proc* 1985;44:341.

26. Allison JB, Bird JC. Elimination of nitrogen from the body. In: Munro HN, Allison JB (eds). *Mammalian protein metabolism.* Vol 1. New York: Academic Press; 1964.

27. Munro HN. Historical introduction: the origin and growth of our present concepts of protein metabolism. In: Munro HN, Allison JB (eds). *Mammalian protein metabolism.* Vol 1. New York: Academic Press;1964.

28. Waterlow JC, Garlick PJ, Millward DJ. *Protein turnover in mammalian tissues and in the whole body.* New York: North-Holland; 1978.

29. Kurzer MS, Calloway DH. Nitrate and nitrogen balances in men. *Am J Clin Nutr* Jul 1981;34(7):1305-13.

30. Piatti PM, Monti F, Fermo I, Baruffaldi L, Nasser R, Santambrogio G, Librenti MC, Galli-Kienle M, Pontiroli AE, Pozza G. Hypocaloric high-protein diet improves glucose oxidation and spares lean body mass: comparison to hypocaloric high-carbohydrate diet. *Metabol* Dec 1994;43(12):1481-7.

31. Minghelli G, Schutz Y, Charbonnier A, Whitehead R, Jequier E. Twenty-four-hour energy expenditure and basal metabolic rate measured in a whole-body indirect calorimeter in Gambian men. *Am J Clin Nutr* Apr 1990;51(4):563-70.

32. Spruce N. Plateaus and energy expenditure. Increased difficulty in attending fat or weight loss goals in healthy subjects. *J Nat Intramur Recreat Sports Ass* Fall 1997;22(1):24-8.

33. Spiller GA, Jensen CD, Pattison TS, Chuck CS, Whittam JH, Scala J. Effect of protein dose on serum glucose and insulin response to sugars. *Am J Clin Nutr* Sep 1987;46(3):474-80.

34. Zawadzki KM, Yaspelkis BB III, Ivy JL. Carbohydrate-protein complex increases the rate of muscle glycogen storage after exercise. *J Appl Physiol* May 1992;72(5):1854-9.

35. Roy BD, Tarnopolsky MA. Influence of differing macronutrient intakes on muscle glycogen resynthesis after resistance exercise. *J Appl Physiol* Mar 1998; 84(3):890-6.

36. Roy B, Tarnopolsky M, MacDougall J, Fowles J, Yarasheski K. Effect of glucose supplement timing on protein metabolism after resistance training. *J Appl Physiol* Jun 1997;82(6):1882-8.

37. Anderson GH, Li ET, Glanville NT. Brain mechanisms and the quantitative and qualitative aspects of food intake. *Brain Res Bull* Feb 1984;12(2):167-73.

38. Gellebter AA. Effects of equicaloric loads of protein, fat and carbohydrate on food intake in the rat and man. *Physiol Behav* 1979;22:267-73.

39. Van Zeggeren A, Li ET. Food intake and choice in lean and obese Zucker rats after intragastric carbohydrate preloads. *J Nutr* Mar 1990;120(3):309-16.

40. Li ET, Anderson GH. Meal composition influences subsequent food selection in the young rat. *Physiol Behav* Nov 1982;29(5):779-83.

41. Booth DA, Chase A, Campbell AT. Relative effectiveness of protein in the late stages of appetite suppression in man. *Physiol Behav* Nov 1970;5(11):1299-302.

42. Barkeling B, Rossner S, Bjorvell H. Effects of a high-protein meal (meat) and a high-carbohydrate meal (vegetarian) on satiety measured by automated computerized monitoring of subsequent food intake, motivation to eat and food preferences. *Int J Obes* Sep 1990;14(9):743-51.

43. Wurtman RJ, Wurtman JJ. Carbohydrate craving, obesity and brain serotonin. *Appet* 1986;7 Suppl:99-103.

44. Drewnoski A, [Oomura Y, Tarui S, Inoue S, Shmazu T (eds)]. *Progress in obesity research.* London: John Libbey; 1990.

45. Lichtenstein AH, Kennedy E, Barrier P, Danford D, Ernst ND, Grundy SM, Leveille GA, VanHorn L, Williams CL, Booth SL. Dietary fat consumption and health. *Nutr Rev* 1998;56(5 pt 2):S3-19.

46. Hu FB, Stampfer MJ, Manson JE, Rimm E, Colditz GA, Rosner BA, Hennekens CH, Willett WC. Dietary fat intake and the risk of coronary heart disease in women. *N Engl J Med* 1997;337(21):1491-9.

47. Leiberman B. Avoiding the fracture zone: calcium. *Nutr Act Heal Letter* Apr 1998;25(2):3-7.

48. Hegsted M, Linkswiler HM. Long-term effects of level of protein intake on calcium metabolism in young adult women. *J Nutr* Feb 1981;111(2):244-51.

49. Kerstetter JE, Mitnick ME, Gundberg CM, Caseria DM, Ellison AF, Carpenter TO, Insogna KL. Changes in bone turnover in young women consuming different levels of dietary protein. *J Clin Endocrinol Metab* Mar 1999;84(3):1052-5.

50. Allen LH, Oddoye EA, Margen S. Protein-induced hypercalciuria: a longer term study. *Am J Clin Nutr* Apr 1979;32(4):741-9.

51. Smolin LA, Grosvenor MB. *Nutrition science and applications.* Orlando, FL: Saunders College Publishing;1994. pp. 576.

52. Curtis D. Pump up your protein powder? *Muscl Fitn* 1991;52(10):75.

53. Parraga IM. Determinants of food consumption. *J Am Diet Assoc* 1990 May;90(5):661-3.

54. Douglas PD, Douglas JG. Nutrition knowledge and food practices of high school athletes. *J Am Diet Assoc* Oct 1984;84(10):1198-202.

55. Perron M, Endres J. Knowledge, attitudes, and dietary practices of female athletes. *J Am Diet Assoc* May 1985;85(5):573-6.

56. Werblow JA, Fox HM, Henneman A. Nutritional knowledge, attitudes, and food patterns of women athletes. *J Am Diet Assoc* Sep 1978;73(3):242-5.

57. Kraemer WJ, Volek JS, Bush JA, Putukian M, Sebastianelli WJ. Hormonal responses to consecutive days of heavy-resistance exercise with or without nutritional supplementation. *J Appl Physiol* Oct 1998;85(4):1544-55.

58. Chandler RM, Byrne HK, Patterson JG, Ivy JL. Dietary supplements affect the anabolic hormones after weight-training exercise. *J Appl Physiol* Feb 1994;76(2):839-45.

59. Tarnopolsky MA, MacDougall JD, Atkinson SA. Influence of protein intake and training status on nitrogen balance and lean body mass. *J Appl Physiol* Jan 1988;64(1):187-93.

60. Staron RS, Karapondo DL, Kraemer WJ, Fry AC, Gordon SE, Falkel JE, Hagerman FC, Hikida RS. Skeletal muscle adaptations during early phase of heavy-resistance training in men and women. *J Appl Physiol* Mar 1994;76(3):1247-55.

61. Tarnopolsky MA, Atkinson SA, MacDougall JD, Chesley A, Phillips S, Schwarcz HP. Evaluation of protein requirements for trained strength athletes. *J Appl Physiol* Nov 1992;73(5):1986-9.

62. Thissen JP, Ketelslegers JM, Underwood LE. Nutritional regulation of the insulin-like growth factors. *Endocr Rev* Feb 1994;15(1):80-101.

63. Volek JS, Kraemer WJ, Bush JA, Incledon T, Boetes M. Testosterone and cortisol in relationship to dietary nutrients and resistance exercise. *J Appl Physiol* Jan 1997;82(1):49-54.

64. Webb KE Jr. Intestinal absorption of protein hydrolysis products: a review. *J Anim Sci* Sep 1990;68(9):3011-22.

65. Poullain MG, Cezard JP, Roger L, Mendy F. Effect of whey proteins, their oligopeptide hydrolysates and free amino acid mixtures on growth and nitrogen retention in fed and starved rats. *J Parenter Enteral Nutr* Jul-Aug 1989;13(4):382-6.

66. Boza JJ, Martinez-Augustin O, Baro L, Suarez MD, Gil A. Protein v. enzymic protein hydrolysates. Nitrogen utilization in starved rats. *Br J Nutr* Jan 1995;73(1):65-71.

67. Demling RH, DeSanti L. Increased protein intake during the recovery phase after severe burns increases body weight gain and muscle function. *J Burn Care Rehabil* Mar-Apr 1998;19(2):161-8.

68. Stegink LD, Peptides in parenteral nutrition. In: Greene HL, Holliday MA, Munro HM (eds). *Clinical nutrition update: amino acids.* Chicago: American Medical Association; 1977.

69. Rolls BJ, Hill JO. *Carbohydrate and weight management.* Washington, DC: ILSI Press; 1998. pp. 60.

70. Jenkins DJ, Vuksan V, Kendall CW, Wursch P, Jeffcoat R, Waring S, Mehling CC, Vidgen E, Augustin LS, Wong E. Physiological effects of resistant starches on fecal bulk, short chain fatty acids, blood lipids and glycemic index. *J Am Coll Nutr* Dec 1998;17(6):609-16.

71. Lewis SJ, Heaton KW. Increasing butyrate concentration in the distal colon by accelerating intestinal transit. *Gut* Aug 1997;41(2):245-51.

72. Jarvi AE, Karlstrom BE, Granfeldt YE, Bjorck IM, Vessby BO, Asp NG. The influence of food structure on postprandial metabolism in patients with non-insulin-dependant diabetes mellitus. *Am J Clin Nutr* 1995;61(4):837-42.

73. Anderson JW, Smith BM, Gustafson NJ. Health benefits and practical aspects of high-fiber diets. *Am J Clin Nutr* 1994;59(5 suppl):1242S-47S.

74. Wolk A, Manson JE, Stampfer MJ, Colditz GA, Hu FB, Speizer FE, Hennekens CH, Willett WC. Long-term intake of dietary fiber and decreased risk of coronary heart disease among women. *JAMA* 1999;281(21):1998-2004.

73. Aldoori WH, Giovanucci EL, Rockett HR, Sampson L, Rimm EB, Willett WC. A prospective study of dietary fiber types and symptomatic divertivular disease in men. *J Nutr* Apr 1998;128(4):714-9.

74. Rimm EB, Ascherio A, Giovannucci E, Spiegelman D, Stampfer MJ, Willett WC. Vegetable, fruit, and cereal fiber intake and risk of coronary heart disease among men. *JAMA* Feb 1996; 275(6):447-51.

75. Anderson JW, Smith BM, Gustafson NJ. Health benefits and practical aspects of high-fiber diets. *Am J Clin Nutr* May 1994;59(5 Suppl):1242S-47S.

78. Howe GR, Benito E, Castelleto R, Cornee J, Esteve J, Gallagher RP, Iscovich JM, Deng-ao J, Kaaks R, Kune GA, et al. Dietary intake of fiber and decreased risk of cancers of the colon and rectum: evidence from the combined analysis of 13 case-controlled studies. *J Natl Canc Inst* Dec 1992;84(24):187-96.

79. Fernstrom JD, Miller GD. *Appetite and body weight regulation.* Boca Raton, FL: CRC Press; 1994. pp. 208.

80. Romijn JA, Coyle EF, Sidossis LS, Gastaldelli A, Horowitz JF, Endert E, Wolfe RR. Regulation of endogenous fat and carbohydrate metabolism in relation to exercise intensity and duration. *Am J Physiol* Sep 1993;265(3 Pt 1):E380-91.

81. Berning JR, Steen SN. *Nutrition for sport and exercise.* Githersburg, MD: Aspen Publishers, Inc.; 1998. pp. 297.

82. Turcoatte LP, Hespel PJ, Graham TE, Richter EA. Impaired plasma FFA oxidation imposed by extreme CHO deficiency in contracting rat skeletal muscle. *J Appl Physiol.* Aug 1994;77(2):517-25.

83. Sahlin K, Katz A, Broberg S. Tricarboxyclic acid cycle intermediates in human muscle during prolonged exercise. *Am J Physiol* Nov 1990;259(5 Pt. 1):C834-41.

84. McArdle WD, Katch FI, Katch VL. *Sports & exercise nutrition.* Baltimore, MD: Lippincott Williams & Wilkins; 1999. pp. 750.

85. Phinney SD, Bistrian BR, Evans WJ, Gervino E, Blackburn GL. The human metabolic response to chronic ketosis without caloric restriction: preservation of submaximal exercise capability with reduced carbohydrate oxidation. *Metabol* 1983(32);769-76.

86. Lambert EV, Speechly DP, Dennis SC, Noakes, TD. Enhanced endurance in trained cyclists during moderate intensity exercise following 2 weeks adaptation to a high-fat diet. *Eur J Appl Physiol* 1994:69(4);287-93.

87. Pendergast DR, Horvath PJ, Leddy JJ, Venkatraman JT. The role of dietary fat on performance, metabolism, and health. *Am J Sports Med* 1996 24(6 Suppl):S53-8.

88. Fallowfield JL, Williams C. Carbohydrate intake and recovery from prolonged exercise. *Int J Sports Nutr* Jun 1993;3(2):150-64.

89. Simonsen JC, Sherman WM, Lamb DR, Dernbach AR, Doyle JA, Strauss R. Dietary carbohydrate, muscle glycogen, and power output during rowing training. *J Appl Physiol* Apr 1991;70(4):1500-5.

90. Lambert EV, Hawley JA, Goedecke J, Noakes TD, Dennis SC. Nutritional strategies for promoting fat utilization and delaying the onset of fatigue during prolonged exercise. *J Sports Sci* Jun 1997;15(3):315-24.

91. Langfort J, Zarzeczny R, Pilis W, Nazar K, Kaciuba-Uscitko H. The effect of a low-carbohydrate diet on performance, hormonal and metabolic responses to a 30-s bout of supramaximal exercise. *Eur J Appl Physiol* 1997; 76(2):128-33.

92. Balsom PD, Gaitanos GC, Soderlund K, Ekblom B. High intensity exercise and muscle glycogen availability in humans. *Acta Physiol Scand* Apr 1999;165(4):337-45.

93. Helge JW, Richter EA, Kiens B. Interaction of training and diet on metabolism and endurance during exercise in man. *J Physiol (Lond)* Apr 1996;492(pt 1):293-306.

94. Sherman WM, Brodowicz G, Wright DA, Allen WK, Simonsen J, Dernbach A. Effects of 4 hr preexercise carbohydrate feedings on cycling performance. *Med Sci Sports Exerc* 1989:(12);598-604.

95. Sherman WM, Brodowicz G, Wright DA, Allen WK, Simonsen J, Dernbach A. Effects of 4 hr preexercise carbohydrate feedings on cycling performance. *Med Sci Sports Exerc* 1989:(12);598-604.

96. Karlsson J, Saltin B. Diet, muscle glycogen, and endurance performance. *J Appl Physiol* 1971;31:203-6.

97. Sherman WM, Costill DL, Fink WJ, Miller JM. The effect of exercise and diet manipulation on muscle glycogen and its subsequent use during performance. *Int J Sports Med* May 1981;2(2):114-8.

98. Coyle EF, Hagberg JM, Hurley BF, Martin WH, Ehsani AA, Holloszy JO. Carbohydrate feeding during prolonged strenuous exercise can delay fatigue. *J Appl Physiol* Jul 1983;55(1 Pt 1):230-5.

99. Coyle EF, Coggan AR, Hemmert WK, Ivy JL. Muscle glycogen utilization during prolonged strenuous exercise when fed carbohydrate. *J Appl Physiol* Jul 1986;61(1):165-72.

100. Wilber RL, Moffatt RJ. Influence of carbohydrate ingestion on blood glucose and performance in runners. *Intl J Sports Nutr* Dec 1992;2(4):317-27.

101. American College of Sports Medicine. Position stand: exercise and fluid replacement. *Med Sci Sports Exerc* 1996(28);i-vii.

102. Below PR, Coyle EF. Fluid and carbohydrate ingestion independently improve performance during 1 hr of intense exercise. *Med Sci Sports Exerc* Feb 1995;27(2);200-10.

103. Ivy JL, Lee MC, Broznick JT, Reed MJ. Muscle glycogen storage after different amounts of carbohydrate ingestion. *J Appl Physiol* Nov 1988;65(5);2018-23.

104. Ivy JL, Katz AL, Cutler CL, Sherman WM, Coyle EF. Muscle glycogen synthesis after exercise: effect of time of carbohydrate ingestion. *J Appl Physiol* Apr 1988;64(4); 1480-5.

105. Liljeberg HG, Akergerg AK, Bjorck IM. Effect of the glycemic index and content of indigestible carbohydrates of cereal-based breakfast meals on glucose tolerance at lunch in healthy subjects. *Am J Clin Nut* Apr 1999;69(4): 647-55.

106. Raben A, Tagliabue A, Christensen NJ, Madsen J, Holst JJ, Astrup A. Resistant starch: the effect on postprandial glycemia, hormonal response, and satiety. *Am J Clin Nutr* Oct 1994;60(4):544-51.

107. Raben A, Christensen NJ, Madsen J, Holst JJ, Astrup A. Decreased postprandial thermogenesis and fat oxidation but increased fullness after a high-fiber meal compared with a low-fiber meal. *Am J Clin Nutr* Jun 1994;59(6):1386-94.

108. Yang MU, Van Itallie TB. Composition of weight lost during short-term weight reduction. Metabolic responses of obese subjects to starvation and low-calorie ketogenic and nonketogenic diets. *J Clin Invest* 1976;58(3):722-30.

109. Karlsson J, Saltin B. Lactate ATP, and CP in working muscles during exhaustive exercise in man. *J Appl Physiol* Nov 1970;29(5):596-602.

110. Shick SM, Wing RR, Klem ML, McGuire MT, Hill JO, Seagle H. Persons successful at long-term weight loss and maintenance continue to consume a low-energy, low-fat diet. *J Am Diet Assoc* Apr 1998;98(4):408-13.

111. McDowell MA, Briefel RR, Alaimo K, Bischof AM, Caughman CR, Carroll MD, Loria CM, Johnson CL. Energy intakes of persons ages 2 months and over in the United States: third national health and nutrition examination survey, phase 1, 1988-91. *Adv Data* Oct 1994;24(255):1-24.

112. Ernst ND, Obarzanek E, Clark MB, Briefel RR, Brown CD, Donato K. Cardiovascular health risks related to overweight. *J Am Diet Assoc* Jul 1997;97(7 Suppl):S47-51.

113. US Department of Agriculture, Center for Nutrition Policy and Promotion (1997) *Nutrient content of the US food supply, 1909-94.* Home Economics Research Report No. 53. Washington, DC: U.S. Government Printing Office.

114. US Department of Health and Human Services. *Physical activity and health: a report of the Surgeon General.* Atlanta, GA: Centers for Disease Control and Prevention; 1996.

115. Flegal KM, Carroll MD, Kuczmarski RJ, Johnson CL. Overweight and obesity in the United States: prevalence and trends, 1960-1994. *Int J Obes Relat Metab Disord* Jan 1998;22(1):39-47.

116. Whitney EN, Rolfes SR. *Understanding nutrition.* St. Paul, MN: West Publishing Company; 1996. 757p.

117. Groff JL, Gropper SS, Hunt SM. *Advanced nutrition and human metabolism.* St. Paul, MN: West Publishing Company; 1995. 575p.

118. Simopoulos AP. Omega-3 fatty acids in health and disease and in growth and development. *Am J Clin Nutr* Sep 1991;54(3):438-63.

119. Simopoulos AP. Omega-3 fatty acids in the prevention-management of cardiovascular disease. *Can J Physiol Pharmacol* Mar 1997;75(3):234-9.

120. Lichtenstein AH, Ausman LM, Jalbert SM, Schaefer EJ. Effects of different forms of dietary hydrogenated fats on serum lipoprotein cholesterol levels. *N Engl J Med* Jun 1999;340(25):1933-40.

121. Tato F. Trans-fatty acids in the diet: a coronary risk factor? *Eur J Med Res* Nov 1995;1(2):118-22.

122. Ascherio A, Willett WC. Health effects of trans fatty acids. *Am J Clin Nutr* Oct 1997;66(4 Suppl):1006S-10S.

123. [NRC] National Research Council. *Recommended dietary allowances.* 10th ed. Washington, DC: National Academy Press; 1989. pp. 285.

124. Lissner L, Levitsky DA, Strupp BJ, Kalkwarf HJ, Roe DA. Dietary fat and the regulation of energy intake in human subjects. *Am J Clin Nutr* Dec 1987;46(6):886-92.

125. Lissner L, Heitmann BL. The dietary fat: carbohydrate ratio in relation to body weight. *Curr Opin Lipidol* Feb 1995;6(1):8-13.

126. Horton TJ, Drougas H, Reed GW, Peters JC, Hill JO. Fat and carbohydrate overfeeding in humans: different effects on energy storage. *Am J Clin Nutr* Jul 1995;62(1):19-29.

127. Leveille GA. Isocaloric diets: effects of dietary changes. *Am J Clin Nutr* Jan 1987;45(1 Suppl):158-63.

128. Stubbs RJ, Ritz P, Coward WA, Prentice AM. Covert manipulation of the ration of dietary fat to carbohydrate and energy density: effect on food intake and energy balance in free-living men eating ad libitum. *Am J Clin Nutr* Aug 1995;62(2):330-7.

129. Groff JL, Gropper SS, Hunt SM. *Advanced nutrition and human metabolism.* Minneapolis/St. Paul: West Publishing Co.; 1995. pp 575.

130. Jeukendrup AE, Saris WH, Schrauwen P, Brouns F, Wagenmakers AJ. Metabolic availability of medium-chain triglycerides coingested with carbohydrate during prolonged exercise. *J Appl Physiol* Sep 1995;79(3):756-62.

131. Van Zyl CG, Lambert EV, Hawley JA, Noakes TD, Dennis SC. Effects of medium-chain triglyceride ingestion on fuel metabolism and cycling performance. *J Appl Physiol* Jun 1996;80(6):2217-25.

132. Epstein F (ed), Shepherd PR, Kahn BB. *New Eng J Med* Jul 1999;341(4):248-57.

133. Buemann B, Tremblay A. Effects of exercise training on abdominal obesity and related metabolic complications. *Sports Med* 1996:21(3):191-212.

134. Pandolfi C, Pellegrini L, Sbalzarini G, Mercantini F. Obesity and insulin resistance. *Minerva Med* 1994:85(4): 167-71.

135. Bloomgarden ZT. Insulin resistance: current concepts. *Clin Ther* 1998;20(2):216-31.

136. Schraer CD, Risica PM, Ebbesson SO, Go OT, Howard BV, Mayer AM. Low fasting insulin levels in Eskimos compared to American Indians: are Eskimos less insulin resistant? *Intl J Circump Heal* Oct 1999; 58(4):272-80.

137. Beck-Nielsen H. General characteristics of the insulin resistance syndrome: prevelance and heritability. European Group for the study of Insulin Resistance (EGIR). *Drugs* 1999;58 Suppl 1:7-10.

138. Pi-Sunyer FX. Medical hazards of obesity. *Ann Intern Med* Oct 1993;119(7 Pt 2): 655-60.

139. Grundy SM. Multifactorial causation of obesity: implications for prevention. *Am J Clin Nutr* 1998:67(3S): 563S-569S.

140. Vaag A. On the pathophysiology of late onset non-insulin dependant diabetes mellitus. Current controversies and new insights. *Dan Med Bull* 1999;46(3):197-234.

141. Parekh PI, Petro AE, Tiller JM, Feinglos MN, Surwit RS. Reversal of diet-induced obesity and diabetes in C57BL/6J mice. *Metabol* 1998;47(9):1089-96.

142. Barnard RJ, Ugianskis EJ, Martin DA, Inkeles SB. Role of diet and exercise in the management of hyperinsulinemia and associated atherosclerotic risk factors. *Am J Cardiol* 1992;69(5):440-4.

143. Wolinsky I, Hickson JF. *Nutrition in exercise and sport.* Boca Raton, FL: CRC Press; 1994. pp 508.

144. Walsh RM, Noakes TD, Hawkey JA, Dennis SC. Impaired high-intensity cycling performance time at low levels of dehydration. *Int J Sports Med* Oct 1994;15(7):392-8.

145. Broad E, Burke LM, Heely P, Grundy M. Body weight changes and ad libitum fluid intakes during training and competition sessions in team sports. *Int J Sport Nutr* Sep 1996;6(3):307-20.

146. Berning JR, Steen SN. *Nutrition for sport and exercise.* Gaithersburg, MD: Aspen Publishers; 1998. pp 297.

147. Convertino VA, Armstrong LE, Coyle EF, Mack GW, Sawka MN, Senay LC Jr, Sherman WM. American College of Sports Medicine position stand. Exercise and fluid replacement. *Med Sci Sports Exerc* Jan 1996;28(1):i-vii.

148. Apex Fitness Group. *Apex Training System: Nutritional Guidelines for Altering Body Composition.*

Supplementation

MODULE 16-1: Dietary Supplements

Introduction to Supplementation

During the first half of the twentieth century, the discovery that vitamins are essential components of food (along with tremendous growth in the understanding of human nutrient needs) set the foundation for the development of dietary supplements containing vitamins and minerals.

The traditional reason for use of a dietary supplement is to provide the body with nutrients that might not be supplied adequately by a person's typical diet. Around the middle of the twentieth century, the use of dietary supplements was primarily in the form of a "one-a-day" type of vitamin-mineral supplement. Although this continues to be the most commonly used type, the rapid growth of the dietary supplement industry has led to the development of a great variety of different types of supplements. Today, dietary supplements are much more than a low-dosage vitamin-mineral pill taken by a small percentage of the population. Contemporary dietary supplements often contain numerous chemical compounds other than nutrients, and people take dietary supplements for a wide variety of reasons other than meeting nutrient needs.

The popularity of dietary supplements has grown steadily in the United States, with sales in the supplement industry booming during the 1990s. Estimates put total sales at $3.3 billion for 1990, growing to 17.7 billion in 2002.[1,2] Associated with this rapid growth, the Dietary Supplement Health and Education Act (DSHEA) was passed in 1994, providing a detailed legal definition of the term "dietary supplement." There are now new regulations for dietary supplements that are separate from the regulations for foods and drugs.[3]

What is a Dietary Supplement?

Based on the DSHEA, the U.S. Food and Drug Administration (FDA) states that a **dietary supplement** is:

DIETARY SUPPLEMENT:
A substance that completes or makes an addition to daily dietary intake.

- A product (other than tobacco) that is intended to supplement the diet and that bears or contains one or more of the following dietary ingredients: a vitamin, a mineral, an herb or other botanical, an amino acid;

- A dietary substance for use by man to supplement the diet by increasing the total daily intake;

- A concentrate, metabolite, constituent, extract, or combinations of these ingredients;

- Intended for ingestion in pill, capsule, tablet or liquid form;

- Not represented for use as a conventional food or as the sole item of a meal or diet; and

- Labeled as a "dietary supplement".

Thus, most anything that is not already classified as a drug can be put into a pill and sold as a dietary supplement.[4]

Inadequate Food Intake
(Especially Diets Less Than 1,000 Calories per Day)

Disordered eating patterns

- Consuming mostly "junk" (nutrient deficient) foods
- Avoidance of foods from specific food groups
- Eating only one major meal each day
- Irregular eating patterns (low-calorie diet one day, high-calorie the next)
- Eating too much or too little protein or carbohydrate
- Food phobias and "picky" eating
- Financial limitations on access to a variety of wholesome foods

Figure 16-1: Common Reasons Why Diets Do Not Contain Adequate Nutrients

Rationale for the Use of Dietary Supplements

People take supplements for many reasons. Some use them to deal with or help prevent specific health problems. Others use supplements in hopes of enhancing performance in physical or mental tasks, altering body composition, stimulating metabolism, controlling appetite, or dealing with age-related changes in body structure and function.

The use of dietary supplements that contain a broad spectrum of micronutrients (in low to moderate doses) can be especially beneficial for individuals consuming diets that do not meet their needs for all nutrients.[5,6] In addition, various studies have reported that people taking a multivitamin supplement experience a reduced risk of chronic disease development.[6]

Additionally, there are specific groups who may have greater need for dietary supplements. For example, older people often do not make proper adjustments in their diets when energy needs decline with age. Although calorie needs generally drop with age, the need for protein, vitamins and minerals does not decline.[7,8] Another group that can benefit from supplemented nutrients is women who are pregnant or breastfeeding. However, due the potential for supplement toxicity or interactions with prescribed medications, it is extremely important for these groups to seek guidance on supplementation from qualified health professionals.[9] Whatever the goal for using a dietary supplement, the considerations for appropriate use are similar.

Supplementation Guidelines

General Guidelines for Responsible Use of Nutritional Dietary Supplements

Dietary supplements usually contain potent natural chemicals. Although these substances are generally safer than drugs, some precautions should be kept in mind. This section will give common guidelines for determining what quantity of a supplemental nutrient is likely to be adequate, safe and beneficial, and how much may be potentially excessive or detrimental to health.

Dietary Reference Intakes

In the United States, the Food and Nutrition Board (FNB) of the Institute of Medicine, National Academy of Sciences periodically reviews the current research on nutrient needs to provide authoritative, updated recommendations for nutrient intake. In 1997, the FNB released the first in a series of publications called "Dietary Reference Intakes." At the time of this writing, five of six major volumes had been published (Table 16-1).

Table 16-1: Dietary Reference Intake Publications	
Nutrients Reviewed	**Year of Publication**
Calcium, Phosphorus, Magnesium, Vitamin D, and Fluoride[12]	1997[10]
Thiamin, Riboflavin, Niacin, Vitamin B-6, Folate, Vitamin B-12, Pantothenic Acid, Biotin, and Choline[13]	1998[11]
Vitamin C, Vitamin E, Selenium, and Carotenoids[14]	2000[12]
Vitamin A, Vitamin K, Arsenic, Boron, Chromium, Copper, Iodine, Iron, Manganese, Molybdenum, Nickel, Silicon, Vanadium, and Zinc[15]	2002[13]
Energy, Carbohydrate, Fiber, Fat, Fatty Acids, Cholesterol, Protein, and Amino Acids[16]	2002[14]
Electrolytes and Water	Expected early 2004

Dietary Reference Intake (DRI) values for nutrients provide good guidelines for what constitutes an adequate intake of a nutrient. For many nutrients, values also have been set for the amount considered to be excessive and potentially harmful. The DRIs are designed to estimate the nutrient needs of healthy people in various age and gender groups. The values also are adjusted for the special needs of women during pregnancy and lactation.

Figure 16-2 describes the DRI terminology used by the Food and

Nutrition Board. The DRIs most commonly used to evaluate or plan diets for individuals are the RDA, AI and UL values (described below).[15] The overall goal in designing a healthy diet is to provide nutrients at levels that represent a high probability of adequate intake (meeting RDA or AI levels) and also a low probability of excessive intake (not exceeding UL levels).

Estimated Average Requirement (EAR):
The average daily nutrient intake level that is estimated to meet the requirement of half the healthy individuals who are in a particular life stage and gender group.

Recommended Dietary Allowance (RDA):
The average daily nutrient intake level that is sufficient to meet the nutrient requirement of nearly all (97 to 98 percent) healthy individuals who are in a particular life stage and gender group.

Adequate Intake (AI):
A recommended average daily nutrient intake level, based on observed (or experimentally determined) approximations or estimates of nutrient intake that are assumed to be adequate for a group (or groups) of healthy people. This measure is used when an RDA cannot be determined.

Tolerable Upper Intake Level (UL):
The highest average daily nutrient intake level likely to pose no risk of adverse health effects to almost all individuals in a particular life stage and gender group. As intake increases above the UL, the potential risk of adverse health effects increases.

Figure 16-2: Dietary Reference Intake Terminology

Dietary Reference Intake Values and Guidelines

Table 16-2 summarizes the currently established adult DRI values for vitamins and minerals, including UL values and possible signs of excess intake of a nutrient. Except for vitamin E and magnesium, the UL values are set for total intake of each nutrient from food and supplements. The ULs for vitamin E and magnesium are set for levels of intake from supplements or pharmacological sources only and do not include dietary intake.

Even essential nutrients are potentially toxic at some level of intake. For some nutrients, the level of intake that causes serious adverse effects is not presently known. For others, the adverse effects of excess have been documented. The effects of some nutrients can be extremely serious. Among the vitamin category of nutrients, excess vitamin A, D and B-6 can produce serious adverse effects and are commonly available in dietary supplement form. Excess vitamin A, for example, can cause birth defects when a woman is taking too much at conception and during early pregnancy.[13] Vitamin D excess can result in the calcification of blood vessels and eventually damage the function of the kidneys, heart and lungs.[10] Excessive intake of vitamin B-6 can cause permanent damage to sensory nerves.[11]

Excess intake of mineral elements also can cause health problems. For example, excess (and inadequate) calcium intake can increase the risk of developing kidney stones. Excess intake of iron can interfere with the absorption of other minerals (such as zinc) and can cause gastrointestinal irritation.[13]

It is important to remember that nutrient requirements and Upper Limits are set for normal, healthy individuals. In some cases, a drug may increase or decrease the need for a nutrient. Anyone that is taking a medication may no longer fit into these DRI parameters. For example, large doses of anti-inflammatory drugs like aspirin and ibuprofen may interfere with folic acid function and potentially increase folic acid requirement.[11,16]

With respect to ULs, the nutrient levels that are perfectly safe for normal, healthy people can be life threatening for those with specific health problems. For example, supplementation with vitamins E and K can complicate conditions for people on anticoagulant therapy (or "blood thinners").[14,15] Consequently, the use of various drugs can contraindicate the use of specific nutrient supplements, as well as the consumption of some foods high in the specific nutrient. Therefore, people with serious health problems, and especially those taking drugs for health problems, should use dietary supplements only with guidance and monitoring by a physician, pharmacist, or other health professional knowledgeable in drug-nutrient interactions.

When no UL has been established for a nutrient, it does not mean that there is no potential for adverse effects from high intake. Rather, it may just mean that too little information is currently available to establish a UL value. Complete tables of the DRI values are available at the Food and Nutrition Board Web site (http://www.iom.edu/board). The tables include the UL values and brief descriptions of the adverse effects of excessive intake.

Another authoritative publication on upper levels for nutrient intake was recently released by the Expert Group on Vitamins and Minerals of the Food Standards Agency in the United Kingdom. This publication, *Safe Upper Levels for Vitamins and Minerals*, provides "Safe Upper Levels" (SUL) for eight nutrients and "Guidance Levels" for the 22 vitamins and minerals, for which data were inadequate to set a SUL.[17] These recommended upper levels of intake refer specifically to intake in the form of dietary supplements. The Expert Group on Vitamins and Minerals describes these terms as follows:

The determination of SULs or Guidance Levels entails the determination of doses of vitamins and minerals that potentially susceptible individuals could take daily on a life-long basis, without medical supervision in reasonable safety. The setting of these levels provides a framework within which the consumer can make an informed decision about intake, having confidence that harm should not ensue. The levels so set will therefore tend to be conservative, and it is possible that for some vitamins and minerals larger amounts could be consumed for shorter periods without risk to health. However, there would be difficulties in deriving SULs for shorter term consumption because the available data are limited and relate to differing time periods. Although less susceptible individuals might be able to consume higher levels without risk to health, separate advice for susceptible individuals would be appropriate only if those individuals could recognize their own potential susceptibility. (Safe Upper Levels for Vitamins and Minerals, 2003)[17]

Values for SULs and Guidance Levels are included in Table 16-2, for comparison with DRI values. It is interesting to note similarities and differences in the values set by the two different approaches. Guidance Levels are based on very limited data and are not meant to be confused with, or used as SULs. However, when no UL or SUL is available, Guidance Levels can provide a reasonable frame of reference.

Obviously, the bottom line is that it is preferable to consume nutrients within a range that is adequate to meet the body's needs. The optimal level of intake within this adequate range is not known. Whether "optimal" is closer to the RDA/AI or to the UL for a nutrient is unknown and likely differs for the various nutrients and also may differ from one individual person to another.

Table 16-2: Comparison of Dietary Reference Intake Values (for adult men and women) and Daily Values for Micronutrients with the Tolerable Upper Intake Levels (UL)[a,c] Safe Upper Levels (SUL)[d] and Guidance Levels[d]

Nutrient	RDA/AI[b] (men/women) ages 31-50	Daily Value (Food Labels)	UL[c]	SUL or Guidance Level[d]	Selected Potential Effects of Excess Intake
Vitamin A (mcg)	900 / 700	1,500 (5,000 IU)	3,000	1,500** (5,000 IU)	Liver damage, bone and joint pain, dry skin, loss of hair, headache, vomiting
beta-Carotene (mg)				7 (11,655 IU)	Increased risk of lung cancer in smokers and those heavily exposed to asbestos
Vitamin D (mcg)	5*	10 (400 IU)	50	25 (1,000 IU)	Calcification of brain, arteries, increased blood calcium, loss of appetite, nausea
Vitamin E (mg)	15	20 (30 IU)	1,000	540 (800 IU)	Deficient blood clotting
Vitamin K (mcg)	120 / 90*	80	-	1,000**	Red blood cell damage/ anemia, liver damage
Thiamin (B-1) (mg)	1.2 / 1.1	1.5	-	100**	Headache, nausea, irritability, insomnia, rapid pulse, weakness (7,000+ mg dose)
Riboflavin (B-2) (mg)	1.3 / 1.1	1.7	-	40**	Generally considered harmless; yellow discoloration of urine
Niacin (mg)	16 / 14	20	35	500**	Liver damage, flushing, nausea, gastrointestinal problems
Vitamin B-6 (mg)	1.3	2	100	10	Neurological problems, numbness and pain in limbs
Vitamin B-12 (mcg)	2.4	6	-	2,000**	No reports of toxicity from oral ingestion
Folic acid (mcg)	400	400	1,000	1,000**	Masks B-12 deficiency (which can cause neurological problems)
Pantothenic acid (mg)	5*	10	-	200**	Diarrhea and gastrointestinal disturbance (10,000+ mg/day)
Biotin (mcg)	30*	300	-	900**	No reports of toxicity from oral ingestion
Vitamin C (mg)	90 / 75	60	2,000	1,000**	Nausea, diarrhea, kidney stones
Boron (mg)			20	9.6	Adverse effects on male and female reproductive system
Calcium (mg)	1,000*	1,000	2,500	1,500**	Nausea, constipation, kidney stones
Chromium (mcg)	35*	120	-	10,000**	Potential adverse effects on liver and kidneys; picolinate form possibly mutagenic
Cobalt (mg)				1.4**	Cardiotoxic effects; not appropriate in a dietary supplement except as vitamin B-12

Table 16-2: **Comparison of Dietary Reference Intake Values**
(Continued) **(for adult men and women) and Daily Values for Micronutrients**
with the Tolerable Upper Intake Levels (UL)[a,c] Safe Upper Levels (SUL)[d] and Guidance Levels[d]

Nutrient	RDA/AI[b] (men/ women) ages 31-50	Daily Value (Food Labels)	UL[c]	SUL or Guidance Level[d]	Selected Potential Effects of Excess Intake
Copper (mcg)	900	2	10,000	10,000	Gastrointestinal distress, liver damage
Fluoride (mg)	4 / 3*		10		Bone, kidney, muscle, and nerve damage; supplement only with professional guidance
Germanium				zero**	Kidney toxin; should not be in a dietary supplement
Iodine (mcg)	150	150	1,100	500**	Elevated thyroid hormone concentration
Iron (mg)	8 / 18	18	45	17**	Gastrointestinal distress, increased risk of heart disease, oxidative stress
Magnesium (mg)	420 / 320	400	350e	400**	Diarrhea
Manganese (mg)	2.3 / 1.8*	2	11	4**	Neurotoxicity
Molybdenum	45	75	2,000	zero**	Gout-like symptoms, joint pains, increased uric acid
Nickel (mcg)				260**	Increased sensitivity of skin reaction to nickel in jewelry
Phosphorus (mg)	700	1,000	4,000	250**	Alteration of parathyroid hormone levels, reduced bone mineral density
Potassium (mg)				3,700**	Gastrointestinal damage
Selenium (mcg)	55	70	400	450	Nausea, diarrhea, fatigue, hair and nail loss
Silicon (mg)				700	Low toxicity, possibility of kidney stones
Vanadium (mg)			1.8	zero	Gastrointestinal irritation; fatigue
Zinc (mg)	11 / 8	15	40	25	Impaired immune function, low HDL-cholesterol

a   Food and Nutrition Board, Institute of Medicine (U.S.). Dietary Reference Intakes Tables.
    Available at http://www4.nationalacademies.org/IOM/IOMHome.nsf/Pages/Food+and+Nutrition+Board

b   RDA = Recommended Dietary Allowance, AI = Adequate Intake, indicated with *

c   UL = Tolerable Upper Intake Level

d   SUL = Safe Upper Levels; SULs and Guidance Levels (incidated by **) set by the Expert Group on Vitamins and Minerals of the Food Standards Agency, United Kingdom.
       These are intended to be levels of daily intake of nutrients in dietary supplements that potentially susceptible individuals could take daily on a life-long basis without medical supervision in reasonable safety. When the evidence base was considered inadequate to set a SUL, Guidance Levels were set based on limited data. SULs and Guidance Levels tend to be conservative and it is possible that, for some vitamins and minerals, greater amounts could be consumed for short periods without risk to health. The values presented are for a 60 kg (132 lb) adult. Consult the full publication for values expressed per kg body weight. This FSA publication, *Safe Upper Levels for Vitamins and Minerals,* is available at: http://www.foodstandards.gov.uk/multimedia/pdfs/vitmin2003.pdf

e   The UL for magnesium represents intake specifically from pharmacological agents and/or dietary supplements in addition to dietary intake.

MODULE 16-1 Summary

Vitamins (and many minerals) are essential components of food and are required in very small amounts by the body. The popularity of dietary supplements has boomed in recent years. In 1994 the Dietary Supplement Health and Education Act (DSHEA) was passed, providing a detailed legal definition of the term "dietary supplement." The U.S. Food and Drug Administration (FDA) states that a dietary supplement is, basically, a labeled pill, capsule, tablet, or liquid intended to supplement the diet and contains one or more vitamin, mineral, botanical or amino acid. Almost anything not already classified as a drug can be sold as a dietary supplement. Taking low-to-moderate dose, broad-spectrum vitamin-mineral supplements is beneficial, especially for those whose diets do not meet all micronutrient requirements. There is also a reduced risk for chronic diseases in people taking a multivitamin supplement.

Most dietary supplements contain potent natural chemicals that are generally considered safer than drugs. However, some precautions for appropriate use should still be taken and guidelines should be followed. The most recent updated recommendations for nutrient intake are presented in a series of publications called "Dietary Reference Intakes."

Dietary Reference Intake (DRI) values are good guidelines for adequate, excessive and potentially harmful intakes of a nutrient for normal, healthy individuals. The overall goal in designing a healthy diet is to provide nutrients that meet Recommended Daily Allowance or Adequate Intake levels and also have a low probability of exceeding Tolerable Upper Intake Levels. Optimal intake may differ for the various nutrients and also may differ from one individual person to another.

Even essential nutrients and minerals are potentially toxic at some level of intake. Nutrient levels that are perfectly safe for normal, healthy people can be altered for those taking medication and even life threatening for those with specific health problems. These clients should use dietary supplements only with guidance and monitoring by a physician, pharmacist, or other health professional knowledgeable in drug-nutrient interactions.

MODULE 16-1 Quiz

1. Today there are separate regulations for dietary supplements from the regulations for foods and drugs.

   ☐ True   ☐ False

2. According to the U.S. Food and Drug Administration, a dietary supplement must be a product (other than tobacco) that contains one or more of the which dietary ingredients (choose all that apply):

   ☐ Protein   ☐ Amino acid

   ☐ Vitamin   ☐ Herb

   ☐ Lipid   ☐ Mineral

3. Give two common reasons why diets do not contain adequate nutrients.

   _____

   _____

4. Give the terms for the following Dietary Reference Intake terminology:

   EAR _____

   RDA _____

   AI   _____

   UL   _____

5. An excess of which vitamin can cause calcification of blood vessels and eventually damage the function of kidneys, heart and lungs?

   _____

6. Large doses of anti-inflammatory drugs like aspirin and ibuprofen may interfere with folic acid function and potentially _____ folic acid requirement.   ☐ Increase   ☐ Decrease

7. Which of the following nutrients are not advised as a dietary supplement (choose all that apply)?

   ☐ Riboflavin   ☐ Germanium   ☐ Biotin

   ☐ Cobalt   ☐ Nickel   ☐ Vitamin B-12

MODULE 16-2:
Vitamins and Mineral Supplements

Labels of Dietary Supplements

Units of Measure Used on Dietary Supplement Labels

Dietary supplement labels contain product information on "Supplement Facts" panels similar to the "Nutrition Facts" on food products (Figure 16-3). Protein, carbohydrate and fat are generally expressed in gram quantities, whereas, vitamins, minerals, amino acids and fatty acids are generally present and expressed in milligram (mg) or microgram (mcg or µg) quantities.

Supplement Facts
Serving Size 1 Capsule

Amount Per Capsule	% Daily Value
Calories 20	
Calories from Fat 20	
Total Fat 2 g	3%*
Saturated Fat 0.5 g	3%*
Polyunsaturated Fat 1 g	†
Monounsaturated Fat 0.5 g	†
Vitamin A 4250 IU	85%
Vitamin D 425 IU	106%
Omega-3 fatty acids 0.5 g	†

* Percent Daily Values are based on a 2,000 calorie diet.
† Daily Value not established.

Ingredients: Cod liver oil, gelatin, water, and glycerin.

Figure 16-3: Sample Supplement Facts Panel Used on a Dietary Supplement Label

In addition to the nutrient amounts required on the "Supplement Facts" panel, dietary supplements must provide a "% Daily Value" for each nutrient listed. Daily Values (DVs) were established specifically for food labeling and are intended to provide the consumer with a frame of reference that indicates how the amount of the nutrient present in a food or supplement compares with approximate levels of recommended intake. The DVs for vitamins and minerals are based on the 1968 RDAs for adults (using the highest of two recommended amounts, when there are differences between males and females). Thus, if a product indicates that the % DV for a nutrient is 50, it means that an adult will obtain about 50 percent of the amount commonly recommended on a daily basis for that nutrient.

The amounts and DVs for nutrients listed on a Supplement Facts panel are the amounts present in the serving size indicated at the top of the label. In Figure 16-3, the serving size is one capsule. However, some products may indicate more than one capsule, pill, tablet, etc., as the serving size. Many components of supplements do not have DVs. When this is the case, there is an indication "Daily Value not established" at the bottom of the panel.

Although the RDAs have been revised several times since 1968, the DVs have not changed, at the request of the food industry. When DVs are used as a general ballpark guide, they still work reasonably well. However, some issues have evolved that will likely lead to a revision in the DVs to more closely match current nutritional recommendations. For example, the DV for iron is 18 mg/day, which was based on a menstruating woman's requirement. The current RDA for a man is 8 mg/day. Consequently, when a dietary supplement provides 100 percent of the DV for iron, it provides more than twice the RDA for a man.

The amounts of vitamins A, D and E are expressed on supplement labels as International Units (IUs). Table 16-3 compares the RDA values for these three nutrients expressed in µg or mg amounts to equivalent amounts expressed in IUs. This table also illustrates that the Daily Values (DV) that are used as reference amounts on food and supplement nutrition labels do not equal the most current RDA values for men and women. The DV for each of these three vitamins exceeds the current RDA for adult males and females. Of particular interest, the DV for vitamin A is actually equal to the SUL value recently set by the Expert Committee on Vitamins and Minerals in the United Kingdom. Comparisons of other micronutrient DVs with current recommendations are shown in Table 16-3.

Table 16-3: Comparison of RDA Adult Values for vitamins A, D and E with Tolerable Upper Intake Levels (UL), Safe Upper Levels (SUL) and Daily Values Used for Food and Supplement Labels				
Vitamin	**Men's RDA**	**Women's RDA**	**Adult UL/SUL**	**Label DV**
Vitamin A µg*	900	700	3,000/1,500	---
Vitamin A IU*	3,000	2,333	10,000/5,000	5,000
Vitamin D µg	5	5	50/25	---
Vitamin D IU	200	200	2,000/1,000	400
Vitamin E µg	15	15	1,000/540	---
Vitamin E IU**	22	22	1,490/800	30

* In the form of retinol (typically as retinyl palmitate)
** Based on natural vitamin E (*d*-α-Tocopherol)

Vitamin and Mineral Supplements

A great variety of dietary supplements are used to enhance overall health and/or reduce the risk of various diseases. The most commonly used supplement is a multiple vitamin and mineral supplement that is intended to compensate for nutrients that may be limited in a person's diet. The amounts of the various nutrients in a multiple vitamin/mineral supplement (multi-Vit/Min) that are reasonable and sensible depend upon an individual's needs and their intake of nutrients from other sources. As a general rule of thumb, the safe level of most nutrients in a multi-Vit/Min should be around 100 percent of the Daily Value. However, there are some notable exceptions to this general rule.

Vitamin A, if present in a supplement only as retinol (usually indicated as retinyl palmitate or vitamin A palmitate), rather than carotene, should be less than 100 percent of the DV. A recent study indicates that high intake of retinol, but not beta-carotene, is associated with increased incidence of hip fracture in older women.[18] Also, as mentioned above, excess intake of retinol at conception and during early pregnancy increases the risk of birth defects.[20]

Concerns also exist for including large doses of beta-carotene in a dietary supplement.[19] Two large intervention trials reported an increased incidence of lung cancer in smokers who were taking 20 to 30 mg/day supplements of beta-carotene.[20,21] However, a large study of 22,071 physicians reported no effect on cancer incidence or mortality in those taking 50 mg/day of beta-carotene and found that supplementation in those with initially low blood levels of beta-carotene helped reduce the incidence of prostate cancer.[22] Still, another large study conducted in China found that daily supplementation with 15 mg beta-carotene in combination with 50 mcg selenium and 30 mg alpha-tocopherol was associated with a 13-percent reduction in cancer risk, mainly due to decreased incidence of gastric cancer.[23] Consequently, supplementation with beta-carotene remains controversial and appears to be most clearly contraindicated in smokers.

Calcium should be at low levels or absent in a multi-Vit/Min because taking 100 percent of the RDA, which is one gram (1,000 mg) of elemental calcium. Common forms of calcium would make the supplement pill too large to swallow easily. Secondly, for best absorption, it is preferable to consume calcium, with meals, spaced throughout the day, rather than to ingest 100 percent of daily needs at one time.[24] Thirdly, excess calcium consumed with other minerals can decrease the absorption of some important trace minerals.[10]

Among the B vitamins, niacin, B-6 and folic acid have UL values. For niacin and folic acid, the adult ULs are only 2.2 and 2.5 times their respective RDA values. The

UL for vitamin B-6 of 100 mg is 77 times the RDA. However, the FSA Expert Group on Vitamins and Minerals SUL value for daily consumption of supplemental vitamin B-6 is only 10 mg/day.[17] At one-tenth the UL value set by the U.S. Food and Nutrition Board, this value is based on the assumption that this SUL level of intake for supplemental B-6 is reasonably safe to consume over the lifetime of an adult.[13]

Some B vitamins (B-1, B-2, B-12, pantothenic acid and biotin) do not have UL values, due to a lack of data on adverse effects.[13] For these nutrients, the FSA Expert Group on Vitamins and Minerals established Guidance Levels that can at least provide a reasonable frame of reference (Table 16-2).[17]

Deficiencies of vitamins and minerals can impair the ability and desire to perform physical activity. In addition, many nutrient deficiencies can cause mental and emotional problems. Clearly, iron deficiency has been shown to affect both physical and mental function adversely.[25,26] Also, a deficiency of some B vitamins can affect mental functions and emotional state. Perhaps the most common example of this is due to vitamin B-12 deficiency which is most commonly seen in the elderly and in those who avoid consuming animal foods.[27,28] In the elderly, mental and emotional changes due to B-12 deficiency are often mistaken for Alzheimer's disease and other dementias. The condition can be reversed, if corrected early in the deficiency state. If not, nerve damage

Vitamin A:	If a dietary supplement contains 100% of the Daily Value, it contains an amount of vitamin A that is more than twice the RDA for a woman, only half of the UL and is equal to the Guidance Level.
Vitamin D:	If a dietary supplement contains 100% of the Daily Value, it contains an amount of vitamin D that is twice the AI value. The UL is only 5 times the DV, and the SUL is only 2.5 times the DV.
Iron:	If a dietary supplement contains 100% of the Daily Value, it contains an amount of iron that is equal to the RDA for women, more than twice the RDA for men. The UL is only a little over twice the DV and the Guidance Level is one milligram less than the DV.
Zinc:	If a dietary supplement contains 100% of the Daily Value, it contains an amount of zinc that is almost twice the RDA for women. The UL is just a little over twice the DV and the SUL is a little less than twice the DV.

Figure 16-4: Nutrients with the Greatest Potential for Excess Dosage in Dietary Supplements

and dementia symptoms can be irreversible. However, correcting the deficiency will prevent further progression of the problems and potentially cause some reversal of symptoms. Since malabsorption is the usual cause of vitamin B-12 deficiency, the usual treatment is to receive monthly injections of the vitamin. However, some research indicates that high dose oral supplementation in the range of 200-2000 µg/day may be as effective as injections.[29-31]

Selecting a multiple vitamin and mineral supplement with reasonable levels of each nutrient for an individual is not a simple task. It is not unusual to find multi-Vit/Mins with some nutrient levels that exceed the UL or SUL values. The information in Table 16-2 can provide some reasonable guidelines. Note that the upper level numbers (UL, SUL and Guidance Level) for some nutrients are much closer to the RDA or AI than they are for others.

Figure 16-4 compares the Daily Value amounts (the reference values on food and dietary supplement labels) for four nutrients to current levels of recommended intake and upper limits. Since the recommended intakes for these nutrients are relatively close to common recommendations for upper limits, people are more likely to consume excessive amounts of these nutrients from supplements and fortified foods combined.

The amount of each nutrient in a supplement that is most appropriate for an individual depends upon the amount of nutrients in his/her diet. Despite claims to the contrary, today's food supply is not devoid of nutrients. Certainly, it is possible to select a diet composed mostly of overly refined foods that provide limited amounts of vitamins and minerals and plenty of calories. However, with the plethora of fortified foods (breakfast cereals, energy bars, protein powders and just about everything with a calcium-fortified option), it is quite possible to consume excessive amounts of some nutrients even without taking dietary supplements. Consequently, decisions to use dietary supplements should be made in the context of a typical diet, with special attention to use of foods fortified with vitamins and minerals.

Position Statements on Dietary Supplements
Used for Specific Applications

1. Everyone should investigate the use of a multivitamin and mineral formula (in addition to a separate calcium supplement) in order to complement his/her best efforts to define and consume a proper diet.

2. Specific compounds, when ingested and manufactured properly, can allow the body to operate at full capacity, without disturbing its natural physiology.

3. Individual results during usage may be based on the physiology and psychological state of the recipient. Manufacturing methods and ingredients used may also affect results. Please refer to NASM's nutrition partner, Apex Fitness Group (www.apexfitness.com), for further information regarding use of dietary supplements.

4. The general population should not use dietary supplements for medicinal purposes, unless recommended by a qualified health professional. Such a practitioner will have experience in treating diseases and symptoms with both prescription drugs and natural compounds and will have performed the research to choose the safest and most effective therapy.

MODULE 16-2 Summary

Dietary supplement labels contain product information on "Supplement Facts" panels, expressed in quantities of milligram (mg) or microgram (mcg or μg) or international units (IU). Also provided are "% Daily Value" (DVs) for each nutrient listed. DVs for vitamins and minerals are based on the 1968 RDAs for adults, which still work reasonably well. However, some nutrients may not match current nutritional recommendations (such as A, D, E and iron).

The most commonly used supplement is a multiple vitamin and mineral supplement (multi-Vit/Min) that is intended to compensate for nutrients that may be limited in a person's diet. Deficiencies of vitamins and minerals can impair ability and desire to perform physical activity and also cause mental and emotional problems.

As a general rule of thumb, the safe level of most nutrients in a multi-Vit/Min should be around 100 percent of the Daily Value. However, there are some exceptions, including:

- Vitamin A (present only as retinol) should be less than 100 percent of the DV,
- Beta-carotene is contraindicated in smokers and
- Calcium should be at low levels or absent in a multi-Vit/Min.

People are more likely to consume excessive amounts of the following nutrients from supplements and fortified foods combined:

- Vitamin A,
- Vitamin D,
- Iron and
- Zinc.

With the plethora of fortified foods available, it is quite possible to consume excessive amounts of some nutrients even without taking dietary supplements. Consequently, decisions to use dietary supplements should be made in the context of a typical diet, with special attention to use of foods fortified with vitamins and minerals.

MODULE 16-2 Quiz

1. What does "IU" mean on a Supplement Facts label?

   _____

2. For components of supplements that do not have DVs, what does it say at the bottom of the panel?

   _____

3. The DV for vitamin A is _____ the SUL value recently set by the Expert Committee on Vitamins and Minerals in the United Kingdom?

   ☐ Less than   ☐ Equal to   ☐ Greater than

4. If a dietary supplement contains 100 percent of the Daily Value of iron, it contains an amount of iron that is ☐ **less than** ☐ **equal to** ☐ **greater than** the RDA for women and ☐ **less than** ☐ **more than twice** the RDA for men.

5. In the elderly, mental and emotional changes due to _____ deficiency are often mistaken for Alzheimer's disease and other dementias.

7. Excess calcium consumed with other minerals inhibits the absorption of some important trace minerals.

   ☐ True   ☐ False

References

1. Kurtzweil P. An FDA guide to dietary supplements. *FDA Consum* 1998;32:28-35.

2. Supplement Business Report 2002. *Nutrition business journal.* Penton Media, Inc.; 2002.

3. U.S. 103rd Congress. Dietary Supplement Health and Education Act of 1994. Public Law 103-417. [http://www.fda.gov/opacom/laws/dshea.html]

4. U. S. Food and Drug Administration, Center for Food Safety and Applied Nutrition. Dietary Supplement Health and Education Act of 1994. December 1, 1995. [http://www.cfsan.fda.gov/~dms/dietsupp.html]

5. Fletcher RH, Fairfield KM. Vitamins for chronic disease prevention in adults: clinical applications. *JAMA* 2002 Jun 19;287(23):3127-9.

6. Fairfield KM, Fletcher RH. Vitamins for chronic disease prevention in adults: scientific review. *JAMA* 2002 Jun 19;287(23):3116-26.

7. Drewnowski A, Shultz JM. Impact of aging on eating behaviors, food choices, nutrition, and health status. *J Nutr Health Aging* 2001;5(2):75-9.

8. Bidlack WR, Smith CH. Nutritional requirements of the aged. *Crit Rev Food Sci Nutr* 1988;27(3):189-218.

9. Gunderson EP. Nutrition during pregnancy for the physically active woman. *Clin Obstet Gynecol* 2003 Jun;46(2):390-402. Review.

10. Food and Nutrition Board, Institute of Medicine. *Dietary reference intakes for calcium, phosphorus, magnesium, vitamin D, and fluoride.* Washington, DC: National Academy Press; 1997.

11. Food and Nutrition Board, Institute of Medicine. *Dietary reference intakes for thiamin, riboflavin, niacin, vitamin b-6, folate, vitamin b-12, pantothenic acid, biotin, and choline.* Washington, DC: National Academy Press; 1998.

12. Food and Nutrition Board, Institute of Medicine. *Dietary reference intakes for vitamin C, vitamin E, selenium, and carotenoids.* Washington, DC: National Academy Press; 2000.

13. Food and Nutrition Board, Institute of Medicine. *Dietary reference intakes for vitamin A, vitamin K, arsenic, boron, chromium, copper, iodine, iron, manganese, molybdenum, nickel, silicon, vanadium, and zinc.* Washington, DC: National Academy Press; 2001.

14. Food and Nutrition Board, Institute of Medicine. *Dietary reference intakes for energy, carbohydrate, fiber, fat, fatty acids, cholesterol, protein, and amino acids* (prepublication copy/uncorrected proofs). Washington, DC: National Academy Press; 2002.

15. Food and Nutrition Board, Institute of Medicine. *Dietary reference intakes: applications in dietary planning* (prepublication copy/uncorrected proofs) Washington, DC: National Academy Press; 2003.

16. Baggott JE, Morgan SL, Ha T, Vaughn WH, Hine RJ. Inhibition of folate-dependent enzymes by non-steroidal anti-inflammatory drugs. *Biochem J* 1992;282 (Pt 1):197-202.

17. Expert Group on Vitamins and Minerals. *Safe upper levels for vitamins and minerals.* United Kingdom: Food Standards Agency; May 2003. http://www.foodstandards.gov.uk/multimedia/pdfs/vitmin2003.pdf

18. Feskanich D, Singh V, Willett WC, Colditz GA. Vitamin A intake and hip fractures among postmenopausal women. *JAMA* 2002 Jan 2;287(1):47-54.

19. Pryor WA, Stahl W, Rock CL. Beta carotene: from biochemistry to clinical trials. *Nutr Rev* 2000 Feb;58(2 Pt 1):39-53.

20. Albanes D, Heinonen OP, Taylor PR, et al. Alpha-tocopherol and beta-carotene supplements and lung cancer incidence in the alpha-tocopherol, beta-carotene cancer prevention study: effects of baseline characteristics and study compliance. *J Natl Cancer Inst* 1996;88:1560-70.

21. Omen GS, Goodman G, Thornquist M, et al. The beta-carotene and retinol efficacy trial (CARET) for chemoprevention of lung cancer in high risk populations: smokers and asbestos-exposed workers. *Cancer Res* 1994;54:2038-43.

22. Cook N, Lee IM, Manson J, et al. Effects of 12 years of beta-carotene supplementation on cancer incidence in the physician's health study (PHS). *Am J Epidemiol* 1999;149:270-9.

23. Blot WJ, Li JY, Taylor PR, et al. Nutritional intervention trials in Linxian, China: supplementation with specific vitamin/mineral combinations, cancer incidence, and disease specific mortality in the general population. *J Natl Cancer Inst* 1993;85:1483-92.

24. Heaney RP, Weaver CM, Fitzsimmons ML. Influence of calcium load on absorption fraction. *J Bone Miner Res* 1990 Nov;5(11):1135-8.

25. Benton D, Donohoe RT. The effects of nutrients on mood. *Public Health Nutr* 1999 Sep;2(3A):403-9.

26. Risser WL, Lee EJ, Poindexter HB, West MS, Pivarnik JM, Risser JM, Hickson JF. Iron deficiency in female athletes: its prevalence and impact on performance. *Med Sci Sports Exerc* 1988 Apr;20(2):116-21.

27. Carmel, R. Current concepts in cobalamin deficiency. *Ann Rev Med* 2000;51:357-75.

28. Carmel R, Melnyk S, James SJ. Cobalamin deficiency with and without neurologic abnormalities: differences in homocysteine and methionine metabolism. *Blood* 2003 Apr 15;101(8):3302-8.

29. Andres E, Kaltenbach G, Noel E, Noblet-Dick M, Perrin AE, Vogel T, Schlienger JL, Berthel M, Blickle JF. Efficacy of short-term oral cobalamin therapy for the treatment of cobalamin deficiencies related to food-cobalamin malabsorption: a study of 30 patients. *Clin Lab Hematol* 2003 Jun;25(3):161-6.

30. Andres E, Perrin AE, Demangeat C, Kurtz JE, Vinzio S, Grunenberger F, Goichot B, Schlienger JL. The syndrome of food-cobalamin malabsorption revisited in a department of internal medicine. A monocentric cohort study of 80 patients. *Eur J Intern Med* 2003 Jul;14(4):221-6.

31. Oh R, Brown DL. Vitamin B12 deficiency. *Am Fam Phys* 2003 Mar 1;67(5):979-86.

CHAPTER SEVENTEEN

Behavior Modification

Objectives

After studying this chapter, you will be able to:

■ Describe the five steps to helping clients achieve more.

■ Understand positive psychology and the importance of setting goals.

Key Terms

■ Root cause analysis

Introduction to Positive Psychology

How to Use the New Science of Success to Help Clients Achieve More

Successful health and fitness professionals have not only mastered exercise science, they also have a working knowledge of psychology (or the science of behavior and mind). They can keep clients motivated, they understand the psychology of peak performance and they can help clients make lasting lifestyle changes, both inside and outside the gym. Fortunately, psychology has more tools and techniques to offer health and fitness professionals than ever before. Psychology's century-long, Freud-inspired focus on deficits and dysfunction is increasingly giving way to "positive psychology" (the scientific study of happy, successful, highly achieving people).

This chapter synthesizes the latest research on positive psychology in a very practical way. It presents a straightforward, science-based, five step process that health and fitness professionals can use to help their clients achieve more. At each step, it offers proven tools and techniques for enhancing performance and facilitating lasting lifestyle changes.

MODULE 17-1: Step One — Vision

The Science of Clarifying Your Ultimate Ambitions

Successful people know what they want from life. Their lives are characterized by a sense of passion, purpose and meaning. Research confirms the physical and psychological benefits of the "vision thing." Those who are certain about what they want to accomplish are up to *six times* more likely to successfully make life changes than those who are less certain.[1] Conversely, those with conflicting goals, or those who are ambivalent about their goals, are significantly more likely to:[2,3]

- Experience depression and anxiety;
- Be less happy and less satisfied with their lives;
- Have more physical illnesses and doctor's visits;
- Be indecisive, uncertain and rebellious;
- Be easily distracted and procrastinate;
- Spend more time thinking about their goals; and
- Spend less time taking action toward their goals.

Successful health and fitness professionals, therefore, must be adept at helping clients clarify what they really want, both in and out of the health club. When asking clients about their goals, health and fitness professionals must be able to break through top-of-mind answers, such as "get in shape," that aren't helpful to health and fitness professionals or inspiring to clients. They must also be able to "reinterpret" unintentionally misleading responses. Many clients, for example, will say their goal is to "lose weight" and emphasize their need for cardiovascular workouts, when in fact they really want their bodies proportioned differently and need a regimen more focused on weight training. Clarifying a client's ultimate objectives will lead to longer, more mutually satisfying relationships for health and fitness professionals and clients alike.

Helping Clients Achieve More by Helping Them Figure out What They Really Want

Keep Asking "Why?"

ROOT CAUSE ANALYSIS:
A method of asking questions on a step-by-step basis to discover the initial cause of a fault.

This process, sometimes called **root cause analysis**, helps uncover the true motivations underlying superficial answers. It's simple: just keep asking "why." Consider the health and fitness professional with two new clients, each of whom says their goal is to "lose weight." When asked, "Why?" Bob answers, "So I'll look better." The health and fitness professional may then ask Bob, "Why do you want to look better?" to which he might answer, "So I'll get more dates." When asked why she wants to lose weight, Karen answers, "So I'll have more energy." The health and fitness professional may then ask Karen, "Why do you want more energy?" to which she may answer, "So I can play sports with my kids and go hiking in Peru this summer." In this very simple example, differences in motivation and orientation become clear after asking "why" just twice. The benefits are obvious. The health and fitness professional is now better equipped to customize the fitness programs (emphasizing toning and bulk versus stamina and energy). He can better target the fitness-related articles that he regularly e-mails to his clients. When the going gets tough, he can more effectively motivate clients by reminding them of their ultimate ambitions. He can also communicate the benefits of additional sessions more persuasively. The list goes on.

Vision Quest-ions

In addition to asking "why," try asking Vision Quest-ions like these:

- What would you try to accomplish if you knew you couldn't fail?
- What would you do if you won the lottery?
- Who are your role models?
- What kinds of experiences do you find so engrossing that, when you engage in them, you forget about everything around you?

A few clients may find questions like these odd, so start by asking permission to pose a few "outside the box" questions and communicate the proven benefits of the "vision thing."

MODULE 17-1 Summary

Successful people are certain about what they want from life and have grasped the "vision thing." Thus, health and fitness professionals must be able to help clients clarify what they truly desire, both in and out of the health club. This can be done through asking "why?" in a process called *root cause analysis*, which uncovers motivations behind superficial answers. In addition, ask "outside the box" questions about clients' vision. Clarifying a client's real objectives will lead to longer, more mutually satisfying relationships for health and fitness professionals and clients alike.

MODULE 17-1 Quiz

1. Those who are certain about what they want to accomplish are up to
   _____ times more likely to successfully make life changes than those who are less certain.

   ☐ Two   ☐ Six   ☐ Ten

2. In the process of "root cause analysis," a health and fitness professional can uncover the true motivations underlying superficial answers by asking clients what question about their goals?

MODULE 17-2: Step Two — Strategy

The Science of Turning Lofty Ambitions into Consistent Action

Success requires a strategy for making one's vision a reality. "Flexible" thinkers who engage in higher-level visionary thinking, as well as lower-level strategic thinking, accomplish more than those who consistently think at either level alone. These "flexible" thinkers also tend to be physically healthier, with lower rates of drug and alcohol abuse.[4] In contrast, a lofty vision without a compelling strategy is associated with perfectionism, procrastination, and labels such as "a hopeless romantic." Properly set, personal goals channel effort, boost motivation and enhance performance, but perhaps most importantly, they intensify the broader process of strategy refinement. After setting challenging goals, people think longer, harder, and more creatively about how to accomplish them.[5]

The challenge with the goal setting literature is separating fact from fiction. Consider this goal setting "study" described by many popular self-improvement experts. The 1953 graduating class at Yale was interviewed, and three percent had written specific goals. When re-interviewed 20 years later, the three percent who wrote goals were worth more, financially, than the other 97 percent combined. It's a compelling story, with one drawback: this "study" was never conducted.[6] It is a self-improvement urban legend, repeated uncritically, until accepted as truthful. In recent years, the legend has morphed; the best-selling popular fitness manual *Body for Life* recently recounted this legend as the "Harvard" study of goals.

Urban legends get repeated because they convey deeper truths and there are, in fact, hundreds of real studies documenting the beneficial effects of goals. To maximize performance, it is best to help clients understand and use the six principles of effective goal setting summarized by the acronym *SMAART*.

Helping Clients Achieve More by Helping Them Set SMAART Goals

Specific

More than 100 published studies document that specific, challenging goals result in better performance than easy goals, no goals or simply trying to "do your best."[7] Encourage specific goals based on the number of workouts per week, the amount of time engaging in cardiovascular exercise, etc.

Measurable

Measuring progress toward goals allows one to ascertain whether the strategy is working.[8] Measurable goals also encourage steady progress by minimizing the tendency to conceptualize success in all-or-none terms, a tendency that leaves clients vulnerable to the "snowball effect" or letting a minor setback "snowball" into a major relapse and a total collapse.[9]

Aggressive

People who set aggressive goals tend to accomplish more than those setting more modest goals.[10] Setting achievable goals at the upper end of a client's ability will inspire more effort, and build more confidence when accomplished.

Approach

Client goals should focus on desired ends to move toward, rather than negative states to avoid. Avoidance goals conjure up memories of accidents or failures, and people with many avoidance goals are less happy, healthy and motivated than others.[11,12]

Relevant

Goals should be relevant in the sense that they are consistent with a client's own ideals and vision. People strive toward relevant goals with greater interest and confidence, leading to enhanced performance, persistence, creativity and self-esteem.

Set expectations for daily performance and outcomes. These should be as specific as the execution of each exercise to how a client desires to feel at the end of each workout. The client should understand how each session and exercise is relevant to his/her higher vision of what he/she desires to achieve. Explain how each component of the OPT™ model is progressing the client toward his/her highest health and fitness aspirations, one exercise at a time.

Time-bound

Time-bound means that the health and fitness professional should assist clients in setting a specific timeframe around their plan for achieving health and fitness goals, both short- and long-term. Supplementing a long-term vision with near-term, proximal goals leads to better performance, as well as a heightened sense of confidence, determination and happiness.[12,13] A client who resolves to lose 20 pounds in the next year, for example, should set more proximal eating and exercise goals that can be reached in a week or two.

Finally, goals should be inspirational in the sense that they are consistent with a client's own ideals and ambitions. People strive toward inspirational goals with greater interest and confidence, leading to enhanced performance, persistence, creativity and self-esteem.[13]

MODULE 17-2 Summary

Vision is important. But, more important is the strategy to make that vision a reality. Those who think on both levels tend to achieve more and be physically healthier. Strategy (and goal-setting) channels effort, boosts motivation and enhances performance.

There are six useful principles of effective goal setting, summarized by the acronym *SMAART*.

S — **Specific** goals result in better performance.

M — **Measurable** goals let a client know if the strategy is working.

A — **Aggressive** goals tend to create greater performance than modest ones.

A — **Approach** to goal setting should be on desired ends to move toward.

R — **Relevant** goals maintain focus and motivation by demonstrating how each component of the OPT™ model correlates with the client's overall goals.

T — **Time-bound** proximal, short-term goals raise sense of confidence and determination.

MODULE 17-2 Quiz

1. What was the flaw with the success study done of Yale's 1953 graduating class?

   _____

2. What does the acronym SMAART stand for?

   _____

   _____

   _____

3. Setting achievable goals at the _____ end of a client's ability will inspire more effort, and build more confidence when accomplished.

   ☐ Upper   ☐ Lower

MODULE 17-3: Step Three — Belief

Science of Minimizing FUD (Fear, Uncertainty and Doubt)

Clients must truly believe that they can implement their strategies and achieve their visions. Belief comes in many "flavors," including self-confidence, self-efficacy, sense of control and hope. Regardless of the label, the findings are clear: belief is one of the most powerful predictors of change and success. Those who truly believe they will be successful are more likely to:[14]

- Work harder, achieve more and perform better in many domains (from academics to sports to keeping their New Year's resolutions).

- Be happy, while more effectively tackling problems of depression, anxiety, burnout, alcoholism, smoking and obesity.

- Set more goals and set them more effectively.

- Persist vigorously in the face of obstacles and view setbacks as a source of motivation.

- Attribute failures to changeable causes (e.g., poor strategies) rather than unchangeable ones (e.g., not being smart enough).

- React better to difficult circumstances, including bad test scores, career setbacks, stressful jobs, paralyzing accidents, and chronic illnesses.

- Use more effective coping habits, such as humor, regular exercise, and preventative care.

Helping Clients Achieve More by Helping Them Believe in Themselves

Think Baby Steps

Encourage clients to start with modest goals and increase them in small increments. Remember that goals should be challenging, but attainable.

Visualization

World-class athletes are routinely trained to visualize performing well in competitive situations, and research suggests that "mental practice" can help everyday athletes as well.[15,16] Visualization must be vivid and detailed to be effective. Envisioning broad ends like "being thinner" or "feeling stronger" may temporarily boost motivation, but greater benefits (reduced anxiety, greater confidence and enhanced performance) result from envisioning the specific means to those ends.[17]

Of course, one must also visualize proper form and technique. Visualization enhances the performance of elite athletes, but can hamper the performance of novices because they mentally practice the wrong skills (e.g., novice basketball players mentally rehearse poor form in free throw shooting).[18]

Schedule Negativity

Many techniques can help clients battle the negative thoughts and attitudes that often undermine belief. Suggest "scheduling" negativity, perhaps setting aside time from 8:00 - 8:30 p.m. for self-doubt. If they find negative thoughts recurring during workouts, they should remind themselves that there will be plenty of time to plague themselves with self-doubt at 8:00 p.m. Another variation involves limiting negativity to a very specific location. Although these techniques may seem "out there," research has shown that anxiety can be lessened by limiting it to 30 minutes a day and only in a "worry chair;" similarly, smoking can be reduced by limiting it to an inconvenient and uncomfortable "smoking chair."[19]

MODULE 17-3 Summary

Belief is extremely important implementing strategies and achieving visions. It is one of the most powerful predictors of change and success. Those who truly believe they will be successful are more likely to be happy, work harder, perform better, set more effective goals, persist in the face of obstacles, handle failure better and achieve more.

Belief can be fostered by having clients start with modest attainable goals, increasing them in small increments. They should also use vivid and detailed visualizations of success. Visualizing proper form and technique is important too. Finally, it may help to "schedule" negativity or confine it to a specific location.

MODULE 17-3 Quiz

1. Those with a high level of belief view setbacks as a source of motivation.

☐ True   ☐ False

MODULE 17-4: Step Four — Persistence

The Science of Drive and Determination

Research confirms the conventional wisdom that successful people work hard, and rebound from setbacks. In short, they persist. People who successfully maintain their New Year's resolutions for two years report an average of 14 slips, but they use those setbacks to strengthen their commitment.[20] Persistence is obviously crucial to weight loss, but it drives weight gain as well. The average person gains only one pound during holiday season, and only a pound and a half over the course of a whole year. The problem is persistence: weight goes on each year, typically staying on permanently, leading to a 10-pound weight gain in only seven years.[21]

Helping Clients Achieve More by Helping Them Persist

Reward Success

Rewarding oneself for success is a rarely used, but powerful technique for change. It has proven effective in aiding weight loss, smoking cessation, battling depression, boosting self-efficacy and adhering to prescribed medical regimens.[22,23,24] It can start as simply as clients treating themselves to smoothies if they work out individually before their next session with you. Increase the goals and rewards gradually. For a more formal system, try the *deposit-and-refund* technique. A client who wants to lose ten pounds could write a check to a friend for $500. The friend refunds the deposited money at the rate of $50 per pound lost. This self-reward system makes instant gratification a positive force for change ("If I lose just one pound, I'll get an immediate reward"), and can facilitate lasting weight loss, even after the formal reward period ends.[25]

Facilitate Networks of Excellence

Those with supportive friends and family achieve more, live longer and feel happier than those who are more isolated.[26,27] They also exhibit greater persistence, as supportive people close to them reward their progress, help celebrate successes and aid in recovery from setbacks.[28,29] Encourage clients to ask for support from friends and family. They should also attempt to surround themselves with excellence, perhaps by finding equally committed workout partners (the deposit-and-refund method described above is even more effective when done as a group).[30] This will also encourage clients to publicly commit to goals, which is another potent predictor of success.

Have a Strategy for Setbacks

Encourage clients to expect success, but prepare them for setbacks. A setback plan might involve identifying a friend to call in the event of a slip. Another technique involves carrying a "reminder card." Smokers who lapse while trying to quit, for example, are encouraged to look at a reassuring card which reads (in part): "Just because you slipped once does not mean that you are a failure, that you have no willpower or that you are a hopeless addict. Look upon the slip as a single, independent event, something which can be avoided in the future with an alternative coping response."[31]

MODULE 17-4 Summary

Successful people succeed by working hard and rebounding from setbacks. In short, they persist. Persistence can by encouraged by rewarding success. Rewards for change may start out simply and gradually increase as goals do. A more formal system is the deposit-and-refund technique, which is best achieved with friends and groups.

Tell clients to ask for support from friends and family and find equally committed workout partners. Publicly committing to goals is another potent predictor of success. This will aid in persistence, achievement and happiness. Their supportive network can reward their progress, help celebrate successes and aid in recovery from setbacks. While expecting success, clients should prepare for setbacks. To help, a setback plan is useful. The plan might be to call a friend in the event of a slip or to carry a "reminder card."

MODULE 17-4 Quiz

1. What is a good formal reward system?

_____

MODULE 17-5: Step Five — Learning

The Science of Making Course Corrections

Clients must learn whether they are persisting in the right direction, and whether course corrections are necessary. The best tool for this type of learning is a process psychologists call *self-monitoring*, which simply means recording aspects of behavior and measuring progress toward goals. Keeping records of eating and exercise habits, for example, is one of the few predictors of lasting weight loss.[32] Similarly, students who keep records of their studying get better grades than those who don't. In clinical situations, self-monitoring has reduced alcohol consumption, smoking, disruptive classroom behavior, nail biting and even hallucinations![33,34] Simply recording behavior has modest effects that diminish over time, but it can be a powerful performance-enhancing tool when combined with the first four steps of the process.[35]

Recording progress serves as a small reward when clients are doing well and as a gentle, but thought-provoking punishment when they are doing poorly. It encourages clients to celebrate success and counteracts the natural tendency to overlook progress (as when dieters focus on times they broke their diets, overlooking all their successes). It enhances accountability and keeps clients focused on their ultimate objectives. But most of all, self-monitoring enhances learning by providing feedback on whether a client's strategy is taking her toward her vision, and it makes clear whether course corrections are necessary.

Helping Clients Achieve More by Helping Them Measure Their Progress

Use What You Already Have

Virtually all health and fitness professionals already record the amount of time clients spend doing cardiovascular workouts, or the amount of weight lifted in various exercises. However, most would admit they could spend more time sharing and discussing this information with clients. Jointly reviewing past data helps clients build confidence by seeing the progress they have made, and helps motivate them to achieve more. Try creating charts and graphs of a client's data that display progress visually. All the data in the world won't help clients if it only exists on a health and fitness professional's clipboard. It needs to get in clients' heads on a regular basis.

Go Further

Encourage clients to take their self-monitoring to the next level by recording progress toward each of their goals on a zero-to-10 scale every day, with zero denoting no progress and 10 representing outstanding progress. This intuitive technique works with any kind of goal and is ideal for computer graphing.

Focus on "Controllable Behaviors"

Initially measure behaviors and avoid tracking physiological "outcome measures," such as changes in weight, blood pressure, body fat or medication needs. These measures are obviously important, and should be tracked over the long-term as appropriate, but they don't change immediately. Clients who measure these variables daily can quickly become discouraged and lose self-efficacy. For clients trying to lose weight, for example, encourage them not to weigh themselves for two or three weeks after beginning exercise programs.

Analyze the Data

Analyzing a client's progress data helps them to quickly ascertain which goals they are progressing toward, and which goals require new strategies or additional effort. Examining trends over time may reveal additional patterns such as "weekend snowballs" (or making solid progress toward eating and exercise goals during the week, but letting one slip snowball into periods of inactivity and overeating on weekends). This knowledge enables "course corrections;" on weekends, a client can redouble his efforts to work out, or cook healthy meals at home, rather than eat out. Goal-setting software programs enable even more sophisticated analyses with point-and-click simplicity, and simplify the entry of progress data as well.

Summing It Up

True success in life isn't rare due to the fact that people are weak or lazy or lack willpower or fear success. Rather, true success is rare because too often people use flawed strategies for success. Across different areas of life, from weight loss to smoking cessation, from academic success to athletic excellence, those who achieve more use the best processes for change. These individuals identify more techniques for change, while using those techniques longer, more frequently, more consistently, and more thoughtfully.[36,37] The process outlined in this chapter synthesizes the most powerful tools for change known to science. Using them with clients, and with yourself, will lead to greater success for all.

MODULE 17-5 Summary

It is important to know whether persistence is paying off or if course corrections are necessary. Self-monitoring (by recording aspects of behavior and measuring progress toward goals) is an excellent way to track this. Clients should keep records of things such as eating and exercise habits and may even want to take self-monitoring to the next level, by recording progress on a zero-to-10 scale every day. These steps encourage celebrating success and also enhance accountability. Clients stay focused on their ultimate objectives and know whether course corrections are necessary.

Health and fitness professionals should share recorded workout data with clients. It may help to create charts and graphs of a data that displays progress visually. Initially, measure behaviors and avoid tracking physiological measures, since they don't change immediately. Analyzing progress data helps to quickly ascertain which goals clients are progressing toward, and which goals require new strategies or additional effort.

MODULE 17-5 Quiz

1. Self-monitoring involves recording aspects of _____ and measuring _____ toward goals.

2. Jointly reviewing past workout data helps clients build confidence by seeing the progress they have made and helps motivate them to achieve more.

   ☐ True ☐ False

3. Clients who are trying to lose weight should be encouraged not to weigh themselves for how long?

   _____

4. Success in life is rare because most people are lazy, lack willpower or have a fear success.

   ☐ True ☐ False

References

1. Heatherton TF, Nichols PA. Personal accounts of successful versus failed attempts at life change. *Pers Soc Psy Bul* 1994;20:664-75.

2. Emmons RA, King LA. Conflict among personal strivings: immediate and long-term implications for psychological and physical well-being. *J Pers Soc Psy* 1988;54:1040-8.

3. Van Hook E, Higgins ET. Self-related problems beyond the self-concept: motivational consequences of discrepant self-guides. *J Pers Soc Psy* 1988;55:625-33.

4. Pennebaker JW. *Opening up.* New York: Morrow; 1994.

5. Latham GP, Locke EA. Self-regulation through goal setting. *Org Beh Hum Decis Proces* 1991;50:212-47.

6. www.fastcompany.com/online/06/cdu.html

7. Tubbs ME. Goal setting: a meta-analytic examination of the evidence. *J App Psy* 1986;71:474-83.

8. Becker LJ. Joint effect of feedback and goal setting on performance: a field study of residential energy conservation. *J App Psy* 1978;63:428-33.

9. Marlatt GA. Relapse prevention: theoretical rationale and overview of the model. In GA Marlatt, Gordon JR (eds). *Relapse prevention.* New York: Guilford Press; 1985. pp. 3-70.

10. Latham GP, Locke EA. Self-regulation through goal setting. *Org Beh Hum Decis Proces* 1991;50:212-47.

11. Elliot A, Sheldon K. Avoidance achievement motivation: a personal goals analysis. *J Pers Soc Psy* 1997;73:171-85.

12. Singer JA, Salovey P. Motivated memory: Self-defining memories, goals, and affect regulation. In: Martin LL, Tesser A (eds). *Striving and feeling: interactions among goals, affect and self-regulation.* Mahwah, NJ: Lawrence Erlbaum Associates; 1996. pp. 229-50.

13. Ryan RM, Deci EL. Self-determination theory and the facilitation of intrinsic motivation, social development, and well-being. *Am Psychol* 2000;55:68-78.

14. Bandura A. *Self-efficacy: the exercise of control.* New York: W.H. Freeman; 1997.

15. Suinn RM. Psychological approaches to performance enhancement. In: Asken M, May J (eds). *Sports psychology: the psychological health of the athlete.* New York: Spectrum; 1987. pp. 41-57.

16. Watson DL, Tharp RG. *Self-directed behavior: self-modification for personal adjustment.* Pacific Grove, CA: Brooks/Cole; 1993.

17. Pham LB, Taylor SE. From thought to action: effects of process-versus outcome-based mental simulations on performance. *Pers Soc Psy Bul* 1999;25:250-60.

18. Suinn RM. Psychological approaches to performance enhancement. In: Asken M, May J (eds). *Sports psychology: the psychological health of the athlete.* New York: Spectrum; 1987. pp. 41-57.

19. Watson DL, Tharp RG. *Self-directed behavior: self-modification for personal adjustment.* Pacific Grove, CA: Brooks/Cole; 1993.

20. Norcross JC, Vangarelli DJ. The resolution solution: longitudinal examination of new year's change attempts. *J Substan Abuse* 1989;1:127-34.

21. You are what you eat. *Psy Today* Mar/Apr 2001.

22. Stall R, Biernacki P. Spontaneous remission from the problematic use of substances: an inductive model derived from a comparative analysis of the alcohol, opiate, tobacco, and food/obesity literatures. *Int J Addict* 1986;21:1-23.

23. Brownell KD, Marlatt GA, Lichtenstein E, Wilson GT. Understanding and preventing relapse. *Am Psychol* 1986;41:765-82.

24. Epstein LH, Cluss PA. A behavioral medicine perspective on adherence to long-term medical regimens. *J Consult Clini Psy* 1982;50:950-71.

25. Jeffery RW, Gerber WM, Rosenthal BS, Lindquist RA. Monetary contracts in weight control: effectiveness of group and individual contracts of varying size. *J Consult Clin Psy* 1983;51:242-8.

26. House JS, Landis KR, Umberson D. Social relationships and health. *Sci* 1988;241;540-5.

27. Kaprio J, Koskenvou M, Rita H. Mortality after bereavement: a prospective study of 95,647 widowed persons. *Am J Pub Heal* 1987;77:283-7.

28. Cohen S, Lichtenstein E. Partner behaviors that support quitting smoking. *J Consult Clin Psy* 1990;58:304-9.

29. Clifford PA, Tan SY, Gorsuch RL. Efficacy of a self-directed behavioral health change program: weight, body composition, cardiovascular fitness, blood pressure, health risk, and psychosocial mediating variables. *J Beh Med* 1991;14:303-23.

30. Jeffery RW, Gerber WM, Rosenthal BS, Lindquist RA. Monetary contracts in weight control: effectiveness of group and individual contracts of varying size. *J Consult Clin Psy* 1983;51:242-8.

31. Marlatt GA, Gordon JR. *Relapse prevention: maintenance strategies in addictive behavior change.* New York: Guilford; 1985.

32. National Weight Control Registry: http://www.lifespan.org/services/bmed/wt_loss/nwcr/

33. Kirschenbaum DS. Self-regulatory failure: a review with clinical implications. *Clin Psy Rev* 1987;7:77-104.

34. Kazdin AE. Reactive self-monitoring: the effects of response desirability, goal setting, and feedback. *J Consult Clin Psy* 1974;42:704-16.

35. Kazdin AE. Reactive self-monitoring: the effects of response desirability, goal setting, and feedback. *J Consult Clin Psy* 1974;42:704-16.

36. Perri MG. Self-change strategies for the control of smoking, obesity, and problem drinking. In: Shiffman S, Wills TA (eds). *Coping and substance use.* Orlando: Academic Press; 1985. pp. 295-317.

37. Heffernan T, Richards CS. Self-control of study behaviors: identification and evaluation of natural methods. *J Counsel Psy* 1981;28:361-4.

CHAPTER EIGHTEEN

Professional Development

Objectives

After studying this chapter, you will be able to:

- Provide uncompromising customer service.
- Approach members and find prospective clients.
- Justify the costs of products and services.
- Know how to READ clients.
- Ask for and close a sale.

Key Terms

- Rapport
- Empathy
- Assessment

MODULE 18-1: Customer Service

The Purpose of a Business

It is often assumed that the primary purpose of a business is to generate a profit. While profit is a measure for how effectively a business is run, it is not the purpose of the business itself. Rather, the purpose of a business is always to create and keep a customer.

When profit alone becomes the sole focus of the business, the source of that profit (or the customer) becomes neglected, which threatens the future of the business. Conversely, organizations (and individuals) that possess a fanatical customer focus reinvent themselves continually in order to provide an ever-growing level of value to their customers. Long-term profit generation is largely the result of creating and keeping customers.

The system presented in this chapter provides the health and fitness professional with a progressive, customer-focused process for creating a distinctive level of value and developing a highly successful client base. By mastering the OPT™ model, completing NASM's CPT certification and applying the tools and solutions learned with clients, you will be able to create or greatly increase your personal level of success.

Providing Uncompromising Customer Service

Success depends, to a great degree, on reputation. Those known for excellence and distinction in their profession gain a competitive advantage over everyone else working in the same position.

It is essential to have a strong commitment to excellence, knowledge and professionalism in order to be thought of with high regard. The best health and fitness professionals operate with the utmost level of integrity and refuse to settle for anything less than their personal best.

Establish a reputation for being adept as a health and fitness professional, then develop a reputation for uncompromising customer service. *Uncompromising customer service* means being adamant about providing an experience and level of assistance that is rarely, if ever, experienced anywhere else. Develop an obsession for becoming artistic in your approach to helping people.

All buying decisions are based on emotion. Clients have many choices regarding where to exercise. Thus, a client's choice is based on how he/she *feels* about a certain facility and its health and fitness professionals. This feeling is often based on the level of customer service received and that client's perception of the value offered. Those who adapt to uncompromising customer service as the minimum acceptable standard of professionalism will give clients positive feelings. It is clear that relationships are the most powerful competitive advantage in a service profession.

Guidelines for Uncompromising Customer Service

In everyday business, there is a tendency to get caught up in tasks and details. However, it is important to ensure that every moment is adding to clients' experience. Clients should never be thought of as an interruption of work; they are the entire purpose behind it! Keys to embodying this philosophy include:

1. Taking every opportunity to meet and greet each club member at all times, while on or off shift. Every contact is an opportunity to create a professional relationship and, eventually, make a sale.

2. Remembering to represent a positive image and high level of professionalism every minute of the day.

3. Never giving the impression that any question is inconvenient, unnecessary or unintelligent.

4. Expressing ideas well through verbal communication, vocal tonality, and body language. All of these work together to convey a message.

5. Obsessing on opportunities to create moments that strengthen professional relationships.

6. Not merely receiving complaints, but taking ownership of them.

Successful health and fitness professionals ask themselves: "If my entire future were based on the way this one client evaluated his experience with me right now, would I change anything?" They may also ask, "Did I exceed this client's expectations?" If the answer to either of these questions is "No," committed health and fitness professionals would continue to look for ways to improve themselves. NASM's education, application, integrity, solutions and tools are the foundation for creating "Yes" answers to these questions and providing optimum performance and results for clients.

MODULE 18-1 Summary

The primary purpose of a business is to create and keep customers. A customer-focused process, utilizing the keys to uncompromising customer service, will create a distinctive level of value and develop success in finding, building and resigning clients. Establish a reputation for excellence and distinction as a health and fitness professional, then develop a reputation for uncompromising customer service. Leave each club member with a positive impression.

A client's buying decisions are based on how he/she feels about a certain facility and its health and fitness professionals. These feelings are influenced by the level of customer service received and perception of value offered. As such, clients are never an interruption of work, but rather the entire purpose behind it. Each client's experience should be treated as if it affects the entire career of the health and fitness professional, because it does.

MODULE 18-1 Quiz

1. Success depends largely on what factors?

_____

2. What are all buying decisions based on?

☐ Price   ☐ Emotion   ☐ Recommendation

3. A successful health and fitness professional should not merely receive complaints, but do what?

_____

4. Every contact with someone should be thought of as what?

_____

MODULE 18-2: The Customer

Who is the Customer?

Clients utilize the services of health and fitness professionals for a variety of reasons. These range from cosmetic augmentation (appearance) and improved performance (sports-specific) to general health and increased physical capacity in activities of daily living. Whatever their reasons, the motivation is the desire to improve quality of life.

In the past decade, technology has created a lifestyle paradox. While technology enables people to complete daily activities with greater efficiency, it has replaced everyday movement. This decline has resulted in increased dysfunction and obesity. It is obvious that the need for professional, personalized physical training is increasing. Fitness training can be a luxury, but it is moving toward becoming a necessity. In the very near future, healthcare will play a pivotal role in the success and growth of the health and fitness industry. NASM's Certified Personal Trainers will be qualified to deliver the OPT™ system and tools, producing remarkable results for clients.

In today's sedentary culture, who is a potential client? Everybody! It is difficult to imagine anyone who does not have a desire to look and feel better, perform at a higher level, be healthier and more confident, enjoy a better quality of life and reduce chronic pain.

Approaching Potential Clients

Don't be afraid to approach clients. Remember that the health and fitness professional can change the life of a client. Openly provide that service be doing any of the following:

- Say "Hello" to every member while working each shift.
- Offer very active members a towel or water, if the club has it available.
- Roam the floor, clean up equipment and make sure that the workout floor is impeccable and represents the highest standard of appearance.
- Do not hide behind the fitness desk, a computer or a newspaper. Be sure to get out there and greet people, at the very least.
- Simply introduce yourself by name and ask members for their names as well.
- Let members know that you are there to enrich the club experience, by attending to any need. Then, do it!
- By resisting the temptation to educate, your first interaction with a member is professional, pleasant and most important, non-threatening.

- During the next encounter, having already met, you will be in a better position to offer valuable assistance. If a member is performing an exercise incorrectly, approach the member and tell him/her about a positive benefit of that exercise. Then, offer to help that person "maximize the exercise." State that you have just attended a seminar or read a book (which should always be true) that offers an alternative to what he/she is already doing. If the member says "No, thanks," leave them alone. However, if he/she says "Yes," provide specific help with the exercise, articulate the benefit that the member will receive, related directly to his/her goal. Continue to offer him/her assistance through the workout.

There are also ways that have been shown to be immediately unfavorable to members. Potential clients are very unreceptive to any approach that may challenge their belief systems, judgments regarding an exercise or competencies. Avoid any of the following opening lines:

- May I make a suggestion?
- Can I recommend a better way of doing that?
- Can I show you a different technique?
- Let me show you the right way.
- Can I help you with that?
- What's your goal for that exercise?

Creating Value

The increased need for personal training does not guarantee the success of all health and fitness professionals. Just because people have a need or a desire, does not mean that they will take action. In the clients' minds, the value of the service must outweigh the cost. *Cost* refers to the price of the services as well as the time, effort and commitment involved in training. In addition, individuals may have reservations created by the potential for failure. It is the health and fitness professional's personal responsibility to create and display the value of their services.

In order to secure a client, the health and fitness professional must use the systematic approach learned in this text to:

- Be excellent at using fitness **assessments** (including subjective and objective information) and various **movement observations** to accurately assess the needs and goals of the individual.
- Have the ability to **design an OPT**™ **training program** and correctly fill **out an OPT**™ **template**.

- Explain to a client how each component of the program focuses on his/her personal goals and needs.

- Be able to safely **demonstrate exercises** and **implement the program** for a client.

- Demonstrate that the OPT™ system offers the highest benefit and explain how a clients needs will be met by it.

Clients need to believe in the health and fitness professionals they choose to work with and trust that those professionals will achieve results. OPT™ system is a map to success and a systematic approach that ensures results.

MODULE 18-2 Summary

Clients utilize the services of health and fitness professionals for a variety of reasons, but all with the motivation to improve quality of life. In today's sedentary culture, everyone can be considered a potential client. There are countless people who desire to look and feel better, be healthier and more confident, perform better, enjoy a higher quality of life and reduce chronic pain. Personal training is moving toward becoming a necessity and healthcare will soon play a pivotal role in the success and growth of the industry.

However, simply because someone has a desire to do so, does not mean that person will take action. The value of personal training services must outweigh their price, time, effort and commitment. It is the health and fitness professional's personal responsibility to create and display that value. Be proactive about approaching clients. Avoid making members feel uncomfortable by saying things such as, "Can I recommend a better way of doing that?" Instead, do things such as:

- Roaming the floor and saying "Hello" to every member, while offering towels and water and making sure that everything is tidy.

- Introducing yourself and asking members for their names, letting them know that you can help them with *any* of their needs.

- Avoid educating an individual, at first. However, if a member is performing an exercise incorrectly, find out what it is about the exercise that is important to him/her. Then, offer to help that person "maximize the exercise." Use movement and postural observations for screening and the OPT™ model to customize the exercise and other recommendations. Continue to offer the potential client assistance through the workout.

In order to secure a client, the health and fitness professional must use the OPT™ model as a map to success and utilize its systematic approach, which ensures results by:

- Using fitness assessments and movement observations to accurately assess the needs and goals of the individual.

- Designing an OPT™ training program and correctly filling out an OPT™ template.

- Explaining how the OPT™ system offers the highest benefit and how each program component focuses on personal goals and needs.

- Demonstrating exercises and implementing programs.

MODULE 18-2 Quiz

1. What is the motivation behind all of the reasons that clients utilize the services of health and fitness professionals?

_____

2. In the client's mind, the value of a health and fitness professional's services must outweigh their cost.

☐ True   ☐ False

MODULE 18-3: The READ System

The READ system was developed by NASM to guide health and fitness professionals through the process of acquiring a new client. Learning the READ system will enable you to be effective in the selling skills described in the previous module.

The acronym READ stands for:

Rapport — Establishing positive relationships

Empathy — Understanding what motivates each individual

Assessment — Identifying the goals and needs of an individual

Development — Developing the program that best meets those needs

The following text will review these components and give the health and fitness professional guidelines that make getting (and keeping) clients easier, by providing systematic steps and professional tips.

Rapport

> **RAPPORT:**
> Aspect of a relationship characterized by similarity, agreement or congruity.

Rapport is the first step in the READ system. In the beginning phases of the relationship between a health and fitness professional and client, interpersonal dynamics are more important than scientific expertise. If trust is established, communication will be open, which enables the health and fitness professional to assess the goals and needs of the client. Only then can the health and fitness professional effectively design a systematic, progressive OPT™ program and help the client reach their goals using proven solutions and tools.

Establishing Trust to Build Rapport

How is trust established? It is done by being honest, caring and effective. Always keep the clients' best interest first and foremost by maintaining integrity and producing results. Once trust is established, rapport can be built.

Effective Communication to Build Rapport

Studies have shown that a mere seven percent of the messages that we communicate to others are transmitted by the words we use verbally. Instead, 55 percent of communication is based on physiology: the way a person stands, whether or not he smiles, degree of eye contact (or lack thereof), etc.[1] The remaining 38 percent of communication is in tone of voice (Figure 18-1). What is said must be consistent with *how* it is said. Incongruent communication is not believable and therefore cannot produce a positive outcome.

People instinctively and spontaneously tend to mirror nonverbal communication patterns.[2] Body language and facial expressions affect emotions.[3] By subconsciously mirroring the physiology of others, a sensory message is sent to the brain, creating a similar emotional state. Therefore, health and fitness professionals who love their work, company and clients and exhibit the body language that corresponds with these emotions, positively affect the people around them.[4] Because all sales decisions are ultimately made on emotion, having this effect on people can open the door to initiating the relationships that a successful career is built on.

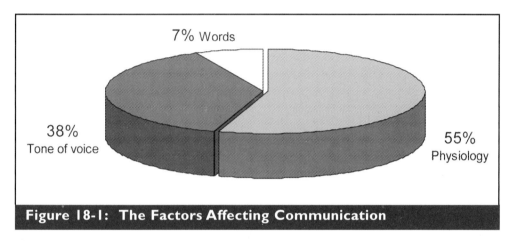

7% Words

38%
Tone of voice

55%
Physiology

Figure 18-1: The Factors Affecting Communication

Creating a Presence to Build Rapport

Communication occurs constantly in a way that affects what people perceive. The most positive messages that a health and fitness professional can send (to influence the perception that people have) are represented by level of confidence, enthusiasm and professionalism.

Confidence

Confident health and fitness professionals convey an image that it is safe to trust them, because they have the experience and expertise to effectively solve problems and produce results. They keep the focus off of themselves and on the needs and goals of the client. Ethical, friendly, knowledgeable, well-spoken health and fitness professionals who have commanding presence, provide reassurance to clients that they have made the right decision. This replaces anxiety with excitement.

Enthusiasm

In addition to confidence, enthusiasm is one of the primary components of building rapport. Enthusiasm is a positive transfer of emotion that is infectious. When every individual that a health and fitness professional comes in contact with has the impression that he is happy to see them, loves helping them and is a friendly person, that professional becomes very approachable.

Enthusiasm means that every client should feel that the health and fitness professional is excited about the time spent with him/her and wouldn't rather be any place else. The client should feel that the professional looks forward to (and is grateful for) every opportunity to assist him/her with anything.

Professionalism

In order to present a manner that is congruent with the level of professionalism desired, appearance, tone of voice and articulation are important. Driven health and fitness professionals make sure that they:

- Are dressed and groomed like highly esteemed professionals.
- Stand or sit like someone who is approachable, and do not lean on a wall, piece of equipment, sit back in a chair or hide behind a computer.
- Smile, make eye contact, greet as many members as possible and genuinely appear to be friendly, considerate and happy to see clients.
- Speak clearly and deliberately, with a cheerful tone of voice.
- Feel confident in their ability to deliver OPT™ solutions.
- Truly believe that the OPT™ tools they have will accomplish any goal.

Empathy

EMPATHY: Action of awareness, understanding and sensitivity of the thoughts, emotions and experience of another without personally having gone through the same.

The power to positively change lives starts with the realization that it's not *what* an individual wants to achieve but *why* they want to achieve it that motivates. The second step in the READ system is **empathy**, which involves understanding and identifying with the thoughts or feelings of another person. This is a process of figuratively stepping in the shoes of someone else to understand their thoughts, emotions and experiences. The process is an excellent way to shed light on a person's motivations. Thus, empathy and understanding the motivation of another person are intimately intertwined.

Motivation

Motivation is based on the forces that affect behavior. Simply stated, motivation is "a reason for doing something or behaving in some way."[5]

Primary Emotions Governing Behavior

All decisions and actions are the result of motivation. Motivation is directed by thoughts, past experiences, interpretation of events and circumstances, what is valued, emotions and so on.[6]

There are four essential questions to ask a client in the initial appointment:
1. What are you trying to achieve?
2. How long has this been a goal?
3. What is most important to you about achieving that?
4. What has prevented you from achieving it in the past?

The first question identifies a goal, directing the path along which each aspect of the appointment must travel. For example, a client may say that she would like to lose weight and "tone up." Her health and fitness professional would first conduct an assessment. He/she would inform her that the assessment will allow him to gather information necessary to individualize each component of her program to the goals of losing weight and "toning up." The health and fitness professional could explain to her how each aspect of the assessment (feet, knee, hip, shoulders and head) helps to customize solutions that will expedite the rate and degree of changes she will experience. If, after performing the assessment and receiving the results, it is revealed that she has an anterior pelvic tilt and tight hip flexors, the health and fitness professional can explain to her that by individualizing the proper foam rolling and flexibility techniques for her hip flexors, there will be a profound change, increasing the "tone" in her glutes (when combined with the other components of her program).

The second question quantifies the desired result and lets the health and fitness professional know just how important the outcome may be.

The third question reveals the outcome that the client hopes to experience when that goal is achieved. The understanding of this requires empathy and understanding on the part of the health and fitness professional. It is the answer to the third question that determines why the client's goal motivates him/her. This insight is essential to having the most positive influence on a client's motivation and actions. If the client says that she has a reunion coming up and wants to look her best, integrate each component of her program with the motivation that led her want to train in the first place. For, example: "Karen, balance training is an essential part of your program. Among other important benefits, this portion will help you to burn more calories in one workout, which will give you the potential to lose more weight in less time. So, you'll absolutely look your best in your new dress the night of your reunion."

The fourth question will help the health and fitness professional identify any foreseeable roadblocks or obstacles and a plan can be implemented to specifically avoid them.

In addition to these questions, work on root cause analysis (explained in Chapter 17) and keep asking "Why?" The follow-up on all of these questions will help in creating a clear strategy that will achieve results.

Motivational Strategies

It is easy to identify which emotions (positive or negative) motivate a client the most. A client may answer the first question by saying, "I want to lose weight." When prompted to answer the second question, she may respond, "Because I'm tired of feeling miserable every time I look in the mirror." She is obviously motivated to alleviate feelings of emotional suffering. However, the client may have responded to the second question by instead saying, "Because I have a family reunion coming up and I want to look great." In that case, she obviously desires to move toward the feeling of satisfaction (success, attractiveness and admiration).

Typically, individuals who want to alleviate discontent are:

- Motivated by a fear of ridicule, rejection, failure, being unattractive, etc.

- Motivated by the fear of the situation becoming even worse.

- Directed more by the need to avoid the feared consequences, than by the attainment of the desired benefits

Conversely, individuals who want to experience satisfaction are:

- Motivated by stated benefits.

- Driven by a desire to be better off tomorrow than they are today.

- In search of achievement, recognition and self-satisfaction.

The bottom line is, those who utilize the services of a health and fitness professional do so to transform some aspect of their lives from the current state to what they desire in the future.[7,8] It is essential to get to the root cause of why they are retaining the services of a fitness professional in order to discover how to be of the most assistance to them.

Essentially, clients buy transformational experiences, rather than a service.[9] It's the outcome they believe those services will produce for them that matters most. The health and fitness professional who doesn't empathize with a client will not understand his/her specific goals, nor what motivates that individual. That health and fitness professional without empathy will fail to be able to deliver the desired results or offer any value for his services.

Assessment

So far the rapport and empathy components of the READ system have been discussed. In the rapport phase of the sale, trust and a relationship were built. By empathizing, goals and the motivation behind them were understood. In the assessment phase of the sale, the objective is to uncover as many of the client's goals and needs as possible, in order to appropriately present benefits and solutions.

The Importance of Questions

In the **assessment** process, direct focus on to the client and his/her specific needs and desires. The more questions are asked, the more involved a client becomes in the assessment process. In turn, the more involved he/she is in the assessment, the more ownership he/she will feel in the development of a program.[10,11,12]

It is important to:

1. Ask directive and non-directive questions (discussed below) that follow a systematic thought process to acquire information.

2. Listen carefully to the response. Show care and concern by being involved.

3. Repeat client's response and paraphrase, to ensure a comprehensive understanding of their needs.

4. Take detailed notes to review later.

> **ASSESSMENT:
> A process of determining the importance, size or value of something.**

Non-directive Questions

Non-directive questions cannot be answered with a simple "Yes" or "No." These types of questions are also referred to as *open-ended questions*, which encourage someone to talk and give more information. Non-directive questions (such as "Why?") are perfect use in root cause analysis. By identifying what a client wants to accomplish, the health and fitness professional can direct every component of a presentation towards the client's goal. Knowing what is most important to a client about his/her goal, allows the health and fitness professional to identify the best motivational strategy.

Directive Questions

Directive questions can only be answered with a "Yes" or a "No" response. The purpose of these questions is to establish agreement within the presentation and make sure that it stays focused on the client's goals. These questions reiterate the importance of repeating a client's responses aloud to ensure understanding.

Paraphrasing

Paraphrasing shows a client that the health and fitness professional is listening and understands what the client is saying, which builds rapport. For example:

Fitness Professional:	Sarah, so what I hear you saying is that losing 10 pounds for your upcoming reunion is your most important goal at this time. Is that right?
Client:	*Yes.*
Fitness Professional:	Wonderful. I can create an OPT™ program that will make that goal easy to accomplish. I am so pleased that we will be working together.

Developing Individualized Program Recommendations

The health and fitness professional's job is to demonstrate how each component of the OPT™ model is related to the client's wants, goals and needs. Clients care about the integration of knowledge and skills that will solve their problems. Solutions, results and retention are the products really being sold.

Each component of the OPT™ program must correlate with the solution it provides. In order to offer compelling solutions, health and fitness professionals must have a superior understanding of the assessments, program design, solutions and tools that make up the OPT™ model.

Features vs. Benefits

Most health and fitness professionals love the technical aspect of what they do because exercise science is the tool of the trade. However, clients are not likely to care as deeply about the technical information (or features). Their focus lies in getting results (or benefits). Health and fitness professionals must focus on benefits that specifically relate to client's goals.

The *features* of personal training programs and products are the number of sessions that they include, what materials come with the product, which assessments will be taken, etc. The benefits are how the features help a client get from where they are now to where they want to be. Every time a feature is explained to the client, be sure to correlate it back to answering his/her mental question: "What's in it for me?" Clearly explain how a feature will help the client reach his/her goals.

Fitness Professional:	Sarah, I am so happy that we are training together. The OPT™ method is a revolutionary training model that will produce great results and get you in shape for your 10-year reunion. You are going to look great!

Once an individual's goals have been identified, use the following chart to correlate each component of the OPT™ program with the features it provides as well as the benefits each component will enable clients to achieve (Table 18-1).

Table 18-1: OPT™ Program Features and Benefits

Goal	Component	Features	Benefits
Activities of Daily Living/ Quality of Life	Flexibility	■ Improved arthrokinematics ■ Decreased synergistic dominance ■ Decreased relative flexibility ■ Decreased reciprocal inhibition and arthrokinematic inhibition of stabilizers ■ Optimal proper movement and range of motion throughout the kinetic chain	■ Decreased risk of injury ■ Lowered risk of missing work, quality time with family, etc.
	Core	■ Inner and outer unit synergy provides proper spinal stability and movement ■ Decreased synergistic dominance provides optimum neuromuscular efficiency which results in acceleration, deceleration and dynamic stabilization ■ Attenuation of forces away from spine prevents excessive, uncontrolled inter-vertebral movement that can lead to injury	■ Greater core stability results in greater strength ■ Lowered risk of joint injury and greater, easier movement ■ Makes daily activities easier, less strenuous
	Balance	■ Improved balance and neuromuscular control during all daily activities ■ Controlled instability transference to Activities of Daily Living	■ Balance, power and strength are all components of physical capacity, needed to meet the requirements of Activities of Daily Living, with optimum safety and effectiveness
	Reactive	■ Develop ability to rapidly change direction and meet demands of Activities of Daily Living	
	Resistance	■ Optimal strength ■ Functional strength ■ Stabilization strength	
Tone	Flexibility	■ Decreased reciprocal inhibition of target areas ■ Decrease arthrokinematic inhibition of target areas	■ Permits greater tone in target areas (such as the glutes)
	Core	■ Proper functioning of inner unit, transversus abdominis, related to "tone"	■ Potential for greater tone, less circumference in mid-section
	Balance	■ Increased motor unit recruitment	■ Challenges and helps properly utilize target areas
	Reactive	■ Heightened excitability of nervous system	■ Potential for greater activation of desired muscles
	Resistance	■ Endurance strength ■ Stabilization strength ■ Core strength	■ Prepares individual for progression, greater utilization of target muscles

Continued on next page

Table 18-1: OPT™ Program Features and Benefits (Continued)

Goal	Component	Features	Benefits
Hyper-trophy/ Strength	Flexibility	■ Improved length-tension relationships ■ Decreased reciprocal inhibition ■ Decreased arthrokinematic inhibition which results in intramuscular recruitment	■ Greater force production and less inhibition of muscles leads to potential for greater growth
	Core	■ Greater neuromuscular control and stabilization strength is a biomechanically efficient position for the kinetic chain, providing optimal sensory motor integration and neuromuscular efficiency	■ Increased strength and ability to recruit muscles throughout the kinetic chain
	Balance	■ Increased recruitment	
	Reactive	■ Optimized activation of prime movers and synergists ■ Optimum neuromuscular control, recruitment, frequency and synchronization	■ A muscle can only grow if it is recruited
	Resistance	■ Optimal strength ■ Functional strength ■ Stabilization strength	■ Greater joint stabilization permits greater activation of muscles and force production
Performance	Flexibility	■ Integrated flexibility continuum with program design, leading to multiplanar tissue extension, under optimum neuromuscular control, through full range of motion	■ All components of the program condition client for greater performance, control and reduced risk of injury (in multiple recreational and competitive sports activities)
	Core	■ Maintain proper alignment of the kinetic chain during activity allows for proper deceleration of ground reaction force, gravity and momentum ■ Strength, neuromuscular control, endurance and power within the lumbo pelvic hip complex	
	Balance	■ Dynamic joint stabilization during repetitive movement ■ Multisensory training stimulates mechano-receptors and proprioceptors ■ Controlled instability	
	Reactive	■ Develops ability to rapidly change direction and meet demands of sport and all functional activities ■ Increased excitability of nervous system ■ Optimum neuromuscular control, recruitment, frequency and synchronization	
	Resistance	■ Speed strength ■ Core strength ■ Relative strength ■ Functional strength ■ Endurance strength ■ Optimal strength ■ Stabilization strength	

Table 18-1: OPT™ Program Features and Benefits (Continued)

Goal	Component	Features	Benefits
Fat Loss	Flexibility	■ Enables efficiency of inner unit and cardiorespiratory system	■ Potential for greater caloric expenditure; Increased lean tissue enables the body to burn a greater amount of calories, even when not training
	Core	■ Decreased synergistic dominance enables proper activation of prime movers, increasing caloric expenditure	
	Balance	■ Increased caloric expenditure	
	Reactive	■ Greater caloric expenditure	
	Resistance	■ Endurance strength ■ Stabilization strength ■ Core strength	

MODULE 18-3 Summary

The acronym READ stands for Rapport, Empathy, Assessment and Development.

Rapport is the aspect of a relationship characterized by similarity, agreement, or congruity. It is more important in the beginning phases of a relationship than scientific expertise. Establishing trust (by being honest, caring and effective) opens the lines of communication. This enables the health and fitness professional to assess the goals and needs of the client, leading to the design of a systematic, progressive OPT™ program. Most communication is conveyed by physiology and tone of voice. People instinctively tend to mirror these nonverbal communication patterns, which sends a sensory message to the brain, creating a similar emotional state. Therefore, health and fitness professionals who love their work, company and clients, positively affect the people around them. The most positive messages that a health and fitness professional can send are represented by a high level of confidence in themselves and the OPT™ system, approachability, genuine enthusiasm, and professionalism of appearance, tone of voice and articulation.

Empathy involves understanding and identifying with the thoughts or feelings of another person, without personally having experienced the same things. Motivation does not come from *what* an individual wants to achieve but *why* they want to achieve it. Empathy and understanding the motivation of another person are intimately intertwined. The four essential questions to ask a client are:

1. What are you trying to achieve?
2. How long has this been a goal?
3. What is most important to you about achieving that?

4. What has prevented you from achieving it in the past?

In addition to these questions, ask "Why?" questions for root cause analysis. Individuals are either motivated by emotions of desire (the desire to experience satisfaction) or fear-driven emotions (the need to alleviate discontent). The answers to the above questions will help to create a clear strategy that will achieve results.

Clients buy transformational experiences. The outcome they believe those services will produce for them is what matters. It is essential to get to the root cause of why a client is retaining the services of a health and fitness professional in order to discover how to be of the most assistance to that person. This requires empathy and an understanding of motivation to deliver the desired results and offer value for services.

Assessment uncovers as many of the client's goals and needs as possible, in order to appropriately present benefits and solutions. Questions should be asked to get the client involved in the process. It is important to ask directive (yes/no) questions to establish agreement and non-directive (open-ended) questions to get more information. Listen carefully to responses, repeat responses and paraphrase to shows the client an understanding of what he/she is saying, and take notes to review later.

Developing solutions is based on demonstrating how each component of the OPT™ model is related to a client's wants, goals and needs. Solutions, results and retention are the products really being sold. In order to offer compelling solutions, health and fitness professionals must have a superior level of technical knowledge about the OPT™ system (to offer features) and understand the client (to offer benefits). Every time a benefit is explained, clearly explain how a feature will help the client reach his/her goals.

MODULE 18-3 Quiz

1. What percentage of communication is based on physiology?

    ☐ 7

    ☐ 38

    ☐ 55

2. The benefits are how the features help a client get from where they are now to where they want to be.

    ☐ True   ☐ False

MODULE 18-4: Asking for the Sale

Selling

It is probable that a high level of customer service will, in turn, increase sales of personal training. To the health and fitness professional, that means sales to clients. However, there are many negative connotations regarding sales. Many health and fitness professionals are reluctant to ask for a sale because they associate selling with either rejection or doing something that is ethically wrong.

It is not through manipulation, but concern and professionalism that sales are created. There are numerous benefits related to performance, health, self-esteem and quality of life that can be gained though the health and fitness professional's services, utilizing the OPT™ solutions and tools. The fact is that until a potential client makes a purchase, he/she cannot benefit from these services. The sale is the first essential step to helping a client to achieve results.

10 Steps to Success

Developing clientele depends on how well a health and fitness professional can work the floor. Don't make the mistake of relying on sales consultants to schedule all potential client orientations. That philosophy is dependent on the productivity of someone else and causes health and fitness professionals to give up control of how many presentations they are able to make each week.

Set up a plan based on a desired annual income goal. Utilize the following 10 steps and corresponding questions to direct the design of that plan.

Step 1 — What is the Desired Annual Income?

An annual income goal is the achievable desired sum total of monthly earnings over twelve months. After clearly identifying a desired annual income, move on to step 2.

> *Example: Based on her expenses and lifestyle, Christy would like to earn $40,000 annually as a health and fitness professional.*

Step 2 — How Much Must be Earned per Week, in Order to Achieve the Annual Goal?

Divide the desired annual income by 50, in order to figure out what will need to be earned on a weekly basis. (Instead of dividing by the 52 weeks in a year, use the number 50 in order to allow for two weeks of vacation, sick time, jury duty, etc.)

Example: Christy divides $40,000 by 50, which equals $800. She knows that she will need to earn $800 each week to hit her goal.

Step 3 — In Order to Earn the Weekly Goal, How Many Sessions Need to be Performed?

In order to earn the weekly amount, how many clients/sessions are needed each week? To establish this number, take the weekly goal and divide it by the amount earned per session.

Example: Christy divides $800 by $25 per hour. Now, Christy knows that she will need to perform 32 sessions per week in order to hit her goal.

Also, take the current average number of paid sessions performed weekly and divide it by the number of clients currently signed up.

Example: Christy currently performs 20 sessions per week and has 11 regular clients. She divides and gets a number of 1.82. So, Christy now divides her goal 32 sessions by 1.82 and can now estimate that she needs at least 18 clients to hit her income goals.

Step 4 — What is the Closing Percentage?

Health and fitness professionals need to figure out their closing percentage. This number is determined by the total number of people helped on the floor, compared with how many of them purchased training packages.

Example: Christy looks back at her contact log and ascertains that she has spoken to 60 members in the last 30 days. Of those 60 members, she managed to sign up five of them as clients. When she divides five by 60, she sees that her closing rate is eight percent.

Step 5 — In What Timeframe Will New Clients be Acquired?

Unrealistic timeframes will likely lead to frustration and disappointment. However, if a timeframe is set too far in the future, it will not create the sense of urgency necessary to maximize performance.

Example: Since she now has 11 clients and needs to have at least 18 to hit her goals, Christy decides that she wants to gain at least seven more clients. She decides to set a timeframe of three weeks to gain seven new clients.

Step 6 — How Many Potential Clients Need to be Interacted with Overall, in Order to Gain Clients Within the Timeframe?

Take the desired number of new clients and divide that number the closing percentage.

> *Example:* *Christy wants seven new clients and her closing rate is eight percent She divides seven by eight percent and comes up with 87.5. Christy must have excellent contact with at least 88 members over the next three weeks, in order to come close to her goal of seven new clients.*

Break down the number of members that need to be interacted with overall into weekly increments, to make the process more manageable.

> *Example:* *Christy needs to contact at least 88 members over the next three weeks. She divides 88 by three and realizes that she has to contact about 30 members each week.*

Step 7 — How Many Potential Clients Need to be Contacted Each Day?

Further break down the number of members that need to be interacted with on a weekly basis into daily increments, to create concrete goals for each workday.

> *Example:* *Christy is aiming to contact 30 members each week. She works five days per week. So, she divides 30 by five and discovers that she only needs to talk to six members each day. This is a much more manageable number that she originally thought.*

Step 8 — How Many Potential Clients Need to be Contacted Each Hour of the Day?

Once more, break down the number of members that need to be contacted on a daily basis into hourly increments, to form easy, solid plans for each hour on the floor.

> *Example:* *Now that she knows she only needs to approach six members each day, Christy divides that number by her actual floor time. She generally conducts four one-hour sessions each day, during her eight-hour shift. She also takes a half-hour lunch and usually conducts one half-hour orientation. That leaves her with three hours on the floor to contact her goal of six members. Christy now knows that after dividing six by three, she must talk to a member every 30 minutes to achieve her goals.*

For each contact in that hour, provide measurable, personalized assistance that is related to the goal of the person being approached. These contacts, even if they do not develop into sales, add to a valuable future prospect base.

Step 9 — Ask Each Member Spoken to for His/Her Contact Information.

The NASM Certified Personal Trainer possesses core competencies of individualized assessment, OPT™ program design and exercise selection. These health and fitness professionals automatically have the capacity to provide a personalized, results-oriented experience for any member they make a connection with.

If a good level of rapport has been built with a member, don't be afraid to ask him/her for their contact information. Offer to develop a few exercises to help him/her achieve the goals discussed. Contact the member and arrange a time to assist him/her in implementing the new exercises, during his/her next visit to the club.

Step 10 — Follow Up.

It should be clear by now that every exercise is an assessment. Regardless of the exercise that a member was doing on the floor, write down what you saw according to the five kinetic chain checkpoints in general movement and postural observations. Write and keep detailed notes on each member.

Within 24 hours, mail the member a hand-written thank-you card for the time they spent with you in the club. This is classy and considerate, causing members to remember a specific health and fitness professional.

Give the card two to three days to arrive and then call the member one week from initial contact. During the call, work toward the following goals:

- Make sure the member got the card.
- Thank him/her personally for his/her time.
- Let the member know that you have thought about his/her goals and would like to go over some exercises that will by helpful.
- Be clear that it will only take about 10 minutes the next time he/she is in the club.
- Determine the next time he/she is coming to the club.
- Schedule an informal appointment, during his/her next visit.

When you see the member again, be sure to:

- Implement a couple of the exercises on the floor and explain how they relate to the member's goal.

- Offer the member a more thorough assessment, an individualized program design and a single training session to maximize the results he/she is currently seeing.

- Directly ask the member to sign up for a package of sessions.

Asking for the Sale

Most sales are lost, because they're not asked for. Failure to close a sale comes down to one or more of the following four reasons:

1. There was not enough value built into the sale.

2. An insufficient level of rapport makes the potential client hesitant to go ahead.

3. The health and fitness professional did not affirmatively ask for the sale.

4. The potential client legitimately does not have the ability to pay.

The first three can be directly controlled. Many health and fitness professionals are able to offer high value and have outstanding personalities, but do not ask for the sale because they fear rejection.

After following the above ten steps and then directly asking for the sale, nine out of 10 members will say, "No." That may seem incredibly discouraging. However, even with a 10-percent closing ratio, thousands of health and fitness professionals in the industry have been able to develop a steady clientele. If the health and fitness professional has established rapport, had empathy for why the client's goals are important to them, conducted a thorough assessment and made the right program recommendations, then rejection is considerably less likely. For example:

Fitness Professional: Sarah, we have outlined what is most important to you and developed the OPT™ program to get you there. Let's go through the OPT™ template and I'll explain all the parts to you. Ask me any questions that come up. Once you feel like you understand it, let's get started today.

When a potential client says "Yes" to a product, program or personal training package, go through the following steps:

1. Finish the sales transaction.

2. Schedule the client's first appointment within **48** hours.

3. Send the client a thank-you card within **24** hours.

4. Call to confirm before the first appointment.

5. Go over the client's goals again and briefly reiterate how he/she will achieve those goals.

6. Congratulate the client and acknowledge him/her for taking the first step in achieving his/her goals.

If a potential client declines to take the appointment or purchase services:

- Remain professional and helpful.

- Thank the potential client for participating in the session.

- Make sure to have the potential client's contact information.

- Ask to call him/her in a couple of weeks to check on program status.

- Send a thank-you card immediately.

- Schedule a follow-up call in 14 days in a daily planner.

- Every 30 days, send information that pertains to the potential client's goals (such as pertinent points from article clippings, trade journals, fitness Web sites, etc.).

- Make sure to follow through on all of the above tasks.

- Keep a record of all points of contact.

Successful health and fitness professionals keep in consistent contact. They understand that a "No" today is not a "No" indefinitely. They realize that contacts equal opportunity and that the more contacts they make, the more opportunity they will have to change lives. Finally, these individuals know that the greater the number of people who consider them "expert" resources, the larger their referral base will be.

MODULE 18-4 Summary

Health and fitness professionals must work the floor and greet members in order to develop rapport, build relationships, and eventually close sales. Use the 10-step plan to work toward an overall goal:

1. Choose a desired annual income.

2. Determine how much must be earned per week in order to achieve the annual goal.

3. Figure out how many sessions need to be performed in order to earn the weekly goal (and how many clients are needed for those sessions).

4. Calculate closing percentage.

5. Decide in what timeframe new clients will be acquired.

6. Determine the number of potential clients that need to be interacted with overall, in order to gain clients within the timeframe. Figure out a weekly contact rate, based on that number.

7. Break down the weekly contact rate into daily increments.

8. Further break down the daily contact rate into the number of hourly contacts.

9. Ask each contact for his/her contact information.

10. Follow up with a thank-you card and a call and schedule an informal appointment, during the member's next visit.

Most sales are lost, because they're not asked for. The sale is the first essential step to helping a client benefit from the health and fitness professional's services. Rejection is much less likely when the health and fitness professional has established rapport, built a relationship, had empathy for why the client's goals are important to them, conducted a thorough assessment and made the right OPT™ program recommendations. Whether a potential client says "Yes" or "No" to a product, it is important to remain professional and helpful, get the potential client's contact information, send out a thank-you card immediately, call to check in, stay in contact, make sure to follow through and, finally, keep a record of all points of contact. A "No" today is not a "No" indefinitely. Having a large base of people who consider a health and fitness professional an "expert" resource will surely increase his/her referral base. More contacts create more opportunities.

MODULE 18-4 Quiz

1. It is not through _____, but concern and professionalism, that sales are created.

2. What are two of the four reasons that a health and fitness professional might fail to close a sale?

_____

_____

References

1. Richardson J. *The magic of rapport: how you can gain personal power in any situation.* Miami Beach, FL: Meta Publishing; 1987. pp.187.

2. Gray P. *Psychology.* 2nd edition. New York: Worth Publishers; 1994. pp. 234-6.

3. Ekman P. Facial expressions of emotion: new findings, new questions. *Psychol Sci.* 102-5.

4. Goleman D, Boyatzis R, McKee A. *Primal leadership: realizing the power of emotional intelligence.* Boston: Harvard Business School Press; 2002.

5. *Encarta world english dictionary;* 2000.

6. Kassin S. *Psychology* 3rd edition. New York: Prentice-Hall, Inc.; 2001. pp. 299-325.

7. O'Connor J. *Leading with nlp: essential leadership skills for influencing and managing people.* Thorstons Publishers; 1999. pp. 226.

8. Aristotle. *Nicomachean ethics: book one; the highest good: happiness. Classics of western philosophy.* 4th edition. Indianapolis: Hackett Publishing Co.; 1977. pp. 277-81

9. Pine J, Gilmore JH. *The experience economy; work is theatre and every business is a stage.* Boston: Harvard Business School Press; 1999. pp. 165.

10. Tracy B. *The psychology of selling* (audiocassette). Illinois: Nightingale Content; 1985. Cassette 4, track 7, 8.

11. Rackham N. *Spin selling.* New York: McGraw Hill Publishing; 1988. pp. 14-7.

12. Jolles RL. *Customer centered selling; eight steps to success from the world's best sales force.* New York: Fireside Publishers; 2000. pp. 91-101.

Appendix

APPENDIX 1: CPR

When to Perform CPR

CPR is indicated in a person who is not breathing (or is "apneic") and has no pulse. Adult CPR is administered to any person eight years of age or older. Children are classified as one to eight years of age and infants are birth to one year of age. There are differences in the application and procedures of adult, child and infant CPR. This is why instruction on the techniques of CPR is vital to its efficient and effective execution. If the rescuer has difficulty in remembering the steps in CPR, dispatchers can frequently provide this information, as well as what to do in special circumstances.

CPR starts with recognition of the emergency, and then ensuring your own personal safety. Always survey the surroundings for existing hazards *before* helping someone. Anytime blood or body fluids could be present, use appropriate infection control techniques (gloves, masks, eyewear, gowns, etc.). Don't become part of the problem by becoming injured. Avoid being exposed to communicable diseases.

After taking safety precautions, you should check the victim for responsiveness. Determining that the adult victim is indeed unresponsive, 911 should be called. Then, the ABCs should be performed. The ABCs of cardiopulmonary resuscitation stand for Airway, Breathing and Circulation (and are discussed in greater detail below).

The ABCs of CPR

The 'A' step in CPR checks for a victim's open airway. This is accomplished by opening the airway with either a head-tilt/chin-lift (for non-traumatic conditions) or the jaw-thrust when trauma is suspected. The *head-tilt/chin-lift* is performed by placing one hand on the victim's forehead with the fingers of other hand under the mandible (or chin). Make sure to stay off the soft tissues of the chin, and apply gentle pressure to forehead to tilt the victim's head back, thus opening their airway. The *jaw-thrust maneuver* is performed when trauma is suspected. It is accomplished by placing the fingers from both hands under the angles of the jaw and the thumbs on both cheekbones (or mask). Gentle pressure is then applied to push the jaw upward without hyperextending the cervical spine. This process allows the tongue to be lifted off the back of the throat (as it is attached to the jaw) without moving the head or neck. (This technique requires practice.) The rescuer then looks for chest rise, listens for air movement and feels for air exchange.

The 'B' signifies breathing. After the rescuer has determined that no air exchange has occurred, artificial respirations are administered. Mouth-to-mouth or mouth-to-mask respirations involve giving two slow breaths, watching for chest rise and feeling for the ease of airflow. When performing mouth-to-mouth, the rescuer gently pinches closed the nose of the adult or child victim and makes a seal with his/her own mouth over the mouth of the victim (infants require mouth-to-mouth-and-nose). Many different types of barrier devices are available to perform mouth-to-mask. Whatever barrier device is chosen, the rescuer must be familiar with its use prior to real-world application. Artificial respirations for adults are one and one-half to two seconds each; for children and infants, one to one and one-half seconds. If only performing rescue breaths, the ratio in adults is one breath every five seconds. In children and infants, the ratio is one breath every three seconds. If the breaths do not go in (signified by lack of chest rise and resistance), the head is repositioned and administration of breaths is attempted again. If still unsuccessful, a foreign body is most likely blocking the airway. The scenario will then involve the procedures needed for foreign body airway removal.

If the breath is successfully administered, the next step consists of the 'C': checking for signs of circulation (such as coughing, moving, breathing or the presence of a carotid pulse). If no signs of circulation are present, the rescuer provides chest compressions. Adult compressions are given over the lower half of the sternum and artificially cause the flow of blood throughout the body with each compression. Chest compressions can provide up to 30 percent of normal cardiac output. The compression site, depth, rate and ratio to breaths for single-rescuer CPR for adults is on the lower half of the sternum (avoiding the xyphoid process). Use two hands to compress the chest one and one-half to two inches at a rate of about 100 compressions/minute and with a ratio of 15 compressions and two ventilations. For children, apply compressions in same CPR site as adults with one hand at a depth of one to one and one-half inches at a rate of about 100 compressions/minute ratio of five compressions and one ventilation. For infants, the compression site is between the nipples, mid-sternum, using the middle and ring finger, compress the chest between one-half and one inch in depth at a rate of at least 100 per minute with a ratio of five compressions and one ventilation. Becoming comfortable with application and management of age-dependent differences in CPR and Foreign Body Airway Obstruction (or FBAO) requires supervised practice with a qualified instructor.

Adult CPR Performance Checklist

1. Check the scene for hazards.

2. Take personal safety and infection control precautions.

3. Check for responsiveness.
   a. Touch the person and ask, "Are you okay?"
   b. If there is no response, continue on.

4. Activate the EMS system.
   a. You (or another person) should call 911 or another emergency response number.
   b. If available, get an AED. (When the AED arrives, use it in conjunction with CPR, as listed in the AED Performance Checklist below.)

5. Open the airway.
   a. If *no trauma* is suspected, use the *head-tilt/chin-lift* method.
   b. If *trauma* is suspected, use the *jaw-thrust* maneuver.

6. Check for breathing.
   a. Look, listen and feel for chest rise.
   b. If the person is breathing adequately, place them in the 'recovery position.'
   c. If breathing is not present, give two slow breaths.
   d. Watch for chest rise and fall. If there is no chest movement, reposition the head and try again. If still unsuccessful, perform foreign body airway maneuvers.

7. Check for circulation.
   a. Assess carotid pulse or check for other signs of circulation: moving, coughing or talking.
   b. If signs of circulation are present but the person is not breathing, give one breath every five seconds.
   c. Reassess signs of circulation in about one minute. If no signs are present, continue on.

8. Begin compressions.
   a. Place the heel of one hand in the center of the person's chest, over the *lower half of the sternum*. Place the other hand on top of the first and deliver compressions, at a depth of 1.5 to 2 inches.
   b. Perform 15 compressions at a rate of approximately *100 times per minute*.
   c. Perform *four cycles of 15 compressions and two ventilations* (one minute).

9. Reassess circulation.
   a. If no breathing or pulse is present, continue CPR.
   b. If pulse is present but there is no breathing, provide rescue breaths.

APPENDIX 2: Administering First Aid

If possible, obtain vital signs (respiratory rate, pulse and blood pressure) while waiting for responders. Also, attempt to obtain pertinent information (such as patient's full name, date of birth, home address, the events leading up to the injury/illness, what occurred during the event, chief complaint, medicines, allergies, past medical history, etc.). Ask permission to share this information with responders before doing so.

Do not perform any 'interventions' that require special knowledge for which you are not trained (i.e. splinting, etc.). Persons suspected of injuries or illness (such as the ones listed below) should always seek the advice of a physician.

Suspected Injuries or Illnesses

Fractures, Sprains, Strains and Dislocations

Often, it is difficult to determine the extent of an injury in the field. Signs and symptoms can be seen in various combinations: pain, swelling, deformity, tenderness, crepitus (or bone ends grinding together), redness, bruising or discoloration and loss of movement. If any indications of **impaired circulation or nerve damage** exist (such as numbness, tingling, weak or absent pulses, cool, pale skin or inability to sense touch, distal to the injury site), this is a **true emergency**! This information should immediately be relayed to the dispatcher.

1. Expose the area for visualization, unless doing so could cause further injury.
2. Control major bleeding. If possible, cover any open wounds with sterile dressings.
3. Prevent further movement of the injury. If trained to do so, immobilize the joints above and below the injury site using splints, cravats, pillows, etc. Remember to check for signs of adequate distal sensation and circulation before and after applying splints!
4. To reduce pain and swelling, apply ice or cold packs, but do not place them directly on the skin.
5. Cover the patient to preserve body heat, as needed.

If someone is suspected of having a spinal fracture, do not move the person or allow him/her to move, unless he/she needs to be protected from immediate danger. Monitor the ABCs and control life-threatening bleeding (if present). If you must open the person's airway, remember to use the jaw-thrust maneuver rather than the head-tilt/chin-lift method.

External Bleeding

Most external bleeding will be effectively controlled with direct pressure. However, if the bleeding persists despite the use of direct pressure, the following methods can be used. Remember not to remove dressings once they are in place. Removing them will disrupt the clotting process.

1. Apply direct pressure, using a gloved hand and, if possible, a sterile dressing.
2. If the bleeding continues, apply a pressure dressing.
3. If the bleeding continues, continue with pressure and elevate the area.
4. If still unsuccessful, find and use appropriate pressure points.
5. As a last resort, apply a tourniquet.

Shock

Patients can experience 'shock' for many different reasons including problems with the heart, vessels and blood volume. If a person experiences weakness, dizziness, thirst, cool, pale, clammy skin, decreased levels of consciousness, nausea and vomiting, follow the steps below:

1. Assist the person into the 'shock position':
   a. Lying down, with feet above the level of the heart.
   b. Cover with blankets to preserve adequate body temperature.
2. Do not give the person anything by mouth.
3. If he/she becomes unconscious, perform ABCs. Administer rescue breathing or CPR, as needed. If CPR is not needed but the person remains unconscious, place him/her on one side and be alert for vomiting.

Fainting or Syncope

There are many causes of fainting, some serious and some not so serious. It is never normal to faint. Frequently, an underlying problem can be complicated with trauma associated from a resulting fall. If you suspect someone is about to faint, instruct them to sit down on the floor, and place them in the 'shock' position. Monitor their ABCs and preserve body temperature with blankets.

Seizures

Most people who suffer from seizures will have a history of epilepsy or previous head trauma. They will be aware when the seizure is about to begin. First aid for a seizure involves:

1. Protect the person from further harm by helping him/her to the floor and working to prevent injuries while the seizure is occurring.

2. Do not allow anyone to try to place anything in the mouth, such as a bite block.

3. Monitor the ABCs and note the length of the seizure. Also note if the seizure stops and then begins again without the person regaining consciousness. *This constitutes a true emergency!*

4. Preserve modesty by covering the person with sheets or blankets, as seizures often cause a voiding of the bladder or bowels.

Insulin Shock

Persons who experience insulin shock will have a history of diabetes. The onset of insulin shock is quick and causes a variety of signs and symptoms including: irritability, weakness, shakiness, decreased levels of consciousness and cool, pale, moist skin. If left untreated, it will lead to unconsciousness and death. If the person is awake and alert, you can assist him/her by providing non-diet colas, fruit juices, hard candies or tubes of oral glucose. If the person is not conscious or alert, do not give anything by mouth. The best way to avoid a severe reaction is prevention.

Asthma Attacks

Suspect an asthma attack if someone is experiencing labored breathing, shortness of breath, wheezing, tightness in the chest, increased respirations, changes in skin color, restlessness or anxiousness. If someone is suffering an asthma attack and can only speak in one or two word sentences, this indicates a very serious attack, which should be immediately relayed to the dispatcher. It is helpful to pass along what medicine is in a person's inhaler and how many times the person has used it.

1. Confirm that no foreign bodies are causing the breathing difficulty.

2. Confirm the cause is not an existing exposure to an allergen. If this is the case, safely remove the substance or move the patient.

3. Most patients will naturally sit or stand in a tripod position (arms outstretched and leaning forward). Allow them to sit or stand however they feel most comfortable.

4. Be supportive.

5. Monitor ABCs.

Heart Attacks

Suspect someone could be having a heart attack if he/she experiences chest pain; pressure, heaviness or squeezing that radiates to the arms (typically the left), neck, jaw or back; shortness of breath; cool, pale, sweaty skin; nausea or vomiting.

1. Prevent further exertion.
2. Provide a position of comfort.
3. Give emotional support.
4. Ask the person if he/she took any Nitroglycerin. If so, ask how much.
5. Monitor ABCs.

Stroke

Strokes are caused by broken or blocked blood vessels in the brain, causing brain damage. The best way to help someone suffering from a stroke is recognition. If someone has a severe headache, numbness or paralysis on one side of the body, slurred speech, visual disturbances or decreased level of consciousness, call 911 immediately.

1. Place the person in a position of comfort, or the recovery position if he/she is having trouble swallowing.
2. Protect paralyzed limbs from injury.
3. Remain calm and be reassuring.
4. Do not give the person anything by mouth.
5. Monitor ABCs.

Choking

Signs and symptoms of choking include: inability to breathe, talk or cough. People who are choking will typically hold their hands to their throats. For adults and children:

1. Stand behind the person.
2. Wrap your arms under his/her armpits and around the waist.
3. Make a fist and place it just above his/her umbilicus (or just above the belly button). Put your other hand on top of your fist.
4. Deliver deliberate, rapid, upward thrusts.
5. Continue until the object is dislodged or the person becomes unconscious.
6. If they become unconscious, assist them to the floor and place them supine.

7. Use the jaw-thrust maneuver to open the mouth and look for an object. Perform a finger sweep if you see something.

8. Open the airway. Attempt two ventilations.

9. If unsuccessful, reposition the head and try again.

10. Straddle the person. Place your hands one on top of the other in the same location (as in the standing position) and deliver five abdominal thrusts.

11. If still unsuccessful, repeat steps 7, 8, 9 and 10.

Heat Exhaustion and Heat Stroke

The differences in heat exhaustion and heat stroke are outlined below:

Heat Exhaustion	*Heat Stroke*
Moist, pale, normal or cool skin	Hot, dry skin (sometimes moist)
Muscle cramps	Altered level of consciousness
Heavy perspiration	Little or no perspiration
Exhaustion, dizziness	Weakness
Weak pulse	Full, rapid pulse

Someone suffering from heat exhaustion should be removed from the hot environment to a cool area. Place in the 'shock' position or the recovery position (if not alert or nauseated). Loosen or remove clothing. Cool with fanning, but do not induce shivering. Alert persons may sip water. Ease muscle cramps with moist towels or gentle massage if the person has no history of circulatory problems.

Someone suffering heat stroke needs to be cooled, but not so rapidly as to induce shivering. Remove him/her from the hot environment and relocate to a cool environment, placing them in the 'shock' position. Loosen or remove clothing. Pour cool water over wet wrappings. Fan the patient and use wrapped cold packs in the armpits and groin.

APPENDIX 3:
AED (Automated External Defibrillators)

Manual Versus Automated Defibrillators

When the word 'defibrillator' is used, most minds conjure images of manual defibrillators like the ones frequently seen on primetime television. *Manual defibrillators* are used by EMS providers who have received in-depth instruction on cardiac arrhythmia recognition and management. In the pre-hospital field, these individuals are typically paramedics.

First Responders, EMTs and the general public are trained to use *automated external defibrillators*. AEDs can be fully or semi-automated. Semi-automated machines require the rescuer to press buttons to assist the machine in analyzing rhythms and/or delivering shocks, while fully automated machines only require the rescuer to turn the device on and correctly place the pads. Whether fully or semi-automated, these machines are programmed to recognize heart arrhythmias and deliver therapeutic shocks when appropriate.

AEDs and Cardiac Arrhythmias

When operating normally, the heart has its own electrical system that works to induce the pumping function of the heart. Cardiac arrhythmias are abnormalities in this electrical system, which inhibit normal pumping function. Normal electrical rhythms most often produce a heartbeat, but the presence of a normal rhythm does not always equate to mechanical activity.

In cases of cardiac arrest, the most common arrhythmias or electrical disturbances consist of asystole, pulseless electrical activity, ventricular fibrillation and pulseless ventricular tachycardia. All of these rhythms prevent the heart from pumping. Unfortunately, neither pulseless electrical activity nor asystole are shockable rhythms. However, ventricular fibrillation and pulseless ventricular tachycardia are shockable and can be treated with the use of an AED.

When Not to use an AED

Patients under eight years of age and/or less than 55 pounds should not be defibrillated with and adult defibrillator. It is important to note that AED manufacturers are starting to provide special pediatric pads for use in children, but do not assume all AEDs are equipped with children's pads.

AEDs should be applied to those persons who are in cardiac arrest (i.e. unresponsive, no respirations and no pulse). If you suspect that a person might go into cardiac arrest, keep the AED nearby and apply when cardiac arrest is confirmed.

Special circumstances can affect the use of AEDs. This is why it is very important that fitness professionals receive training in the use of AEDs by a qualified instructor, prior to real world application. Contact your local fire department, community college, area hospital, the American Heart Association or the AED Instructor Foundation. All of these agencies either directly offer CPR/AED training or can recommend qualified area instructors.

Adult AED Performance Checklist

1. Check the scene for hazards.

2. Take personal safety and infection control precautions.

3. Confirm unresponsiveness.

4. Activate the EMS system and retrieve the AED.
   a. If possible, send someone else to accomplish these tasks.

5. Perform ABCs.
   a. Confirm that no breathing or circulation is present.

6. Start CPR.

7. When it arrives, turn on the AED.

8. Follow the verbal prompts given by the machine.

9. Attach pads to the patient's bare chest.
   a. Correct placement is often illustrated on the pads.

10. When instructed, stop CPR and allow the machine to analyze.
    a. Some machines require the rescuer press an 'analyze' button and other machines are fully automated.
    b. *Ensure that no one is touching the patient when analyzing or shocking!*

11. If instructed, press the 'shock' button.
    a. Some machines are fully automated and do not require the rescuer to press a button.

12. Repeat this step, as instructed.
    a. The machine may indicate to shock up to three times.

13. Reassess ABCs.

14. If no pulse, perform CPR for one minute.

15. Repeat the analyzing and shock steps, as instructed, while ensuring that no one touches the patient. Follow the voice prompts. Reassess ABCs and provide CPR as needed.

16. If the machine states 'no shock advised', reassess ABCs.
    a. If there is no pulse, continue CPR.
    b. If pulse is regained, ensure adequate breathing.
    c. If inadequate or no breathing is present, perform rescue breaths.
    d. If breathing is adequate and pulse is present, place the patient in the recovery position.

17. Continue to monitor the patient for changes.

References

Bergeron J, Bizjak G. *Brady's first responder.* Sixth edition. Prentice Hall; 2001.

National Safety Council. *CPR and AED.* Fourth edition. Jones and Bartlett Publishers; 2002.

American Heart Association. *BLS instructor's manual.* 2000

APPENDIX 4:
Circumference Measurement Conversions for Body Fat Assessment

Young Women 17-26						Abdomen	
Inches	Constant A	Inches	Constant A	Inches	Constant A	Inches	Constant A
20.00	26.74	32.00	42.78	44.00	58.81	56.00	74.85
20.25	27.07	32.25	43.11	44.25	59.14	56.25	75.18
20.50	27.41	32.50	43.45	44.50	59.48	56.50	75.52
20.75	27.74	32.75	43.78	44.75	59.81	56.75	75.85
21.00	28.07	33.00	44.12	45.00	60.15	57.00	76.18
21.25	28.41	33.25	44.45	45.25	60.48	57.25	76.52
21.50	28.74	33.50	44.78	45.50	60.82	57.50	76.85
21.75	29.08	33.75	45.12	45.75	61.15	57.75	77.19
22.00	29.41	34.00	45.45	46.00	61.48	58.00	77.52
22.25	29.74	34.25	45.79	46.25	61.82	58.25	77.85
22.50	30.08	34.50	46.12	46.50	62.15	58.50	78.19
22.75	30.41	34.75	46.46	46.75	62.49	58.75	78.52
23.00	30.75	35.00	46.79	47.00	62.82	59.00	78.86
23.25	31.08	35.25	47.12	47.25	63.15	59.25	79.19
23.50	31.42	35.50	47.46	47.50	63.49	59.50	79.52
23.75	31.75	35.75	47.79	47.75	63.82	59.75	79.86
24.00	32.08	36.00	48.13	48.00	64.16	60.00	80.19
24.25	32.42	36.25	48.46	48.25	64.49		
24.50	32.75	36.50	48.80	48.50	64.82		
24.75	33.09	36.75	49.13	48.75	65.16		
25.00	33.42	37.00	49.46	49.00	65.49		
25.25	33.76	37.25	49.80	49.25	65.83		
25.50	34.09	37.50	50.13	49.50	66.16		
25.75	34.42	37.75	50.47	49.75	66.49		
26.00	34.76	38.00	50.80	50.00	66.83		
26.25	35.09	38.25	51.13	50.25	67.16		
26.50	35.43	38.50	51.47	50.50	67.50		
26.75	35.76	38.75	51.80	50.75	67.83		
27.00	36.10	39.00	52.14	51.00	68.17		
27.25	36.43	39.25	52.47	51.25	68.50		
27.50	36.76	39.50	52.81	51.50	68.83		
27.75	37.10	39.75	53.14	51.75	69.17		
28.00	37.43	40.00	53.47	52.00	69.50		
28.25	37.77	40.25	53.80	52.25	69.84		
28.50	38.10	40.50	54.13	52.50	70.17		
28.75	38.43	40.75	54.47	52.75	70.50		
29.00	38.77	41.00	54.80	53.00	70.84		
29.25	39.10	41.25	55.14	53.25	71.17		
29.50	39.44	41.50	55.47	53.50	71.51		
29.75	39.77	41.75	55.80	53.75	71.84		
30.00	40.11	42.00	56.14	54.00	72.17		
30.25	40.44	42.25	56.47	54.25	72.51		
30.50	40.77	42.50	56.81	54.50	72.84		
30.75	41.11	42.75	57.14	54.75	73.18		
31.00	41.44	43.00	57.47	55.00	73.51		
31.25	41.78	43.25	57.81	55.25	73.85		
31.50	42.11	43.50	58.14	55.50	74.18		
31.75	42.45	43.75	58.48	55.75	74.51		

| Young Women 17-26 | | | | | Thigh |
Inches	Constant B	Inches	Constant B	Inches	Constant B
14.00	29.13	25.00	52.01	36.00	74.90
14.25	29.65	25.25	52.53	36.25	75.42
14.50	30.17	25.50	53.05	36.50	75.94
14.75	30.69	25.75	53.57	36.75	76.46
15.00	31.21	26.00	54.09	37.00	76.98
15.25	31.73	26.25	54.61	37.25	77.50
15.50	32.25	26.50	55.13	37.50	78.02
15.75	32.77	26.75	55.65	37.75	78.54
16.00	33.29	27.00	56.17	38.00	79.06
16.25	33.81	27.25	56.69	38.25	79.58
16.50	34.33	27.50	57.21	38.50	80.10
16.75	34.85	27.75	57.73	38.75	80.62
17.00	35.37	28.00	58.26	39.00	81.14
17.25	35.89	28.25	58.78	39.25	81.66
17.50	36.41	28.50	59.30	39.50	82.18
17.75	36.93	28.75	59.82	39.75	82.70
18.00	37.45	29.00	60.34	40.00	83.22
18.25	37.97	29.25	60.86		
18.50	38.49	29.50	61.38		
18.75	39.01	29.75	61.90		
19.00	39.53	30.00	62.42		
19.25	40.05	30.25	62.94		
19.50	40.57	30.50	63.46		
19.75	41.09	30.75	63.98		
20.00	41.61	31.00	64.50		
20.25	42.13	31.25	65.02		
20.50	42.65	31.50	65.54		
20.75	43.17	31.75	66.06		
21.00	43.69	32.00	66.58		
21.25	44.21	32.25	67.10		
21.50	44.73	32.50	67.62		
21.75	45.25	32.75	68.14		
22.00	45.77	33.00	68.66		
22.25	46.29	33.25	69.18		
22.50	46.81	33.50	69.70		
22.75	47.33	33.75	70.22		
23.00	47.85	34.00	70.74		
23.25	48.37	34.25	71.26		
23.50	48.89	34.50	71.78		
23.75	49.41	34.75	72.30		
24.00	49.93	35.00	72.82		
24.25	50.45	35.25	73.34		
24.50	50.97	35.50	73.86		
24.75	51.49	35.75	74.38		

Young Women 17-26		Forearm	
Inches	Constant C	Inches	Constant C
6.00	25.86	17.00	73.28
6.25	26.94	17.25	74.36
6.50	28.02	17.50	75.43
6.75	29.10	17.75	76.51
7.00	30.17	18.00	77.59
7.25	31.25	18.25	78.67
7.50	32.33	18.50	79.74
7.75	33.41	18.75	80.82
8.00	34.48	19.00	81.90
8.25	35.56	19.25	82.98
8.50	36.64	19.50	84.05
8.75	37.72	19.75	85.13
9.00	38.79	20.00	86.21
9.25	39.87	20.25	87.29
9.50	40.95	20.50	88.37
9.75	42.03	20.75	89.45
10.00	43.10	21.00	90.53
10.25	44.18	21.25	91.61
10.50	45.26	21.50	92.69
10.75	46.34	21.75	93.77
11.00	47.41	22.00	94.85
11.25	48.49	22.25	95.93
11.50	49.57	22.50	97.01
11.75	50.65	22.75	98.09
12.00	51.73	23.00	99.17
12.25	52.80	23.25	100.25
12.50	53.88	23.50	101.33
12.75	54.96	23.75	102.41
13.00	56.04	24.00	103.49
13.25	57.11	24.25	104.57
13.50	58.19	24.50	105.65
13.75	59.27	24.75	106.73
14.00	60.35	25.00	107.81
14.25	61.42		
14.50	62.50		
14.75	63.58		
15.00	64.66		
15.25	65.73		
15.50	66.81		
15.75	67.89		
16.00	68.97		
16.25	70.04		
16.50	71.12		
16.75	72.20		

Note: Percent fat = Constant A + Constant B - Constant C - 19.6.
For athletic people, the age correction is 22.6.

Older Women 27-50				Abdomen	
Inches	Constant A	Inches	Constant A	Inches	Constant A
25.00	29.69	37.00	43.94	49.00	58.18
25.25	29.98	37.25	44.23	49.25	58.48
25.50	30.28	37.50	44.53	49.50	58.78
25.75	30.58	37.75	44.83	49.75	59.07
26.00	30.87	38.00	45.12	50.00	59.37
26.25	31.17	38.25	45.42	50.25	59.67
26.50	31.47	38.50	45.72	50.50	59.96
26.75	31.76	38.75	46.01	50.75	60.26
27.00	32.06	39.00	46.31	51.00	60.56
27.25	32.36	39.25	46.61	51.25	60.86
27.50	32.65	39.50	46.90	51.50	61.15
27.75	32.95	39.75	47.20	51.75	61.45
28.00	33.25	40.00	47.50	52.00	61.75
28.25	33.55	40.25	47.79	52.25	62.04
28.50	33.84	40.50	48.09	52.50	62.34
28.75	34.14	40.75	48.39	52.75	62.64
29.00	34.44	41.00	48.69	53.00	62.93
29.25	34.73	41.25	48.98	53.25	63.23
29.50	35.03	41.50	49.28	53.50	63.53
29.75	35.33	41.75	49.58	53.75	63.82
30.00	35.62	42.00	49.87	54.00	64.12
30.25	35.92	42.25	50.17	54.25	64.42
30.50	36.22	42.50	50.47	54.50	64.71
30.75	36.51	42.75	50.76	54.75	65.01
31.00	36.81	43.00	51.06	55.00	65.31
31.25	37.11	43.25	51.36	55.25	65.60
31.50	37.40	43.50	51.65	55.50	65.90
31.75	37.70	43.75	51.95	55.75	66.20
32.00	38.00	44.00	52.25	56.00	66.49
32.25	38.30	44.25	52.54	56.25	66.79
32.50	38.59	44.50	52.84	56.50	67.09
32.75	38.89	44.75	53.14	56.75	67.38
33.00	39.19	45.00	53.44	57.00	67.68
33.25	39.48	45.25	53.73	57.25	67.98
33.50	39.78	45.50	54.03	57.50	68.28
33.75	40.08	45.75	54.33	57.75	68.57
34.00	40.37	46.00	54.62	58.00	68.87
34.25	40.67	46.25	54.92	58.25	69.17
34.50	40.97	46.50	55.22	58.50	69.46
34.75	41.26	46.75	55.51	58.75	69.76
35.00	41.56	47.00	55.81	59.00	70.06
35.25	41.86	47.25	56.11	59.25	70.35
35.50	42.15	47.50	56.40	59.50	70.65
35.75	42.45	47.75	56.70	59.75	70.95
36.00	42.75	48.00	57.00	60.00	71.24
36.25	43.05	48.25	57.29		
36.50	43.34	48.50	57.59		
36.75	43.64	48.75	57.89		

Older Women 27-50					Thigh
Inches	Constant B	Inches	Constant B	Inches	Constant B
14.00	17.31	26.00	32.15	38.00	46.98
14.25	17.62	26.25	32.46	38.25	47.29
14.50	17.93	26.50	32.77	38.50	47.60
14.75	18.24	26.75	33.08	38.75	47.91
15.00	18.55	27.00	33.38	39.00	48.22
15.25	18.86	27.25	33.69	39.25	48.53
15.50	19.17	27.50	34.00	39.50	48.84
15.75	19.47	27.75	34.31	39.75	49.15
16.00	19.78	28.00	34.62	40.00	49.46
16.25	20.09	28.25	34.93		
16.50	20.40	28.50	35.24		
16.75	20.71	28.75	35.55		
17.00	21.02	29.00	35.86		
17.25	21.33	29.25	36.17		
17.50	21.64	29.50	36.48		
17.75	21.95	29.75	36.79		
18.00	22.26	30.00	37.09		
18.25	22.57	30.25	37.40		
18.50	22.87	30.50	37.71		
18.75	23.18	30.75	38.02		
19.00	23.49	31.00	38.33		
19.25	23.80	31.25	38.64		
19.50	24.11	31.50	38.95		
19.75	24.42	31.75	39.26		
20.00	24.73	32.00	39.57		
20.25	25.04	32.25	39.88		
20.50	25.35	32.50	40.19		
20.75	25.66	32.75	40.49		
21.00	25.97	33.00	40.80		
21.25	26.28	33.25	41.11		
21.50	26.58	33.50	41.42		
21.75	26.89	33.75	41.73		
22.00	27.20	34.00	42.04		
22.25	27.51	34.25	42.35		
22.50	27.82	34.50	42.66		
22.75	28.13	34.75	42.97		
23.00	28.44	35.00	43.28		
23.25	28.75	35.25	43.58		
23.50	29.06	35.50	43.89		
23.75	29.37	35.75	44.20		
24.00	29.68	36.00	44.51		
24.25	29.98	36.25	44.82		
24.50	30.29	36.50	45.13		
24.75	30.60	36.75	45.44		
25.00	30.91	37.00	45.75		
25.25	31.22	37.25	46.06		
25.50	31.53	37.50	46.37		
25.75	31.84	37.75	46.68		

Older Women 27-50			Calf
Inches	Constant C	Inches	Constant C
10.00	14.46	22.00	31.81
10.25	14.82	22.25	32.17
10.50	15.18	22.50	32.54
10.75	15.54	22.75	32.90
11.00	15.91	23.00	33.26
11.25	16.27	23.25	33.62
11.50	16.63	23.50	33.98
11.75	16.99	23.75	34.34
12.00	17.35	24.00	34.70
12.25	17.71	24.25	35.07
12.50	18.08	24.50	35.43
12.75	18.44	24.75	35.79
13.00	18.80	25.00	36.15
13.25	19.16	25.25	36.51
13.50	19.52	25.50	36.87
13.75	19.88	25.75	37.23
14.00	20.24	26.00	37.59
14.25	20.61	26.25	37.95
14.50	20.97	26.50	38.31
14.75	21.33	26.75	38.67
15.00	21.69	27.00	39.03
15.25	22.05	27.25	39.39
15.50	22.41	27.50	39.75
15.75	22.77	27.75	40.11
16.00	23.14	28.00	40.47
16.25	23.50	28.25	40.83
16.50	23.86	28.50	41.19
16.75	24.22	28.75	41.55
17.00	24.58	29.00	41.91
17.25	24.94	29.25	42.27
17.50	25.31	29.50	42.63
17.75	25.67	29.75	42.99
18.00	26.03	30.00	43.35
18.25	26.39		
18.50	26.75		
18.75	27.11		
19.00	27.47		
19.25	27.84		
19.50	28.20		
19.75	28.56		
20.00	28.92		
20.25	29.28		
20.50	29.64		
20.75	30.00		
21.00	30.37		
21.25	30.73		
21.50	31.09		
21.75	31.45		

Note: *Percent fat = Constant A + Constant B - Constant C - 18.4.*
For athletic people, the age correction is 21.4.

Young Men 17-26			Upper Arm
Inches	**Constant A**	**Inches**	**Constant A**
10.00	37.01	22.00	81.42
10.25	37.94	22.25	82.34
10.50	38.86	22.50	83.26
10.75	39.79	22.75	84.18
11.00	40.71	23.00	85.10
11.25	41.64	23.25	86.03
11.50	42.56	23.50	86.95
11.75	43.49	23.75	87.88
12.00	44.41	24.00	88.81
12.25	45.34	24.25	89.73
12.50	46.26	24.50	90.66
12.75	47.19	24.75	91.58
13.00	48.11	25.00	92.51
13.25	49.04	25.25	93.43
13.50	49.96	25.50	94.36
13.75	50.89	25.75	95.28
14.00	51.82	26.00	96.21
14.25	52.74	26.25	97.13
14.50	53.67	26.50	98.06
14.75	54.59	26.75	98.98
15.00	55.52	27.00	99.91
15.25	56.44	27.25	100.83
15.50	57.37	27.50	101.76
15.75	58.29	27.75	102.68
16.00	59.22	28.00	103.61
16.25	60.14	28.25	104.54
16.50	61.07	28.50	105.46
16.75	61.99	28.75	106.39
17.00	62.97	29.00	107.31
17.25	63.84	29.25	108.24
17.50	64.77	29.50	109.16
17.75	65.69	29.75	110.09
18.00	66.62	30.00	111.01
18.25	67.54		
18.50	68.47		
18.75	69.40		
19.00	70.32		
19.25	71.25		
19.50	72.17		
19.75	73.10		
20.00	74.02		
20.25	74.95		
20.50	75.87		
20.75	76.80		
21.00	77.72		
21.25	78.65		
21.50	79.57		
21.75	80.50		

Young Men 17-26				Abdomen	
Inches	Constant B	Inches	Constant B	Inches	Constant B
28.00	36.74	40.00	52.49	52.00	68.22
28.25	37.07	40.25	52.82	52.25	68.55
28.50	37.40	40.50	53.14	52.50	68.88
28.75	37.73	40.75	53.47	52.75	69.20
29.00	38.05	41.00	53.80	53.00	69.53
29.25	38.38	41.25	54.13	53.25	69.86
29.50	38.71	41.50	54.46	53.50	70.19
29.75	39.04	41.75	54.78	53.75	70.52
30.00	39.37	42.00	55.11	54.00	70.84
30.25	39.69	42.25	55.43	54.25	71.17
30.50	40.02	42.50	55.76	54.50	71.50
30.75	40.35	42.75	56.09	54.75	71.83
31.00	40.68	43.00	56.42	55.00	72.16
31.25	41.01	43.25	56.74	55.25	72.48
31.50	41.33	43.50	57.07	55.50	72.81
31.75	41.66	43.75	57.40	55.75	73.14
32.00	41.99	44.00	57.73	56.00	73.47
32.25	42.32	44.25	58.06	56.25	73.80
32.50	42.65	44.50	58.38	56.50	74.12
32.75	42.97	44.75	58.71	56.75	74.45
33.00	43.30	45.00	59.04	57.00	74.78
33.25	43.63	45.25	59.37	57.25	75.11
33.50	43.96	45.50	59.70	57.50	75.43
33.75	44.29	45.75	60.02	57.75	75.76
34.00	44.61	46.00	60.35	58.00	76.09
34.25	44.94	46.25	60.68	58.25	76.42
34.50	45.27	46.50	61.01	58.50	76.75
34.75	45.60	46.75	61.34	58.75	77.07
35.00	45.93	47.00	61.66	59.00	77.40
35.25	46.25	47.25	61.99	59.25	77.73
35.50	46.58	47.50	62.32	59.50	78.06
35.75	46.91	47.75	62.65	59.75	78.39
36.00	47.24	48.00	62.97	60.00	78.71
36.25	47.57	48.25	63.30		
36.50	47.89	48.50	63.63		
36.75	48.22	48.75	63.96		
37.00	48.55	49.00	64.29		
37.25	48.88	49.25	64.61		
37.50	49.21	49.50	64.94		
37.75	49.54	49.75	65.27		
38.00	49.86	50.00	65.60		
38.25	50.19	50.25	65.93		
38.50	50.52	50.50	66.25		
38.75	50.85	50.75	66.58		
39.00	51.18	51.00	66.91		
39.25	51.50	51.25	67.24		
39.50	51.83	51.50	67.57		
39.75	52.16	51.75	67.89		

Young Men 17-26		Forearm	
Inches	Constant C	Inches	Constant C
10.00	54.30	22.00	119.45
10.25	55.65	22.25	120.80
10.50	57.01	22.50	122.15
10.75	58.37	22.75	123.50
11.00	59.73	23.00	124.85
11.25	61.08	23.25	126.21
11.50	62.44	23.50	127.57
11.75	63.80	23.75	128.92
12.00	65.16	24.00	130.28
12.25	66.51	24.25	131.64
12.50	67.87	24.50	133.00
12.75	69.23	24.75	134.35
13.00	70.59	25.00	135.71
13.25	71.94		
13.50	73.30		
13.75	74.66		
14.00	76.02		
14.25	77.37		
14.50	78.73		
14.75	80.09		
15.00	81.45		
15.25	82.80		
15.50	84.16		
15.75	85.52		
16.00	86.88		
16.25	88.23		
16.50	89.59		
16.75	90.95		
17.00	92.31		
17.25	93.66		
17.50	95.02		
17.75	96.38		
18.00	97.74		
18.25	99.09		
18.50	100.45		
18.75	101.81		
19.00	103.17		
19.25	104.52		
19.50	105.88		
19.75	107.24		
20.00	108.60		
20.25	109.95		
20.50	111.31		
20.75	112.67		
21.00	114.02		
21.25	115.38		
21.50	116.74		
21.75	118.10		

Note: Percent fat = Constant A + Constant B - Constant C - 10.2.
For athletic people, the age correction is 14.2.

Older Men 27-50				Buttocks	
Inches	Constant A	Inches	Constant A	Inches	Constant A
35.00	36.68	47.00	49.26	59.00	61.83
35.25	36.94	47.25	49.52	59.25	62.09
35.50	37.20	47.50	49.78	59.50	62.35
35.75	37.46	47.75	50.04	59.75	62.61
36.00	37.73	48.00	50.30	60.00	62.87
36.25	37.99	48.25	50.56		
36.50	38.25	48.50	50.83		
36.75	38.51	48.75	51.09		
37.00	38.78	49.00	51.35		
37.25	39.04	49.25	51.61		
37.50	39.30	49.50	51.87		
37.75	39.56	49.75	52.13		
38.00	39.82	50.00	52.39		
38.25	40.08	50.25	52.66		
38.50	40.35	50.50	52.92		
38.75	40.61	50.75	53.18		
39.00	40.87	51.00	53.44		
39.25	41.13	51.25	53.70		
39.50	41.39	51.50	53.97		
39.75	41.66	51.75	54.23		
40.00	41.92	52.00	54.49		
40.25	42.18	52.25	54.75		
40.50	42.44	52.50	55.01		
40.75	42.70	52.75	55.28		
41.00	42.97	53.00	55.54		
41.25	43.23	53.25	55.80		
41.50	43.49	53.50	56.06		
41.75	43.75	53.75	56.32		
42.00	44.02	54.00	56.59		
42.25	44.28	54.25	56.85		
42.50	44.54	54.50	57.11		
42.75	44.80	54.75	57.37		
43.00	45.06	55.00	57.63		
43.25	45.32	55.25	57.90		
43.50	45.59	55.50	58.16		
43.75	45.85	55.75	58.42		
44.00	46.12	56.00	58.68		
44.25	46.37	56.25	58.94		
44.50	46.64	56.50	59.21		
44.75	46.89	56.75	59.47		
45.00	47.16	57.00	59.73		
45.25	47.42	57.25	59.99		
45.50	47.68	57.50	60.25		
45.75	47.94	57.75	60.52		
46.00	48.21	58.00	60.78		
46.25	48.47	58.25	61.04		
46.50	48.73	58.50	61.30		
46.75	48.99	58.75	61.56		

Older Men 27-50				Abdomen	
Inches	Constant B	Inches	Constant B	Inches	Constant B
32.00	28.66	44.00	39.41	56.00	50.15
32.25	28.88	44.25	39.63	56.25	50.37
32.50	29.11	44.50	39.85	56.50	50.59
32.75	29.33	44.75	40.08	56.75	50.82
33.00	29.55	45.00	40.30	57.00	51.04
33.25	29.78	45.25	40.52	57.25	51.26
33.50	30.00	45.50	40.74	57.50	51.49
33.75	30.22	45.75	40.97	57.75	51.71
34.00	30.45	46.00	41.19	58.00	51.94
34.25	30.67	46.25	41.41	58.25	52.16
34.50	30.89	46.50	41.64	58.50	52.38
34.75	31.12	46.75	41.86	58.75	52.60
35.00	31.35	47.00	42.09	59.00	52.83
35.25	31.57	47.25	42.31	59.25	53.05
35.50	31.79	47.50	42.54	59.50	53.28
35.75	32.02	47.75	42.76	59.75	53.50
36.00	32.24	48.00	42.98	60.00	53.72
36.25	32.46	48.25	43.21		
36.50	32.69	48.50	43.43		
36.75	32.91	48.75	43.66		
37.00	33.14	49.00	43.88		
37.25	33.36	49.25	44.10		
37.50	33.58	49.50	44.33		
37.75	33.81	49.75	44.55		
38.00	34.03	50.00	44.77		
38.25	34.26	50.25	45.00		
38.50	34.48	50.50	45.22		
38.75	34.70	50.75	45.45		
39.00	34.93	51.00	45.67		
39.25	35.15	51.25	45.89		
39.50	35.38	51.50	46.12		
39.75	35.59	51.75	46.34		
40.00	35.82	52.00	46.56		
40.25	36.05	52.25	46.79		
40.50	36.27	52.50	47.01		
40.75	36.49	52.75	47.24		
41.00	36.72	53.00	47.46		
41.25	36.94	53.25	47.68		
41.50	37.17	53.50	47.91		
41.75	37.39	53.75	48.13		
42.00	37.62	54.00	48.35		
42.25	37.87	54.25	48.58		
42.50	38.06	54.50	48.80		
42.75	38.28	54.75	49.03		
43.00	38.51	55.00	49.25		
43.25	38.73	55.25	49.47		
43.50	38.96	55.50	49.70		
43.75	39.18	55.75	49.92		

Older Men 27-50			Forearm
Inches	**Constant C**	**Inches**	**Constant C**
8.00	24.02	19.00	57.03
8.25	24.76	19.25	57.78
8.50	25.52	19.50	58.53
8.75	26.26	19.75	59.28
9.00	27.02	20.00	60.03
9.25	27.76	20.25	60.78
9.50	28.52	20.50	61.53
9.75	29.26	20.75	62.28
10.00	30.02	21.00	63.03
10.25	30.76	21.25	63.78
10.50	31.52	21.50	64.53
10.75	32.27	21.75	65.28
11.00	33.02	22.00	66.03
11.25	33.77	22.25	66.78
11.50	34.52	22.50	67.53
11.75	35.27	22.75	68.28
12.00	36.02	23.00	69.03
12.25	36.77	23.25	69.78
12.50	37.53	23.50	70.52
12.75	38.27	23.75	71.27
13.00	39.03	24.00	72.02
13.25	39.77	24.25	72.77
13.50	40.53	24.50	73.52
13.75	41.27	24.75	74.27
14.00	42.03	25.00	75.02
14.25	42.77		
14.50	43.53		
14.75	44.27		
15.00	45.03		
15.25	45.77		
15.50	46.53		
15.75	47.28		
16.00	48.03		
16.25	48.78		
16.50	49.53		
16.75	50.28		
17.00	51.03		
17.25	51.78		
17.50	52.54		
17.75	53.28		
18.00	54.04		
18.25	54.78		
18.50	55.53		
18.75	56.28		

Note: Percent fat = Constant A + Constant B - Constant C - 15.0.
For athletic people, the age correction is 19.0.

APPENDIX 5: Percent of One Rep Maximum (1RM) Conversions

Percent of One Rep Maximum										
Weight	30%	40%	50%	55%	60%	65%	70%	75%	80%	85%	90%
5	2	2	3	3	3	3	4	4	4	4	5
10	3	4	5	6	6	7	7	8	8	9	9
15	5	6	8	8	9	10	11	11	12	13	14
20	6	8	10	11	12	13	14	15	16	17	18
25	8	10	13	14	15	16	18	19	20	21	23
30	9	12	15	17	18	20	21	23	24	26	27
35	11	14	18	19	21	23	25	26	28	30	32
40	12	16	20	22	24	26	28	30	32	34	36
45	14	18	23	25	27	29	32	34	36	38	41
50	15	20	25	28	30	33	35	38	40	43	45
55	17	22	28	30	33	36	39	41	44	47	50
60	18	24	30	33	36	39	42	45	48	51	54
65	20	26	33	36	39	42	46	49	52	55	59
70	21	28	35	39	42	46	49	53	56	60	63
75	23	30	38	41	45	49	53	56	60	64	68
80	24	32	40	44	48	52	56	60	64	68	72
85	26	34	43	47	51	55	60	64	68	72	77
90	27	36	45	50	54	59	63	68	72	77	81
95	29	38	48	52	57	62	67	71	76	81	86
100	30	40	50	55	60	65	70	75	80	85	90
105	32	42	53	58	63	68	74	79	84	89	95
110	33	44	55	61	66	72	77	83	88	94	99
115	35	46	58	63	69	75	81	86	92	98	104
120	36	48	60	66	72	78	84	90	96	102	108
125	38	50	63	69	75	81	88	94	100	106	113
130	39	52	65	72	78	85	91	98	104	111	117
135	41	54	68	74	81	88	95	101	108	115	122
140	42	56	70	77	84	91	98	105	112	119	126
145	44	58	73	80	87	94	102	109	116	123	131
150	45	60	75	83	90	98	105	113	120	128	135
155	47	62	78	85	93	101	109	116	124	132	140
160	48	64	80	88	96	104	112	120	128	136	144
165	50	66	83	91	99	107	116	124	132	140	149
170	51	68	85	94	102	111	119	128	136	145	153
175	53	70	88	96	105	114	123	131	140	149	158
180	54	72	90	99	108	117	126	135	144	153	162
185	56	74	93	102	111	120	130	139	148	157	167
190	57	76	95	105	114	124	133	143	152	162	171
195	59	78	98	107	117	127	137	146	156	166	176
200	60	80	100	110	120	130	140	150	160	170	180
205	62	82	103	113	123	133	144	154	164	174	185
210	63	84	105	116	126	137	147	158	168	179	189
215	65	86	108	118	129	140	151	161	172	183	194
220	66	88	110	121	132	143	154	165	176	187	198
225	68	90	113	124	135	146	158	169	180	191	203
230	69	92	115	127	138	150	161	173	184	196	207
235	71	94	118	129	141	153	165	176	188	200	212
240	72	96	120	132	144	156	168	180	192	204	216

Percent of One Rep Maximum

Weight	30%	40%	50%	55%	60%	65%	70%	75%	80%	85%	90%
245	74	98	123	135	147	159	172	184	196	208	221
250	75	100	125	138	150	163	175	188	200	213	225
255	77	102	128	140	153	166	179	191	204	217	230
260	78	104	130	143	156	169	182	195	208	221	234
265	80	106	133	146	159	172	186	199	212	225	239
270	81	108	135	149	162	176	189	203	216	230	243
275	83	110	138	151	165	179	193	206	220	234	248
280	84	112	140	154	168	182	196	210	224	238	252
285	86	114	143	157	171	185	200	214	228	242	257
290	87	116	145	160	174	189	203	218	232	247	261
295	89	118	148	162	177	192	207	221	236	251	266
300	90	120	150	165	180	195	210	225	240	255	270
305	92	122	153	168	183	198	214	229	244	259	275
310	93	124	155	171	186	202	217	233	248	264	279
315	95	126	158	173	189	205	221	236	252	268	284
320	96	128	160	176	192	208	224	240	256	272	288
325	98	130	163	179	195	211	228	244	260	276	293
330	99	132	165	182	198	215	231	248	264	281	297
335	101	134	168	184	201	218	235	251	268	285	302
340	102	136	170	187	204	221	238	255	272	289	306
345	104	138	173	190	207	224	242	259	276	293	311
350	105	140	175	193	210	228	245	263	280	298	315
355	107	142	178	195	213	231	249	266	284	302	320
360	108	144	180	198	216	234	252	270	288	306	324
365	110	146	183	201	219	237	256	274	292	310	329
370	111	148	185	204	222	241	259	278	296	315	333
375	113	150	188	206	225	244	263	281	300	319	338
380	114	152	190	209	228	247	266	285	304	323	342
385	116	154	193	212	231	250	270	289	308	327	347
390	117	156	195	215	234	254	273	293	312	332	351
395	119	158	198	217	237	257	277	296	316	336	356
400	120	160	200	220	240	260	280	300	320	340	360
405	122	162	203	223	243	263	284	304	324	344	365
410	123	164	205	226	246	267	287	308	328	349	369
415	125	166	208	228	249	270	291	311	332	353	374
420	126	168	210	231	252	273	294	315	336	357	378
425	128	170	213	234	255	276	298	319	340	361	383
430	129	172	215	237	258	280	301	323	344	366	387
435	131	174	218	239	261	283	305	326	348	370	392
440	132	176	220	242	264	286	308	330	352	374	396
445	134	178	223	245	267	289	312	334	356	378	401
450	135	180	225	248	270	293	315	338	360	383	405
455	137	182	228	250	273	296	319	341	364	387	410
460	138	184	230	253	276	299	322	345	368	391	414
465	140	186	233	256	279	302	326	349	372	395	419
470	141	188	235	259	282	306	329	353	376	400	423
475	143	190	238	261	285	309	333	356	380	404	428
480	144	192	240	264	288	312	336	360	384	408	432
485	146	194	243	267	291	315	340	364	388	412	437
490	147	196	245	270	294	319	343	368	392	417	441
495	149	198	248	272	297	322	347	371	396	421	446
500	150	200	250	275	300	325	350	375	400	425	450

Percent of One Rep Maximum

Weight	30%	40%	50%	55%	60%	65%	70%	75%	80%	85%	90%
505	152	202	253	278	303	328	354	379	404	429	455
510	153	204	255	281	306	332	357	383	408	434	459
515	155	206	258	283	309	335	361	386	412	438	464
520	156	208	260	286	312	338	364	390	416	442	468
525	158	210	263	289	315	341	368	394	420	446	473
530	159	212	265	292	318	345	371	398	424	451	477
535	161	214	268	294	321	348	375	401	428	455	482
540	162	216	270	297	324	351	378	405	432	459	486
545	164	218	273	300	327	354	382	409	436	463	491
550	165	220	275	303	330	358	385	413	440	468	495
555	167	222	278	305	333	361	389	416	444	472	500
560	168	224	280	308	336	364	392	420	448	476	504
565	170	226	283	311	339	367	396	424	452	480	509
570	171	228	285	314	342	371	399	428	456	485	513
575	173	230	288	316	345	374	403	431	460	489	518
580	174	232	290	319	348	377	406	435	464	493	522
585	176	234	293	322	351	380	410	439	468	497	527
590	177	236	295	325	354	384	413	443	472	502	531
595	179	238	298	327	357	387	417	446	476	506	536
600	180	240	300	330	360	390	420	450	480	510	540
605	182	242	303	333	363	393	424	454	484	514	545
610	183	244	305	336	366	397	427	458	488	519	549
615	185	246	308	338	369	400	431	461	492	523	554
620	186	248	310	341	372	403	434	465	496	527	558
625	188	250	313	344	375	406	438	469	500	531	563
630	189	252	315	347	378	410	441	473	504	536	567
635	191	254	318	349	381	413	445	476	508	540	572
640	192	256	320	352	384	416	448	480	512	544	576
645	194	258	323	355	387	419	452	484	516	548	581
650	195	260	325	358	390	423	455	488	520	553	585
655	197	262	328	360	393	426	459	491	524	557	590
660	198	264	330	363	396	429	462	495	528	561	594
665	200	266	333	366	399	432	466	499	532	565	599
670	201	268	335	369	402	436	469	503	536	570	603
675	203	270	338	371	405	439	473	506	540	574	608
680	204	272	340	374	408	442	476	510	544	578	612
685	206	274	343	377	411	445	480	514	548	582	617
690	207	276	345	380	414	449	483	518	552	587	621
700	210	280	350	385	420	455	490	525	560	595	630
705	212	282	353	388	423	458	494	529	564	599	635
710	213	284	355	391	426	462	497	533	568	604	639
715	215	286	358	393	429	465	501	536	572	608	644
720	216	288	360	396	432	468	504	540	576	612	648
725	218	290	363	399	435	471	508	544	580	616	653
730	219	292	365	402	438	475	511	548	584	621	657
735	221	294	368	404	441	478	515	551	588	625	662
740	222	296	370	407	444	481	518	555	592	629	666
745	224	298	373	410	447	484	522	559	596	633	671
750	225	300	375	413	450	488	525	563	600	638	675
755	227	302	378	415	453	491	529	566	604	642	680
760	228	304	380	418	456	494	532	570	608	646	684
765	230	306	383	421	459	497	536	574	612	650	689

Percent of One Rep Maximum

Weight	30%	40%	50%	55%	60%	65%	70%	75%	80%	85%	90%
770	231	308	385	424	462	501	539	578	616	655	693
775	233	310	388	426	465	504	543	581	620	659	698
780	234	312	390	429	468	507	546	585	624	663	702
785	236	314	393	432	471	510	550	589	628	667	707
790	237	316	395	435	474	514	553	593	632	672	711
795	239	318	398	437	477	517	557	596	636	676	716
800	240	320	400	440	480	520	560	600	640	680	720
805	242	322	403	443	483	523	564	604	644	684	725
810	243	324	405	446	486	527	567	608	648	689	729
815	245	326	408	448	489	530	571	611	652	693	734
820	246	328	410	451	492	533	574	615	656	697	738
825	248	330	413	454	495	536	578	619	660	701	743
830	249	332	415	457	498	540	581	623	664	706	747
835	251	334	418	459	501	543	585	626	668	710	752
840	252	336	420	462	504	546	588	630	672	714	756
845	254	338	423	465	507	549	592	634	676	718	761
850	255	340	425	468	510	553	595	638	680	723	765
855	257	342	428	470	513	556	599	641	684	727	770
860	258	344	430	473	516	559	602	645	688	731	774
865	260	346	433	476	519	562	606	649	692	735	779
870	261	348	435	479	522	566	609	653	696	740	783
875	263	350	438	481	525	569	613	656	700	744	788
880	264	352	440	484	528	572	616	660	704	748	792
885	266	354	443	487	531	575	620	664	708	752	797
890	267	356	445	490	534	579	623	668	712	757	801
895	269	358	448	492	537	582	627	671	716	761	806
900	270	360	450	495	540	585	630	675	720	765	810
905	272	362	453	498	543	588	634	679	724	769	815
910	273	364	455	501	546	592	637	683	728	774	819
915	275	366	458	503	549	595	641	686	732	778	824
920	276	368	460	506	552	598	644	690	736	782	828
925	278	370	463	509	555	601	648	694	740	786	833
930	279	372	465	512	558	605	651	698	744	791	837
935	281	374	468	514	561	608	655	701	748	795	842
940	282	376	470	517	564	611	658	705	752	799	846
945	284	378	473	520	567	614	662	709	756	803	851
950	285	380	475	523	570	618	665	713	760	808	855
955	287	382	478	525	573	621	669	716	764	812	860
960	288	384	480	528	576	624	672	720	768	816	864
965	290	386	483	531	579	627	676	724	772	820	869
970	291	388	485	534	582	631	679	728	776	825	873
975	293	390	488	536	585	634	683	731	780	829	878
980	294	392	490	539	588	637	686	735	784	833	882
985	296	394	493	542	591	640	690	739	788	837	887
990	297	396	495	545	594	644	693	743	792	842	891
995	299	398	498	547	597	647	697	746	796	846	896
1000	300	400	500	550	600	650	700	750	800	850	900

APPENDIX 6:
One Rep Maximum (IRM) Conversions

Repetitions									
Pounds	10	9	8	7	6	5	4	3	2
5	7	6	6	6	6	6	6	5	5
10	13	13	13	12	12	11	11	11	11
15	20	19	19	18	18	17	17	16	16
20	27	26	25	24	24	23	22	22	21
25	33	32	31	30	29	29	28	27	26
30	40	39	38	36	35	34	33	32	32
35	47	45	44	42	41	40	39	38	37
40	53	52	50	48	47	46	44	43	42
45	60	58	56	55	53	51	50	49	47
50	67	65	63	61	59	57	56	54	53
55	73	71	69	67	65	63	61	59	58
60	80	77	75	73	71	69	67	65	63
65	87	84	81	79	76	74	72	70	68
70	93	90	88	85	82	80	78	76	74
75	100	97	94	91	88	86	83	81	79
80	107	103	100	97	94	91	89	86	84
85	113	110	106	103	100	97	94	92	89
90	120	116	113	109	106	103	100	97	95
95	127	123	119	115	112	109	106	103	100
100	133	129	125	121	118	114	111	108	105
105	140	135	131	127	124	120	117	114	111
110	147	142	138	133	129	126	122	119	116
115	153	148	144	139	135	131	128	124	121
120	160	155	150	145	141	137	133	130	126
125	167	161	156	152	147	143	139	135	132
130	173	168	163	158	153	149	144	141	137
135	180	174	169	164	159	154	150	146	142
140	187	181	175	170	165	160	156	151	147
145	193	187	181	176	171	166	161	157	153
150	200	194	188	182	176	171	167	162	158
155	207	200	194	188	182	177	172	168	163
160	213	206	200	194	188	183	178	173	168
165	220	213	206	200	194	189	183	178	174
170	227	219	213	206	200	194	189	184	179
175	233	226	219	212	206	200	194	189	184
180	240	232	225	218	212	206	200	195	189
185	247	239	231	224	218	211	206	200	195
190	253	245	238	230	224	217	211	205	200
195	260	252	244	236	229	223	217	211	205
200	267	258	250	242	235	229	222	216	211
205	273	265	256	248	241	234	228	222	216
210	280	271	263	255	247	240	233	227	221
215	287	277	269	261	253	246	239	232	226
220	293	284	275	267	259	251	244	238	232
225	300	290	281	273	265	257	250	243	237
230	307	297	288	279	271	263	256	249	242
235	313	303	294	285	276	269	261	254	247
240	320	310	300	291	282	274	267	259	253

Repetitions									
Pounds	10	9	8	7	6	5	4	3	2
245	327	316	306	297	288	280	272	265	258
250	333	323	313	303	294	286	278	270	263
255	340	329	319	309	300	291	283	276	268
260	347	335	325	315	306	297	289	281	274
265	353	342	331	321	312	303	294	286	279
270	360	348	338	327	318	309	300	292	284
275	367	355	344	333	324	314	306	297	289
280	373	361	350	339	329	320	311	303	295
285	380	368	356	345	335	326	317	308	300
290	387	374	363	352	341	331	322	314	305
295	393	381	369	358	347	337	328	319	311
300	400	387	375	364	353	343	333	324	316
305	407	394	381	370	359	349	339	330	321
310	413	400	388	376	365	354	344	335	326
315	420	406	394	382	371	360	350	341	332
320	427	413	400	388	376	366	356	346	337
325	433	419	406	394	382	371	361	351	342
330	440	426	413	400	388	377	367	357	347
335	447	432	419	406	394	383	372	362	353
340	453	439	425	412	400	389	378	368	358
345	460	445	431	418	406	394	383	373	363
350	467	452	438	424	412	400	389	378	368
355	473	458	444	430	418	406	394	384	374
360	480	465	450	436	424	411	400	389	379
365	487	471	456	442	429	417	406	395	384
370	493	477	463	448	435	423	411	400	389
375	500	484	469	455	441	429	417	405	395
380	507	490	475	461	447	434	422	411	400
385	513	497	481	467	453	440	428	416	405
390	520	503	488	473	459	446	433	422	411
395	527	510	494	479	465	451	439	427	416
400	533	516	500	485	471	457	444	432	421
405	540	523	506	491	476	463	450	438	426
410	547	529	513	497	482	469	456	443	432
415	553	535	519	503	488	474	461	449	437
420	560	542	525	509	494	480	467	454	442
425	567	548	531	515	500	486	472	459	447
430	573	555	538	521	506	491	478	465	453
435	580	561	544	527	512	497	483	470	458
440	587	568	550	533	518	503	489	476	463
445	593	574	556	539	524	509	494	481	468
450	600	581	563	545	529	514	500	486	474
455	607	587	569	552	535	520	506	492	479
460	613	594	575	558	541	526	511	497	484
465	620	600	581	564	547	531	517	503	489
470	627	606	588	570	553	537	522	508	495
475	633	613	594	576	559	543	528	514	500
480	640	619	600	582	565	549	533	519	505
485	647	626	606	588	571	554	539	524	511
490	653	632	613	594	576	560	544	530	516
495	660	639	619	600	582	566	550	535	521
500	667	645	625	606	588	571	556	541	526

Repetitions									
Pounds	10	9	8	7	6	5	4	3	2
505	673	652	631	612	594	577	561	546	532
510	680	658	638	618	600	583	567	551	537
515	687	665	644	624	606	589	572	557	542
520	693	671	650	630	612	594	578	562	547
525	700	677	656	636	618	600	583	568	553
530	707	684	663	642	624	606	589	573	558
535	713	690	669	648	629	611	594	578	563
540	720	697	675	655	635	617	600	584	568
545	727	703	681	661	641	623	606	589	574
550	733	710	688	667	647	629	611	595	579
555	740	716	694	673	653	634	617	600	584
560	747	723	700	679	659	640	622	605	589
565	753	729	706	685	665	646	628	611	595
570	760	735	713	691	671	651	633	616	600
575	767	742	719	697	676	657	639	622	605
580	773	748	725	703	682	663	644	627	611
585	780	755	731	709	688	669	650	632	616
590	787	761	738	715	694	674	656	638	621
595	793	768	744	721	700	680	661	643	626
600	800	774	750	727	706	686	667	649	632
605	807	781	756	733	712	691	672	654	637
610	813	787	763	739	718	697	678	659	642
615	820	794	769	745	724	703	683	665	647
620	827	800	775	752	729	709	689	670	653
625	833	806	781	758	735	714	694	676	658
630	840	813	788	764	741	720	700	681	663
635	847	819	794	770	747	726	706	686	668
640	853	826	800	776	753	731	711	692	674
645	860	832	806	782	759	737	717	697	679
650	867	839	813	788	765	743	722	703	684
655	873	845	819	794	771	749	728	708	689
660	880	852	825	800	776	754	733	714	695
665	887	858	831	806	782	760	739	719	700
670	893	865	838	812	788	766	744	724	705
675	900	871	844	818	794	771	750	730	711
680	907	877	850	824	800	777	756	735	716
685	913	884	856	830	806	783	761	741	721
690	920	890	863	836	812	789	767	746	726
695	927	897	869	842	818	794	772	751	732
700	933	903	875	848	824	800	778	757	737
705	940	910	881	855	829	806	783	762	742
710	947	916	888	861	835	811	789	768	747
715	953	923	894	867	841	817	794	773	753
720	960	929	900	873	847	823	800	778	758
725	967	935	906	879	853	829	806	784	763
730	973	942	913	885	859	834	811	789	768
735	980	948	919	891	865	840	817	795	774
740	987	955	925	897	871	846	822	800	779
745	993	961	931	903	876	851	828	805	784
750	1000	968	938	909	882	857	833	811	789
755	1007	974	944	915	888	863	839	816	795
760	1013	981	950	921	894	869	844	822	800

Repetitions

Pounds	10	9	8	7	6	5	4	3	2
765	1020	987	956	927	900	874	850	827	805
770	1027	994	963	933	906	880	856	832	811
775	1033	1000	969	939	912	886	861	838	816
780	1040	1006	975	945	918	891	867	843	821
785	1047	1013	981	952	924	897	872	849	826
790	1053	1019	988	958	929	903	878	854	832
795	1060	1026	994	964	935	909	883	859	837
800	1067	1032	1000	970	941	914	889	865	842
805	1073	1039	1006	976	947	920	894	870	847
810	1080	1045	1013	982	953	926	900	876	853
815	1087	1052	1019	988	959	931	906	881	858
820	1093	1058	1025	994	965	937	911	886	863
825	1100	1065	1031	1000	971	943	917	892	868
830	1107	1071	1038	1006	976	949	922	897	874
835	1113	1077	1044	1012	982	954	928	903	879
840	1120	1084	1050	1018	988	960	933	908	884
845	1127	1090	1056	1024	994	966	939	914	889
850	1133	1097	1063	1030	1000	971	944	919	895
855	1140	1103	1069	1036	1006	977	950	924	900
900	1200	1161	1125	1091	1059	1029	1000	973	947
905	1207	1168	1131	1097	1065	1034	1006	978	953
910	1213	1174	1138	1103	1071	1040	1011	984	958
915	1220	1181	1144	1109	1076	1046	1017	989	963
920	1227	1187	1150	1115	1082	1051	1022	995	968
925	1233	1194	1156	1121	1088	1057	1028	1000	974
930	1240	1200	1163	1127	1094	1063	1033	1005	979
935	1247	1206	1169	1133	1100	1069	1039	1011	984
940	1253	1213	1175	1139	1106	1074	1044	1016	989
945	1260	1219	1181	1145	1112	1080	1050	1022	995
950	1267	1226	1188	1152	1118	1086	1056	1027	1000
955	1273	1232	1194	1158	1124	1091	1061	1032	1005
960	1280	1239	1200	1164	1129	1097	1067	1038	1011
965	1287	1245	1206	1170	1135	1103	1072	1043	1016
970	1293	1252	1213	1176	1141	1109	1078	1049	1021
975	1300	1258	1219	1182	1147	1114	1083	1054	1026
980	1307	1265	1225	1188	1153	1120	1089	1059	1032
985	1313	1271	1231	1194	1159	1126	1094	1065	1037
990	1320	1277	1238	1200	1165	1131	1100	1070	1042
995	1327	1284	1244	1206	1171	1137	1106	1076	1047
1000	1333	1290	1250	1212	1176	1143	1111	1081	1053

APPENDIX 7:
OPT™ Templates for Special Populations

NASM
NATIONAL ACADEMY OF SPORTS MEDICINE

Optimum Performance Training™

NAME: YOUTH CLIENT

DATE: _____

TRAINER: _____

PHASE: 2: Integrated Stabilization Training

DAYS/WEEK: _____

GOAL: _____

CARDIO TRAINING: Stage I	TIME: 20 minutes	EQUIPMENT: Elliptical trainer

WARMUP/FLEXIBILITY	Sets	Reps	Duration	Rest	Notes
1. SMR: IT band, piniformis, adductors	1				Hold tender spots 20-30 sec.
2. Cardio: Dynamic Functional Warm-up	1				10-12 dynamic flexibility exercises
3.					

CORE & BALANCE	Sets	Reps	Tempo	Rest	Notes
1. Prone Iso-ab	1-2	20	5-10 sec. hold	0 sec.	
2. Floor Cobra	1-2	20	5-10 sec. hold	0 sec.	
3. Single-leg Balance Reach	1-2	20	5-10 sec. hold	60 sec.	

REACTIVE	Sets	Reps	Tempo	Rest	Notes
1. Box Jump-up with Stabilization	1	8	3 sec. hold	90 sec.	

SPEED, AGILITY, QUICKNESS	Sets	Reps	Tempo	Rest	Notes
1. Speed Ladder	2			0 sec.	6 exercises
2. Box Drill	2-4			60 sec.	

STRENGTH	Exercise	Sets	Reps	Intensity	Tempo	Rest	Notes
TOTAL BODY							
CHEST	Push-up	1-2	20	60%	4-2-1	0	
BACK	Standing Tubing Row	1-2	20	60%	4-2-1	0	
SHOULDERS	Single-leg Scaption	1-2	20	60%	4-2-1	0	
BICEPS							
TRICEPS							
LEGS	Single-leg Squat	1-2	20	60%	4-2-1	90 sec.	

COOL-DOWN	
POST-WORKOUT FLEXIBILITY	Static Stretching: Calves, adductors, hip flexors, lats, pectorals

Optimum Performance Training™

NASM NATIONAL ACADEMY OF SPORTS MEDICINE

NAME: ELDERLY CLIENT

TRAINER: _____

DAYS/WEEK: _____

DATE: _____

PHASE: 1: Corrective Exercise Training

GOAL: _____

CARDIO TRAINING: Stage I, II and III	TIME: 30-60 minutes	EQUIPMENT: Elliptical trainer

WARMUP/FLEXIBILITY	Sets	Reps	Duration	Rest	Notes
1. SMR: IT band, calves, adductors	1				Hold tender spots 20-30 sec.
2. Cardio: Elliptical trainer			5-10 min.		
3. Static Stretching: Calves, hip flexors, lats	1		30 sec.		

CORE & BALANCE	Sets	Reps	Tempo	Rest	Notes
1. Marching	1-2	15	3-10 sec. hold	0 sec.	
2. Floor Bridge	1-2	15	3-10 sec. hold	0 sec.	
3. Single-leg Balance	1-2	15	3-10 sec. hold	60 sec.	

REACTIVE	Sets	Reps	Tempo	Rest	Notes
1. N/A					

SPEED, AGILITY, QUICKNESS	Sets	Reps	Tempo	Rest	Notes
1. N/A					
2.					

STRENGTH	Exercise	Sets	Reps	Intensity	Tempo	Rest	Notes
TOTAL BODY	Step-up, Curl to Overhead Press	1-2	15	40%	4-2-2	0 sec.	
CHEST	Standing Cable Chest Press	1-2	15	40%	4-2-2	0 sec.	
BACK	Standing Cable Row	1-2	15	40%	4-2-2	0 sec.	
SHOULDERS	Standing Dumbbell Scaption	1-2	15	40%	4-2-2	0 sec.	
BICEPS							
TRICEPS							
LEGS	Ball Squat	1-2	15	40%	4-2-2	90 sec.	

COOL-DOWN	
POST-WORKOUT FLEXIBILITY	Static Stretching: Calves, adductors, hip flexors, pectorals

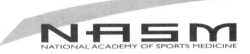

Optimum Performance Training™

NAME: <u>OBESE CLIENT</u>

TRAINER: _____

DAYS/WEEK: _____

DATE: _____

PHASE: <u>1: Corrective Exercise Training</u>

GOAL: _____

CARDIO TRAINING: Stage I and II	TIME: 40-60 minutes	EQUIPMENT: Elliptical trainer

WARMUP/FLEXIBILITY	Sets	Reps	Duration	Rest	Notes
1. SMR: Calves, lats	1				Hold tender spots 20-30 sec.
2. Cardio: Elliptical trainer			5-10 min.		
3. Static Stretching: Calves, hip flexors, lats	1		30 sec.		

CORE & BALANCE	Sets	Reps	Tempo	Rest	Notes
1. Marching	1-2	15	3-10 sec. hold	0 sec.	
2. Floor Bridge	1-2	15	3-10 sec. hold	0 sec.	
3. Single-leg Balance	1-2	15	3-10 sec. hold	60 sec.	

REACTIVE	Sets	Reps	Tempo	Rest	Notes
1. N/A					

SPEED, AGILITY, QUICKNESS	Sets	Reps	Tempo	Rest	Notes
1. N/A					
2.					

STRENGTH	Exercise	Sets	Reps	Intensity	Tempo	Rest	Notes
TOTAL BODY							
CHEST	Seated Machine Chest Press	1-2	15	40%	4-2-2	0 sec.	
BACK	Standing Cable Row	1-2	15	40%	4-2-2	0 sec.	
SHOULDERS	Standing Dumbbell Shoulder Press	1-2	15	40%	4-2-2	0 sec.	
BICEPS	Standing Dumbbell Curl	1-2	15	40%	4-2-2	0 sec.	
TRICEPS	Standing Cable Tricep Extension	1-2	15	40%	4-2-2	0 sec.	
LEGS	Step-up	1-2	15	40%	4-2-2	90 sec.	

COOL-DOWN	
POST-WORKOUT FLEXIBILITY	Static Stretching: Calves, adductors, hip flexors, pectorals

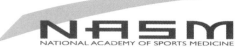

Optimum Performance Training™

NAME:	DIABETIC CLIENT	DATE:
TRAINER:		PHASE: 1: Corrective Exercise Training
DAYS/WEEK:		GOAL:

CARDIO TRAINING: Stage I, II and III	TIME: 20-60 minutes	EQUIPMENT: Elliptical trainer

WARMUP/FLEXIBILITY	Sets	Reps	Duration	Rest	Notes
1. SMR: Calves, IT band, adductors	1				Hold tender spots 20-30 sec.
2. Cardio: Elliptical trainer			5-10 min.		
3. Static Stretching: Calves, hip flexors, lats	1		30 sec.		

CORE & BALANCE	Sets	Reps	Tempo	Rest	Notes
1. Quadruped Arm Raise	1-2	15	3-10 sec. hold	0 sec.	
2. Floor Bridge	1-2	15	3-10 sec. hold	0 sec.	
3. Single-leg Balance	1-2	15	3-10 sec. hold	60 sec.	

REACTIVE	Sets	Reps	Tempo	Rest	Notes
1. N/A					

SPEED, AGILITY, QUICKNESS	Sets	Reps	Tempo	Rest	Notes
1. N/A					
2.					

STRENGTH	Exercise	Sets	Reps	Intensity	Tempo	Rest	Notes
TOTAL BODY							
CHEST	Standing Cable Chest Press	1-2	15	40%	4-2-2	0 sec.	
BACK	Seated Machine Row	1-2	15	40%	4-2-2	0 sec.	
SHOULDERS	Standing Dumbbell Scaption	1-2	15	40%	4-2-2	0 sec.	
BICEPS	Standing Dumbbell Curl	1-2	15	40%	4-2-2	0 sec.	
TRICEPS	Standing Cable Tricep Extension	1-2	15	40%	4-2-2	0 sec.	
LEGS	Step-up	1-2	15	40%	4-2-2	90 sec.	

COOL-DOWN	
POST-WORKOUT FLEXIBILITY	Static Stretching: Calves, adductors, hip flexors, pectorals

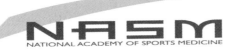

Optimum Performance Training™

NAME: HYPTERTENSIVE CLIENT	**DATE:**	
TRAINER:	**PHASE:** 1: Corrective Exercise Training	
DAYS/WEEK:	**GOAL:**	

CARDIO TRAINING: Stage I and II	**TIME:** 30-60 minutes	**EQUIPMENT:** Elliptical trainer

WARMUP/FLEXIBILITY	Sets	Reps	Duration	Rest	Notes
1. SMR: Calves, IT band, adductors	1				Hold tender spots 20-30 sec.
2. Cardio: Elliptical trainer			5 min.		
3. Static Stretching: Calves, hip flexors, lats	1		30 sec.		

CORE & BALANCE	Sets	Reps	Tempo	Rest	Notes
1. Quadruped Arm Raise	1-2	15	3-10 sec. hold	0 sec.	
2. Floor Cobra	1-2	15	3-10 sec. hold	0 sec.	
3. Single-leg Balance	1-2	15	3-10 sec. hold	60 sec.	

REACTIVE	Sets	Reps	Tempo	Rest	Notes
1. N/A					

SPEED, AGILITY, QUICKNESS	Sets	Reps	Tempo	Rest	Notes
1. N/A					
2.					

STRENGTH	Exercise	Sets	Reps	Intensity	Tempo	Rest	Notes
TOTAL BODY	Ball Squat, Curl, Press	1-2	15	40%	4-1-1	30 sec.	
CHEST	Seated Single-arm Machine Chest Press	1-2	15	40%	4-1-1	30 sec.	
BACK	Standing Cable Row	1-2	15	40%	4-1-1	30 sec.	
SHOULDERS	Seated Ball Dumbbell Scaption	1-2	15	40%	4-1-1	30 sec.	
BICEPS	Optional						
TRICEPS	Standing Cable Tricep Extension	1-2	15	40%	4-1-1	30 sec.	
LEGS	Step-up	1-2	15	40%	4-1-1	30 sec.	

COOL-DOWN	
POST-WORKOUT FLEXIBILITY	Static Stretching: Calves, adductors, hip flexors, pectorals

NASM
NATIONAL ACADEMY OF SPORTS MEDICINE

Optimum Performance Training™

NAME: HEART DISEASE CLIENT

DATE:

TRAINER:

PHASE: 1: Corrective Exercise Training

DAYS/WEEK:

GOAL:

CARDIO TRAINING: Stage I and II	TIME: 30-60 minutes	EQUIPMENT: Elliptical trainer

WARMUP/FLEXIBILITY	Sets	Reps	Duration	Rest	Notes
1. SMR: Calves, IT band, adductors	1				Hold tender spots 20-30 sec.
2. Cardio: Elliptical trainer			5-10 min.		
3. Static Stretching: Calves, hip flexors, lats	1		30 sec.		

CORE & BALANCE	Sets	Reps	Tempo	Rest	Notes
1. Quadruped Arm Raise	1-2	15	3-10 sec. hold	0 sec.	
2. Ball Bridge	1-2	15	3-10 sec. hold	0 sec.	
3. Single-leg Balance	1-2	15	3-10 sec. hold	60 sec.	

REACTIVE	Sets	Reps	Tempo	Rest	Notes
1. N/A					

SPEED, AGILITY, QUICKNESS	Sets	Reps	Tempo	Rest	Notes
1. N/A					
2.					

STRENGTH	Exercise	Sets	Reps	Intensity	Tempo	Rest	Notes
TOTAL BODY							
CHEST	Machine Chest Press	1-2	15	40%	4-2-2	30 sec.	
BACK	Standing Cable Row	1-2	15	40%	4-2-2	30 sec.	
SHOULDERS	Seated Ball Dumbbell Scaption	1-2	15	40%	4-2-2	30 sec.	
BICEPS	Optional						
TRICEPS	Cable Pushdown	1-2	15	40%	4-2-2	30 sec.	
LEGS	Step-up (Frontal)	1-2	15	40%	4-2-2	30 sec.	

COOL-DOWN	
POST-WORKOUT FLEXIBILITY	Static Stretching: Calves, adductors, hip flexors, pectorals

NASM
NATIONAL ACADEMY OF SPORTS MEDICINE

Optimum Performance Training™

NAME: _____OSTEOPOROSIS CLIENT_____   DATE: _____

TRAINER: _____   PHASE: 1: Corrective Exercise Training

DAYS/WEEK: _____   GOAL: _____

CARDIO TRAINING: Stage I and II	TIME: 30-60 minutes	EQUIPMENT: Elliptical trainer

WARMUP/FLEXIBILITY	Sets	Reps	Duration	Rest	Notes
1. Cardio: Elliptical trainer			5 min.		
3. Static Stretching: Calves, hip flexors, lats	1		30 sec.		

CORE & BALANCE	Sets	Reps	Tempo	Rest	Notes
1. Marching	1-2	15	3-10 sec. hold	0 sec.	
2. Floor Bridge	1-2	15	3-10 sec. hold	0 sec.	
3. Single-leg Balance	1-2	15	3-10 sec. hold	60 sec.	

REACTIVE	Sets	Reps	Tempo	Rest	Notes
1. N/A					

SPEED, AGILITY, QUICKNESS	Sets	Reps	Tempo	Rest	Notes
1. N/A					
2.					

STRENGTH	Exercise	Sets	Reps	Intensity	Tempo	Rest	Notes
TOTAL BODY							
CHEST	Seated Machine Chest Press	1-2	15	40%	4-2-2	0 sec.	
BACK	Seated Machine Row	1-2	15	40%	4-2-2	0 sec.	
SHOULDERS	Seated Machine Shoulder Press	1-2	15	40%	4-2-2	0 sec.	
BICEPS							
TRICEPS							
LEGS	Ball Squat	1-2	15	40%	4-2-2	90 sec.	

COOL-DOWN	
POST-WORKOUT FLEXIBILITY	Static Stretching: Calves, adductors, hip flexors, pectorals

Optimum Performance Training™

NASM
NATIONAL ACADEMY OF SPORTS MEDICINE

NAME: ARTHRITIC CLIENT

TRAINER:

DAYS/WEEK:

DATE:

PHASE: 1: Corrective Exercise Training

GOAL:

CARDIO TRAINING: Stage I and II	TIME: 30 minutes	EQUIPMENT: Elliptical trainer

WARMUP/FLEXIBILITY	Sets	Reps	Duration	Rest	Notes
1. SMR: Calves, adductors, lats	1				Hold tender spots 20-30 sec.
2. Cardio: Elliptical trainer			5 min.		
3. Static Stretching: Calves, hip flexors (standing), lats (kneeling)	1		30 sec.		

CORE & BALANCE	Sets	Reps	Tempo	Rest	Notes
1. Quadruped Arm/Opposite Leg Raise	1-2	15	3-10 sec. hold	0 sec.	
2. Ball Bridge	1-2	15	3-10 sec. hold	0 sec.	
3. Single-leg Balance	1-2	15	3-10 sec. hold	60 sec.	

REACTIVE	Sets	Reps	Tempo	Rest	Notes
1. N/A					

SPEED, AGILITY, QUICKNESS	Sets	Reps	Tempo	Rest	Notes
1. N/A					
2.					

STRENGTH	Exercise	Sets	Reps	Intensity	Tempo	Rest	Notes
TOTAL BODY							
CHEST	Standing Cable Chest Press	1-2	12	40%	4-2-2	0 sec.	
BACK	Standing Cable Row	1-2	12	40%	4-2-2	0 sec.	
SHOULDERS	Standing Dumbbell Scaption	1-2	12	40%	4-2-2	0 sec.	
BICEPS							
TRICEPS							
LEGS	Step-up to Balance	1-2	12	40%	4-2-2	90 sec.	

COOL-DOWN	
POST-WORKOUT FLEXIBILITY	Static Stretching: Calves, adductors, hip flexors, pectorals

NASM
NATIONAL ACADEMY OF SPORTS MEDICINE

Optimum Performance Training™

NAME: _____CANCER CLIENT_____   DATE: _____

TRAINER: _____   PHASE: 1: Corrective Exercise Training

DAYS/WEEK: _____   GOAL: _____

CARDIO TRAINING: Stage I and II	TIME: 15-30 minutes	EQUIPMENT: Elliptical trainer

WARMUP/FLEXIBILITY	Sets	Reps	Duration	Rest	Notes
1. SMR: Calves, IT band, adductors	1				Hold tender spots 20-30 sec.
2. Cardio: Elliptical trainer			5-10 min.		
3. Static Stretching: Calves, hip flexors, adductors	1		30 sec.		

CORE & BALANCE	Sets	Reps	Tempo	Rest	Notes
1. Quadruped Arm Raise	1-2	15	3-10 sec. hold	0 sec.	
2. Floor Bridge	1-2	15	3-10 sec. hold	0 sec.	
3. Single-leg Balance	1-2	15	3-10 sec. hold	60 sec.	

REACTIVE	Sets	Reps	Tempo	Rest	Notes
1. N/A					

SPEED, AGILITY, QUICKNESS	Sets	Reps	Tempo	Rest	Notes
1. N/A					
2.					

STRENGTH	Exercise	Sets	Reps	Intensity	Tempo	Rest	Notes
TOTAL BODY							
CHEST	Seated Single-arm Machine Chest Press	1-2	15	40%	4-2-2	0 sec.	
BACK	Standing Cable Row	1-2	15	40%	4-2-2	0 sec.	
SHOULDERS	Seated Dumbbell Shoulder Press	1-2	15	40%	4-2-2	0 sec.	
BICEPS	Seated Alternating-arm Ball Dumbbell Curl	1-2	15	40%	4-2-2	0 sec.	
TRICEPS	Standing Cable Tricep Extension	1-2	15	40%	4-2-2	0 sec.	
LEGS	Ball Squat	1-2	15	40%	4-2-2	90 sec.	

COOL-DOWN	
POST-WORKOUT FLEXIBILITY	Static Stretching: Calves, adductors, hip flexors, pectorals

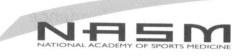

Optimum Performance Training™

NAME: PREGNANT CLIENT

DATE: _____

TRAINER: _____

PHASE: 1: Corrective Exercise Training

DAYS/WEEK: _____

GOAL: _____

CARDIO TRAINING: Stage I, II and III	TIME: 20-60 minutes	EQUIPMENT: Elliptical trainer

WARMUP/FLEXIBILITY	Sets	Reps	Duration	Rest	Notes
1. SMR: Calves, IT band, adductors	1				Hold tender spots 20-30 sec.
2. Cardio: Elliptical trainer			5-10 min.		
3. Static Stretching: Calves, hip flexors, lats	1		30 sec.		

CORE & BALANCE	Sets	Reps	Tempo	Rest	Notes
1. Quadruped Arm Raise	1-2	15	3-10 sec. hold	0 sec.	
2. Floor Bridge	1-2	15	3-10 sec. hold	0 sec.	
3. Single-leg Balance	1-2	15	3-10 sec. hold	60 sec.	

REACTIVE	Sets	Reps	Tempo	Rest	Notes
1. N/A					

SPEED, AGILITY, QUICKNESS	Sets	Reps	Tempo	Rest	Notes
1. N/A					
2.					

STRENGTH	Exercise	Sets	Reps	Intensity	Tempo	Rest	Notes
TOTAL BODY							
CHEST	Standing Cable Chest Press	1-2	15	40%	4-2-2	0 sec.	
BACK	Standing Cable Row	1-2	15	40%	4-2-2	0 sec.	
SHOULDERS	Standing Dumbbell Scaption	1-2	15	40%	4-2-2	0 sec.	
BICEPS	Seated Ball Dumbbell Curl	1-2	15	40%	4-2-2	0 sec.	
TRICEPS	Cable Pressdown	1-2	15	40%	4-2-2	0 sec.	
LEGS	Frontal Step-up	1-2	15	40%	4-2-2	90 sec.	

COOL-DOWN	
POST-WORKOUT FLEXIBILITY	Static Stretching: Calves, adductors, hip flexors, pectorals

NASM
NATIONAL ACADEMY OF SPORTS MEDICINE

Optimum Performance Training™

NAME: ___LUNG DISEASE CLIENT___

TRAINER: _____

DAYS/WEEK: _____

DATE: _____

PHASE: 1: Corrective Exercise Training

GOAL: _____

CARDIO TRAINING: Stage I	TIME: 20-45 minutes	EQUIPMENT: Elliptical trainer

WARMUP/FLEXIBILITY	Sets	Reps	Duration	Rest	Notes
1. SMR: Calves, IT band, adductors	1				Hold tender spots 20-30 sec.
2. Cardio: Elliptical trainer			5-10 min.		
3. Static Stretching: Calves, hip flexors, lats	1		30 sec.		

CORE & BALANCE	Sets	Reps	Tempo	Rest	Notes
1. Marching	1-2	15	3-10 sec. hold	0 sec.	
2. Floor Bridge	1-2	15	3-10 sec. hold	0 sec.	
3. Single-leg Balance	1-2	15	3-10 sec. hold	60 sec.	

REACTIVE	Sets	Reps	Tempo	Rest	Notes
1. N/A					

SPEED, AGILITY, QUICKNESS	Sets	Reps	Tempo	Rest	Notes
1. N/A					
2.					

STRENGTH	Exercise	Sets	Reps	Intensity	Tempo	Rest	Notes
TOTAL BODY							
CHEST	Machine Chest Press	1-2	15	40%	4-2-2	60 sec.	
BACK	Machine Row	1-2	15	40%	4-2-2	60 sec.	
SHOULDERS	Shoulder Press Machine	1-2	15	40%	4-2-2	60 sec.	
BICEPS							
TRICEPS							
LEGS	Ball Squat	1-2	15	40%	4-2-2	60 sec.	

COOL-DOWN	
POST-WORKOUT FLEXIBILITY	Static Stretching: Calves, adductors, hip flexors, pectorals

Optimum Performance Training™

NAME: PAD CLIENT

TRAINER:

DAYS/WEEK:

DATE:

PHASE: 1: Corrective Exercise Training

GOAL:

CARDIO TRAINING: Stage I and II	TIME: 20-45 minutes	EQUIPMENT: Elliptical trainer

WARMUP/FLEXIBILITY	Sets	Reps	Duration	Rest	Notes
1. SMR: Calves, IT band, adductors	1				Hold tender spots 20-30 sec.
2. Cardio: Elliptical trainer			5-10 min.		
3. Static Stretching: Calves, hip flexors, lats	1		30 sec.		

CORE & BALANCE	Sets	Reps	Tempo	Rest	Notes
1. Marching	1-2	15	3-10 sec. hold	0 sec.	
2. Floor Bridge	1-2	15	3-10 sec. hold	0 sec.	
3. Single-leg Balance	1-2	15	3-10 sec. hold	60 sec.	

REACTIVE	Sets	Reps	Tempo	Rest	Notes
1. N/A					

SPEED, AGILITY, QUICKNESS	Sets	Reps	Tempo	Rest	Notes
1. N/A					
2.					

STRENGTH	Exercise	Sets	Reps	Intensity	Tempo	Rest	Notes
TOTAL BODY							
CHEST	Machine Chest Press	1-2	15	40%	4-2-2	60 sec.	
BACK	Machine Row	1-2	15	40%	4-2-2	60 sec.	
SHOULDERS	Shoulder Press Machine	1-2	15	40%	4-2-2	60 sec.	
BICEPS							
TRICEPS							
LEGS	Ball Squat	1-2	15	40%	4-2-2	60 sec.	

COOL-DOWN	
POST-WORKOUT FLEXIBILITY	Static Stretching: Calves, adductors, hip flexors, pectorals

Answer Key

Quiz 1-1 Answers

1. A large number of people who were uneducated about training and the gym environment
2. 33
3. False. Low back pain has been demonstrated to be more prevalent among sedentary societies.
4. True
5. False. The less conditioned it is, the higher the risk of injury.
6. Deconditioned

Quiz 1-2 Answers

1. Integrated training
2. Stabilization, strength and power
3. Strength
4. Phase 6: Elastic Equivalent Training

Quiz 2-1 Answers

1. True
2. Axon
3. Sensory (afferent) neuron
4. Central nervous system and peripheral nervous system
5. Mechanoreceptors
6. Muscle spindles sense over-stretching and cause contraction. Golgi tendon organs sense over-tension and cause relaxation. Joint receptors sense stress and inhibit surrounding muscles.

Quiz 2-2 Answers

1. Appendicular skeleton
2. Tarsals: Short bone
   Vertebrae: Irregular bone
   Femur: Long bone
   Patella: Flat bone
3. Synovial
4. Gliding joint: Vertebrae
   Condyloid joint: Knee
   Hinge joint: Elbow
   Saddle joint: Carpometacarpal joint of thumb
   Pivot joint: Radioulnar
   Ball-and-socket joint: Hip
5. True
6. False. Joints provide stability.
7. False. Joints are connected by ligaments.
8. True

Quiz 2-3 Answers

1. Sarcomere
2. True
3. Sliding Filament Theory
4. Type II
5. Fusiform
   Longitudinal
   Quadrilateral
6. a. Agonist
   b. Synergist
   c. Stabilizer
   d. Antagonist

Quiz 3-1 Answers

1. The heart, blood and blood vessels
2. The sinoatrial node (SA)
3. Right, left
4. Right
5. Oxygen, hormones, nutrients and heat
6. Venule

Quiz 3-2 Answers

1. True
2. Inspiration
3. In the alveolar sacs

Quiz 3-3 Answers

1. 1. Inhalation through the nose and mouth
   2. Through the bronchi
   3. To the lungs and alveolar sacs

4. Blood is pumped through the right ventricle of the heart
5. Through the pulmonary arteries to the lungs
6. Blood becomes oxygenated
7. Pumped out through the pulmonary veins to the heart's left atrium
8. Pumped out to the left ventricle of the heart
9. Pumped out to the body's tissues

2. Carbon dioxide
3. True
4. Oxidative
5. ATP-CP (Creatine Phosphate)
6. Diaphragm

Quiz 4-1 Answers

1. a. Near the middle of the body
   b. Farther away from the middle of the body
   c. On the opposite side of the body
   d. On the same side of the body
   e. On the front of the body
   f. On the back of the body
   g. Nearest the center of the body
   h. Farthest from the center of the body
   i. Below a point of reference
   j. Above a point of reference
2. The frontal plane
3. Eccentric
4. Stabilization
5. Upward rotation of the scapula
6. Rotary motion, torque
7. Increases, decreases

Quiz 4-2 Answers

1. All of the above
2. True
3. External
4. Knowledge of Performance

Quiz 5-1 Answers

1. Acute variable
2. False. It is not designed to diagnose a condition.
3. False. They should provide clients with general information on healthy eating and refer clients to a qualified dietitian or nutritionist for specific diet plans.
4. Subjective

Quiz 5-2 Answers

1. Hip flexors
2. Golfing, skiing, playing tennis
3. True
4. 75

Quiz 5-3 Answers

1. Skin fold calipers, underwater weighing, bio-electrical impedance
2. Right
3. Bicep, tricep, iliac crest, subscapular
4. Moderate

Quiz 5-4 Answers

1. Maximum Heart Rate x 0.80; Maximum Heart Rate x 0.85
2. Stage 1 Program

Quiz 5-5 Answers

1. True
2. Optimum neuromuscular efficiency
3. Lumbo-pelvic-hip and lower-extremity postural distortions
4. Dynamic
5. Dynamic postural assessment

Quiz 5-6 Answers

1. Bench Press Strength Assessment
2. Shark Skill
3. Three

Quiz 6-1 Answers

1. All of the above
2. Externally, dorsiflexion
3. Altered reciprocal inhibition, synergistic dominance,

arthrokinetic dysfunction and decreased neuromuscular efficiency.

4. False. The neural impulses that sense tension are greater than the impulses that cause muscles to contract.

Quiz 6-2 Answers

1. The ability to help correct muscular imbalances.
2. True
3. Cumulative Injury Cycle
4. Davis' Law

Quiz 6-3 Answers

1. Reciprocal inhibition
2. Foam roll
3. Active Flexibility
4. True
5. Static stretching and self-myofascial release
6. Force production
7. Active
8. Functional flexibility

Quiz 6-4 Answers

1. False. An athlete should do controlled, dynamic, functional activities as a warm-up and cool-down unless muscular imbalances are present.
2. Upper-extremity
3. Lower-extremity and lumbo-pelvic-hip

Quiz 7-1 Answers

1. True
2. Dynamic stretches can be performed through a circuit, providing an ample cardiorespiratory warm-up.
3. Lower
4. Decreases, decreases

Quiz 7-2 Answers

1. True
2. By heart rate and/or maximal oxygen consumption (VO$_2$ max)

3. True
4. Lower, higher

Quiz 7-3 Answers

1. Energy
2. Equal to
3. When the body is at rest
4. False. The body must utilize increased amounts of oxygen to replenish energy supplies, lower tissue temperature and return the body to a resting state.

Quiz 7-4 Answers

1. True
2. Anaerobic
3. Because the body will soon adapt
4. It produces greater levels of EPOC. It produces near-identical caloric expenditure for the same give time span, when compared to walking at a fast pace.

Quiz 7-5 Answers

1. False. Bicycles and steppers are ill-advised since the hips are placed in a constant state of flexion, adding to a shortened hip flexor complex.
2. Flatten and externally rotate feet
3. Upper-extremity

Quiz 8-1 Answers

1. All of the above
2. The stabilization system and the movement system
3. Iliopsoas
4. False. The stabilization system should be trained before the movement system.

Quiz 8-2 Answers

1. False. They have a decreased activation of these muscles.
2. Navel, spine
3. The pelvo-occular reflex and muscle imbalances
4. 6-20 seconds

Quiz 8-3 Answers

1. Neuromuscular control, stabilization strength, biomechanically efficient, neuromuscular efficiency
2. Plane of motion, range of motion, type of resistance, body position, speed of motion, duration, frequency or amount of feedback
3. True
4. Back Extension: Strength
   Rotation Chest Pass: Power
   Ball Bridge: Stabilization
   Back Extension Throw: Power

Quiz 8-4 Answers

1. Core strength
2. 8-12
3. None. That client's core exercises are included in the resistance training portion of his/her workout.

Quiz 9-1 Answers

1. Center of gravity
2. True
3. Proprioceptively enriched environment
4. False. Balance is not an isolated activity.

Quiz 9-2 Answers

1. True
2. Dynamic joint stabilization
3. All of the above
4. False. It should only be as unstable as can be controlled by the individual.

Quiz 9-3 Answers

1. Proprioceptively challenging, systematic, progressive
2. Increase
3. Single-leg Balance: Stabilization
   Single-leg Hop with Stabilization: Power
   Single-leg Squat: Strength
   Lunge to Balance: Strength

Quiz 9-4 Answers

1. Balance-strength exercises
2. Five to 20 seconds and hold

Quiz 10-1 Answers

1. Maximal, minimal
2. To react and produce sufficient force to avoid a fall
3. Rate of force production
4. True

Quiz 10-2 Answers

1. Progressive
2. Stabilization
3. Ice Skater: Power
   Box Jump-up with Stabilization: Stabilization
   Tuck Jump: Strength
   Squat Jump with Stabilization: Strength

Quiz 10-3 Answers

1. Reactive-stabilization exercises
2. Explosive

Quiz 11-1 Answers

1. 2.1-2.5
2. True
3. Backside mechanics

Quiz 11-2 Answers

1. None
2. 0-60 seconds

Quiz 12-1 Answers

1. A stressor or some form of stress that creates the need for a response.
2. The Specific Adaptation to Imposed Demands (or SAID Principle).
3. Increase
4. False. Connective tissues do not adapt as fast as muscle, due to their lack of blood supply.

Quiz 12-2 Answers

1. Stabilization
2. Increase
3. False. It uses higher levels of force with lower repetitions (six to 12)

and more sets, often supersets.

Quiz 12-3 Answers

1. Multiple-set
2. False. Compound-sets involve the performance of two exercises for antagonistic muscles.
3. Circuit training system
4. Horizontal
5. The Peripheral Heart Action System is another variation of circuit training that alternates upper body and lower body exercises throughout the circuit.
6. Recovery time

Quiz 13-1 Answers

1. True

Quiz 13-2 Answers

1. False. Beginners should do higher repetition schemes in order to build proper connective tissue strength, stability and endurance.
2. 24-36
3. Three minutes
4. True
5. Russian Deadlift: Strength
Squat Jump: Power
Chest Press on a Stability Ball: Stabilization
Bench Press: Strength
Step-up: Strength
Squat: Strength

Quiz 13-3 Answers

1. Monthly plan
2. True
3. Volume

Quiz 13-4 Answers

1. Three, seven
2. Low, high
3. Phase 3: Stabilization Equivalent Training; Phase 6: Elastic Equivalent Training
4. Velocity

Quiz 13-5 Answers

1. Three
2. 1, 2, 3, 5 and 6
3. False. Once the client has completed Phase 1 and moves on to Phase 2, it will not necessary to return to Phase 1, unless an extended amount of time is taken off.
4. One week

Quiz 14-1 Answers

1. Because children do not exhibit a plateau in oxygen uptake at maximum exercise
2. 10
3. Maximum oxygen uptake, maximum exercise heart rate, bone mass, measures of pulmonary function, lean body mass

Quiz 14-2 Answers

1. Height (in meters squared)
2. Two-thirds
3. 40-70 percent of work capacity

Quiz 14-3 Answers

1. Hyperglycemia
2. It is important to check daily for blisters or skin injury.
3. True

Quiz 14-4 Answers

1. Smoking, a diet high in fat (particularly saturated fat) and excess weight
2. Three, four
3. True

Quiz 14-5 Answers

1. 40
2. True
3. Decreased

Quiz 14-6 Answers

733

1. 70
2. False. A principal observation in Type I osteoporosis is a deficit in estrogen.
3. High

Quiz 14-7 Answers

1. False. Avoid early-morning exercise for clients with rheumatoid arthritis.
2. Anemia, increased body mass, osteoporosis
3. Five

Quiz 14-8 Answers

1. Use intermittent bouts of exercise to accumulate 20-30 minutes of total aerobic exercise.
2. 44%
3. True

Quiz 14-9 Answers

1. True
2. Core-stabilization
3. Prone, supine

Quiz 14-10 Answers

1. Obstructive lung disease
2. Shortness of breath
3. True

Quiz 14-11 Answers

1. Leg pain
2. False. A continuous format of exercise utilizing walking is preferred.

Quiz 15-2 Answers

1. Due to their slower rate of synthesis within the body, these amino acids cannot be manufactured by the body at a rate that will support growth (especially in children).
2. Limiting factor
3. Less
4. 15-30 percent of total caloric intake

Quiz 15-3 Answers

1. a. Compounds containing carbon, hydrogen and oxygen
   b. Sugars
   c. Starches
   d. Storage form of carbohydrates in plants
   e. Storage form of carbohydrates in humans
   f. Single sugar unit
   g. Two sugar units
   h. Blood sugar
   i. Fruit sugar
   j. Common sugar
   k. Milk sugar
2. Carbohydrate
3. False. Weight gain or loss is related to total energy intake, not the source of the food eaten.
4. 50-70

Quiz 15-4 Answers

1. Monounsaturated, polyunsaturated
2. Thermic effect
3. True

Quiz 15-5 Answers

1. 60
2. False. When exercising for fewer than 60 minutes, water is the experts' choice. For exercise exceeding 60 minutes, use of a sports drink is recommended.

Quiz 16-1 Answers

1. True
2. Vitamin, amino acid, herb, mineral
3. ■ Inadequate food intake (especially diets less than 1,000 calories per day)
   ■ Disordered eating patterns
   ■ Consuming mostly "junk" (nutrient deficient) foods
   ■ Avoidance of foods from specific food groups
   ■ Eating only one major meal each day
   ■ Irregular eating patterns (low

ANSWER KEY

calorie diet one day, high calories the next)

- Eating too much or too little protein or carbohydrate
- Food phobias and "picky" eating
- Financial limitations on access to a variety of wholesome foods

4. EAR: Estimated Average Requirement
RDA: Recommended Dietary Allowance
AI: Adequate Intake
UL: Tolerable Upper Intake Level

5. Vitamin D

6. Increase

7. Germanium, cobalt

Quiz 16-2 Answers

1. International Units
2. Daily Value not established
3. Equal to
4. Equal to, more than twice
5. B-12
6. True

Quiz 17-1 Answers

1. Six
2. Why?

Quiz 17-2 Answers

1. It didn't exist.
2. Specific, Measurable, Aggressive, Approach, Relevant, Time-bound
3. Upper

Quiz 17-3 Answers

1. True

Quiz 17-4 Answers

1. The deposit-and-refund technique

Quiz 17-5 Answers

1. Behavior, progress
2. True
3. For two or three weeks after beginning exercise programs
4. False. True success is rare because too often people use flawed strategies
for success.

Quiz 18-1 Answers

1. Reputation, meeting and greeting clients, uncompromising customer service
2. Emotion
3. Take ownership of them
4. An opportunity to create a professional relationship and, eventually, make a sale

Quiz 18-2 Answers

1. A desire to improve their quality of life
2. True

Quiz 18-3 Answers

1. 55
2. True

Quiz 18-4 Answers

1. Manipulation
2. There was not enough value built into the sale. Insufficient level of rapport makes the potential client hesitant to go ahead. The health and fitness professional did not affirmatively ask for the sale. The potential client legitimately does not have the ability to pay.

735

Glossary

Abduction: Movement of a body part away from the middle of the body.

Active-isolated stretch: The process of using agonists and synergists to dynamically move the joint into a range of motion.

Acute variables: Important components that specify how each exercise is to be performed.

Adaptive: Capable of changing for a specific use.

Adduction: Movement of a body part toward the middle of the body.

Adequate Intake (AI): A recommended average daily nutrient intake level, based on observed (or experimentally determined) approximations or estimates of nutrient intake that are assumed to be adequate for a group (or groups) of healthy people. This measure is used when an RDA cannot be determined.

Agility: The ability to accelerate, decelerate, stabilize and change direction quickly, while maintaining proper posture.

Alarm reaction: The initial reaction to a stressor.

Altered reciprocal inhibition: The concept of muscle inhibition, caused by a tight agonist, which inhibits its functional antagonist.

Annual plan: Generalized training plan that spans one year to show when the client will progress between phases.

Anterior (or ventral): On the front of the body.

Arthritis: Chronic inflammation of the joints.

Arthrokinematics: The motions of joints in the body.

Arthrokinetic dysfunction: A biomechanical and neuromuscular dysfunction leading to altered joint motion.

Assessment: A process of determining the importance, size, or value of something.

Autogenic inhibition: The process when neural impulses that sense tension is greater than the impulses that cause muscles to contract, which prevents muscle spindles from contracting.

Biomechanics: A study that uses principles of physics to quantitatively study how forces interact within a living body.

Cancer: Any of various types of malignant neoplasms, most of which invade surrounding tissues, may metastasize to several sites and are likely to recur after attempted removal and to cause death of the patient unless adequately treated.

Cardiorespiratory training: Any physical activity that involves and places stress on the cardiorespiratory system.

Concentric contraction: The shortening of a muscle under the control of the nervous system.

Contralateral: Positioned on the opposite side of the body.

Controlled instability: Training environment that is as unstable as can safely be controlled by an individual.

Core: The central section of the body consisting of the cervical, thoracic and lumbar spine, pelvic girdle and hip joint, and all of the muscles that attach to these specific areas.

Diabetes: Chronic metabolic disorder, caused by insulin deficiency, which impairs carbohydrate usage and enhances usages of fats and protein.

Dietary supplement: A substance that completes or makes an addition to daily dietary intake.

Distal: Positioned farthest from the center of the body, or point of reference.

Drawing-in maneuver: The action of pulling the navel toward the spine.

Dynamic functional flexibility: Multiplanar soft tissue extensibility with optimal neuromuscular efficiency throughout the full range of motion.

Dynamic joint stabilization: The ability of the kinetic chain to stabilize a joint during movement.

Dynamic range of motion: Controlled, accurate movement that utilizes flexibility and neuromuscular efficiency.

Dynamic stretch: The active extension of a muscle, using force production and momentum, in order to move the joint through the full available range of motion.

Eccentric contraction: The lengthening of a muscle under the control of the nervous system.

Empathy: Action of awareness, understanding and sensitivity of the thoughts, emotions and experience of another without personally having gone through the same.

Enjoyment: The amount of pleasure derived from performing a physical activity.

Equilibrium: A condition of balance between opposed forces, influences or actions.

Estimated Average Requirement (EAR): The average daily nutrient intake level that is estimated to meet the requirement of half the healthy individuals who are in a particular life stage and gender group.

Excess post-exercise oxygen consumption (EPOC): Elevation of the body's metabolism following exercise.

Exercise selection: The process of choosing appropriate exercises for a client's program.

Exhaustion: Prolonged stress or stress that is intolerable and will produce exhaustion or distress to the system.

Extensibility: Capability to be elongated or stretched.

Extension: The straightening of a joint, causing the angle to the joint to increase.

External feedback: Information provided by some external source, such as a health and fitness professional, videotape, mirror or heart rate monitor to supplement internal environment

External rotation: Rotation of a joint away from the middle of the body.

Feedback: The use of sensory information and sensorimotor integration to help the kinetic chain in motor learning.

Flexibility training: Physical training of the body that integrates various stretches in all three planes of motion in order to produce the maximum extensibility of tissues.

Flexibility: The normal extensibility of all soft tissues that allow the full range of motion of a joint.

Flexion: The bending of a joint, causing the angle to the joint to decrease.

Force: An influence applied by one object to another, which results in an acceleration or deceleration of the second object.

Force-couple: Muscle groups moving together to produce movement around a joint.

Frequency: The number of training sessions in a given timeframe.

Frontal plane: An imaginary bisector that divides the body into front and back halves.

Functional efficiency: The ability of the neuromuscular system to monitor and manipulate movement during functional tasks using the least amount of energy, creating the least amount of stress of the kinetic chain.

Functional strength: The ability of the neuromuscular system to contract eccentrically, isometrically and concentrically in all three planes of motion.

General Adaptation Syndrome: The kinetic chain's ability to adapt to stresses placed upon it.

General warm-up: Low-intensity exercise consisting of movements that do not necessarily relate to the more intense exercise that is to follow.

Ground Reaction Force (GRF): The equal and opposite force that is exerted back onto the body with every step that is taken.

Homeostasis: The ability or tendency of an organism or a cell to maintain internal equilibrium by adjusting its physiological processes.

Hypertension: Raised systemic arterial blood pressure, which, if sustained at a high enough level, is likely to induce cardiovascular or end-organ damage.

Hypertrophy: Enlargement of skeletal muscle fibers in response to overcoming force from high volumes of tension.

Inferior: Positioned below a point of reference.

Integrated Performance Paradigm: in order to move with precision, forces must be reduced (eccentrically), stabilized (isometrically) and then produced (concentrically).

Intensity: The level of demand that a given activity places on the body.

Intermittent claudication: The manifestation of the symptoms caused by peripheral arterial disease.

Intermuscular coordination: The ability of the neuromuscular system to allow all muscles to work together with proper activation and timing between them.

Internal feedback: The process whereby sensory information is utilized by the body to reactively monitor movement and the environment.

Internal rotation: Rotation of a joint toward the middle of the body.

Intramuscular coordination: The ability of the neuromuscular system to allow optimal levels of motor unit recruitment and synchronization within a muscle.

Ipsilateral: Positioned on the same side of the body.

Isometric contraction: A muscle maintaining a certain length under the control of the nervous system.

Lateral: Positioned farther away from the middle of the body.

Length-tension relationship: The length at which a muscle can produce the greatest force.

Maximal strength: The maximum force that a muscle can produce in a single, voluntary effort, regardless of velocity.

Mechanical specificity: The specific muscular exercises using different weights and movements that are performed to increase strength or endurance in certain body parts.

Medial: Positioned near the middle of the body.

Metabolic specificity: The specific muscular exercises using different levels of energy that are performed to increase endurance, strength or power.

Momentum: The product of the size of the object (mass) and its velocity (speed with which it is moving).

Monthly plan: Generalized training plan that spans one month and shows which phases will be required each day of each week.

Motor behavior: The process of the body responding to internal and external stimuli.

Motor control: The study of posture and movements and the involved structures and mechanisms that the central nervous system uses to assimilate and integrate sensory information with previous experiences.

Motor learning: Repeated practice of motor control processes, which lead to a change in the ability to produce complex movements.

Multisensory condition: Training environment that provides heightened stimulation to proprioceptors and mechanoreceptors.

Muscle imbalance: Alteration of muscle length surrounding a joint.

Muscular endurance: The ability of the body to produce low levels of force and maintain them for extended periods of time.

Neuromuscular efficiency: 1) The ability of the nervous system to communicate effectively with the muscular system. 2) The ability of the neuromuscular system to allow agonists, antagonists, synergists and stabilizers to work synergistically to produce, reduce and dynamically stabilize the entire kinetic chain in all three planes of motion.

Neuromuscular specificity: The specific muscular exercises using different speeds and styles that are performed to increase neuromuscular efficiency.

Obesity: The condition of subcutaneous fat exceeding the amount of lean body mass.

Obstructive lung disease: The condition of altered air flow through the lungs, generally caused by airway obstruction, due to mucous production.

Osteoarthritis: Arthritis in which cartilage becomes soft, frayed or thins out, due to trauma or other conditions.

Osteopenia: A decrease in the calcification or density of bone as well as reduced bone mass.

Osteoporosis: Condition in which there is a decrease in bone mass and density as well as an increase in the space between bones, resulting in porosity and fragility.

Pattern overload: Repetitive physical activity that moves through the same patterns of motion, placing the same stresses on the body over a period of time.

Periodization: Division of a training program into smaller, progressive stages.

Peripheral arterial disease: A condition characterized by narrowing of the major arteries that are responsible for supplying blood to the lower extremities.

Plyometric: Exercise that enhances muscular power through quick, repetitive eccentric and concentric contraction of muscles.

Posterior (or dorsal): On the back of the body.

Postural distortion patterns: Predictable patterns of muscle imbalances.

Postural equilibrium: Maintaining a state of balance in the alignment of the kinetic chain.

Posture: Position and bearing of the body for alignment and function of the kinetic chain.

Power: Ability of the neuromuscular system to produce the greatest force in the shortest time.

Pregnancy: The condition of a female who contains an unborn child within the body.

Principle of Specificity OR **Specific Adaptation to Imposed Demands (SAID Principle):** Principle that states the body will adapt to the specific demands that are placed upon it.

Program design: A purposeful system or plan put together to help an individual achieve a specific goal.

Proximal: Positioned nearest the center of the body, or point of reference.

Quickness: The ability to react and change body position with maximum rate of force production, in all planes of motion, from all body positions, during functional activities.

Rapport: Aspect of a relationship characterized by similarity, agreement or congruity.

Rate of force production: Ability of muscles to exert maximal force output in a minimal amount of time

Reactive training: Exercises that utilize quick, powerful movements involving an eccentric contraction immediately followed by an explosive concentric contraction.

Recommended Dietary Allowance (RDA): The average daily nutrient intake level that is sufficient to meet the nutrient requirement of nearly all (97 to 98 percent) healthy individuals who are in a particular life stage and gender group.

Relative flexibility: The tendency of the body to seek the path of least resistance during functional movement patterns.

Repetition (or rep): One complete movement of a single exercise.

Repetition tempo: The speed with which each repetition is performed.

Resistance development: The body increases its functional capacity to adapt to the stressor.

Rest interval: The time taken to recuperate between sets.

Restrictive lung disease: The condition of a fibrous lung tissue, which results in a decreased ability to expand the lungs.

Rheumatoid arthritis: Arthritis primarily affecting connective tissues, in which there is a thickening of articular soft tissue, and extension of synovial tissue over articular cartilages that have become eroded.

Root cause analysis: A method of asking questions on a step-by-step basis to discover the initial cause of a fault.

Rotary motion: Movement of the bones around the joints.

Sagittal plane: An imaginary bisector that divides the body into left and right halves.

Self-myofascial release: A flexibility technique where muscles are rolled over a cylindrical piece of foam (or foam roll), using body pressure to massage micro-adhesions in the fibrous tissue that surrounds and separates muscle tissue.

Sensorimotor integration: The cooperation of the nervous and muscular system in gathering information, interpreting and executing movement.

Set: A group of consecutive repetitions.

Skin fold caliper: An instrument with two adjustable legs to measure thickness of a skin fold.

Specific warm-up: Low-intensity exercise consisting of movements that mimic those that will be included in the more intense exercise that is to follow.

Speed: The ability to move the body in one intended direction as fast as possible.

Stability: The ability of the body to maintain postural equilibrium and support joints during movement.

Static stretch: Passively taking a muscle to the point of tension and holding for at least 20 seconds.

Strength endurance: The ability of the body to repeatedly produce high levels of force, over prolonged periods of time.

Strength: The ability of the neuromuscular system to produce internal tension in order to overcome an external force.

Structural efficiency: The alignment of the musculoskeletal system that allows our center of gravity to be maintained over our base of support.

Superior: Positioned above a point of reference.

Synergies: Groups of muscles that are recruited by the central nervous system to provide movement.

Synergistic dominance: The neuromuscular phenomenon that occurs when inappropriate muscles take over the function of a weak or inhibited prime mover.

Time: The length of time an individual is engaged in a given activity.

Tolerable Upper Intake Level (UL): The highest average daily nutrient intake level likely to pose no risk of adverse health effects to almost all individuals in a particular life stage and gender group. As intake increases above the UL, the potential risk of adverse health effects increases.

Torque: A force that produces rotation.

Training duration: The timeframe of a workout (including warm-up and cool-down) or the length of time spent in one phase of training.

Training frequency: The number of training sessions performed over a specified time period (usually one week).

Training intensity: An individual's level of effort, compared to their maximal effort, which is usually expressed as a percentage.

Training plan: The specific outline, created by a health and fitness professional to meet a client's goals, that details the form of training, length of time, future changes and specific exercises to be performed.

Training volume: Amount of physical training performed within a specified time period.

Transverse plane: An imaginary bisector that divides the body into top and bottom halves.

Type: The type or mode of physical activity that an individual is engaged in.

Unipenniform Muscle Fiber: Muscle fibers that are arranged with short, oblique fibers that extend from one side of a long tendon. An example would include the tibialis posterior.

Upper-extremity Postural Distortion: An individual, who exhibits a forward head, rounded shoulder posture.

Veins: Vessels that transport blood back to the heart.

Vertical Loading: A circuit style of training that involves a series of exercises being performed in succession.

Ventral: Refers to a position on the front or towards the front of the body.

Ventricles: Larger chambers located inferiorly on either side of the heart.

Ventilation: The actual process of moving air in and out of the body.

Venules: Vessels that collect blood from the capillaries.

Weekly plan: Training plan of specific workouts that spans one week to show which exercises are required each day of the week.

Index

A

B